Register Now for Online Access to Your Book!

SPRINGER PUBLISHING COMPANY
CONNECT™

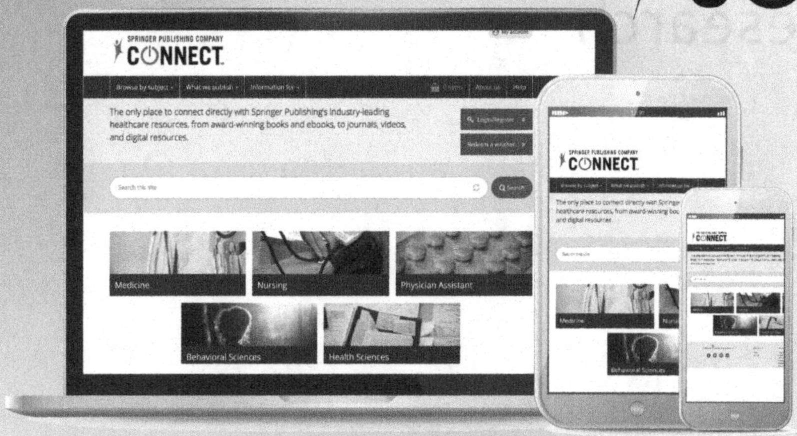

Your print purchase of *Principles of Clinical Cancer Research* **includes online access to the contents of your book**—increasing accessibility, portability, and searchability!

Access today at:

http://connect.springerpub.com/content/book/978-1-6170-5239-2
or scan the QR code at the right with your smartphone
and enter the access code below.

8CXGK71Y

Scan here for quick access.

If you are experiencing problems accessing the digital component of this product, please contact our customer service department at cs@springerpub.com

The online access with your print purchase is available at the publisher's discretion and may be removed at any time without notice.

Publisher's Note: New and used products purchased from third-party sellers are not guaranteed for quality, authenticity, or access to any included digital components.

demosMEDICAL
An Imprint of Springer Publishing
View all our products at springerpub.com/demosmedical

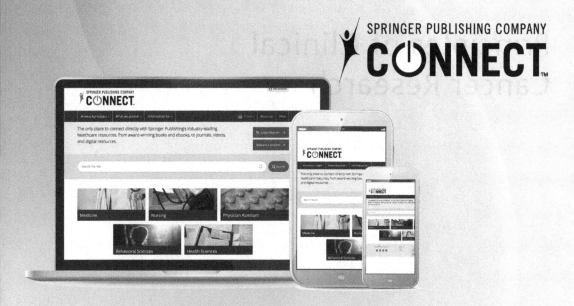

Principles of Clinical Cancer Research

Principles of Clinical Cancer Research

Editors

Loren K. Mell, MD
Professor and Vice Chair of Clinical and Translational Research
Department of Radiation Medicine and Applied Sciences
University of California San Diego, Moores Cancer Center
La Jolla, California

Phuoc T. Tran, MD, PhD
Associate Professor
Departments of Radiation Oncology & Molecular Radiation Sciences, Oncology and Urology
Program in Cellular and Molecular Medicine
The Johns Hopkins School of Medicine
The Sidney Kimmel Comprehensive Cancer Center
Baltimore, Maryland

James B. Yu, MD
Associate Professor of Therapeutic Radiology
Director, Prostate and Genitourinary Cancer Radiotherapy Program
Cancer Outcomes, Public Policy, and Effectiveness Research (COPPER) Center at Yale
Department of Therapeutic Radiology
Yale School of Medicine
New Haven, Connecticut

Qiang (Ed) Zhang, MD, PhD
Research Professor
Department of Ophthalmology
Vision Research Center
Wills Eye Hospital
Department of Pharmacology & Experimental Therapeutics
Division of Biostatistics
Sidney Kimmel Medical College
Thomas Jefferson University
Philadelphia, Pennsylvania

demosMEDICAL
An Imprint of Springer Publishing

Visit our website at www.Springerpub.com

ISBN: 9781620700693
ebook ISBN: 9781617052392

Acquisitions Editor: David D'Addona
Compositor: Exeter Premedia Services Pvt Ltd.
Cover artwork: Nicholette Kominos

Demos Medical Publishing is an imprint of Springer Publishing Company, LLC.

Medicine is an ever-changing science. Research and clinical experience are continually expanding our knowledge, in particular our understanding of proper treatment and drug therapy. The authors, editors, and publisher have made every effort to ensure that all information in this book is in accordance with the state of knowledge at the time of production of the book. Nevertheless, the authors, editors, and publisher are not responsible for errors or omissions or for any consequences from application of the information in this book and make no warranty, expressed or implied, with respect to the contents of the publication. Every reader should examine carefully the package inserts accompanying each drug and should carefully check whether the dosage schedules mentioned therein or the contraindications stated by the manufacturer differ from the statements made in this book. Such examination is particularly important with drugs that are either rarely used or have been newly released on the market.

Library of Congress Cataloging-in-Publication Data

Names: Mell, Loren K., editor. | Tran, Phuoc T., editor. | Yu, James B., editor. | Zhang, Qiang (Biostatistician), editor.
Title: Principles of clinical cancer research / editors, Loren K. Mell, Phuoc T. Tran, James B. Yu, Qiang (Ed) Zhang.
Description: New York : Demos Medical Publishing, [2019] | Includes bibliographical references and index.
Identifiers: LCCN 2018032583 | ISBN 9781620700693 | ISBN 9781617052392 (ebook)
Subjects: | MESH: Neoplasms | Biomedical Research
Classification: LCC RC267 | NLM QZ 206 | DDC 616.99/40072—dc23
LC record available at https://lccn.loc.gov/2018032583

Printed in the United States of America.
18 19 20 21 22 / 5 4 3 2 1

To Mom, who conceived me
To Dad, who catechized me
To Jean and Bus, who crafted me
To Jared, who sings to me
To Jaime, who inspires me
To my patients, who treat me
To Ryan, who keeps me in tempo
To Elliot, who enriches me
And above all to Gina, who makes me want to dance
May this book accomplish one of the above for everyone else.—Loren K. Mell

The inspiration for this work was and is from my brave and gracious patients who elect to enroll on clinical trials and was only made possible by the immense support of my family (DJ, CDT, LTT, and QNT) and trainees (HW, AS, JD, KT, RM, and AM). Lastly, to my fearless and timeline-driven coeditor and friend who was the impetus for this project and for saving my father's life (LKM). Thank you.—Phuoc T. Tran

For Brenna.—James B. Yu

This book is dedicated to my family, especially my sons, H.G. Zhang (Columbia University) and his twin brothers R.G. Zhang and W.G. Zhang.—Qiang (Ed) Zhang

Contents

Contributors

Sanjay Aneja, MD, Assistant Professor, Department of Therapeutic Radiology, Yale School of Medicine, New Haven, Connecticut

Karla V. Ballman, PhD, Chief of Biostatistics and Epidemiology, Professor of Biostatistics, Department of Healthcare Policy and Research, Weill Cornell Medicine, New York, New York

Jeff Burkeen, MD, Resident, Department of Radiation Medicine and Applied Sciences, University of California, San Diego, La Jolla, California

Enoch Chang, BA, Medical Student, Department of Therapeutic Radiology, Yale School of Medicine, New Haven, Connecticut

Mark Chang, PhD, Senior Vice President, Strategic Statistical Consulting, Veristat, Southborough, Massachusetts

Aadel A. Chaudhuri, MD, PhD, Assistant Professor, Department of Radiation Oncology, Washington University, St. Louis, Missouri

Aileen Chen, MD, MPP, Associate Professor, Department of Radiation Oncology, Division of Radiation Oncology, The University of Texas MD Anderson Cancer Center, Houston, Texas

Rishi Deka, PhD, Postdoctoral Fellow, Department of Radiation Medicine and Applied Sciences, University of California, San Diego, La Jolla, California

Xuan Deng, PhD, Research Assistant, Department of Biostatistics, Boston University, Boston, Massachusetts

Benjamin Djulbegovic, MD, PhD, Professor, Department of Supportive Care Medicine, Department of Hematology, Program for Evidence-Based Medicine and Comparative Effectiveness Research, City of Hope, Duarte, California

Mak Djulbegovic, BS (Finance/Biomedical Sciences), MS Candidate in Bioinformatics & Computational Biology, Morsani College of Medicine, University of South Florida, Tampa, Florida

Mia Djulbegovic, MD, Postdoctoral Fellow, National Clinicians Scholars Program, Yale University School of Medicine, and Veterans Affairs Connecticut Healthcare System, New Haven, Connecticut

Jacqueline Douglass, MS, MD-PhD Candidate in Oncology/Cellular and Molecular Medicine, Johns Hopkins University School of Medicine, Baltimore, Maryland

Michael A. Dyer, MD, Assistant Professor of Radiation Oncology, Boston Medical Center, Boston University School of Medicine, Boston, Massachusetts

Sharad Goyal, MD, Professor of Radiology & Division Chief, Department of Radiation Oncology, George Washington University, Washington, District of Columbia

Jona Hattangadi-Gluth, MD, Associate Professor, Department of Radiation Medicine and Applied Sciences, University of California, San Diego, La Jolla, California

Scott Keith, PhD, Assistant Professor, Department of Biostatistics, Thomas Jefferson University, Philadelphia, Pennsylvania

Jack J. Lee, PhD, Professor, Department of Biostatistics, The University of Texas MD Anderson Cancer Center, Houston, Texas

Benjamin E. Leiby, PhD, Associate Professor and Director, Division of Biostatistics, Department of Pharmacology and Experimental Therapeutics, Sidney Kimmel Medical College, Thomas Jefferson University, Philadelphia, Pennsylvania

Swan Lin, Pharm D, Postdoctoral Clinical Pharmacology Fellow, Skaggs School of Pharmacy and Pharmaceutical Sciences, University of California, San Diego, La Jolla, California

Reem A. Malek, PhD, Postdoctoral Fellow, Department of Radiation Oncology and Molecular Radiation Sciences, Johns Hopkins University School of Medicine, Baltimore, Maryland

Ariel E. Marciscano, MD, Assistant Attending Radiation Oncologist, Department of Radiation Oncology, Memorial Sloan Kettering Cancer Center, New York, New York

Loren K. Mell, MD, Professor and Vice Chair of Clinical and Translational Research, Department of Radiation Medicine and Applied Sciences, University of California San Diego, Moores Cancer Center, La Jolla, California

Michael Milligan, MD, MBA, Medical Student, Harvard Medical School, Boston, Massachusetts

James Murphy, MD, MS, Associate Professor, Department of Radiation Medicine and Applied Sciences, University of California, San Diego, La Jolla, California

Tie-Hua Ng, PhD, Mathematical Statistician, Food and Drug Administration, Silver Spring, Maryland

Henry S. Park, MD, MPH, Assistant Clinical Professor, Department of Therapeutic Radiology, Yale School of Medicine, New Haven, Connecticut

Sandip Pravin Patel, MD, Associate Professor, Division of Hematology & Oncology and Center for Personalized Cancer Therapy, UC San Diego Moores Cancer Center, La Jolla, California

Yazdi K. Pithavala, PhD, Senior Director, Global Product Development–Clinical Pharmacology, Oncology, Pfizer, Inc., San Diego, California

Zorimar Rivera-Núñez, PhD, Research Associate, Department of Radiation Oncology, Rutgers Cancer Institute of New Jersey, New Brunswick, New Jersey

Brent S. Rose, MD, Assistant Professor, Department of Radiation Medicine and Applied Sciences, University of California, San Diego, La Jolla, California

Reith Roy Sarkar, MAS, Clinical Research Associate, Department of Radiation Medicine and Applied Sciences, University of California, San Diego, La Jolla, California

Andrew Sharabi, MD, PhD, Assistant Professor, Department of Radiation Medicine and Applied Sciences, University of California, San Diego School of Medicine, La Jolla, California

Hanjie Shen, MS, Biostatistics Shared Resources Manager/Staff Research Associate III, Department of Radiation Medicine and Applied Sciences, University of California, San Diego, La Jolla, California

Paige Sheridan, MPH, Graduate Student Researcher, Department of Radiation Medicine and Applied Sciences, University of California, San Diego, San Diego, California

Aaron B. Simon, MD, PhD, Resident, Department of Radiation Medicine and Applied Sciences, University of California, San Diego, La Jolla, California

Daniel R. Simpson, MD, MAS, Assistant Professor, Department of Radiation Medicine and Applied Sciences, University of California, San Diego, La Jolla, California

Kekoa Taparra, PhD, Doctoral Candidate, Mayo Clinic School of Medicine, Mayo Clinic, Rochester, Minnesota

Phuoc T. Tran, MD, PhD, Associate Professor, Departments of Radiation Oncology & Molecular Radiation Sciences, Oncology and Urology, Program in Cellular and Molecular Medicine, The Johns Hopkins School of Medicine, The Sidney Kimmel Comprehensive Cancer Center, Baltimore, Maryland

Minh Tam Truong, MD, Associate Professor and Chair of Radiation Oncology, Boston Medical Center, Boston University School of Medicine, Boston, Massachusetts

Brandon E. Turner, MSc, Medical Student, Radiation Oncology, Stanford School of Medicine, Stanford, California

Hailun Wang, PhD, Instructor, Department of Radiation Oncology and Molecular Radiation Sciences, Johns Hopkins University School of Medicine, Baltimore, Maryland

James B. Yu, MD, Associate Professor of Therapeutic Radiology, Director, Prostate and Genitourinary Cancer Radiotherapy Program, Cancer Outcomes, Public Policy, and Effectiveness Research (COPPER) Center at Yale, Department of Therapeutic Radiology, Yale School of Medicine, New Haven, Connecticut

Ying Yuan, PhD, Professor, Department of Biostatistics, The University of Texas MD Anderson Cancer Center, Houston, Texas

Kaveh Zakeri, MD, MAS, Resident Physician, Department of Radiation Medicine and Applied Sciences, University of California, San Diego, La Jolla, California

Nicholas G. Zaorsky, MD, Assistant Professor, Department of Radiation Oncology; Assistant Professor, Department of Public Health Sciences, Penn State Cancer Institute, Hershey, Pennsylvania

Qiang (Ed) Zhang, MD, PhD, Research Professor, Department of Ophthalmology, Vision Research Center, Wills Eye Hospital, Department of Pharmacology & Experimental Therapeutics, Division of Biostatistics, Sidney Kimmel Medical College, Thomas Jefferson University, Philadelphia, Pennsylvania

Yanhong Zhou, MS, Graduate Student, Department of Biostatistics, The University of Texas MD Anderson Cancer Center, Houston, Texas

Foreword

Drs. Mell, Tran, Yu, and Zhang have written a readable yet comprehensive textbook on various aspects of clinical cancer research. They cover valuable information relating to clinical research in cancer. Important aspects, such as basic science in the context of translational research, principles of molecular biology, cell cycle, metastasis, mechanisms of resistance, preclinical models, and prognostic and predictive biomarkers, are introduced in a comprehensive way. They then move on to describe population and outcomes research in the context of statistical modeling, cancer epidemiology with a focus on longitudinal and observational analysis, time-to-event models, and machine learning, followed by two important chapters on health disparities and cost-effectiveness analysis. Toward the end of the book they deal with clinical trials, including early and late phase trials, quality of life analysis, screening and prevention, imaging, adaptive trials, noninferiority trials, and finally meta-analysis. The conclusion of the book leads into "omics" research, an exciting area at the forefront of clinical cancer research.

It is unusual to find such diverse topics covered in depth for a book focused on clinical research. Usually wide searching is required to bring each of these important topics into a specific, concentrated research focus. Although this book is geared toward trainees and junior investigators, this senior investigator found the book highly informative, covering topics that were no longer familiar and I needed to reacquaint myself with. The general organization of the chapters proceeds from simplicity to complexity as appropriate to the topics under investigation. The wide range of topics covered under this book is extremely valuable, with comprehensive coverage of nearly all aspects of clinical cancer research.

I plan to keep this book handy as I assist junior faculty in designing and implementing clinical research, especially those with translational aspects. I particularly enjoyed the first chapter, which focuses on careers in clinical cancer research, elements of running a lab, writing protocols, and obtaining funding. Many diagrams throughout the book assist the reader in following the more complex concepts. I congratulate the authors on an outstanding book, with its unification of many diverse topics. I am sure it will find a place in many investigators' libraries.

Ralph R. Weichselbaum, MD
Daniel K. Ludwig Distinguished Service Professor and Chairman
Department of Radiation and Cellular Oncology
Co-Director, Ludwig Center for Metastases Research
UChicago Medicine
Chicago, Illlinois

Preface

In the long run men hit only what they aim at. Therefore, though they should fail immediately, they had better aim at something high.

—Henry David Thoreau

Clinical cancer research is the scientific discipline concerned with advancing knowledge to benefit cancer patients. The field encompasses a broad spectrum of subdisciplines and methods, including wet and dry laboratory sciences, controlled and uncontrolled experiments, and retrospective and prospective study designs. The cohesive bond these subdisciplines share is their common quest. What makes "clinical cancer research" different from other kinds of research is the meaning we attach to its purpose—a quest that is not simply for our, or even knowledge's, own sake, but for the sake of patients afflicted with the insidious assortment of diseases we collectively call cancer.

Stemming from this motivation, we proffer this book, which endeavors to address a gap in the existing tertiary literature. Although several textbooks about clinical research exist, few have specifically and simultaneously addressed the needs of both clinicians and physician-scientists in oncology. Other popular textbooks have predominantly focused on either a broad range of disciplines not specific to oncology, or on technical statistics of clinical research, or solely on issues related to cancer clinical trials. Clinical cancer research, however, involves much more than clinical trials, encompassing branches ranging from developmental or translational preclinical and retrospective modeling studies, to clinical trials, to population-based studies and meta-analyses designed to answer questions that clinical trials cannot. In that sense, it represents a set of interwoven and integrally dependent physical and humanitarian sciences, uniting to form the translational research spectrum[1]:

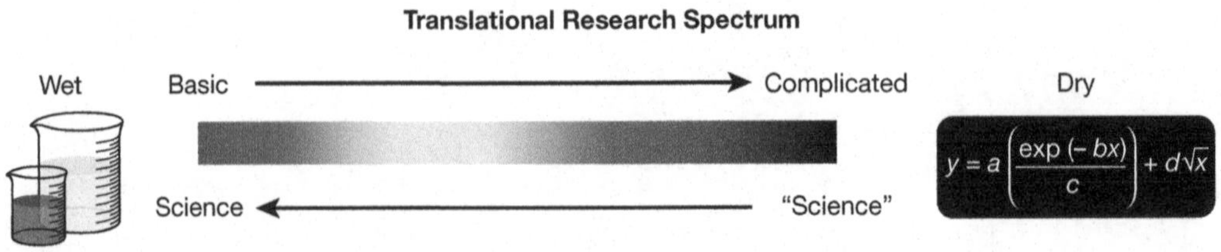

[1] Readers can view the color version of this figure in the free ebook that accompanies the purchase of the print version of this book.

In this book, we provide a wider perspective on the clinical oncologic sciences. We have written this book primarily for trainees and junior faculty interested in careers in clinical and translational research. It has three principal aims. The first is to introduce readers to the fundamentals of clinical cancer research, including the basic methodologies used in our field, and, in doing so, arm them with the skills to recognize, produce, and disseminate quality clinical science in oncology. The second is to guide trainees who aspire to careers in this field, by offering a mix of practical advice and analytical tools, and references to resources that address areas falling outside the scope of our handbook. The third is to assist educators, by providing them with an organizational structure and a set of practical examples upon which they can build an effective curriculum. In short, this is a book by clinical scientists, for current and future clinical scientists. However, we also hope that general medical professionals will find this book helpful in navigating the vast and often bewildering nomenclature used in clinical cancer research, and that it will facilitate their application of evidence-based medicine, ultimately benefiting the patients they treat.

The translational research spectrum exists, representing the trade-off between idealized models with controlled experimental conditions and real-world implementation in patients, where ideals may fall short and pure experimentation becomes infeasible, with increasing reliance on mathematical representations of biologic processes. At its best, clinical cancer research marries the extremes of this spectrum to produce advances in knowledge that benefit patients.

Loren K. Mell, MD

I Introduction

1

Introduction to Clinical Cancer Research

LOREN K. MELL

OVERVIEW

Welcome to the wonderful world of clinical cancer research! Over the past century, we have made tremendous strides in the understanding of cancer biology, opening doors to novel paradigms and effective therapies that give us greater hope than ever before in our fight against the disease. In addition, unprecedented technology is enabling us to capitalize on massive troves of data to advance patient care in increasingly creative and sophisticated ways. One of the most exciting yet frustrating aspects of cancer research, however, is how much there is still to learn.

The book you are about to read is designed to help individuals build careers dedicated to the advancement of cancer care through research. Our editorial team and authors have created a compendium of the fundamental information we believe one should know to be successful in this field. With a foundation in cancer biology and preclinical methods, one can better appreciate how new therapies develop from bench to bedside, ultimately translating into better patient care. To complement this knowledge, exposure to study design and analytic methods helps investigators draw proper inferences from their findings and reverse-transcribe them, as it were, back to their laboratory. Moreover, throughout a career in academic oncology, one is frequently called upon to evaluate work that is outside the narrow domain of one's expertise. Often you will find yourself the reigning biologist, physicist, clinician, or statistician in the room, with others depending on you to judge the value of a given proposal. Therefore, this book's territorial range is purposely broad, with emphasis on the key principles spanning diverse subdisciplines, to serve as an introductory learning tool and reference guide.

Within each chapter, we have attempted to provide a basic theoretical framework and heuristic explanation, coupled with a moderate degree of technicality and real-world examples. However, as with any broad treatment of a subject, what we do not cover could fill more than a book. For example, the field of bioinformatics is important in clinical research, but is not something we had room to treat in detail. Many advanced statistical and biological methods also could not be given thorough attention. Wherever possible, however, we attempt to broach advanced topics and refer readers to available tertiary sources that expand upon them in depth. Many source manuals for software and statistical packages provide additional methodological details related to specific procedures.

Although many investigators outsource their data analysis, we recommend investing the time to learn programming in at least one of the common statistical packages, such as R (www.r-project.org), SAS (www.sas.com), or STATA (www.stata.com). For example, a list of packages for design, monitoring, and analysis of clinical trial data is available within R (cran.r-project.org/web/views/ClinicalTrials.html). This effort will provide investigators a level of familiarity with data structure and analysis that can help them anticipate needs when designing new projects. Some software packages, such as JMP for SAS, have user-friendly interfaces that can facilitate more technical analysis (www.jmp.com). Many simple statistical calculations also can be done within spreadsheet applications, such as Microsoft Excel, or with the help of online calculators, such as can be found at www.vassarstats.net. Several data capture systems are useful for collecting and organizing data, as well as generating data collection forms (e.g., case report forms [CRFs]) and exporting data into analyzable formats. Examples of such systems include Research Electronic Data Capture (REDCap; www.project-redcap.org), Velos (velos.com), and VisionTree (www.visiontree.com).

The first phase of this book is dedicated to translational research, including principles of molecular and cell biology, mechanisms of tumor growth, therapeutic strategies, and preclinical research methods. Later in the section, biomarker development and collaborations with industry are discussed as a segue into clinical applications. The second phase of this book focuses on fundamentals of human subjects research, including basic study designs and statistical methods. Gradually, more sophisticated methods such as generalized linear modeling, time-to-event analysis, and machine learning are introduced, as well as introductions to critical branches of the population sciences, including cancer epidemiology, disparities research, and cost-effectiveness analysis. The final phase of the book deals with prospective human subjects research (i.e., clinical trials), including classic early and late phase trial designs, innovative adaptive trial designs, and meta-analysis. Special applications in the context of imaging, screening and prevention, quality of life, and comparative effectiveness research are also considered, to round out the volume.

THE HIERARCHY OF EVIDENCE

The hierarchy of clinical evidence is often depicted in a pyramidal structure, with expert opinion and case reports representing the lowest tier, retrospective and prospective cohort studies occupying middle tiers, and rarer well-designed randomized trials and meta-analyses (so-called level I evidence) representing the highest tier of evidence. This categorical model has inarguable utility in certain contexts, such as defining practice guidelines. For example, the National Comprehensive Cancer Network (NCCN) uses a categorical system to support their treatment recommendations, ranging from category 3 (major disagreement whether the intervention is appropriate), to 2 (general consensus that the intervention is appropriate based on lower level evidence), to 1 (uniform consensus that the intervention is appropriate based on high-level evidence) (1). An advantage of this model is that it attributes a certain rigor to the grade of a treatment recommendation, which can help adjudicate which recommendations should take precedence (especially if the evidence is contradictory).

This hierarchy naturally extends to the archetypal bench-to-bedside framework of developmental therapeutics, in which a (brilliant) scientist, working in isolation, develops a theory and a testable hypothesis, subjects it to rigorous in vitro and in vivo experimentation, develops a novel therapy based on the experimental results, performs early clinical testing of the said therapy to refine the therapeutic scheme, confirms its efficacy in a prospective study, and then establishes its clinical benefit in a gold standard, definitive, practice-changing, randomized controlled phase III trial. Amazingly, as discussed in Chapter 9, there are several notable examples that roughly mimic this progression, resulting in blockbuster therapeutic advances, such as trastuzumab for breast cancer and imatinib for chronic myeloid leukemia. While triumphs such as these are laudable and serve as an aspirational model or gold standard for clinical cancer research, they are also unusual and represent a relatively small fraction of the studies that affect medical decision making.

When it comes to regarding clinical oncologic sciences on the whole and how they affect patient management, a wider purview is required. First, because *all* studies have ineluctable scientific flaws, the notion of a "gold standard" study is somewhat specious. Take for example, a phase III trial. Ostensibly, such a design allows one to make inferences about the effects of a treatment in a population. However, in order to do so, one must invoke assumptions that invariably could be called into question and affect the study's validity. The most fundamental of these is the assumption of random sampling, since participation in trials, for ethical reasons, must be voluntary—an unquestionably nonrandom process. In addition, phase III trials often combine heterogeneous subpopulations of patients accrued over many years with follow-up in uncontrolled experimental conditions of dubious reproducibility, occasionally haunted by the specter of bias from special interests. In this way, such trials deviate substantially from the "gold standard" scientific experimental design, which aims to isolate the intervention under study as the sole source of variation. This is a long way of saying that a phase III trial is the worst possible study design (except for all the others).

In truth, there is not necessarily a best study design, except perhaps for the particular question at hand. Often, this will be a randomized trial. In other instances, it may be a patient-derived xenographic murine model, or a large institutional case series. The validity of inferences depends on the level of agreement regarding the validity of the assumptions—an inherently subjective fly in the pristine ointment of objectivity. Some study designs will be infeasible, impractical, unfundable, or unfunded, and the answers to some questions will be inherently unknowable, forcing us to rely on lower standards of evidence for decision making, including, occasionally, gut feeling. In many cases, the application of scientific knowledge in clinical settings (i.e., evidence-based medicine) degenerates to a binary decision (treat or do not treat) determined through a combination of physicians' gestalt and patients' willingness to comply.

A different way to view scientific contributions to the evidence base, then, is feeding a cycle of knowledge (Figure 1.1). In a way, this cycle might be seen as a union between the ends of the spectrum introduced in the preface to this book. In the central core of the cycle is the canonical, idealized linear representation of progressive scientific experimentation and its application to practice. In the peripheral shell lie the other forms scientific contributions can take that influence medical decision making in the aggregate. All of the nodes represent a model, in one form or another, with varying robustness. The goal of a scientist or team of scientists is to examine these models, seeking to define the contexts in which they function or fail to explain observed phenomena.

ETHICS IN CLINICAL SCIENCE

Chapter 2 rounds out the introductory section of our book with an in-depth discussion of the various biases that can contaminate a research study and undermine its conclusions. Formally, in a simplified manner, the absence of **bias** means that the **expected value** of an **estimator** (β) is equal to the true value of the theoretical parameter (b) that it is supposed to represent

$$E(\beta) = b. \qquad [1]$$

If we accept that all science, in some sense, comes down to generating an unbiased measure to model some phenomenon, then informally, the absence of bias indicates that the value of our experimental measure means what we think it means. If whatever errors exist in our measurement process are random, then the results come out in the wash, so to speak. But if there is systematic error (e.g., a broken gauge), then of course unbiased measurement is impossible.

Scientists are tremendously influential, so it is the responsibility of all scientists to ensure that their "gauges" are working properly, to control for and mitigate the effects of bias in rendering conclusions from their research. The power to influence is also the power to mislead. Scientists can mislead in both subtle and not-so-subtle ways. An example of the former is the use of prejudicial language in scientific writing, such as "demonstrating" or "showing" results (especially if the measurement is stochastic or inconclusive in nature), or remarking that results "trend

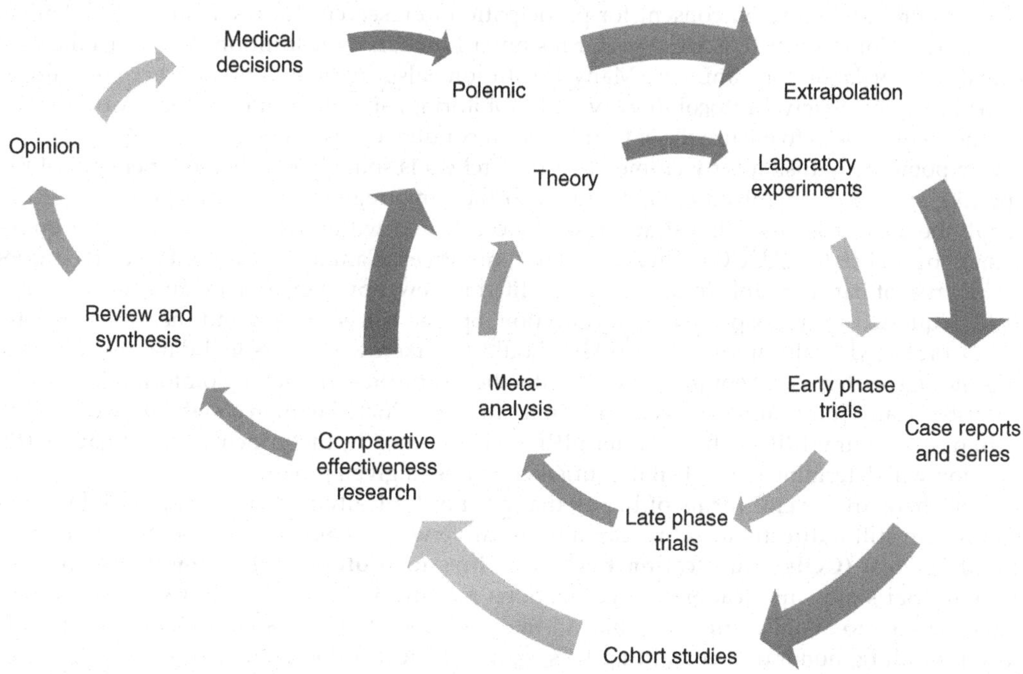

FIGURE 1.1 Schematic representation of evidence-based practice.

toward" statistical significance, which typically means the data are actually consistent with the null hypothesis (supposedly defined a priori). Sometimes it is simply the overzealous interpretation of relatively primitive or premature data. As an indicator of its importance to clinical cancer research, several chapters in this book address various nonmalicious forms of bias, the apotheosis being **selection bias**. Indeed, there is no better cancer therapy than selection bias; nothing else can make results look so impressive—except perhaps for malignant bias.

Malignant bias, in its assorted forms, is typically characterized by the conscious production of false research results and/or intentional harm to human or animal subjects, usually for the sake of personal advancement. Its practitioners are akin to denizens of the sundry corners of the dark web: all are bad, some are abominable. An example of a relatively minor infraction is engineering results to satisfy a predetermined p-value threshold or otherwise fitting data to a preformed hypothesis, rather than the converse. You should not do this. It is misleading and unethical. Outright plagiarism is also clearly verboten, but a subtler and likely more prevalent form is attaching one's name to publications one has not contributed to as an author. Fortunately, most reputable journals now require all authors at least to attest to their specific contribution(s). Predatory publishing and collusive publishing rings also constitute obvious academic misconduct; for further discussion, see Zietman (2). Last, fabrication of data constitutes an especially dastardly class of academic malfeasance. Famous examples include Andrew Wakefield, who falsely published a link between the measles, mumps, and rubella (MMR) vaccine and autism, and Werner Bezwoda, who fabricated data indicating that breast cancer patients could be cured with high-dose chemotherapy with bone marrow transplant. The ongoing ripple effects of Wakefield's misconduct have doubtless led to millions of children going unvaccinated and spikes in measles fatalities.

Institutional Review Boards (IRBs), established by the 1975 Helsinki Declaration governing ethical human subjects research, now largely prevent the especially heinous forms of academic malfeasance seen with the infamous Tuskegee incident or the case of Chester Southam, who injected the skin of patients with cancer cells, without their consent, to study the effect of the immune system on cancer cells. These boards, among other mandates, establish the need for patients to provide informed consent for participation in research studies. Institutional Animal Care and Use Committees (IACUCs) perform similar functions at institutions to govern the ethical treatment of laboratory animals. Many institutions also involve various other committees such as Biological Safety, Protocol Review and Monitoring, and Human Exposure (for radiation and other biohazards) to ensure the safe and ethical conduct of research.

One point of confusion for well-meaning researchers is sometimes whether oversight of retrospective and/or anonymized data is subject to the same regulations as prospective trials. In general, the answer is yes—almost any research conducted within an academic center requires oversight by an IRB (or IACUC or an equivalent committee for animal subjects). Typically, studies with low risk of harm are able to undergo expedited review, however, and a waiver of consent is usually requested for retrospective data collection. Special consideration and measures for handling of protected health information (PHI) should be taken when personal data are collected; secure storage systems are required, and are often best coordinated with a bioinformatics and/or biostatistics team. Some human subjects research can be conducted with oversight of a Central IRB (CIRB) or extramural IRB, such as Western IRB (WIRB). Usually, the principal investigator's (PI) institution will determine which IRB has jurisdiction over a given project.

Last, there are several forms of biases that are not typically malicious in nature but nevertheless can still indirectly affect research in negative ways. Among these are pecuniary **conflicts of interest (COIs)**, **publication bias**, and "**bias of professional accomplishment** (3)." Most editorial staffs and academic organizations require the disclosure of COIs on the part of investigators to avoid commercial bias in the presentation of research. COIs might include research funding, honoraria, consulting fees, speaker's bureau fees, stock or stock options, or direct ownership of companies sponsoring research. COI disclosures often extend to immediate family as well. Publication bias is a well-established phenomenon that refers to the situation when the results of a study influence its probability of publication, or the impact factor (IF) of the resulting publication. Publication bias is of particular concern for meta-analysts, as investigators often will not bother to publish unfinished trials, trials that failed to meet their accrual target, or trials that yield "negative" results (i.e., fail to reject the null hypothesis). Unfortunately, it also creates perverse incentives to whitewash or selectively present results that tend to make experimental therapies look more favorable, in order to achieve a more visible level of publication.

The latter ties into an important and increasingly recognized problem called bias of professional accomplishment. Many markers of academic success exist, including being promoted to professor rank, garnering tenure, achieving leadership positions within the academic community, publishing research in reputable and high-IF journals, procuring sizable research grants, gaining membership to exclusive academic societies, and gaining public recognition through awards or media coverage. These and other status markers in academia are duly set up to reward and acknowledge hard work and creativity in research, and distinguish those whose impact on the field has been especially remarkable. An unfortunate consequence is that this practice can introduce incentives to behave unethically in ways that ultimately do not serve the scientific community or patients. Examples might be sabotaging or downgrading others' work, failing to recuse oneself when COIs arise, or massaging results to make them publishable. Some PIs operate on the principle of "least publishable unit (LPU)," referring to the partitioning of findings into separate manuscripts in order to increase the length of one's curriculum vitae. Such shenanigans rarely serve the perpetrator but do tend to contribute to a large volume of noncontributory and me-too publications that dilute the scientific canon.

A CAREER IN CLINICAL CANCER RESEARCH

The first thing to mention is that a successful research career can be defined by one good paper. If Watson and Crick only published one study, their impact would still be reverberating. Keeping one's eyes trained downfield on the bigger picture is important when navigating the numerous obstacles in one's career path. Another way to say this is not to use aforementioned *markers* of success, or your **h-index**[1], as *definitions* of success; that definition depends on grander goals.

For junior investigators, the importance of establishing a mentor–mentee relationship cannot be overemphasized. This can and should be done at several different levels: with those 5, 10, 15, and even 20 years more experience, with those who can spend time with you to develop and hone your ideas, and those who have the career standing to pave roads and generate unique opportunities. Most science done today is done by teams, and most grant and publication reviewers will expect members of the research team to have pertinent and complementary expertise. So, reaching out to investigators and establishing collegial working relationships within and outside your department and institution is also essential.

Yet, this should not crowd out the role of individual thinking. Before embarking on a research career, you should ask yourself certain questions. What problems do I think are important? Will I still think this problem is important in a decade? Two decades? How will future generations benefit from this knowledge? What unique skills can I bring to bear on this problem? What new skills can I develop? How will I leverage the particular strengths and capabilities of my institution to generate novel insights? After that, what question should I drive at next? And finally, what dogma doesn't sit right with me? Agitates me? Angers me?

Regarding these skills, there is nothing sadder than an investigator who keeps applying the same techniques over and over again without evolving over the course of his or her career. As science and research methods evolve and improve, you should evolve and improve as well. Take classes in research methods that you are curious about. Attend symposia where the latest research is being discussed. Look at other fields outside of your own discipline for ideas and innovations. Listen to young people and their crazy ideas about how to answer questions about which you have been wondering. Remain curious and never stop reading.

Remember that everything you need to know about the scientific method you learned in your elementary school science fair. You would be shocked to realize how few scientific manuscripts and grant applications lack a single mention of the word "**hypothesis**." Remembering the fifth grade will give you a leg up on the competition. So, to review:

1. Do your background research. Why is this question so important?
2. Articulate your hypothesis or question. What specific aim can I achieve?
3. Describe your methods in a reproducible way. How will I measure my outcome?
4. Explain how you will control your experiment. What other factors could influence my results?
5. Present your results. What outcome did you measure?
6. Discuss any pitfalls. Did the experiment go as expected?
7. Draw your conclusions. Are the results consistent with or do they conflict with your hypothesis?
8. Envision next steps. What were the strengths and limitations of your analysis? What should the next experiment look like?

An especially important part of describing research methodology is describing how you plan to **control** the experiment, in order to isolate the effect and outcome of interest. In particular, an experiment that implements both **positive control** (to show the effect is present when it is expected to be present) and **negative control** (to show the effect is not present when it is expected not to be present) has greater scientific validity.

PRACTICAL ASPECTS OF RUNNING A LAB

For many PIs, running a laboratory will be their first experience hiring and managing personnel. Being responsible for employees can be both an enjoyable and a stressful aspect of the job, yet many PIs do not receive specialized management training. New PIs must simultaneously play

[1] Your h-index is 10, for example, if you have published 10 papers that have been cited 10 times or more.

the role of mentee while transitioning into the role of mentor for their students, trainees, and staff who will be seeking their guidance. An effective PI is able, affable, and available for his or her staff. PIs must work with human resources to understand specific job classifications and pay scales, the impact of collective bargaining agreements, and criteria for fair hiring practices. Taking active steps to ensure diversity and a healthy workplace environment free from discrimination and harassment is also the responsibility of PIs. PIs must be prepared to handle personnel turnover and unforeseen shocks such as medical or family leave, or visa requirements for foreign workers. Sharing personnel, equipment, and space with other PIs can often provide a buffer against sudden shifts in staffing that could jeopardize the pace or conduct of one's research. Also, new PIs must be prepared to negotiate reasonable space for their laboratories to thrive and grow, which is often tied to indirect costs associated with extramural grants. Ultimately, each PI is expected to exhibit professionalism in the workplace when interacting with his or her staff. As a boss, it is okay to be demanding, but not demeaning. Several great resources are available to orient young PIs to running their own laboratory (4–6).

WRITING MANUSCRIPTS AND PROTOCOLS

Most journals have particular quirks in their style but generally conform to a classic presentation of an Abstract followed by Background, Methods and Materials, Results, and Discussion. Many basic science publications present the Methods and Materials at the end. In general, lengthy introductions (more than three or four paragraphs, preferably two or three) should be avoided. Second, one should write in a way that others can easily reproduce what was done. Clearly defining your population, sampling methods, primary and secondary hypotheses, and statistical methods (including power and sample size calculations, and coding methods) is a must. Results should correlate directly with the stated hypothesis(es), and graphs and figures should illuminate that which cannot be conveyed easily in text form. Interpretations of results in the discussion should be duly cautious and emphasize both strengths and novelty as well as weaknesses and limitations of the study. Whenever possible, the presentation should conform to established editorial guidelines (e.g., CONSORT, PRISMA) governing quality scientific presentation (7–30); see Table 1.1. A careful read of the relevant guideline in advance of conducting a study can help with templating the manuscript for publication.

Similarly, clinical trial protocols tend to follow a standard format including a Table of Contents, Schema, Objectives, Background, Eligibility, Schedule or Table of Assessments/Events, Treatment Plan, Requirements for Treatment Modifications, Adverse Event Reporting Requirements, Registration Procedures, Pathology/Biospecimen Procedures, Quality Assurance Plan, Data Collection and Management Procedures, and Statistical Considerations. In addition, the Informed Consent Form (ICF) must explain in plain language (typically, eighth-grade reading level) the usual approach or standard of care, the voluntary nature of consent and the patient's choices if he or she does not wish to participate, purpose and design of the study, length of time the patient will be on study, extra tests and procedures involved with participation, expected risks and potential benefits (if any) associated with participation, costs of participation, rights and options for withdrawing from the study, plan for disseminating information, processes in the event of patient injury, and contact information for study personnel. Clinical trials should be registered at clinicaltrials.gov and assigned a protocol number for tracking trial results.

For research protocols, it is important to balance specificity in the interest of scientific rigor with simplicity in the interest of practical execution. Study coordinators are obliged to follow a protocol to the letter, so often the less said the better, particularly when a requirement is not directly pertinent to the research question. In some sections, it is acceptable to allow normal practice variation per institutional standards (such as for treatment modifications). Regulatory processes at most institutions can take several months or more, so multiple protocol amendments can significantly delay a study's conduct. Often, outside agencies (e.g., Food and Drug Administration [FDA]) and study sponsors (National Institutes of Health [NIH], industry partners) will also need

TABLE 1.1 COMMON GUIDELINES FOR STUDY DESIGN AND PUBLICATION

Acronym	Guideline	Purpose	Reference
AGREE	**A**ppraisal of **G**uidelines, **Re**search and **E**valuation	Improve reporting of clinical practice guidelines	(8)
ARRIVE	**A**nimal **R**esearch: **R**eporting of **I**n **V**ivo **E**xperiments	Improve reporting of research based on animals	(9)
BRISQ	**B**iospecimen **R**eporting for **I**mproved **S**tudy **Q**uality	Standardized information specific to the preanalytical conditions relating to biospecimens	(10)
CARE	Consensus-based Clinical **Ca**se **Re**porting	Improve completeness and transparency of case reports and case series	(11)
CONSORT	**Cons**olidated **S**tandards **o**f **R**eporting **T**rials	Establish reporting guidelines for parallel group randomized trials	(12)
COREQ	**Co**nsolidated Criteria for **Re**porting **Q**ualitative Research	Help researchers report important elements of qualitative research, including interviews and focus groups	(13)
EQUATOR	**E**nhancing the **Qu**ality **a**nd **T**ransparency **o**f Health **R**esearch	Monitor use of guidelines, improve quality of scientific publications, promote accurate reporting of medical research	(14)
GNOSIS	**G**uidelines for **N**euro-**O**ncology: **S**tandards for **I**nvestigational **S**tudies	Standardize reporting of clinical trials in neuro-oncology	(15)
MIAME	**M**inimum **I**nformation **A**bout a **M**icroarray **E**xperiment	Outline the minimum information required to ensure that microarray-based gene expression data can be easily interpreted and independently verified	(16)
MOOSE	**M**eta-analysis **o**f **O**bservational **S**tudies in **E**pidemiology	Describe specifications for reporting meta-analyses of observational studies in epidemiology	(17)
PRISMA	**P**referred **R**eporting **I**tems for **S**ystematic Reviews and **M**eta-**A**nalyses	Standardize guidelines for reporting systematic reviews and meta-analyses	(18)
QUOROM	**Qu**ality **o**f **R**eporting **o**f **M**eta-analyses	Improve the quality of reports of meta-analyses of randomized controlled trials	(19)
REMARK	**Re**porting Recommendations for Tumor **Mark**er Prognostic Studies	Establish guidelines for reporting tumor marker studies, including relevant information about the study design, preplanned hypotheses, patient and specimen characteristics, assay methods, and statistical analysis methods	(20)

(continued)

TABLE 1.1 COMMON GUIDELINES FOR STUDY DESIGN AND PUBLICATION (*continued*)

Acronym	Guideline	Purpose	Reference
RIGHT	Reporting Tool for Practice Guidelines in Healthcare	Improve quality of reporting practice guidelines in healthcare including basic information, background, evidence, recommendations, quality assurance, funding, and declaration and management of interests	(21)
SISAQOL	Setting International Standards in Analyzing Patient-Reported Outcomes and Quality of Life Endpoints Data	Standardize the reporting and inclusion of patient-reported outcome and quality of life instruments on clinical trials	(31)
SPIRIT	Standard Protocol Items: Recommendations for Interventional Trials	Provides recommendations for scientific, ethical, and administrative elements that should be addressed in a clinical trial protocol in order to promote proper trial implementation and facilitate appraisal of scientific and ethical considerations	(22)
SPIRIT-PRO	Standard Protocol Items: Recommendations for Interventional Trials—Patient Reported Outcomes	Provides recommendations for elements that should be addressed in a clinical trial protocol involving patient-reported outcome instruments	(23)
SQUIRE	Standards for Quality Improvement Reporting Excellence	Establish guidelines for conducting and reporting studies on quality improvement	(24)
STARD	Standards for the Reporting of Diagnostic Accuracy Studies	Improve design and conduct of diagnostic accuracy studies	(25)
STREGA	Strengthening the Reporting of Genetic Association Studies	Enhances transparency of studies reporting genetic associations, particularly concerning population stratification, genotyping errors, replication, selection of participants, treatment effects, statistical methods, and reporting of outcome data	(26)
STROBE	Strengthening the Reporting of Observational Studies in Epidemiology	Improve design and reporting of observational studies in epidemiology, including cohort, case-control, and cross-sectional studies	(27)
STROGAR	Strengthening the Reporting of Genetic Association Studies in Radiogenomics	Increase the transparency and completeness of reporting studies involving radiogenomics	(28)

(*continued*)

TABLE 1.1 COMMON GUIDELINES FOR STUDY DESIGN AND PUBLICATION (*continued*)

Acronym	Guideline	Purpose	Reference
TREND	Transparent Reporting of Evaluations with Nonrandomized Designs	Improve reporting standards for nonrandomized evaluations of behavioral and public health interventions	(29)
TRIPOD	Transparent Reporting of a Multivariable Prediction Model for Individual Prognosis or Diagnosis	Improve quality of reporting for studies involving prediction models	(30)

to weigh in on study changes. In addition to regulatory committees and sponsors, an institution's budget or contracts office often will need to approve the protocol to ensure there is adequate financial coverage for the proposed study procedures, taking into account what procedures are considered the standard of care versus experimental.

FUNDING YOUR RESEARCH

Applying for funding can be one of the more intimidating processes for young investigators. The time-consuming nature of grant preparation and fear of rejection and exposing oneself to criticism pose common barriers to prospective applicants. Fortunately, many funding agencies have special mechanisms such as seed grants and career development awards to support early stage investigators and protect time to focus on research. During training, seeking opportunities to apply for small grants can initiate one to the process and build practice, as well as an early track record if one happens to be successful. Many departments will also provide start-up funding for newly hired junior faculty.

Ultimately, it is important to get comfortable with rejection, because if your career is long, it will happen often. The process is sort of like asking someone to go on a date. There is a considerable degree of randomness and subjectivity, and sometimes things do not work out. However, certain behaviors that constitute good **grantsmanship** can increase the likelihood of success over the long run. It is also morally acceptable to "date" multiple prospective sponsors simultaneously, at least until things get serious (i.e., your project is funded). Most importantly, you need to make a good first impression in order to convince reviewers that your idea is important and novel.

One helpful approach is to try to regard your own writing through a reviewer's eyes. Volunteering to serve on review committees is a great way to gain practice and perspective. For example, one thing to understand is that reviewers will usually be experts in their field, but not necessarily yours. Typically they are busy, impatient people with declining eyesight who find crammed pages and compressed figures painful to read. Therefore, clarity, simplicity, and organization in writing are cardinal virtues. Pleasurably written applications with under-reliance on acronyms are frequently rewarded with better scores.

When following the NIH scoring system, reviewers grade applications according to five key features: Significance, Innovation, Approach, Investigators, and Environment. Each element is important and rather self-explanatory, but the greatest variation in scoring usually occurs in the first three areas, which form the core of the Research Strategy. The NIH scoring system grades applications from 1 (best) to 9 (worst), with scores of 1 to 3 indicating no or only minor weaknesses, 4 to 6 indicating one or more moderate weaknesses, and 7 to 9 indicating one or more major weaknesses. These are combined into an overall score for the application. A study section usually convenes to discuss the top-scored grants, and a summary statement reflecting the commentary (regardless of whether it was discussed) is issued to the PI.

Typically, grant applications include several standard elements: Specific Aims, Research Strategy, Investigator Biosketches, Facilities/Environment, and Budget/Budget Justification. Other elements may include letters of support, abstracts, or other documents that can bolster the application. The most crucial sections are the Research Strategy and the Specific Aims. However, the grant application cannot proceed without all the elements. Because tracking down and preparing supporting documents can be tedious and time-consuming, collecting these when you start the application can save last-minute headaches and prevent missed deadlines. Other general tips are to develop a document checklist and carefully follow the directions pertinent to the funding announcement to which you are responding. Being mindful of key deadlines for internal institutional review, which may precede the grant deadline by days or even weeks, is also crucial. Finally, as PI of a grant, you need to be prepared to track down and review your coinvestigators' biosketches, letters of support, and personal statements, to ensure they support and enhance the application, as these will affect its score.

The Specific Aims section is a one-page synopsis of the application, designed to succinctly convey why your research is significant and innovative, what you plan to do, and how you will go about it. There are many different strategies but generally two aims (primary and exploratory) are sufficient for smaller grants (R03, R21, etc.) and three aims (primary, secondary, and exploratory) are ideal for larger grants (R01, etc.). More aims are appropriate for very large grants (center awards, etc.). A grant can have more than one primary aim, but too many can raise feasibility questions and distract from the core objectives one is trying to achieve. A primary aim should address a critical question or hypothesis that is definitely answerable given the methods proposed. Often the primary aim will principally determine the sample size and cost of the study. A secondary aim may address a related but distinct hypothesis that can be answered as a consequence of collecting data to achieve the primary aim. A tertiary or **exploratory aim** usually is designed as a hypothesis-generating strategy to collect novel preliminary data to seed future work along the same research line. A key piece of advice is not to make your aims dependent on one another; that is, Aim 2 should not depend critically on the results you obtain in Aim 1. This is a classic pitfall that will cause many reviewers to downgrade applications.

The Research Strategy section is the meat of the application. It is your opportunity to showcase why the research is significant and innovative, and explain in detail the approach you will use to achieve your specific aims. The Background section should carefully review the pertinent literature and explain the existing state of knowledge, and what crucial gaps this new research will fill. The Innovation section should emphasize what is novel about your approach and techniques, and may include any preliminary data *you and your research group* have collected; you should not cite others' work as your preliminary data. The Approach section should provide an in-depth, point-by-point explanation of how you intend to achieve each specific aim, and what methods you will employ. In this section it is also important to address any statistical considerations, including power analysis, as well as to provide a schedule or table of data collection and other study events. Many PIs include a timeline for study execution as well. Finally, it is wise to briefly address any potential pitfalls, limitations, or obstacles you anticipate and how you envision managing them.

Making sure the prospective sponsor is likely to be receptive to your ideas is also a helpful strategy. For example, the largest sponsor of medical research, the NIH, currently comprises 21 institutes, each with a different emphasis and focus (visit grants.nih.gov for further information). The National Cancer Institute (NCI), National Institute of Biomedical Imaging and Bioengineering (NIBIB), National Institute of Neurological Disorders and Stroke (NINDS), and National Institute on Aging (NIA) are examples of institutes that support funding initiatives relevant to oncology. The U.S. Department of Defense (DOD), National Science Foundation (NSF), and Agency for Healthcare Research and Quality (AHRQ) are other federal agencies that support cancer research. Each institute issues its particular funding programs, requests for applications (RFAs), requests for proposals (RFPs), and contract initiatives that may align with your research direction and scale of project. Many clinical trials are funded through cooperative groups, such as Southwest Oncology Group (SWOG), NRG Oncology, Alliance, and Eastern Cooperative Oncology Group (ECOG), with support from the NCI. Most state governments and numerous nonprofit entities and foundations, such as Howard Hughes Medical Institute (HHMI), Burroughs Wellcome Fund, Bill and Melinda Gates Foundation, and the Patient-Centered Outcomes Research Institute (PCORI) operate research funding programs. Medical societies such as the American Society of Clinical Oncology (ASCO) and Radiological Society of North America (RSNA) typically offer grant programs as well. Last, the private industry plays a vital role in sponsoring cancer research, particularly in supporting large registration clinical trials of novel cancer therapies (see Chapter 9).

Asking for support from key individuals who can advocate for your application is also useful. Ideally, one should seek input from mentors and coinvestigators in designing the study and provide them a chance to review any materials and gather feedback. In addition, many institutions have support staff that can assist with preparing and collecting ancillary documents crucial to the application. In particular, working with administrative staff to review the proposed budget is an essential and often overlooked aspect of grant application preparedness. Having the Specific Aims, Key Personnel, and Schedule of Events handy will greatly assist in properly budgeting your and your colleagues' effort on the project, staffing needs, and equipment and other resources you will need to execute your research. When working through nonprofit funding agencies, often it is helpful to identify the Program Officer (PO) and Scientific Review Officer (SRO) throughout the process for advice on your application. You can also find out who is on the study section roster for your application, but it is not permissible to contact members of the study section to discuss your grant. When proposing concepts through a cooperative group mechanism, it is often instructive to contact the committee leaders or other members to learn the procedures and deadlines for submitting a Letter of Intent (LOI). Last, private companies often designate medical science liaisons (MSLs) to assist with applications and advocate for new study concepts. MSLs are also helpful for predicting which strategies and concepts are likely to be reviewed favorably, saving tremendous amounts of work.

Becoming a successful academic is a lot like becoming a good poker player. Luck plays a significant role, but over the long run, savvy players will come out ahead. For despite the finer gradations of scoring systems, most grants fall into three more or less evenly distributed categories: "Great," "Pretty Good," and "Has Issues." Roughly the top 15% to 20% of NIH grants in a given cycle will ultimately be funded, and approximately 25% of investigators who apply for funding in a given year will be successful (Figure 1.2). This means that many great proposals will not be funded, indicating a large component of random noise in the system, which can be demonstrated using the **pigeonhole principle**. This principle dictates that if there are m bins (e.g., funding slots) each with room for one object (e.g., a grant), and there are n objects (e.g., applications) with $n > m$, then at least one object will not get assigned to a bin. If the n objects are indistinguishable, then the probability of not being assigned a bin is $\frac{n-m}{n}$. This is where the benefits of repeated sampling become manifest, since the probability (P) of repeatedly not being assigned to a bin after k (independent) tries is

$$P = \left(\frac{n-m}{n}\right)^k. \quad [2]$$

Note that since $0 < \left(\frac{n-m}{n}\right) < 1$, $P \rightarrow 0$ as $k \rightarrow \infty$. Thus, we arrive at a Bernoullian exposition of the value of perseverance in grant writing. Your goal, therefore, should be to enter as many tournaments as possible.

CONCLUSIONS

Let us end this introductory chapter with a few additional pieces of general advice. First, never design an experiment to *confirm* your hypothesis. Design an experiment to *interrogate* your hypothesis. You should be equally interested in your findings regardless of whether they appear to confirm

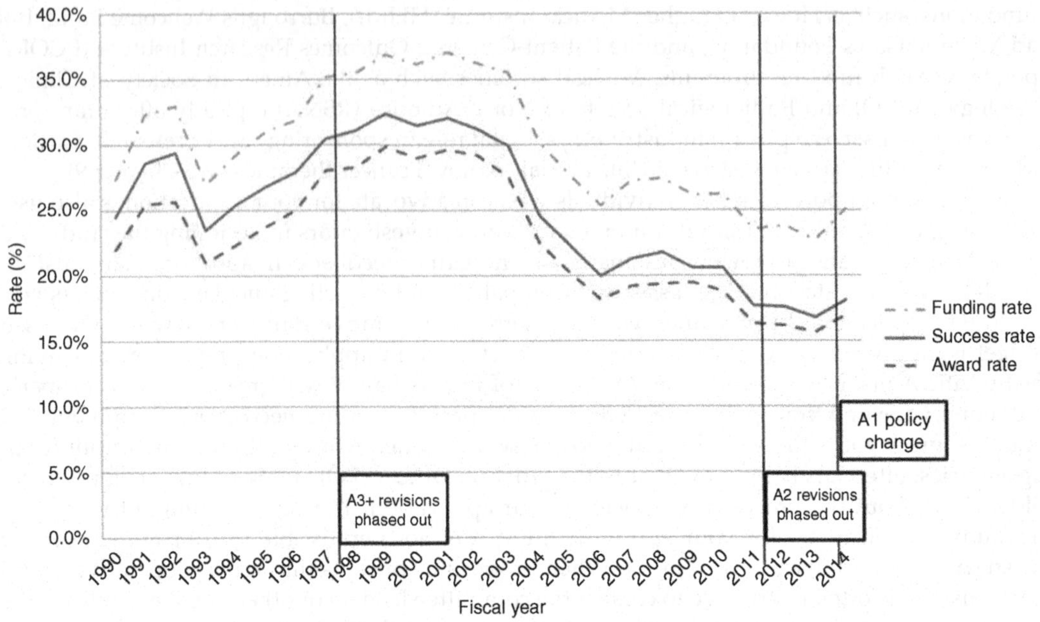

FIGURE 1.2 Current National Institutes of Health award, success, and funding rates* for research project grants (fiscal years 1990–2014).

*Excludes awards made with American Recovery and Reinvestment Act (ARRA) funds, and ARRA-solicited applications.

or deny your suppositions. If you cannot say that, you need to redesign your study. Second, never wholly trust anyone's data—least of all your own. Allowing others' research to inform but not define your thinking will put you in a better position to question assumptions. Moreover, you should be the least forgiving critic of your results; that way everyone else's critiques will seem nicer.

Last, a great scientist is both creative and trustworthy. Present your results dispassionately and in good faith. Your colleagues will appreciate it when you expose truths rather than espouse beliefs. Ultimately, however, the greatest asset you can bring to the field is your curiosity, which motivates the steady drive toward scientific enlightenment.

GLOSSARY

bias: a systematic deviation from the truth due to research design, conduct, analysis, or reporting.

bias of professional accomplishment: value skewing created by reputation and publication(s).

conflict of interest (COI): a usually nonmalicious form of bias created by monetary or other influences.

control: (verb) to isolate the effect and outcome of interest; (noun) a factor or experimental condition that allows one to isolate an effect or outcome of interest.

estimator: a statistic or method for acquiring an estimate of a given quantity based on observed data.

expected value: a predicted value of a variable, calculated as the sum of all possible values each multiplied by the probability of its occurrence.

exploratory aim: usually, a hypothesis-generating strategy to collect novel preliminary data to seed future work along the same research line.

grantsmanship: behaviors that can increase the possibility that a project will be funded.

h-index: a measure of both the productivity and impact of a scholar, defined as the highest number of a scholar's publications for which each have h or more citations.

hypothesis: theory to be tested/proven or question to be answered by research.

negative control: a factor or condition that shows that an effect is not present when it is expected not to be present.

pigeonhole principle: principle which dictates that if there are m bins, each with room for one object, and there are n objects, with n > m, then at least one object will not get assigned to a bin.

positive control: a factor or condition that shows that an effect is present when it is expected to be present.

publication bias: a situation when the results of a study influence its probability of publication.

selection bias: a distortion in a measure of association or effect that is due to sample selection which does not accurately reflect the target population.

REFERENCES

1. National Comprehensive Cancer Network. NCCN guidelines & clinical resources. https://www.nccn.org/professionals/physician_gls/categories_of_consensus.aspx
2. Zietman AL. Falsification, fabrication, and plagiarism: the unholy trinity of scientific writing. *Int J Radiat Oncol Biol Phys.* 2013;87(2):225–227. doi:10.1016/j.ijrobp.2013.07.004
3. Trifiletti DM, Showalter TN. Bias of professional accomplishment: another important concept for the ethics of clinical research. *Int J Radiat Oncol Biol Phys.* 2018;100(2):297–298. doi:10.1016/j.ijrobp.2017.10.035
4. Barker K. *At The Helm: A Laboratory Navigator.* 2nd ed. New York, NY: Cold Spring Harbor Laboratory Press; 2010.
5. Barker K. *At the Bench: A Laboratory Navigator.* New York, NY: Cold Spring Harbor Laboratory Press; 2004.
6. Burroughs Wellcome Fund, Howard Hughes Medical Institute. *Making the Right Moves: A Practical Guide to Scientific Management for Postdocs and New Faculty.* 2nd ed. Chevy Chase, MD: Howard Hughes Medical Institute; 2006. http://www.hhmi.org/developing-scientists/making-right-moves
7. Vandenbroucke JP. STREGA, STROBE, STARD, SQUIRE, MOOSE, PRISMA, GNOSIS, TREND, ORION, COREQ, QUOROM, REMARK... and CONSORT: for whom does the guideline toll? *J Clin Epidemiol.* 2009;62(6):594–596. doi:10.1016/j.jclinepi.2008.12.003
8. Brouwers MC, Kerkvliet K, Spithoff K. The AGREE Reporting Checklist: a tool to improve reporting of clinical practice guidelines. *BMJ.* 2016;352:i1152. doi:10.1136/bmj.i1152
9. Kilkenny C, Browne WJ, Cuthill IC, et al. Improving bioscience research reporting: the ARRIVE guidelines for reporting animal research. *PLoS Biol.* 2010;8(6):e1000412. doi:10.1371/journal.pbio.1000412
10. Moore HM, Kelly A, Jewell SD, et al. Biospecimen reporting for improved study quality. *Biopreserv Biobank.* 2011;9(1):57–70. doi:10.1089/bio.2010.0036
11. Gagnier JJ, Kienle G, Altman DG, et al. The CARE guidelines: consensus-based clinical case reporting guideline development. *J Clin Epidemiol.* 2014;67(1):46–51. doi:10.1016/j.jclinepi.2013.08.003
12. Schulz KF, Altman DG, Moher D. CONSORT 2010 statement: updated guidelines for reporting parallel group randomised trials. *BMJ.* 2010;340:c332. doi:10.1136/bmj.c332
13. Tong A, Sainsbury P, Craig J. Consolidated criteria for reporting qualitative research (COREQ): a 32-item checklist for interviews and focus groups. *Int J Qual Health Care.* 2007;19(6):349–357. doi:10.1093/intqhc/mzm042
14. EQUATOR Network. Home page. https://www.equator-network.org
15. Chang SM, Reynolds SL, Butowski N, et al. GNOSIS: guidelines for neuro-oncology: standards for investigational studies-reporting of phase 1 and phase 2 clinical trials. *Neuro Oncol.* 2005;7(4):425–434. doi:10.1215/S1152851705000554
16. Brazma A, Hingamp P, Quackenbush J, et al. Minimum information about a microarray experiment (MIAME)-toward standards for microarray data. *Nat Genet.* 2001;29(4):365–371. doi:10.1038/ng1201-365
17. Stroup DF, Berlin JA, Morton SC, et al. Meta-analysis of observational studies in epidemiology: a proposal for reporting. *JAMA.* 2000;283(15):2008–2012. doi:10.1001/jama.283.15.2008
18. Moher D, Liberati A, Tetzlaff J, et al. Preferred reporting items for systematic reviews and meta-analyses: the PRISMA statement. *Ann Intern Med.* 2009;151(4):264–269, W64. doi:10.7326/0003-4819-151-4-200908180-00135
19. Moher D, Cook DJ, Eastwood S, et al. Improving the quality of reports of meta-analyses of randomised controlled trials: the QUOROM statement. Quality of Reporting of Meta-analyses. *Lancet.* 1999;354(9193):1896–1900. doi:10.1016/S0140-6736(99)04149-5

20. McShane LM, Altman DG, Sauerbrei W, et al. Reporting recommendations for tumor marker prognostic studies (REMARK). *J Natl Cancer Inst.* 2005;97(16):1180–1184. doi:10.1093/jnci/dji237
21. Chen Y, Yang K, Marušić A, et al. A reporting tool for practice guidelines in health care: the RIGHT statement. *Ann Intern Med.* 2017;166(2):128–132. doi:10.7326/M16-1565
22. Chan A-W, Tetzlaff JM, Gøtzsche PC, et al. SPIRIT 2013 explanation and elaboration: guidance for protocols of clinical trials. *BMJ.* 2013;346:e7586. doi:10.1136/bmj.e7586
23. Calvert M, Kyte D, Mercieca-Bebber R, et al. Guidelines for inclusion of patient-reported outcomes in clinical trial protocols: the SPIRIT-PRO extension. *JAMA.* 2018;319(5):483–494. doi:10.1001/jama.2017.21903
24. Ogrinc G, Davies L, Goodman D, et al. SQUIRE 2.0—Standards for Quality Improvement Reporting Excellence: revised publication guidelines from a detailed consensus process. *J Am Coll Surg.* 2016;222(3):317–323. doi:10.1016/j.jamcollsurg.2015.07.456
25. Bossuyt PM, Reitsma JB, Bruns DE, et al. STARD 2015: an updated list of essential items for reporting diagnostic accuracy studies. *BMJ.* 2015;351:h5527. doi:10.1136/bmj.h5527
26. Little J, Higgins JP, Ioannidis JP, et al. STrengthening the REporting of Genetic Association studies (STREGA)—an extension of the STROBE statement. *Eur J Clin Invest.* 2009;39(4):247–266. doi:10.1111/j.1365-2362.2009.02125.x
27. von Elm E, Altman DG, Egger M, et al. The Strengthening the Reporting of Observational Studies in Epidemiology (STROBE) Statement: guidelines for reporting observational studies. *Lancet.* 2007;370(9596):1453–1457. doi:10.1016/S0140-6736(07)61602-X
28. Kerns SL, de Ruysscher D, Andreassen CN, et al. STROGAR–STrengthening the Reporting of Genetic Association studies in Radiogenomics. *Radiother Oncol.* 2014;110(1):182–188. doi:10.1016/j.radonc.2013.07.011
29. Fuller T, Peters J, Pearson M, Anderson R. Impact of the transparent reporting of evaluations with nonrandomized designs reporting guideline: ten years on. *Am J Public Health.* 2014;104(11):e110–e117. doi:10.2105/AJPH.2014.302195
30. Collins GS, Reitsma JB, Altman DG, Moons KG. Transparent reporting of a multivariable prediction model for individual prognosis or diagnosis (TRIPOD): the TRIPOD statement. *Br J Cancer.* 2015;112(2):251–259. doi:10.1038/bjc.2014.639
31. Bottomley A, Pe M, Sloan J, et al. Analysing data from patient-reported outcome and quality of life endpoints for cancer clinical trials: a start in setting international standards. *Lancet Oncol.* 2016;17(11):e510–e514. doi:10.1016/S1470-2045(16)30510-1

2

Bias and Pitfalls in Cancer Research

MAK DJULBEGOVIC ■ MIA DJULBEGOVIC ■ BENJAMIN DJULBEGOVIC

The rise of the evidence-based medicine (EBM) movement (1) has forced physicians and clinical researchers to realize the "scandal of poor medical research" (2), which is associated with many avoidable pitfalls. Numerous influential studies have shown that most research "findings" are false (3). As such, approximately 50% of research efforts are wasted at each stage of generation and reporting of research, resulting in more than 85% of all research being considered wasteful (4). Human suffering due to poorly done research has been enormous (5), resulting in avoidable morbidity and mortality, as in the case of biased research being used to promote bone marrow transplantation for the treatment of breast cancer (6). Not surprisingly, the past several years have increasingly witnessed calls for improvements in standards for clinical research (5).

In this chapter, we address the most common pitfalls and summarize the main sources of bias affecting the production of clinical research evidence. We explain how these pitfalls are often committed by clinical researchers' ***bias***, which is defined as *a systematic deviation from the truth due to research design, conduct, analysis, or reporting* (7). Key sources of bias include (a) choosing an inappropriate control intervention (***comparator bias***); (b) systematic differences in comparison groups (***selection bias***); (c) systematic differences in the care provided (apart from the intervention being evaluated; ***performance bias***); (d) systematic errors in the measurement of information on exposure or outcomes (***information bias***); (e) systematic differences in withdrawal of participants from the trial (***attrition bias***); and (f) systematic differences in outcome assessment (***detection, recall,*** and ***observer biases***). We provide examples of each pitfall and strategies to avoid it, with emphasis on therapeutic research, which arguably dominates research practice in oncology.

ARCHITECTURE OF CLINICAL RESEARCH: A BRIEF OVERVIEW

Figure 2.1 provides an overview of the types of clinical research (8). In general, the key question in designing and conducting a clinical research study revolves around the investigators' involvement in the assignment of exposure (e.g., treatment). If the investigator has control over the treatment assignment, the study is called an ***experimental*** study. An investigator can, however, divorce

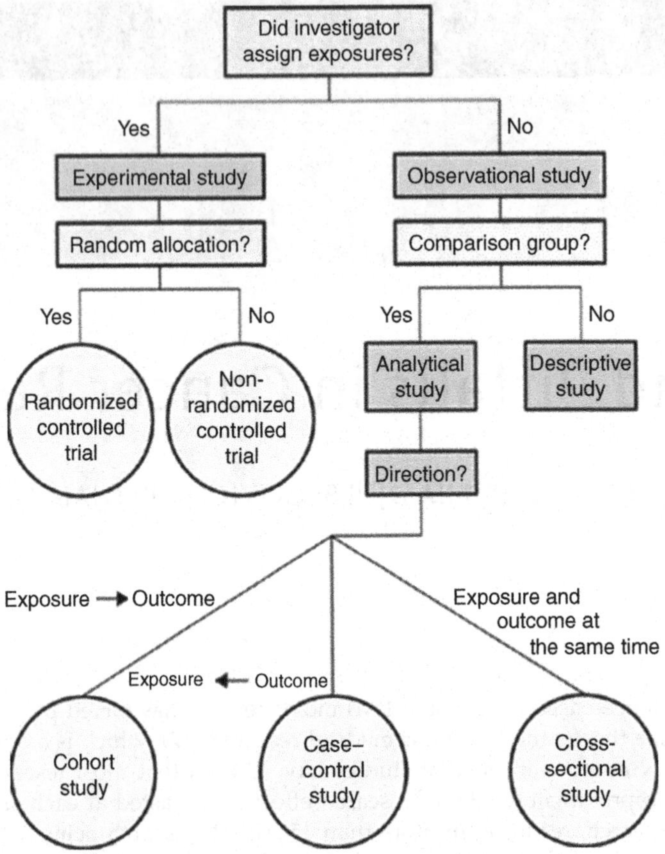

FIGURE 2.1 The architecture of clinical research.

Source: Grimes DA, Schulz KF. An overview of clinical research: the lay of the land. *Lancet.* 2002;359:57–61. doi:10.1016/S0140-6736(02)07283-5

herself/himself from assigning the treatment exposure, as in the case of a randomized controlled trial (RCT), when treatment allocation is performed randomly. If the researcher fully controls the exposure, the research design is considered a nonrandomized experimental study. For example, this would be the case if a treatment was given on alternative days with the investigator's full knowledge of treatment allocation. If, however, the investigator does not control the exposure (such as the treatment assignment) but instead just records the outcomes (as they would otherwise occur without the investigation), the research design is considered ***observational***.

When investigators first assess patient outcomes, followed by retrospectively assessing the exposure (i.e., treatments), this research design is referred to as a ***case–control study***. If, however, researchers first determine the exposure and then over time follow the outcomes in each exposure (i.e., treatment) group, the study is referred to as a ***cohort study***. Cohort studies can be prospective or retrospective, depending on the way the data are collected. When the exposure and outcome occur at about the same time, such a study is often called a cross-sectional study. Controversy exists about the proper classification of cross-sectional studies, but this design is typically used to assess the value of diagnostic tests and rarely to evaluate the effect of treatments in an oncology setting. Hence, it is not further considered here.

A fundamental concept in the field of therapeutic research is that treatment evaluation should always be an exercise in ***comparison***. Even if a study does not include a comparator (such as what is often seen in ***case series***) (9), implicit counterfactual comparisons exist.

BIAS IN THERAPEUTIC RESEARCH

Any research results can only be explained in one of three ways: (a) The findings represent correct results, that is, they represent the "truth"; (b) they reflect a play of chance (random error); or (c) they are due to systematic error or deviation from the "truth" (10). The results should be accepted only when the treatment effect (effect size) is greater than the combined effect of biases and random errors. In this chapter, we focus on bias that can creep into the conduct of clinical research. Bias can occur at each step of conduct, such as at the level of research idea conception, performance, analysis, publication, or citation (11) (Figure 2.2). It is estimated that about $200 billion is lost annually worldwide from wasteful generation and reporting of flawed research (4). Here, we focus on assessing and avoiding the risk of bias in the way studies are carried out. By applying correct research methodology, avoidable waste could be reduced by 42% (12).

The contrast between **precision** and **accuracy** is discussed further in Chapter 23. For example, a well-conducted, small study with a low risk of bias (high accuracy) may provide results with a wide confidence interval (low precision). In contrast, the results of a large study may generate very narrow confidence intervals (high precision) but have a high risk of bias (low accuracy) due to inadequate internal validity (7).

Reporting bias also plagues the current literature (13,14). A classic example is the **Texas sharpshooter fallacy**. A "Texas sharpshooter" jokingly refers to one who first fires shots into the side of a barn, then draws the target around the bullet holes. Fallacies of this type occur in analysis when an investigator fits the data to the hypothesis, rather than the converse. This fallacy commonly results from multiple hypothesis testing (Chapter 11), which raises the probability of spurious findings and "p-value hacking," where data are reanalyzed until a statistically significant finding emerges. Similarly, **confirmation bias** can result when investigators continue to interrogate data up until the point that the data appear to support the hypothesis, then stop. In general, investigators should avoid selective reporting and, in particular, they should declare all prespecified outcomes (7,15) (see Figure 2.2). Finally, bias or confounding resulting from *nonspecificity*, which is a particular problem in survival analysis, is treated later in Chapter 16.

BIAS IN RANDOMIZED TRIALS

Figure 2.3 depicts how an RCT is conducted and the points where bias can occur at each step of the trial. Historically, bias has been considered in the context of ***internal validity***—the extent to

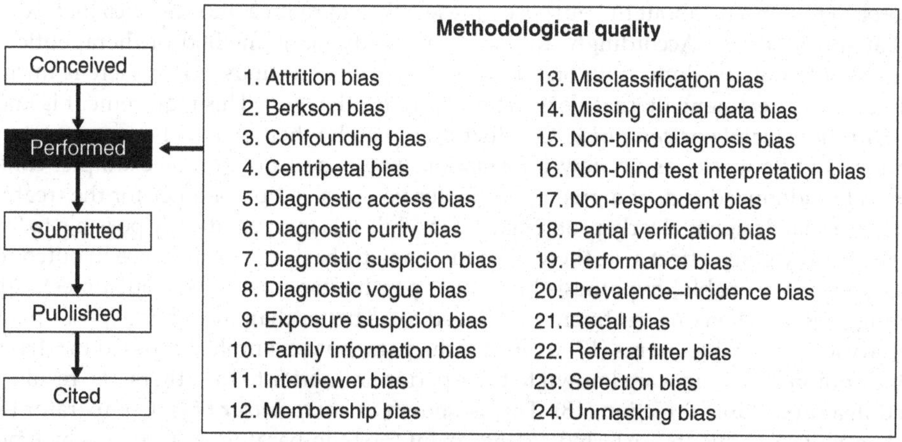

FIGURE 2.2 Sources of bias in the production and dissemination of evidence.

Source: Courtesy of Dr. Mike Clarke.

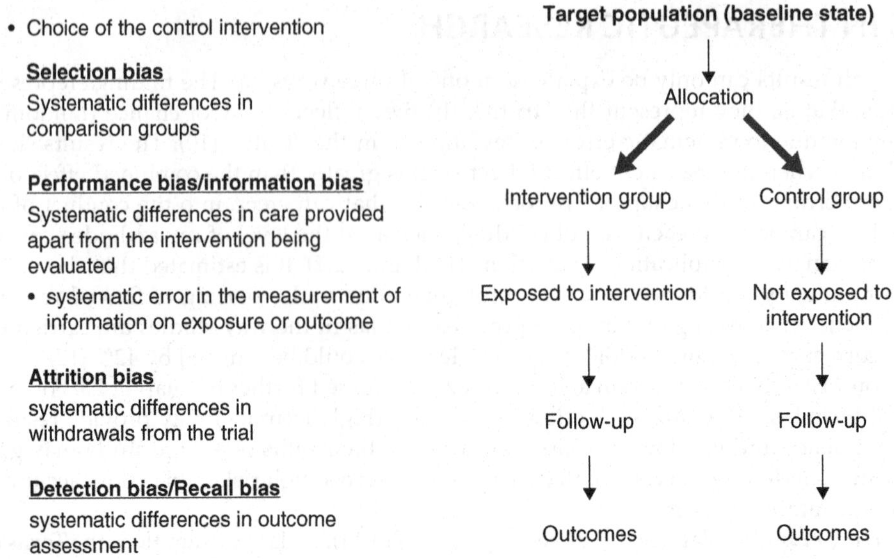

FIGURE 2.3 The main sources of bias during the conduct of clinical study. The first term typically refers to randomized controlled studies, whereas the second term is most commonly used in observational research.

which a trial provides valid information under the current trial conditions. In other words, internal validity refers to how confident we are that an estimate of effect is correct (free from bias) (7). This should be distinguished from ***external validity***—the extent to which the study findings can be applied (generalized) to another clinical setting (i.e., your patient) (7). Obviously, trials with poor internal validity (biased trials) cannot have adequate external validity. However, the opposite can be true: trials with excellent internal validity can have poor generalizability. This occurs, for example, when the results of an RCT that enrolled patients with narrow eligibility criteria and no comorbidities are applied to older patients with multiple comorbidities (16).

COMPARATOR BIAS

One approach to thinking about the purpose of research is to reduce uncertainties that exist in the world that surrounds us. Accordingly, RCTs—as a paradigmatic method of therapeutic clinical research—should only be done, both on ethical and scientific grounds, when there is uncertainty as to whether one treatment alternative is better than the other (17). This requirement is known as the ***uncertainty principle*** or ***equipoise***. Conducting research when there is no uncertainty would amount to scientific waste, as no new information would be learned. For example, consider a hypothetical randomized trial of a green peashooter versus a red peashooter for the treatment of cancer. Such a trial design is clearly problematic, for while it is mathematically possible to "power" such a trial for any given effect size, there is no mechanistic basis for a difference in outcomes (the essential [and unreasonable] hypothesis being that peashooter color affects outcomes). Ethically, performing an RCT when one treatment is believed to be better than the other exposes patients to unnecessary and avoidable harms (17) (consider the parachute example discussed in Chapter 10).

If one or more treatments are known to be superior or inferior to the others, the results would be biased in a predictable direction (18). This is known as ***comparator bias***. Comparator bias can occur when active treatments are tested against an inferior comparator or placebo, which predominantly happens in industry-sponsored trials (18–21). For example, in 1995, after conducting five trials that enrolled a total of 656 patients, researchers demonstrated that exogenous erythropoietin administration improved cancer-related anemia compared to placebo. However, investigators continued to test the effects of exogenous erythropoietin in 13 additional placebo-controlled RCTs that were reported well beyond 1995, thus denying effective treatment to patients who were inappropriately administered placebo (22). Interestingly, uncertainty remains regarding the effect of exogenous erythropoietin administration on overall survival, even though the drug was originally approved in 1989 after testing its effects on anemia. Comparator bias can also occur when researchers inappropriately select an active comparator: for example, when new drug regimens are compared to lower (and thus less effective) doses of the same drug (18). Such pitfalls can be significantly reduced if the investigators and regulatory agencies undertake RCTs only when equipoise exists, thus enabling the choice of a correct and fair comparator (17).

Methods of assessing whether uncertainty exists about treatment effects include surveying experts, consulting practice guidelines, or relying on systematic reviews of relevant existing evidence to inform choice of control intervention (18,23). Unfortunately, less than 50% of therapeutic research investigators are aware of existing studies that could inform their choice of an appropriate comparator. Comparator bias can be significantly reduced when RCTs are conducted under conditions of true epistemic uncertainty (17).

SELECTION BIAS

Proper or fair comparisons should be based on comparing "like with like." *Selection bias* refers to systematic differences between comparison groups (apart from the treatment that is being compared) (24). Selection bias is pervasive in medicine and is a major cause of biased inferences and treatment effect overestimation. For example, when high-dose chemotherapy and stem cell transplant were compared to standard chemotherapy using two well-matched, standardized databases, the investigators found a 72% relative risk reduction of death due to breast cancer in favor of stem cell transplant (25). This large effect helped established stem cell transplant as the standard of care for the treatment of breast cancer in the late 1990s and early 2000s. However, subsequent randomized trials showed no difference between these two treatment modalities (6), proving that even when using well-matched patients, observational studies can lead to biased assessments. Apparently, women who received stem cell transplants had markedly different risk profiles (i.e., were healthier at baseline and/or had more indolent disease) than those who did not, and the observed differences were due to important but uncollected covariates that were not adjusted for in the comparison (i.e., confounders). For example, data on genomic profiles, which are now known to profoundly impact patients' prognosis and response to treatment, were not collected in the late 1980s and early 1990s (26). As a result, stem cell transplant—one of the major hyped treatments for breast cancer in the late 1990s and early 2000s—virtually disappeared from the cancer treatment lexicon.

Although many analytical methods have been developed, randomization remains the best method for controlling selection bias (27). However, RCTs are not automatically immune from selection bias. In RCTs, selection bias is controlled by making sure that (a) random allocation is properly done through adequate generation of random assignments, which is typically computer generated (e.g., using block randomization); and (b) treatment allocation is adequately concealed, that is, treatment assignment is concealed until after the treatment has been allocated (7). Failure to adequately implement random assignment and ensure ***allocation concealment*** can lead to biased treatment effect estimates in up to 35% to 45% of RCTs, respectively (12,28). Of note, allocation concealment is not the same as ***masking*** or ***blinding***: It refers to the technique of ensuring that the treatment assignment is unknown to the involved parties—typically patients and physicians—until after treatment assignment itself. In contrast, blinding and masking refer to concealing information about the assignment throughout the trial and different phases of conduct and analysis. In practice, completing the process of informed consent prior to randomization and, subsequently, adhering to the actual treatment assignment usually ensures adequate allocation concealment.

A common form of selection bias that has been difficult to eradicate from oncology is the retrospective analysis of health outcomes (e.g., survival) according to the observed response (29,30).

For example, when patients whose tumor responded to treatment live longer than those whose tumor has not responded, this is often interpreted to mean that treatment is efficacious. However, comparing responders to nonresponders is biased and should not be employed (29,30). Bias occurs because responders may live longer due to other favorable risk factors and, importantly, they must live long enough for treatment response to be observed, while there is no such requirement for nonresponders (29,30). There are, however, valid statistical methods for analyzing survival by response; common techniques include the ***Mantel-Byar method*** and the ***"landmark method,"*** which evaluate the response to all patients at some fixed time following treatment onset (29,30). Nevertheless, they are not substitutes for randomization, where survival is preferably measured from the date of randomization.

PERFORMANCE BIAS

Performance bias refers to systematic differences in the care provided to the groups of participants being studied apart from the intervention being evaluated (7). Typically, this is due to the effects of cointerventions or temporal shifts in practice that contaminate the results. Such contamination can occur in multicenter trials when various participating centers practice different standards of care with respect to common ancillary interventions, such as antibiotics, transfusions, and pain control. Wheatley et al. report a particularly vivid example that illustrates the effects of performance bias (31). The authors analyzed two induction regimens for the treatment of acute myeloid leukemia: daunorubicin-cytosine arabinoside-thioguanine (DAT) and another regimen called SAB (SAB stands for *same-as-before* treatment), which was introduced later on in the investigators' institutions. They found that SAB reduced mortality in relative terms by 50% (from 30% to 15%; $p = .00007$)! Treatments with such large effects are rarely seen in oncology and if they are true, are typically touted as "breakthrough treatments." Obviously, the reason for observing such dramatic effects in this study was, however, not due to the superiority of DAT as a treatment for leukemia. Rather, mortality dramatically dropped because different supportive care protocols, including more liberal use of antibiotics and growth factors, were introduced into practice (31).

Pitfalls due to performance bias can be avoided by standardizing the management protocols across the institutions participating in a trial, which should be nearly identical (apart from the intervention that is being randomized). Blinding and masking of participants and trial personnel also help prevent this common pitfall (7,24).

ATTRITION BIAS

Attrition bias refers to systematic differences in withdrawals (dropouts) from the trial (7,24). This occurs if the characteristics of those who were lost to follow-up differ between the groups being compared, particularly if these characteristics correlate with the trial's outcome measures (32). This can cause an imbalance among prognostic factors, which will then affect the internal validity of the trial. Attrition bias occurs so commonly that more than 50% of trials have some loss to follow-up or missing data (32). Although some authors suggest that 5% to 20% of data loss is inconsequential, there is no minimum dropout rate that is not associated with bias. This is particularly true if there is a differential dropout rate between the treatment groups. Although complex statistical models can be used to impute missing data, the only way to avoid attrition bias is to assure completeness of follow-up (7,24). The authors should also report the baseline characteristics of those who were included in the analysis and those who were lost to follow-up, in order to allow readers to better assess the extent of attrition bias (32).

DETECTION (OBSERVER) BIAS

Detection bias refers to systematic differences in outcome assessment (7). Knowledge of the allocated intervention can predispose to bias among those who may assess outcomes in favor of a particular intervention. In oncology, this commonly occurs when investigators (or radiologists who read the radiographic response to treatment) are aware of the treatment assignment. This pitfall can be avoided both by blinding outcome assessors to the treatment allocation and by implementing a standardized approach to the assessment of treatment responses, such as through central review, and standard guidelines, such as the Response Evaluation Criteria In Solid Tumors (RECIST) or the World Health Organization's response criteria (33). Detection bias can be especially problematic in the assessment of "soft" or qualitative outcomes, such as pain, in contrast to "hard" or quantitative outcomes, such as deaths (34,35). Masking and blinding are particularly important in the assessment of soft outcomes.

BIAS IN OBSERVATIONAL STUDIES

Observational studies are predisposed to more pitfalls than RCTs. In general, the internal validity of RCTs is superior to that of observational studies. This is because of the so-called ***confounding by indication***, whereby treatment assignment is a function of prognosis or other factors that influence the physicians' treatment assignment or the patients' reasons to accept or decline the intervention (36). For example, patients with more aggressive or extensive disease may be at higher risk for recurrence and thus referred for additional (adjuvant) therapy following a primary treatment, such as surgery. This effect tends to diminish observed differences in survival according to the administration of adjuvant therapy.

Confounding by indication cannot be controlled in the observational studies (36). Additionally, knowledge of the probability distribution of unmeasured covariates allows for their adjustment in the analysis of results of RCTs, whereas this is not possible with an **observational study** design (36). Similarly, treatment allocation that would be similar to randomized assignments is not possible in case–control or cohort studies: in these study designs, the patient decides to accept or not accept the intervention, which in turn is subjected to the study evaluation (36).

It is important for investigators to realize that there are no alternative methods—including the popular Cox multivariate regression models, propensity score, or instrumental variable analysis—that can replace randomization. Randomization remains the only method that can reduce or even eliminate the pitfall of confounding by indication (36).

Additional pitfalls can be avoided if the investigators consider potential traps that occur in observational studies, by attempting to mimic the design of a target RCT (37). A confounding variable, or ***confounder***, is associated with both the outcome and the factor(s) of interest, without being an intermediate link in the chain of causation between exposure and outcome (37,38). Improperly controlling for confounders (not to be confused with confounding by indication) results in a type of selection bias known as ***case-mix bias***, or ***channeling bias***, referring to the mixing or blurring of effects (37,38). For example, carrying matches is associated with a 9.1 odds of developing lung cancer; but it is smoking, not the matches, that causes lung cancer (38). Carrying matches blurs (confounds) the effect of smoking. Limiting selection bias due to confounders is best done by controlling for all measurable confounders in cohort studies or by matching in case–control studies (39). Unlike confounding by indication (a true bias), this type of confounding can be controlled by using techniques such as restriction, matching, stratification, and various multivariate methods either prior to or after the study's completion.

A particularly common bias that occurs in cohort studies conducted in the field of oncology is the so-called ***immortal bias*** (also known as ***inception bias*** or ***lead-time bias***) (37,40). This pitfall occurs when additional (survival) time is incorrectly added to the treated group, while no such attribution is made in the control group. For example, Emilsson et al. compared the effect of immortal bias on survival in studies of statins in patients with active cancer. They concluded that statins' apparent prolongation of survival can be explained by immortal bias (41). The survival advantage occurred because many studies compared the combined start date of follow-up time and time after first prescription in the treated group versus time recorded only from the beginning of follow-up in the control group. However, the patients had to survive (i.e., be immortal) to receive the treatment, while no such requirement was made for the control group (40). When time was excluded from the analysis, statins had no effect on survival (41). Notably, this type of bias commonly arises in studies of postoperative radiation therapy, because patients who get postoperative radiation live longer than those who die before they can get it (41).

In general, investigators should avoid the biased selection of participants by ensuring equal prognosis, utilization of interventions, and attribution of follow-up time (37). Investigators can avoid immortal bias in cohort studies by relying on time-dependent analysis, including a time-matched, nested case–control analysis of the cohort studies (40).

Performance bias is also known as ***information bias, measurement bias,*** or ***recall bias*** in observational studies (37,38). It is best controlled by ensuring that data (for outcome assessment) are collected the same way in the exposed and unexposed group (cohort study). In a case–control study, the researchers should strive to obtain information about exposure in the same way for cases and controls.

Attrition bias and missing data commonly occur in observational studies. The strategy used to mitigate this pitfall in RCTs also applies to observational research. For both cohort and case–control studies, investigators should do their best to ensure thorough data collection and completeness of follow-up. Investigators should separately report the baseline characteristics of participants who were both included in the analysis and lost to follow-up (7,37). Several strategies to handle missing data are discussed in Chapter 11, Chapter 15, and Chapter 22.

In observational studies, differences in outcome measurement between cases and controls can lead to differences in outcome assessment, leading to detection bias (37). Detection bias may be controlled using similar strategies as for RCTs; however, this can be more challenging for cohort studies, since the exposure is not managed in the same fashion. Thus, blinding is often impossible. In addition, under-detection of treatment utilization is a recognized problem in some epidemiologic databases, such as the Surveillance Epidemiology and End Results (SEER) registry (42). To avoid bias in detecting outcomes, investigators should ensure that the same methods are used to collect and identify outcomes and exposures. Table 2.1 summarizes the main sources of bias that can occur in both observational and experimental research and the key strategies for avoiding them.

TABLE 2.1 A SUMMARY OF THE MAIN SOURCES OF PITFALLS (BIASES) THAT CAN OCCUR IN OBSERVATIONAL AND EXPERIMENTAL RESEARCH AND THE KEY STRATEGIES FOR AVOIDING THEM

Source of Bias	Cohort Studies	Case–Control Studies	Randomized Trial
Selection Bias	Control for confounders	Matching	Adequate allocation concealment
Performance Bias	Measurement of exposure (treatment of intervention)	Measurement of exposure (treatment of intervention)	Avoiding cointerventions/ contamination
Attrition Bias	Completeness of follow-up	Completeness of follow-up	Completeness of follow-up
Detection Bias	Blinding	Case definition	Blinding
Reporting Bias (Publication Bias and Outcome Reporting Bias)	Reporting of outcomes as specified in protocol	Reporting of outcomes as specified in protocol	Study registration and reporting of outcomes as specified in protocol

CONCLUSION: METHODOLOGICAL QUALITY VERSUS QUALITY OF REPORTING

Although we referred to tools used to assess the risk of bias throughout this chapter (7,37), in order to detect these biases in the reports of clinical studies, it is important to distinguish between the methodological quality of study design (and execution) and the quality of reporting (42). In other words, as Altman at al. explained: "High quality reporting cannot transform a poorly designed or analyzed study into a good one" (43). Similarly, "Bad reporting does not mean bad methods" (43). For example, when comparing publication reports with research protocols, we found that adequate allocation concealment was achieved in all trials, but reported in only 42% of the corresponding manuscripts (44). Awareness of these potential pitfalls and instituting the appropriate measures during the protocol phase of research design are crucial to avoiding problems later, even if one adheres to high-quality reporting (45).

GLOSSARY

accuracy: the degree to which given entity of interest (such as clinical characteristics or variables) represent what it is supposed to represent; it can be affected by bias (NB accuracy in diagnostic research refers to the percent of patients correctly classified as having or not having disease)

allocation concealment: the technique of ensuring that the treatment assignment is unknown to the involved parties—typically patients and physicians—until after treatment assignment itself.

attrition bias: bias that results from systematic differences in withdrawal of participants from a trial (dropouts).

blinding: concealing information about assignment throughout the trial and different phases of conduct and analysis.

case series: research or study in which there are no comparators.

case–control study: research design in which investigators first assess patient outcomes, then retrospectively assess the exposure.

case-mix bias: a type of selection bias that results from improperly controlling for confounders, and refers to the mixing or blurring of effects.

channeling bias: a type of selection bias that results from improperly controlling for confounders, and refers to the mixing or blurring of effects.

cohort study: design in which researchers first determine the exposure and then over time follow the outcomes in each exposure (i.e., treatment) group.

comparator bias: bias in a predictable direction when a treatment is known to be superior or inferior to others.

comparator bias: bias that results from choosing an inappropriate control intervention.

comparison: judgment of two or more items of study.

confirmation bias: bias that results when investigators continue to interrogate data up until the point that the data appear to support the hypothesis, then stop.

confounder: a confounding variable.

confounding by indication: bias that occurs when treatment assignment is a function of prognosis or other factors that influence the physicians' treatment assignment or the patients' reasons to accept or decline the intervention.

detection bias: results from systematic differences in outcome assessment.

equipoise: see uncertainty principle.

experimental study: research in which the investigator has control over the treatment assignment.

external validity: the extent to which study findings can be applied (generalized) to another clinical setting.

immortal bias: (also known as **inception bias** or **lead-time bias**) Performance bias is also known as information bias, measurement bias, or recall bias in observational studies occurs when additional (survival) time is incorrectly added to the treated group, while no such attribution is made in the control group.

inception bias: occurs when additional (survival) time is incorrectly added to the treated group, while no such attribution is made in the control group.

information bias: bias that results from systematic errors in the measurement of information on exposure or outcomes.

internal validity: the extent to which a trial provides valid information under the current trial conditions; refers to confidence that an estimate of effect is correct.

landmark method: statistical method for analyzing survival by response, which evaluates the response to all patients at some fixed time following treatment onset.

lead-time bias: occurs when additional (survival) time is incorrectly added to the treated group, while no such attribution is made in the control group.

Mantel-Byar method: statistical method for analyzing survival by response, which evaluates the response to all patients at some fixed time following treatment onset.

masking: see *blinding*.

measurement bias: see *performance bias*

observational study: research in which the investigator does not control the exposure (such as the treatment assignment) but instead just records the outcomes.

observer bias: results from systematic differences in outcome assessment.

performance bias: (information bias, measurement bias, or **recall bias**) bias that occurs in observational studies; results from systematic differences in the care provided to the groups of participants being studied apart from the intervention being evaluated.

precision: refers to the degree to which measurement generates identical or nearly identical value when repeatedly measured

recall bias: results from systematic differences in outcome assessment.

reporting bias: bias that results from reporting errors.

selection bias: results from systematic differences between comparison groups (apart from the treatment that is being compared).

Texas sharpshooter fallacy: analytical fallacy that occurs when an investigator fits the data to the hypothesis (based on the "sharpshooter" one who first fires shots into the side of a barn, then draws the target around the bullet holes).

uncertainty principle: states that RCTs should be done only when there is uncertainty as to whether one treatment alternative is better than the other.

REFERENCES

1. Djulbegovic B, Guyatt GH. Progress in evidence-based medicine: a quarter century on. *Lancet.* 2017;390(10092):415–423. doi:10.1016/S0140-6736(16)31592-6
2. Altman D. The scandal of poor medical research. *BMJ.* 1994;308:283–284. doi:10.1136/bmj.308.6924.283
3. Ioannidis J. Why most published research findings are false. *PLoS Med.* 2005;2:e124. doi:10.1371/journal.pmed.0020124
4. Macleod MR, Michie S, Roberts I, et al. Biomedical research: increasing value, reducing waste. *Lancet.* 2014;383(9912):101–104. doi:10.1016/S0140-6736(13)62329-6
5. Chalmers I, Bracken MB, Djulbegovic B, et al. How to increase value and reduce waste when research priorities are set. *Lancet.* 2014;383(9912):156–165. doi:10.1016/S0140-6736(13)62229-1
6. Rettig RA, Jacobson PD, Farquhar CM, Aubry WM. *False Hope: Bone Marrow Transplantation for Breast Cancer.* New York, NY: Oxford University Press; 2007.
7. Higgins JPT, Altman DG, Gøtzsche PC, et al. The Cochrane Collaboration's tool for assessing risk of bias in randomised trials. *BMJ.* 2011;343:d5928. doi:10.1136/bmj.d5928
8. Grimes DA, Schulz KF. An overview of clinical research: the lay of the land. *Lancet.* 2002;359:57–61. doi:10.1016/S0140-6736(02)07283-5
9. Mathes T, Pieper D. Clarifying the distinction between case series and cohort studies in systematic reviews of comparative studies: potential impact on body of evidence and workload. *BMC Med Res Methodol.* 2017;17(1):107. doi:10.1186/s12874-017-0391-8
10. Higgins J, Hopewell S. *Bias Susceptibility in Cochrane Reviews.* vol 34. 2005:1,5.
11. Higgins J, Green S. *Cochrane Handbook for Systematic Reviews of Interventions, Version 5.1.0.* Oxford, UK: Wiley-Blackwell; 2011.
12. Yordanov Y, Dechartres A, Porcher R, et al. Avoidable waste of research related to inadequate methods in clinical trials. *BMJ.* 2015;350:h809. doi:10.1136/bmj.h809
13. Chalmers I, Glasziou P, Godlee F. All trials must be registered and the results published. *BMJ.* 2013;346:f105. doi:10.1136/bmj.f105
14. McGauran N, Wieseler B, Kreis J, et al. Reporting bias in medical research–a narrative review. *Trials.* 2010;11:37. doi:10.1186/1745-6215-11-37
15. Armstrong R, Waters E, Doyle J, eds. Reviews in public health and health promotion. In: Higgins JPT, Green S, eds. *Cochrane Handbook for Systematic Reviews of Interventions.* Chichester, UK: John Wiley & Sons; 2008:593–606.
16. Kumar A, Soares HP, Balducci L, Djulbegovic B. Treatment tolerance and efficacy in geriatric oncology: a systematic review of phase III randomized trials conducted by five National Cancer Institute-sponsored cooperative groups. *J Clin Oncol.* 2007;25(10):1272–1276. doi:10.1200/JCO.2006.09.2759
17. Djulbegovic B. Articulating and responding to uncertainties in clinical research. *J Med Philosophy.* 2007;32:79–98. doi:10.1080/03605310701255719
18. Mann H, Djulbegovic B. Comparator bias: why comparisons must address genuine uncertainties. *J R Soc Med.* 2013;106(1):30–33. doi:10.1177/0141076812474779
19. Djulbegovic B, Bennet CL, Adams JR, Lyman GH. Industry-sponsored research. *Lancet.* 2000;356:2193–2194. doi:10.1016/s0140-6736(05)67271-6
20. Djulbegovic B, Lacevic M, Cantor A, et al. The uncertainty principle and industry-sponsored research. *Lancet.* 2000;356:635–638. doi:10.1016/S0140-6736(00)02605-2
21. Djulbegovic B, Kumar A, Miladinovic B, et al. Treatment success in cancer: industry compared to publicly sponsored randomized controlled trials. *PLoS One.* 2013;8(3):e58711. doi:10.1371/journal.pone.0058711
22. Clark O, Adams JR, Bennett CL, Djulbegovic B. Erythropoietin, uncertainty principle and cancer related anaemia. *BMC Cancer.* 2002;2(1):23. doi:10.1186/1471-2407-2-23
23. Mann H, Djulbegovic B. Comparator bias: why comparisons must address genuine uncertainties. 2012. http://www.jameslindlibrary.org/articles/comparator-bias-why-comparisons-must-address-genuine-uncertainties
24. Higgins JPT, Green S, eds. *Cochrane Handbook for Systematic Reviews of Interventions.* Chichester, UK: Wiley-Blackwell; 2011.
25. Peters WP, Ross M, Vredeburgh JJ, et al. High-dose chemotherapy and autologous bone marrow support as consolidation after standard-dose adjuvant therapy for high-risk primary breast cancer. *J Clin Oncol.* 1993;11:1132–1143. doi:10.1200/JCO.1993.11.6.1132
26. Djulbegovic M, Djulbegovic B. Implications of the principle of question propagation for comparative-effectiveness and "data mining" research. *JAMA.* 2011;305(3):298–299. doi:10.1001/jama.2010.2013
27. Kunz R, Oxman A. The unpredictability paradox: review of empirical comparisons of randomized and non-randomized trials. *BMJ.* 1998;317:1185–1190. doi:10.1136/bmj.317.7167.1185
28. Schulz KF, Altman DG, Moher D. Allocation concealment in clinical trials. *JAMA.* 2002;288:2406–2409. doi:10.1001/jama.288.19.2406-JLT1120-4-1

29. Anderson JR, Cain KC, Gelber RD. Analysis of survival by tumor response. *J Clin Oncol.* 1983;1(11):710–719. doi:10.1200/JCO.1983.1.11.710
30. Anderson JR, Cain KC, Gelber RD. Analysis of survival by tumor response and other comparisons of time-to-event by outcome variables. *J Clin Oncol.* 2008;26(24):3913–3915. doi:10.1200/JCO.2008.16.1000
31. Wheatley K. SAB–a promising new treatment to improve remission rates in AML in the elderly? *Br J Haematol.* 2002;118(2):432–433. doi:10.1046/j.1365-2141.2002.03620.x
32. Dumville JC, Torgerson DJ, Hewitt CE. Reporting attrition in randomised controlled trials. *BMJ.* 2006;332(7547):969–971. doi:10.1136/bmj.332.7547.969
33. Jaffe CC. Measures of response: RECIST, WHO, and new alternatives. *J Clin Oncol.* 2006;24(20):3245–3251. doi:10.1200/JCO.2006.06.5599
34. Wood L, Egger M, Gluud LL, et al. Empirical evidence of bias in treatment effect estimates in controlled trials with different interventions and outcomes: meta-epidemiological study. *BMJ.* 2008;336:601–605. doi:10.1136/bmj.39465.451748.AD
35. Savovic J, Jones HE, Altman DG, et al. Influence of reported study design characteristics on intervention effect estimates from randomized, controlled trials. *Ann Intern Med.* 2012;157(6):429–438. doi:10.7326/0003-4819-157-6-201209180-00537
36. La Caze A, Djulbegovic B, Senn S. What does randomisation achieve? *Evid-Based Med.* 2012;17(1):1–2. doi:10.1136/ebm.2011.100061
37. Sterne JA, Hernan MA, Reeves BC, et al. ROBINS-I: a tool for assessing risk of bias in non-randomised studies of interventions. *BMJ.* 2016;355:i4919. doi:10.1136/bmj.i4919
38. Grimes DA, Schulz KF. Bias and causal associations in observational research. *Lancet.* 2002;359:248–252. doi:10.1016/S0140-6736(02)07451-2
39. Wells GA, Shea B, O'Connell D, et al. The Newcastle-Ottawa Scale (NOS) for assessing the quality of nonrandomised studies in meta-analyses. http://www.ohri.ca/programs/clinical_epidemiology/oxford.asp
40. Lévesque LE, Hanley JA, Kezouh A, Suissa S. Problem of immortal time bias in cohort studies: example using statins for preventing progression of diabetes. *BMJ.* 2010;340:b5087. doi:10.1136/bmj.b5087
41. Emilsson L, García-Albéniz X, Logan RW, et al. Examining bias in studies of statin treatment and survival in patients with cancer. *JAMA Oncol.* 2018;4(1):63–70. doi:10.1001/jamaoncol.2017.2752
42. Park HS, Gross CP, Makarov DV, Yu JB. Immortal time bias: a frequently unrecognized threat to validity in the evaluation of postoperative radiotherapy. *Int J Radiat Oncol Biol Phys.* 2012;83:1365–1373. doi:10.1016/j.ijrobp.2011.10.025
43. Walker GV, Grant SR, Jagsi R, Smith BD. Reducing bias in oncology research: the end of the radiation variable in the surveillance, epidemiology, and end results (SEER) program. *Int J Radiat Oncol Biol Phys.* 2017;99(2):302–303. doi:10.1016/j.ijrobp.2017.05.018
44. Altman DG, Sauerbrei W, McShane LM. Importance of the distinction between quality of methodology and quality of reporting. *HPB.* 2017;19(7):649–650. doi:10.1016/j.hpb.2017.02.444
45. Soares HP, Daniels S, Kumar A, et al. Bad reporting does not mean bad methods for randomised trials: observational study of randomised controlled trials performed by the Radiation Therapy Oncology Group. *BMJ.* 2003;328:22–25. doi:10.1136/bmj.328.7430.22

3

Principles of Molecular Biology

REEM A. MALEK ■ PHUOC T. TRAN

Understanding the unique nature of cancer cells and the process of malignant transformation is heavily dependent on advances in molecular biology. A working knowledge of molecular biology concepts is essential to clinical oncology in order to stay informed of the latest findings, assays of prognostic and predictive factors, and potential new therapies to deliver or enhance current treatments. Insights resulting from molecular biology research are crucial for developing newer and more specific targets. This principle forms the basis for "precision medicine."

CENTRAL DOGMA

The central dogma of molecular biology describes the flow of cellular genetic information within biological organisms. As first published by James Watson in 1968, it simply states that genetic information flows from DNA, which undergoes replication, to ribonucleic acid (RNA) by the process of transcription and finally to proteins by the process of translation (1). All of these steps are highly coordinated in eukaryotic cells and occur in a temporally and spatially specific manner that is also dependent on a sequence of events known as the cell cycle. Of importance in cancer are alterations in the structure as well as the transcription of DNA and the disruption of critical processes essential to the cell cycle.

DNA encodes the basic unit of inheritance—the gene. DNA is a double-helical polymer of the four bases adenine (A), guanine (G), cytosine (C), and thymine (T), and their arrangement defines the genetic code. The linear sequence of the bases, in sets of three, dictates each amino acid to be translated and consequently, the protein sequence (primary structure) and folding (secondary structure). While there are over three billion base pairs in the human genome, only approximately 1% to 2% are coding, resulting in an estimated 30,000 to 40,000 genes (2). The structure of genes can be divided functionally into two components—a coding region and a promoter region. A gene *coding* region specifies the structure of the cognate protein product. It contains all the information necessary for cellular machinery to assemble amino acids in proper order to make specific proteins. The *promoter* region is upstream of the coding region and, in concert with other "enhancer" and "silencing" regions of DNA and numerous associated proteins, controls gene transcription (3). This regulation depends on a number of contextual factors including, but not limited to, cell type, extracellular signals, and stressors.

All of the DNA contained within a cell is present in a tightly wound form inside the nucleus. The DNA is present in close association with different accessory proteins, such as the histones, and this form of condensed DNA is called chromatin (4). These accessory proteins such as the histones are mostly involved in packaging of the DNA. Others proteins such as the topoisomerases and histone-modifying enzymes are responsible for regulating chromatin structure during replication and transcription. This interaction of DNA and accessory proteins adds another considerable layer of complex regulation to gene expression and is referred to as "epigenetics" (5).

Genetic changes, like those that result in cancer, can result from de novo mutations in the coding region of a gene. DNA can be damaged from a variety of sources including inherent instability, exposure to environmental and toxic stresses, and a natural limit to replicative accuracy, necessitating repair mechanisms to maintain genetic integrity. DNA repair genes themselves can be altered early in carcinogenesis leading to a greater propensity for mutations (6). In extreme cases, double-stranded DNA breaks occurring in two different places and their subsequent joining can lead to a completely different arrangement of genes on the same or different chromosomes. These chromosomal rearrangements can lead to loss or abnormal gene activation of critical growth regulatory genes with resultant tumorigenic effects. These alterations are frequently seen in some cancers, such as the Philadelphia chromosome (*BCR-ABL* fusion) in leukemia, wherein the *BCR* gene on chromosome 22 is juxtaposed to *ABL* on chromosome 9. This results in a hybrid tyrosine kinase signaling protein that is always active, leading to and maintaining the neoplastic phenotype (7).

Gene expression changes that lead to cancer can also result from changes to the promoter region and other indirect processes. For example, defects in mechanisms regulating posttranscriptional and translational control or other epigenetic changes can result in aberrant gene expression or silencing. Some of these are discussed in greater detail in the next section.

CANCER GENETICS AND EPIGENETICS

CANCER GENETICS

There is a general consensus that cancer is broadly a genetic disease, even though our knowledge of this disease is constantly being updated. Molecular alterations can accumulate in the genome of somatic cells and is the basis for cancer initiation and progression. These alterations confer a selective advantage to the cells, leading not only to uncontrolled proliferation and clonal expansion but ultimately also to invasion of surrounding tissues and metastasis to distant sites. Genetic changes that promote cancer can be inherited from parents if these mutations are present in germ cells (germline changes). They can also be acquired in somatic cells during the lifetime as a result of spontaneous mutations that may occur due to errors in cell division and aging or from exposure to carcinogens that damage DNA, such as tobacco smoke and radiation.

Hereditary cancer syndromes resulting from germline changes underlie 3% to 10% of all cancers (8). They are characterized by early onset of neoplasms in specific organ systems in multiple members of the same family. The most common ones include hereditary breast-ovarian cancer syndrome (HBOC) and hereditary non-polyposis colon cancer (HNPCC, Lynch syndrome) (9). An increased impetus for a clearer understanding of the tumor genetics in some hereditary syndromes has led to better screening strategies, molecular diagnostics, and therapeutics.

Nongenetic factors that influence cancer development include environmental factors such as carcinogens. These affect the genetic evolution in the life of a cell, leading directly to mutations in key tumor-promoting genes, such as *KRAS*, or inactivation of tumor suppressor genes, like *TP53*. Cancer incidence following exposure to radiation also demonstrates the link between environmental factors and genetic damage that lead to tumorigenesis.

Oncogenes and Tumor Suppressors

Cancer genes can be broadly grouped into two types—***oncogenes*** and ***tumor suppressor genes***. Activating or gain-of-function mutations in oncogenes can accelerate tumor development and progression; in contrast, inactivating mutations in tumor suppressor genes are required for neoplastic progression. Oncogene and tumor suppressor genes can be differentiated by the nature of mutation in tumors. Mutations occurring in oncogenes will oftentimes occur at hot spots within the same codon in a tumor or within neighboring codons in different tumors. Tumor suppressor genes, however, are mutated throughout the gene, generally resulting in a truncated protein. This may affect both alleles, resulting in **loss of heterozygosity** (LOH).

Vogelstein et al. in 2013 proposed a "20/20" rule for classification of genes as oncogenes or tumor suppressors. If more than 20% of the mutations in the gene are at recurrent positions and are missense mutations (i.e., the resulting codon encodes a different amino acid), it would be classified as an oncogene. If more than 20% of the mutations in the gene are inactivating, it would be classified as a tumor suppressor (10).

By definition, oncogenes are genes with somatic mutations that result in constitutive activation of signaling circuits triggered normally by upstream activation of a broad array of cell surface receptor proteins. From high-throughput DNA sequencing analyses of cancer cell genomes we now know that ~40% of human melanomas have mutations in the oncogene *BRAF*, resulting in constitutive activation of the **mitogen-activated protein kinase (MAPK) pathway** (11). Similarly, mutations in **phosphoinositide 3-kinase (PI3K) pathway** and KRAS have been detected in various tumor types (12). In general, these mutations serve to hyperactivate the downstream growth signaling pathways and/or repress cell death pathways that ultimately contribute to tumor development.

On the other hand, tumor suppressor genes generally code for proteins that normally operate to restrain cell proliferation, by dampening various types of signaling. Tumor suppressor genes also ensure homeostatic regulation of signals in the intracellular machinery, functioning as cell cycle checkpoint proteins that govern the decision of cells to activate senescence and apoptotic programs in response to cellular stresses (13,14). A prominent example of the first type is the phosphatase and tensin homolog (PTEN) phosphatase, which antagonizes PI3K signaling. Loss-of-function mutations in *PTEN* amplify PI3K signaling and promote tumorigenesis in a variety of experimental models of cancer. An important example of the second type of tumor suppressor, cell cycle checkpoint protein, is the tumor suppressor p53. It is one of the most commonly mutated proteins in cancer. The so-called guardian of the genome, p53, controls proliferation and stress signals such as DNA damage response, senescence, and apoptosis.

Cancer Genomics

In the past few decades, progress in DNA sequencing technologies leading to the human genome sequencing and subsequent cancer genome sequencing has dramatically improved our knowledge of this disease (15). In a major push toward this, in the past decade, The Cancer Genome Atlas (TCGA) project was established by the U.S. National Institutes of Health (NIH). The goal was to generate a comprehensive, multidimensional map of the key genomic changes in major types and subtypes of cancer. The insights gleaned from these studies are transforming the field of cancer research and oncology practice at multiple levels. Genomic maps are redesigning the tumor taxonomy by incorporating genetic information to supplement clinical information. Success of cancer drugs designed to target specific molecular alterations underlying tumorigenesis (e.g., imatinib to target *BCR-ABL* fusions in leukemia) has proven that somatic genetic alternations are legitimate targets for therapy (16). Additionally, genetic alterations represent highly sensitive biomarkers for disease detection and monitoring. Ongoing analyses of multiple cancer genomes will identify additional targets whose diagnostic and pharmacological exploitation will undoubtedly result in new therapeutic approaches.

One of the important facts uncovered by large-scale, genome-wide sequencing studies for various cancers is that despite the complexity in cancer genomes, only a few of these alterations are significant in terms of cancer development and progression. Mutations that result in a selective growth advantage to the cell are the "**driver**" mutations. Although each tumor may have hundreds or thousands of mutations, most of these are "**passengers**" and—depending on the tumor type—perhaps only two to eight are legitimate "driver mutations." Although the selective advantage offered by driver mutations is small, over a period of years, it can result in a large tumor mass made up of billions of cells. In most cases, passenger and driver mutations occur at similar frequencies, and the identification of mutations as passenger versus driver is an ongoing challenge in cancer genetics (10). Mutations commonly observed in cancers may be of different types: **point mutations** (*KRAS*^{G12V}, where the amino acid at the 12th position, glycine, is replaced with valine), **deletions** (*PTEN*), **inversions**, or **amplifications** (*MYC*). LOH often affects tumor suppressors like *RB* and *TP53* (12).

Another interesting feature revealed from the overall tumor "genomic landscape" is that specific sets of cancer genes are found to be mutated in a tissue-specific fashion (10). The alterations observed in colorectal, lung, or breast tumors are very different from one another. This indicates that specific genetic alterations cause tumors at specific sites or are associated with specific stages of development, cellular differentiation, tumorigenesis, or regulation of the microenvironment. Furthermore, different histologic tumor types tend to follow specific patterns of gene mutations in oncogenes and tumor suppressors. They also have different combinations of gene mutations. To illustrate, *KRAS* mutations are present in a large majority of pancreatic cancers, but are very rare in breast cancer. Similarly, *BRAF* mutations are prevalent in melanomas, but infrequent in lung cancers. The molecular basis for occurrence of cancer mutations in tissue-specific profiles is still largely unknown. Tissue-specific expression and cell-specific transformation are believed to be the most common causes for this phenomenon. Identification of cancer-specific mutation patterns is important as it may allow for the development of individualized therapeutics.

Conversely, when similar gene mutations are identified across different cancer types, the tumors tend to show similar vulnerabilities. TCGA studies across cancer types have identified the possible convergence of cancer types based on the underlying driver mutations in ~10% of cancer cases (17). This opens the doors for customizing treatments based on the underlying molecular driver rather than tissue of origin. In May 2017, the U.S. Food and Drug Administration (FDA), in a first-of-its kind decision, approved the immunotherapeutic drug Keytruda (pembrolizumab) to treat any metastatic solid tumors with specific defects in DNA-repair pathways regardless of the tumor site (18). Similarly, poly (ADP-ribose) polymerase (PARP) inhibitors, a class of drugs that exploit defects in another DNA-repair pathway, showed promise in the treatment of ovarian and breast cancer linked to mutations in *BRCA1* and *BRCA2* genes. Cancer researchers are now taking a closer look at the application of PARP inhibitors in other cancers such as prostate cancer with similar gene variants.

There is a nationwide trial underway through the National Cancer Institute (NCI) called NCI-MATCH (Molecular Analysis for Therapy Choice) that seeks to identify whether targeted therapies for people with tumors harboring specific gene mutations will be effective regardless of cancer type. The trial combines more than 20 different study drugs or drug combinations and matches each patient with a therapy that targets a molecular abnormality in the tumor. Results from these studies may direct mutation-specific cancer treatment in the coming years (19).

Due to the significant advances in DNA sequencing technology including the rise of "next-generation" sequencing, it is now possible to do large-scale sequencing, including whole-genome sequencing (WGS) and whole-exome sequencing (WES) (20). Based on these technologies, there is considerable interest in offering genomic sequencing–based tests on a clinical basis (21). This offers many advantages over classic methods in which genes are analyzed individually, which can be time-consuming, relatively expensive, and biased. The use of WGS/WES in the clinical setting has already begun, and there is heightened interest surrounding the availability of such testing. These approaches have great potential to improve our ability to determine the molecular causation in most Mendelian diseases like hereditary cancer syndromes. In fact, guidelines for clinical applications have been published by the American College of Medical Genetics and Genomics (22). Furthermore, in more complex disorders such as sporadic cancers, patients may harbor multiple variants that modify their cancer risk, where WGS/WES can provide a more comprehensive risk assessment. This complexity has been demonstrated in *BRCA*-mutant ovarian cancers, where two novel germline mutations were identified in 3 of 360 ovarian cancer patients

(23). This information is not only helpful for individual patients, who may be at increased risk for other cancers, but also critical for family members, since these mutations may be missed by standard genetic testing.

CANCER EPIGENETICS

Cancer research has focused largely on genetic defects found in cancer cells; however, during the past decade, epigenetic changes have been recognized as another hallmark of cancer (24). Epigenetic mechanisms are defined as the mechanisms that maintain heritable patterns of gene regulation and function without affecting the sequence of the genome. This also serves to explain a previous question in molecular biology—how two identical genotypes can lead to different phenotypes in response to the environmental stimulus. There are four general mechanisms of epigenetic regulation: DNA methylation, posttranslational modification of histone proteins, chromatin remodeling, and non-coding RNAs (25). While evidence for DNA methylation has been accumulating over the past decade, the contribution of other mechanisms to cancer formation are an emerging area of interest to understand cancer etiology as diagnostic and treatment germane biomarkers and also as direct targets for cancer therapy.

DNA Methylation

An important method by which gene transcription is regulated in cancer is methylation of the promoter region leading to gene silencing (26). This was the first epigenetic marker to be associated with cancer (27). Aberrant DNA methylation can be of three types: hypermethylation, hypomethylation, and loss of imprinting. DNA hypermethylation occurs when a cytosine before a guanosine (CpG), especially in the area of the genome known as CpG island (CGI), is methylated while remaining unmethylated in normal conditions. It occurs frequently in the promoter region of genes and has been associated with transcriptional inhibition. It appears to play a significant role in the disruption of tumor suppressor genes (28). For some genes, for example, the gene encoding tumor suppressor p16, *CDKN2A*, this form of epigenetic silencing is even more common than gene mutations, underscoring the fact that DNA methylation is a crucial mechanism by which epigenetic dysregulation can cause cancer (25,29).

Losses of DNA methylation in genome-wide regions are found in genes of cancer cells compared to normal counterparts in several tumor types such as colorectal, gastric, melanoma, and others (30). This global DNA hypomethylation, in the context of cancers, occurs in non-coding genomic areas that include repetitive elements, retrotransposons, and introns, where it leads to genomic instability. In tumor progression, DNA hypomethylation has been observed to increase from benign proliferative lesions to invasive cancers (31). Loss of imprinting refers to the loss of parental allele–specific expression of genes occurring as a result of aberrant hypomethylation at either of the two parental alleles. For example, the loss of *IGF2* imprinting is observed in various types of neoplasia and associated with increased risk of some cancers like colorectal cancer (32).

Histone Modification

Histone proteins can undergo posttranslational covalent modifications that result in activation or repression of transcription, depending on which amino acids are modified, and the type and number of modifications (5). Atypical patterns of histone modifications are now recognized as a hallmark of cancer as well as biomarkers of cancer recurrence following definitive treatment. In prostate cancer, global analysis of histone modifications reveal altered dimethyl-lysine 4 (K4) and acetyl-K18 of histone H3 (33). Lesions in genes encoding for components of histone-modifying complexes are also associated with an aberrant epigenetic landscape in cancer cells that can arise from chromosomal translocations that involve histone modifier complexes (34). Additionally, overexpression of histone deacetylases (HDAC), components of histone methyltransferases (like BMI1 and EZH2), and lysine demethylases have been associated with cancer development and progression (25).

Non-Coding RNAs

Non-coding RNAs are transcribed from genes that do not code for proteins but nonetheless have specific functions in the cell, and many examples have been submitted for their role in cancer. In fact, the majority of the transcription that occurs in the cell results in these non-coding transcripts. Two that we highlight with relevance to cancer are the so-called microRNAs (miRNAs) and long non-coding RNAs (lncRNAs). Small non-coding RNAs (19–25 nucleotides long) that regulate gene expression in a sequence-specific manner are known as miRNAs. Many miRNA families have been implicated in cancer etiology. Several studies have revealed differences in miRNA profiles of normal and tumor tissues (35). Application of genome-wide approaches has enabled production of miRNA fingerprints in various tumors and identification of new potential tissue-specific and stage-specific biomarkers (25). Much less is known regarding lncRNAs, defined as transcripts that are longer than 200 nucleotides, but they seem to be composed of a large number of species with diverse roles in transcriptional, posttranscriptional, epigenetic, and translational machinery. Although still a new area, some lncRNAs have already been demonstrated to be involved in tumorigenesis, tumor progression, and cancer treatment response.

CROSS TALK BETWEEN GENETICS AND EPIGENETICS IN CANCER

It is now accepted that the process of tumorigenesis is a multistep process whereby the cells undergo multiple genetic and epigenetic alterations that contribute to the progressive transformation of normal cells toward malignancy (25). Methylation of CGIs can directly cause genetic changes in cancer by the generation of mutational hot spots within the genome. Conversely, mutations in epigenetic regulators that regulate cellular programs, like DNMT1 and TET1 that control DNA methylation or EZH2, SETD2, and KDM6A that are histone-modifying enzymes, are seen in cancers (5,29). Therefore, cancer is both a genetic and epigenetic disease. Epigenetic changes are reversible and therefore there is considerable interest in developing therapies that work by reversing epigenetic effects.

SIGNAL TRANSDUCTION PATHWAYS

In spite of the genetic and epigenetic complexity present in tumors, the majority of the alterations in tumors are passenger changes that accumulate over time. Only a few of these alterations cause a selective growth advantage that drives cancer growth. Moreover, these alterations impinge on an even more limited number of signaling pathways that can provide a growth advantage. Most of the driver mutations can be classified as effecting a limited number of signal transduction pathways that can be organized into the fundamental cellular process of cell fate, cell survival, and genome maintenance (10).

CELL SURVIVAL

While cancer cells divide abnormally due to cell intrinsic defects, different components of the tumor microenvironment, like the stromal cells and tumor vasculature, are still largely normal and cannot keep pace with tumor growth. This results in an environment of limited nutrients and potential activation of death signaling or quiescence. Accumulation of mutations that allow cells to grow in low glucose concentrations, inhibit apoptotic signaling, or stimulate vasculature can provide an important selective advantage (10).

Epidermal Growth Factor Receptor (EGFR) Signaling Pathway

Growth factors and their receptors are involved in proliferation, differentiation, and survival. Not surprisingly, they are often overexpressed in cancers. Many growth factors work through their cognate **receptor tyrosine kinases (RTKs)** that, when activated, lead to signaling cascades that can have various effects on protein expression.

One of the most well studied of the growth factor receptor system and RTKs is the HER/Erb-B family, which consists of EGFR (HER1/ErbB-1), HER2/Erb-B2, HER3/Erb-B3, and HER4/Erb-B4. EGFR is a transmembrane receptor that binds to several ligands such as the epithelial growth factor (EGF), transforming growth factor-α (TGF-α), epiregulin, and neuregulin. Ligand binding triggers receptor dimerization and tyrosine kinase (TK) autoactivation, resulting in a cascade of intracellular signaling pathways (Figure 3.1). HER2 is an orphan receptor and usually heterodimerizes with EGFR or HER3, after binding to their respective ligands for activation. Activation of these receptors results in multiple, integrated biological responses such as proliferation, inhibition of apoptosis, motility, angiogenesis, and regulation of differentiation (36). Activation of EGFR/HER2 triggers downstream propagation of two major pathways—RAS-/MAPK–dependent pathways and PI3K-dependent pathways.

RAS/MAPK Signaling Pathway

Growth factor receptors, cytokines (IL2, IL3, GM-CSF), and hormones (insulin, insulin-like growth factor [IGF]) activate signal transduction cascade through 21-kDa, guanine-nucleotide binding proteins, RAS proteins. Key members of this family include H-RAS, N-RAS, and K-RAS. Aberrant activation of RAS protein has been implicated in almost all aspects of malignant progression including mutagenesis, transformation, invasion, and metastasis. Activity of RAS proteins is regulated by cycling between inactive GDP-bound and active GTP-bound forms. In its GTP-bound active form, RAS further activates downstream effector pathways that mediate cell proliferation and

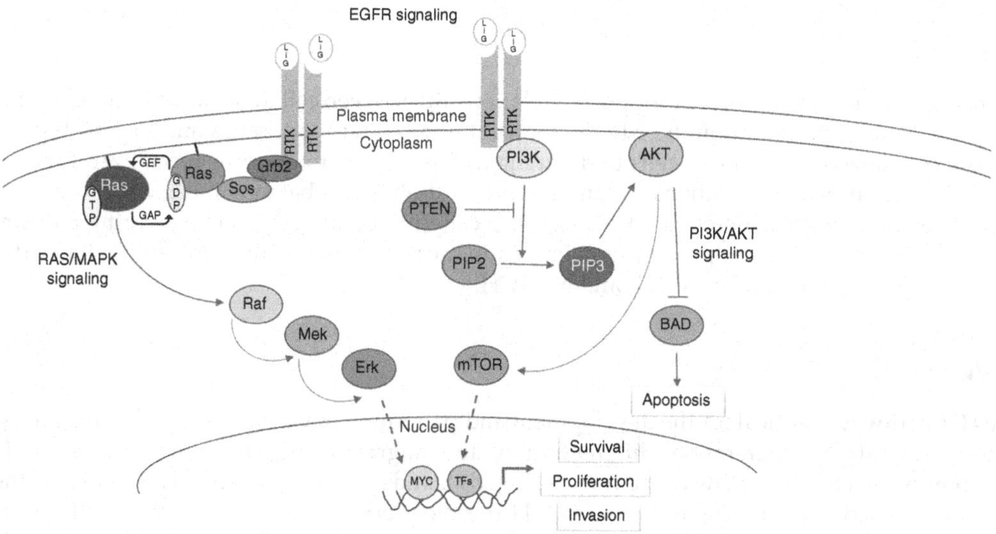

FIGURE 3.1 Growth signaling pathways in cancer—EGFR signaling, RAS/MAPK signaling, and PI3K/AKT signaling.

EGFR, epidermal growth factor receptor; Lig, ligand (e.g., EGF, heregulin, IGF); MAPK, mitogen-activated protein kinase; PI3K, phosphoinositide 3-kinase; PTEN, phosphatase and tensin homolog; RTK, receptor tyrosine kinase (e.g., EGFR/Erb-B1, Erb-B2, Erb-B3, IGFR); TF, transcription factor.

suppression of apoptosis. Hydrolysis of GTP by GTPase-activating proteins (GAPs) like p120GAP and NF1 attenuates this signaling (37).

Point mutations in *RAS* at amino acid 12, 13, or 61 are oncogenic as they make the resulting protein insensitive to GAP stimulation, resulting in a permanently active GTP-bound RAS form even in the absence of upstream stimulation (Figure 3.1). Additionally, aberrant activation of continuous upstream signals (like activation of EGFR/HER receptors) can cause continuous activation of RAS even in the absence of mutations in *RAS*. Active RAS activates multiple effector molecules including components of the following pathways: RAF-MAPK, PI3K-AKT, and RAC-RHO. An important target of the RAS/RAF/MAPK pathway is MYC, which is phosphorylated by MAPK, leading to its stabilization by suppression of ubiquitylation (ubiquitination). MYC stimulates cell proliferation by inducing genes that promote proliferation, such as those encoding G1/S cyclins, cyclin-dependent kinases (CDKs), and the E2F family of transcription factors (38). In addition, it represses cell cycle inhibitors (e.g., CKIs) and blocks the activity of transcription factors that promote differentiation.

PI3K/AKT/mTOR Pathway

AKT is a serine/threonine protein kinase, which is a critical regulator of cell survival and proliferation. AKT interacts with the membrane phospholipid, phosphatidyl-inositol-triphosphate (PIP3) produced by PI3K upon activation by growth factor receptors. Activation of AKT is attenuated by PTEN, a phosphatase that catalyzes the removal of PIP3 (39). AKT itself activates the mammalian target of rapamycin (mTOR), a chief controller of cell growth, cellular metabolism, and proliferation. AKT phosphorylates and inactivates mTOR inhibitors like tuberin (TSC2; Figure 3.1) (40). AKT is activated by many growth signals including IGF and RAS activation. Activation of AKT allows cells to withstand apoptotic stimuli through phosphorylation and inactivation of proapoptotic proteins like BAD and Caspase9. AKT is commonly overexpressed and the negative regulator of AKT, and PTEN is frequently lost in human cancer (39). Moreover, increased levels of PI3K and AKT activation downstream of growth factor receptors like IGF-1 receptor (IGF-1R) is a mechanism for failure of EGFR-/HERtargeted drugs in some cancers.

CELL FATE

There is a consensus regarding the opposing relationship between cell division and differentiation. Cells undergoing proliferation in order to contribute to the bulk of tissues and organs typically are less specialized. Conversely, cells undergoing differentiation to perform specialized functions divide less often. Many alterations in cancer serve to abolish this balance and favor proliferation over differentiation, as differentiated cells are typically more quiescent, some entering a postmitotic state never to divide. Important signaling pathways that function in controlling cell fate decisions include Hedgehog (HH), WNT, and NOTCH.

Hedgehog (HH) Pathway

The **HH pathway** is critical for the development and patterning of various organs during embryogenesis. It controls proliferation, differentiation, and migration of many progenitor cells. The key components of HH pathway are three secreted ligands (Desert, Indian, and Sonic) and their receptor Patched (PTCH). The unbound PTCH receptor serves as a constitutive inhibitor of the transmembrane protein Smoothened (SMO). In this state, the HH effectors GLI proteins, GLI3 and GLI2-repressor repress transcription of target genes. On binding of HH to PTCH, the repression of SMO is relieved, allowing the transcriptional activators GLI1 and GLI2-activator to initiate transcription of target genes (41) (Figure 3.2A). Activation of aberrant HH signaling has been identified in over a dozen types of cancer. The role of HH signaling has been studied in basal cell carcinoma, multiple myeloma, glioblastoma, medulloblastoma, leukemia, and colon cancer.

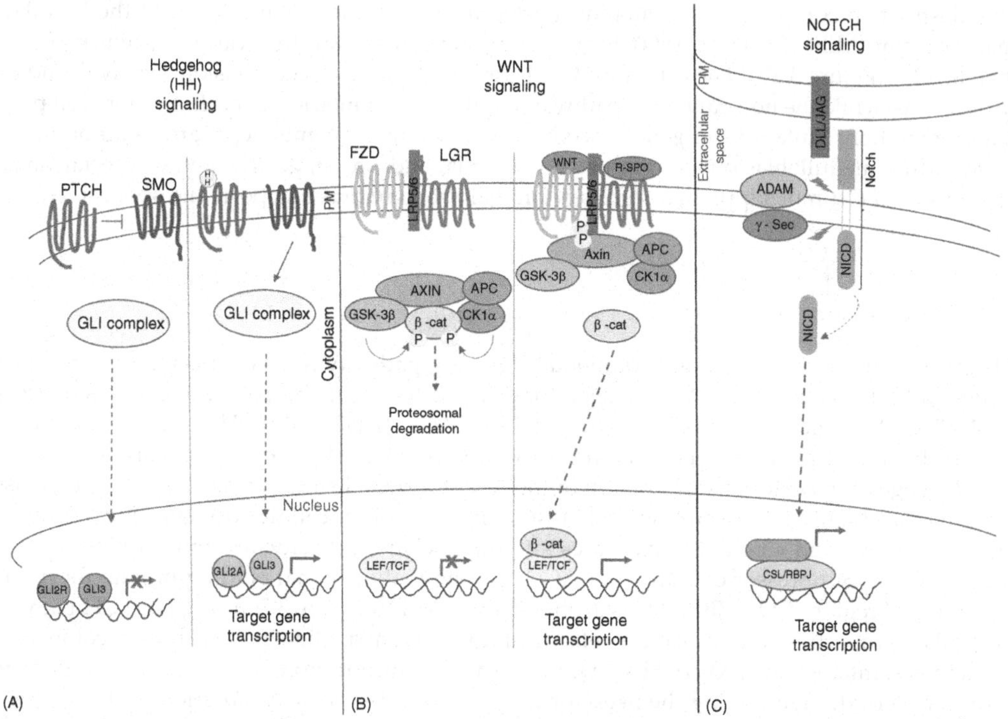

FIGURE 3.2 Cell fate signaling in cancer. (A) Inactive (left panel) and active (right panel) HH signaling. (B) Inactive (left panel) and active (right panel) WNT signaling, (C) NOTCH signaling.

ADAM, a disintegrin and metalloproteinase; APC, adenomatous polyposis coli; AXIN, Axis inhibition protein; β-cat, β-catenin; CK1α, casein kinase 1α; FZD, Frizzled; GLI, Glioma associated oncogene; GSK3-β, glycogen synthase kinase 3-β; LEF, LEF lymphoid enhancer factor; LGR, Leucine-rich repeat-containing G-protein coupled receptor; PM, plasma membrane; NICD, Notch intracellular domain; PTCH; Patched; SMO Smoothened; RBPJ, recombining binding protein suppressor of hairless; TCF, T-cell factor; β-cat, β-catenin; γ-Sec, γ-secretase.

Mutations in PTCH1 gene in humans, *PTCH1,* cause Gorlin syndrome and are associated with increased risk of basal cell carcinoma and medulloblastoma (42). Importantly, the HH pathway is an important therapeutic target in cancer where targeted agents have shown considerable promise and have been awarded regulatory approval.

WNT Pathway

The **WNT pathway** is a complex signaling pathway that has been evolutionarily conserved. It comprises of 19 WNT ligands and over 15 receptors (43). WNTs are secreted factors that regulate cell growth, motility, and differentiation during embryonic development. The WNT pathway encompasses two signaling pathways—canonical (mediated by the transcription factor β-catenin) and non-canonical (independent of β-catenin) (43). Canonical WNT signaling is activated by binding of Frizzled (FZD) receptors to WNT ligands and/or low-density lipoprotein–related protein (LRP) 5 and 6 co-receptors on a neighboring cell. Without WNT ligand binding, β-catenin levels are kept low in the cell through a destruction complex. This complex is made up of scaffolding proteins AXIN and adenomatous polyposis coli (APC), the kinase glycogen synthase kinase 3-β (GSK3-β), and casein kinase 1α (CK1α). GSK3-β and CK1α phosphorylate β-catenin, targeting it to ubiquitination and proteasomal degradation.

Binding of WNT to FZD/LRP phosphorylates the intracellular domain of LRP, causing it to sequester GSK3-β and AXIN and recruiting the scaffolding protein Disheveled (DVL). In the absence of the destruction complex, free β-catenin translocates to the nucleus and binds to the lymphoid enhancer factor (LEF)/T-cell factor (TCF) transcription factors, activating various downstream target genes (44) (Figure 3.2B). The canonical WNT pathway regulates cell division, survival, and cell fate decisions, while the non-canonical pathway regulates asymmetric stem cell division, cell polarity, and migration. Mutations in genes encoding WNT pathway components are common in cancers including medulloblastoma, lymphoma, leukemia, and breast, gastric, and colorectal cancer. Mutations in *APC* tumor suppressor results in familial adenomatous polyposis and sporadic colorectal cancer (45).

NOTCH Pathway

NOTCH is a highly conserved developmental signaling pathway that is critical in cell fate specification and differentiation of stem/progenitor cells. Notch signaling pathway consists of receptors (NOTCH1-4) and ligands (DLL1, DLL3, DLL4, JAG1, JAG2). NOTCH pathway is activated when the ligand produced by one cell binds to a receptor on a neighboring cell. This binding activates cleavage of the cytoplasmic domain of the receptor by a disintegrin and metalloproteinases (ADAMs) and finally by γ-secretase. This results in Notch intracellular domain (NICD) release in the cytoplasm from where it translocates into the nucleus and activates transcription of target genes via CBF1, Suppressor of Hairless, LAG-1/recombination signal binding protein for immunoglobulin κ J region (CSL/RBPJ) transcription factor (46,47) (Figure 3.2C). The NOTCH pathway can regulate properties of many cancer cells including leukemia, glioblastoma, breast, colon, lung, and pancreas. Interestingly, NOTCH signaling can act as a tumor promoter or suppressor depending on the context, highlighting the need for tissue- and cell-specific exploration of this pathway and its contribution to tumorigenesis (48). This contextual cancer-related duality of the NOTCH pathway has made cancer therapeutic targeting a more complicated endeavor.

GENOME MAINTENANCE

Mutations and damage accumulate in the DNA during cell division and from internal and external stressors. Cell cycle checkpoint proteins detect stressors and slow down damaged cells to allow for repair, or help direct cells that are too far gone toward cell death or senescence. Signals that induce these DNA damage checkpoints include activation of oncogenes, DNA damage, aberrant stroma–cell and cell–cell interactions, and hypoxia. In addition to the increased rate of cell division, cancer cells also reside in unfavorable microenvironments that increase the likelihood of DNA damage. Tumor cells must typically evade these inherent cell cycle checkpoints and also survive this damage in order to have a selective growth advantage.

RETINOBLASTOMA (RB) PATHWAY

First identified in retinoblastoma, RB aberrations have been identified in many different human cancers due to the central role RB plays during initiation of cell division. The RB protein has a central role in inhibiting the G1/S transition by physically restraining and inhibiting transcriptional activation, through direct binding to the E2F family of transcription factors. As the cell progresses from G1 to the S phase, RB becomes increasingly hyperphosphorylated and disassociates from the E2F transcription factor. Once unbound, E2F can induce transcription of the genes necessary for normal DNA synthesis. Cyclin D–CDK complexes control phosphorylation of RB and are regulated by multiple factors including MYC and E2F (49) (covered in more detail in Chapter 4).

P53 PATHWAY

As mentioned before, the guardian of the genome, p53 is a key factor in the cellular response to internal and external stresses in cancer. The p53 transcription factor is mutated in over half of all human cancers. Nearly all cancers evolve a way to circumvent this pathway, pointing to its pivotal role in preventing cancer development. p53 responds to a host of stress signals and regulates cellular processes such as maintenance of genomic integrity, metabolism, cell fate, cell death, migration, and cell signaling. This regulation of cellular processes is through transcriptional activation, interaction with other signaling pathways, and a role in DNA repair.

The protein HDM2 (also called MDM2), which itself is transcribed by p53, regulates p53 activity through ubiquitination and proteasomal degradation, thus creating an autoregulatory loop. Inhibition of HDM2 can occur when p53 is phosphorylated in response to stress or the binding of HDM2 by p14(ARF), a protein upregulated by oncogenes such as MYC, RAS, and E2F. The active form of p53 is a tetramer that allows transcriptional activation of genes involved in apoptosis, cell cycle arrest, and DNA repair (50). A large number of human cancers directly inactivate p53 through mutations or deletions in the *TP53* locus. Germline mutations in *TP53* are associated with the classic cancer predisposition disorder, Li-Fraumeni syndrome (LFS). LFS is characterized by a high frequency of diverse cancer types in adults and children. Additionally, cancers may upregulate HDM2 or HDM4 and amplification of *HDM2* locus is seen in sarcomas, glioblastoma, bladder urothelial carcinoma, and lung adenocarcinoma. *HDM4* amplifications have been associated with breast and hepatocellular carcinoma (51).

DNA REPAIR PATHWAYS

DNA damage response is mediated by multiple signal transduction process, the major ones being **ATM-CHK2** and **ATR-CHK1 pathways**. ATM and CHK2 are strongly activated by radiation and genotoxins that cause double-strand breaks (DSBs). In contrast, ATR-CHK1 is activated potently if DNA replication fork machinery is stalled either because of nucleotide depletion or replication blocks. Activation of these DNA damage response pathways ensures proper coordination of cell cycle checkpoint and DNA repair processes. In addition, they modulate other outcomes such as senescence and apoptosis. Inherited defects in DNA damage response pathways predispose individuals to cancer by allowing accumulation of oncogenic mutations.

Genomic instability is also a common occurrence in sporadic cancers (52). Inherited and sporadic mutations in *ATM* and *CHK2* have been found in human cancer; however, *ATR* and *CHK1* mutations are rare. Mutations in genes encoding for proteins involved in **homologous recombination (HR)** repair such as *BRCA1* and *BRCA2* can predispose individuals to a host of cancers including breast, ovarian, prostate, and pancreatic cancer. Genomic instability resulting from HR deficiency is thought to play an important role in development of these cancers. However, the absence of DNA repair proficiency also provides an exploitable therapeutic target. An inherent deficiency in HR makes cancer cells exquisitely sensitive to PARP1 inhibition. The basis of this is explained by synthetic lethality, where genes or pathways when individually lost can be tolerated, but the combined loss results in cellular lethality (52).

GLOSSARY

oncogenes: genes with somatic mutations that result in constitutive activation of signaling circuits triggered normally by upstream activation of a broad array of cell surface receptor proteins; genes in which activating or gain-of-function mutations can accelerate tumor development and progression.

tumor suppressor genes: genes that generally code for proteins that normally operate to restrain cell proliferation, by dampening various types of signaling; genes in which inactivating mutations can result in neoplastic progression.

loss of heterozygosity: occurs when a mutation throughout the gene affects both alleles.

mitogen-activated protein kinase (MAPK) pathway: in which mutations serve to hyperactivate the downstream growth signaling pathways and/or repress cell death pathways that ultimately contribute to tumor development.

phosphoinositide 3-kinase (PI3K) pathway: pathway in which mutations serve to hyperactivate the downstream growth signaling pathways and/or repress cell death pathways that ultimately contribute to tumor development.

driver mutation: mutation that results in a selective growth advantage to the cell.

passenger mutation: mutation that does not necessarily result in a selective growth advantage to the cell.

point mutations: type of mutation commonly observed in cancer cells.

deletions: type of mutation commonly observed in cancer cells.

inversions: type of mutation commonly observed in cancer cells.

amplifications: type of mutation commonly observed in cancer cells.

receptor tyrosine kinases (RTKs): growth factor cognates that, when activated, lead to signaling cascades that can have various effects on protein expression.

hedgehog (HH) pathway: genetic pathway critical for the development and patterning of various organs during embryogenesis.

WNT pathway: a complex genetic signaling pathway that has been evolutionarily conserved.

ATM-CHK2 pathway: a DNA damage response mediator pathway.

ATR-CHK1 pathway: a DNA damage response mediator pathway.

homologous recombination (HR): a DNA repair pathway.

REFERENCES

1. Watson JD, ed. *Molecular Biology of the Gene*, vol. 1, 4th ed. Menlo Park, CA: Benjamin Cummings; 1987.
2. Lander ES, Linton LM, Birren B, et al. Initial sequencing and analysis of the human genome. *Nature*. 2001;409(6822): 860–921. doi:10.1038/35057062
3. Polyak K, Meyerson M. Molecular biology, genomics, and proteomics. In: Kufe DW, Pollock RE, Weichselbaum RR, et al., eds. *Holland-Frei Cancer Medicine*. 6th edition. Hamilton, ON, Canada: BC Decker; 2003. Chapter 2. Available from: https://www.ncbi.nlm.nih.gov/books/NBK13922/
4. Laskey RA, Earnshaw WC. Nucleosome assembly. *Nature*. 1980;286(5775):763. doi:10.1038/286763a0
5. Sharma S, Kelly TK, Jones PA. Epigenetics in cancer. *Carcinogenesis*. 2010;31(1):27–36. doi:10.1093/carcin/bgp220
6. Ronen A, Glickman BW. Human DNA repair genes. *Environ Mol Mutagen*. 2001;37(3):241–283. doi:10.1002/em.1033
7. Hasty P, Montagna C. Chromosomal rearrangements in cancer. *Mol Cell Oncol*. 2014;1(1):e29904. doi:10.4161/mco.29904
8. Garber JE, Offit K. Hereditary cancer predisposition syndromes. *J Clin Oncol*. 2005;23(2):276–292. doi:10.1200/JCO.2005.10.042
9. Nagy R, Sweet K, Eng C. Highly penetrant hereditary cancer syndromes. *Oncogene*. 2004;23(38):6445–6470. doi:10.1038/sj.onc.1207714
10. Vogelstein B, Papadopoulos N, Velculescu VE, et al. Cancer genome landscapes. *Science*. 2013;339(6127):1546–1558. doi:10.1126/science.1235122
11. Davies MA, Samuels Y. Analysis of the genome to personalize therapy for melanoma. *Oncogene*. 2010;29(41):5545–5555. doi:10.1038/onc.2010.323
12. Sever R, Brugge JS. Signal transduction in cancer. *Cold Spring Harb Perspect Med*. 2015;5(4):a006098. doi:10.1101/cshperspect.a006098
13. Wertz IE, Dixit VM. Regulation of death receptor signaling by the ubiquitin system. *Cell Death Differ*. 2010;17(1):14–24. doi:10.1038/cdd.2009.168
14. Amit I, Citri A, Shay T, et al. A module of negative feedback regulators defines growth factor signaling. *Nat Genet*. 2007;39(4):503–512. doi:10.1038/ng1987

15. DeVita VT, Lawrence TS, Rosenberg SA. *Cancer Principles & Practice of Oncology: Primer of the Molecular Biology of Cancer*, 2nd ed. Philadelphia, PA: Wolters Kluwer Health; 2015.
16. An X, Tiwari AK, Sun Y, et al. BCR-ABL tyrosine kinase inhibitors in the treatment of Philadelphia chromosome positive chronic myeloid leukemia: a review. *Leuk Res*. 2010;34(10):1255–1268. doi:10.1016/j.leukres.2010.04.016
17. Hoadley KA, Yau C, Wolf DM, et al. Multiplatform analysis of 12 cancer types reveals molecular classification within and across tissues of origin. *Cell*. 2014;158(4):929–944. doi:10.1016/j.cell.2014.06.049
18. U.S. Food and Drug Administration.. FDA approves first cancer treatment for any solid tumor with a specific genetic feature. 2017.https://www.fda.gov/newsevents/newsroom/pressannouncements/ucm560167.htm
19. National Cancer Institute. NCI-MATCH Trial (Molecular Analysis for Therapy Choice). 2018. https://www.cancer.gov/about-cancer/treatment/clinical-trials/nci-supported/nci-match
20. Metzker ML. Sequencing Technologies—the next Generation. *Nat Rev Genet*. 2010;11(1):31. doi:10.1038/nrg2626
21. O'Daniel JM, Lee K. Whole-genome and whole-exome sequencing in hereditary cancer: impact on genetic testing and counseling. *Cancer J*. 2012;18(4):287–292. doi:10.1097/PPO.0b013e318262467e
22. ACMG Board of Directors. Points to consider in the clinical application of genomic sequencing. *Genet Med*. 2012;14(8):759–761. doi:10.1038/gim.2012.74
23. Walsh T, Casadei S, Lee MK, et al. Mutations in 12 genes for inherited ovarian, fallopian tube, and peritoneal carcinoma identified by massively parallel sequencing. *Proc Natl Acad Sci USA*. 2011;108(44):18032–18037. doi:10.1073/pnas.1115052108
24. Hanahan D, Weinberg RA. Hallmarks of cancer: The next generation. *Cell*. 2011;144(5):646–674. http://www.cell.com/cell/fulltext/S0092-8674(11)00127-9
25. Sandoval J, Esteller M. Cancer epigenomics: beyond genomics. *Curr Opin Genet Dev*. 2012;22(1):50–55. doi:10.1016/j.gde.2012.02.008
26. Herman JG, Baylin SB. Gene silencing in cancer in association with promoter hypermethylation. *N Engl J Med*. 2003;349(21):2042–2054. doi:10.1056/NEJMra023075
27. Feinberg AP, Vogelstein B. Hypomethylation distinguishes genes of some human cancers from their normal counterparts. *Nature*. 1983;301(5895):89. doi:10.1038/301089a0
28. Bird A. The essentials of DNA methylation. *Cell*. 1992;70(1):5–8. doi:10.1016/0092-8674(92)90526-I
29. Suvà ML, Riggi N, Bernstein BE. Epigenetic reprogramming in cancer. *Science*. 2013:339(6127):1567–1570. doi:10.1126/science.1230184
30. Kulis M, Esteller M. DNA methylation and cancer. In: Herceg Z, Ushijima T, eds. *Advances in Genetics. Epigenetics and Cancer, Part A*. San Deigo, CA: Academic Press; 2010:27–56.
31. Fraga MF, Herranz M, Espada J, et al. A mouse skin multistage carcinogenesis model reflects the aberrant DNA methylation patterns of human tumors. *Cancer Res*. 2004;64(16):5527–5534. doi:10.1158/0008-5472.CAN-03-4061
32. Lim DHK, Maher ER. 6–Genomic imprinting syndromes and cancer. In: Herceg Z, Ushijima T, eds. *Advances in Genetics: Epigenetics and Cancer, Part A*. San Diego, CA: Academic Press; 2010:145–175.
33. Seligson DB, Horvath S, Shi T, et al. Global histone modification patterns predict risk of prostate cancer recurrence. *Nature*. 2005;435(7046):1262. doi:10.1038/nature03672
34. Esteller M. Epigenetics provides a new generation of oncogenes and tumour-suppressor genes. *Br J Cancer*. 2006;94(2):179. doi:10.1038/sj.bjc.6602918
35. Lu J, Getz G, Miska EA, et al. MicroRNA expression profiles classify human cancers. *Nature*. 2005;435(7043):834. doi:10.1038/nature03702
36. Yarden Y, Sliwkowski MX. Untangling the ErbB signalling network. *Nat Rev Mol Cell Biol*. 2001;2(2):127. doi:10.1038/35052073
37. Shields JM, Pruitt K, McFall A, et al. Understanding RAS: "it ain't over 'til it's over." *Trends Cell Biol*. 2000;10(4):147–154. doi:10.1016/S0962-8924(00)01740-2
38. Duronio RJ, Xiong Y. Signaling pathways that control cell proliferation. *Cold Spring Harb Perspect Biol*. 2013;5(3):a008904. doi:10.1101/cshperspect.a008904
39. Sansal I, Sellers WR. The biology and clinical relevance of the PTEN tumor suppressor pathway. *J Clin Oncol*. 2004;22(14):2954–2963. doi:10.1200/JCO.2004.02.141
40. Bjornsti M-A, Houghton PJ. The TOR pathway: a target for cancer therapy. *Nat Rev Cancer*. 2004;4(5):335–348. doi:10.1038/nrc1362
41. Clevers H, Loh KM, Nusse R. Stem cell signaling. An integral program for tissue renewal and regeneration: Wnt signaling and stem cell control. *Science*. 2014;346(6205):1248012. doi:10.1126/science.1248012
42. Matsui WH. Cancer stem cell signaling pathways. *Medicine*. 2016;95(Suppl 1):S8–S19. doi:10.1097/MD.0000000000004765
43. Merchant AA, Matsui W. Targeting hedgehog—a cancer stem cell pathway. *Clin Cancer Res*. 2010;16(12):3130–3140. doi:10.1158/1078-0432.CCR-09-2846
44. Clement V, Sanchez P, de Tribolet N, et al. HEDGEHOG-GLI1 signaling regulates human glioma growth, cancer stem cell self-renewal, and tumorigenicity. *Curr Biol*. 2007;17(2):165–172. doi:10.1016/j.cub.2006.11.033
45. Kahn M. Can we safely target the WNT pathway? *Nat Rev Drug Discov*. 2014;13(7):513–532. doi:10.1038/nrd4233
46. Karamboulas C, Ailles L. Developmental signaling pathways in cancer stem cells of solid tumors. *Biochim Biophys Acta*. 2013;1830(2):2481–2495. doi:10.1016/j.bbagen.2012.11.008
47. Takebe N, Miele L, Harris PJ, et al. Targeting Notch, Hedgehog, and Wnt pathways in cancer stem cells: clinical update. *Nat Rev Clin Oncol*. 2015;12(8):445–464. doi:10.1038/nrclinonc.2015.61
48. Ranganathan P, Weaver KL, Capobianco AJ. Notch signalling in solid tumours: a little bit of everything but not all the time. *Nat Rev Cancer*. 2011;11(5):338. doi:10.1038/nrc3035
49. Beier R, Bürgin A, Kiermaier A, et al. Induction of cyclin E-Cdk2 kinase activity, E2F-dependent transcription and cell growth by Myc are genetically separable events. *EMBO J*. 2000;19(21):5813–5823. doi:10.1093/emboj/19.21.5813

50. Haupt Y, Robles AI, Prives C, Rotter V. Deconstruction of p53 functions and regulation. *Oncogene.* 2002;21(54):8223–8231. doi:10.1038/sj.onc.1206137
51. Wasylishen AR, Lozano G. Attenuating the p53 pathway in human cancers: many means to the same end. *Cold Spring Harb Perspect Med.* 2016;6(8):a026211. doi:10.1101/cshperspect.a026211
52. Smith J, Mun Tho L, Xu N, Gillespie AD. The ATM–Chk2 and ATR–Chk1 pathways in DNA damage signaling and cancer. In: Vande Woude GF, Klein G, eds. *Advances in Cancer Research*, vol. 108. Academic Press, Cambridge, MA; 2010:73–112.

4

The Cell Cycle, Cellular Death, and Metabolism

JACQUELINE DOUGLASS ■ ANDREW SHARABI ■ PHUOC T. TRAN

THE CELL CYCLE

Cancers are universally characterized by dysregulation of the cell cycle, allowing for uninhibited and inappropriate cell growth. Thus, cell cycle analysis tools are commonly used by cancer researchers to ask specific questions about the underlying cancer biology. For example, in elucidating signaling pathways, one may want to determine how overexpression or knockdown of a particular gene influences cell growth. Alternatively, in the identification of novel drug targets, one may need to characterize the mechanism by which cancer cells escape cell cycle checkpoints. A number of antineoplastic agents influence the cell cycle. Thus, cell cycle analysis provides critical tools for drug development. Cell cycle analysis is also used by clinicians; for instance, mitotic dye staining of pathologic specimens can help determine the grade and prognosis of patients' tumors. The optimal choice and implementation of a cell cycle assay will depend on the question being asked and the system under study.

BACKGROUND

The cell cycle is a conserved series of steps leading to cell division and two daughter cells (Figure 4.1). There are four main phases in the cell cycle: ***G1 phase, S phase, G2 phase,*** and ***M phase*** (1,2). G1 phase is a period of growth during which proteins and organelles are synthesized. During G1, or gap 1, the cell integrates a variety of external and internal cues to determine the suitability of cell division. Such signals include nutrient availability, cell crowding, and DNA integrity. Under favorable conditions, the cell will continue into S phase, the synthesis phase, during which the cell's genome is duplicated. Following S phase is G2 phase, the second gap phase, when the cell continues to grow and prepare for division. Collectively, the G1, S, and G2 periods are known as ***interphase***.

The cell divides during M, or ***mitotic***, phase, first with division of the nucleus (mitosis), followed by division of organelles and cell membrane to form two new cells (***cytokinesis***). Cells not actively in the process of dividing are said to be in G0 phase, referring to both senescent and quiescent cells. In fact, most cells in the adult human (e.g., neurons, myocytes) are senescent cells that are terminally differentiated and never re-enter the cell cycle (2). Some cells are ***quiescent*** (e.g.,

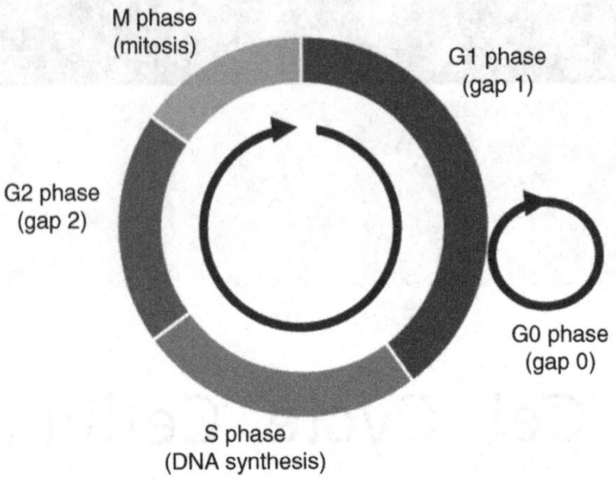

FIGURE 4.1 Diagram of cell cycle with restriction points.

hepatocytes, renal tubular epithelium), meaning they are in the resting G0 phase but can under certain circumstances reenter the cell cycle (2,3). Only a small fraction of human cells are actively in the cell cycle. These cells tend to be stem cells or stemlike cells that divide to replace lost or damaged cells, for example, hematopoietic cells in bone marrow or epithelial cells of the skin or gut (4).

Regulation of the cell cycle is a tightly controlled process with redundant pathways converging on key checkpoints to prevent inappropriate cell division, important for the health of both the cell and the entire organism. The master regulators of the cell cycle are ***cyclins*** and ***cyclin-dependent kinases*** (CDKs) (5). Different cyclin–CDK pairs control different portions of the cell cycle, with the presence of the cyclin necessary for the activity of its cognate CDK. For example, the cyclin D–CDK4 pair regulates early G1 progression, while the cyclin A–CDK2 and cyclin B–CDK1 pairs control the G2 to M phase progression (6,7).

Although CDKs are constitutively expressed in the cell, cyclin levels vary during the cell cycle. Each cyclin promotes its own degradation and the expression of downstream cyclins, thereby forcing the cell cycle forward (8). The activity of CDKs is further modulated by CDK inhibitors (CKIs), which collectively act to prevent cell cycle progression (2). There are two broad classes of CKIs, the *Ink4 family*, which includes p16, and the *cip/kip family*, which includes p21, p27, and p57. The complex balance of cyclin and CKI activity is critical for tight regulation of CDKs.

Three discrete checkpoints serve as potential halting points during the cell cycle, ensuring the proper order of events and fitness of the cell for division. The G1/S checkpoint, or restriction point, is the major checkpoint controlling entry into the cell cycle from a resting phase (9). Passing the restriction checkpoint commits a cell to division, making it insensitive to external stimuli. In the presence of mitogenic signaling, such as growth factor-receptor ligation, the canonical *MAPK signaling* pathway is triggered, increasing cyclin D levels. Cyclin D-CDK4 phosphorylates retinoblastoma protein (*Rb*), thereby inhibiting Rb's sequestration of the transcription factor *E2F*. The free E2F activates transcription of proteins responsible for further cell cycle progression, such as cyclins E and A. However, if internal signals are not favorable, the cell will not pass the restriction point. For instance, if DNA damage is detected by *p53*, p53 activates the CKI p21 to dephosphorylate Rb, allowing continued Rb-mediated sequestration of E2F and halting progression of the cell cycle (10). This pause gives the cell time to try to fix the damage; however, irreparable cell death can induce cell senescence or even death via apoptosis.

The second checkpoint is the G2/M checkpoint or DNA damage checkpoint, in which the cell confirms that complete and accurate genome duplication has occurred during S phase (11). The cyclin B–CDK1 complex drives progression through the G2/M checkpoint. CDK1 is normally inhibited by *Wee1* and other kinases. At the G2/M transition, another kinase, *Plk1*, phosphorylates Wee1, targeting it for degradation, thereby relieving inhibition on the cyclin B–CDK1 complex. As in the G1/S checkpoint, DNA damage can trigger a halt in the cell cycle by inhibition of cyclin B–CDK1 activity. The third checkpoint is the spindle assembly checkpoint occurring during mitosis, to confirm proper alignment of the chromosomes and attachment of the mitotic spindle (12).

In cancer, pro-growth signals outweigh anti-growth signals, and this imbalance can occur at multiple points in the regulation of the cell cycle. Elevated pro-growth signals can manifest as enhanced growth factor receptor activity (e.g., *Her2* in certain breast cancers, *EGFR* in lung cancers), MAPK and other pro-growth pathways mutations (e.g., *Braf* mutations in melanomas), or direct mutations in cell cycle proteins (e.g., cyclin D mutations in breast cancer) (2,13). Such proteins responsible for pro-growth signals are proto-oncogenes; with activating mutations or enhanced expression, they drive tumor growth.

Diminished anti-growth signaling is the result of loss of function of tumor suppressor proteins. Tumor suppressors can act at upstream points in cell cycle regulation, such as inhibition of growth pathway signaling (e.g., *PTEN* mutations in breast cancer), or can be directly involved in the cell cycle (e.g., the CKIs p16 found in a range of cancer types or Rb mutations in retinoblastoma) (14,15). Due to redundancy in cell cycle regulation, cancers display several driver mutations in oncogene and tumor suppressor proteins (16).

Premalignant lesions have genetic or epigenetic alterations resulting in a proliferative growth advantage, allowing those cells to out-divide their neighbor cells. Higher proliferation rates increase the probability of further mutations in these cells over their normal neighbors, even if the baseline mutation rate is unchanged (17). However, aberrant cell cycle regulation and lack of responsiveness to normal checkpoint controls further increases genetic instability, resulting in daughter cells with errors in DNA replication or gross chromosomal abnormalities. For example, if the cell becomes unresponsive to lack of proper chromosome-mitotic spindle assembly, the chromosomes may unevenly segregate, resulting in aneuploidy, a common feature of many cancers (18). Such genomic and chromosomal instability dramatically increases the evolution rate of daughter tumor cell clones. As more mutations arise, tumor cell clones with mutations conferring a selective growth advantage become dominant, resulting in a progressively more aggressive tumor.

While dysfunctional cell cycle checkpoint regulation gives cancer cells a proliferative advantage and higher rates of genetic evolution, this ubiquitous attribute opens a therapeutic window for specific targeting of cancer cells, while minimizing harm to normal tissue. Dysregulation at specific cell cycle stages is frequently targeted in anti-neoplastic therapy (19,20). For instance, DNA ***alkylating agents*** (e.g., cyclophosphamide) and other drugs that damage DNA (e.g., cisplatin) have been used for years in the clinic and take advantage of the increased proliferation rate and poor DNA replication fidelity of cancers. ***Antimitotic*** chemotherapies (i.e., docetaxel, vincristine) disrupt the microtubules that form the mitotic spindle, interrupting cell division. Growth factor signaling blockade using ***monoclonal antibodies*** (e.g., trastuzumab against Her2, cetuximab against EGFR) is an effective method to starve cancers dependent on growth signals. More details about how cell cycle aberrations can be targeted for anticancer therapies are discussed in Chapter 7.

CELL CYCLE ANALYSIS

One of the most commonly asked questions by cancer researchers and clinicians is the fraction of cells undergoing mitosis at a particular time, known as the ***mitotic index***. Pathologists often grade cancers in part based on the number of observed mitotic cells in a given field, as this metric reflects the aggressiveness of the cancer and thus prognosis for the patient and predicted response to chemotherapy. Similarly, cancer researchers may want to compare mitotic rates for ***in vitro*** cell cultures or ***in vivo*** animal models under an experimental condition, such as in the presence of drug targeting a mutated gene or cell cycle. To answer this question, one can quantify the amount of DNA present in the cell, with duplication of the genome reflecting a mitotic state, or use mitosis-specific markers.

During mitosis, the genome condenses to form visible chromosomes. Thus, the mitotic index is defined as the fraction of cells observed with visible chromosomes. Typically pathological specimens are formalin-fixed and paraffin-embedded (FFPE) and stained with hematoxylin and eosin (H&E). Hematoxylin is a dark blue dye that stains acidic or negatively charged substances, such as DNA and ribonucleic acid (RNA); eosin is a red dye staining basic or positively charged substances, including many proteins (21). Mitotic figures (compacted chromatin) are visible as dense blue hematoxylin staining, and the number counted per high-power field is often a criterion in the grading of certain cancers (22,23). One important protocol note regardless of the dye used is that the specimen must be rapidly fixed or else the mitotic count may be overestimated. Biopsied or resected tumor cells that are not rapidly fixed continue to undergo cell cycle progression, but tend to arrest midway through mitosis due to lack of oxygen and energy supply (24).

Alternatively, detection of markers uniquely associated with cell proliferation can be used to determine the fraction of dividing cells in a population. Specifically, the nuclear antigens ***Ki67*** and ***PCNA*** are strictly expressed in the cell during mitosis, and validated antibodies for each exist (25). Immunohistochemistry (IHC) on tumor specimens can be performed using, for instance, an anti-Ki67 primary antibody and an enzyme-conjugated secondary. Enzymes such as horseradish peroxidase (HRP) and alkaline phosphatase (AP) can be conjugated to secondary antibodies and produce a colorimetric change upon addition of particular substrates. Alternatively, immunofluorescence using a fluorophore-conjugated secondary followed by microscopy is frequently used in research settings. Like with the mitotic index, the fraction of Ki-67+ or PCNA+ cancer cells in a pathology specimen is frequently used to gauge cancer aggressiveness and predict clinical course (26,27).

DNA binding dyes are frequently used in cancer research to distinguish cells undergoing mitosis. DAPI is a blue dye commonly used for immunofluorescence of fixed cells; however, DAPI has poor permeability to live cell membranes (28). Fixing can introduce artifacts and in some experiments, live cell imaging may be desired. Other DNA binding dyes, namely, Hoeschst dyes (33258 and 33342) and DRAQ5, will stain the DNA of live cells and exhibit low cytotoxicity, an important factor for live cell studies (29,30). Alternatively, other DNA binding dyes are particularly well suited for ***flow cytometry*** analysis of stained cell populations (31,32). When using these dyes, the fluorescence of cells in S, G2, and M phases will be greater than the baseline fluorescence of either resting or G1 phase cells, due to duplication of the genome that occurs during S phase.

Propidium iodide (PI) is a red fluorescent dye that binds all nucleic acids, preferentially of dead or fixed cells. Cells can be fixed with paraformaldehyde or methanol and treated with RNaseA prior to staining, which will degrade RNA in the cell, reducing background RNA staining (33). The fraction of cells undergoing division is determined by comparing relative area under the peak of the lower staining population (2N) with that under higher staining population (>2N to 4N). Aneuploidy, an abnormal chromosome number, is common in cancer and can also be observed using DNA binding dyes (32). Because PI staining does not clearly distinguish between S, G2, and M phase cells, staining the fixed cells simultaneously for a mitosis-specific marker (e.g., phosphorylated serine 10 of histone H3) can allow one to quantify the fraction of mitotic cells (34). Flow cytometry has the added benefit over traditional microscopy and IHC of allowing the investigator to quickly and consistently analyze a large number of cells (typically on the order of 10,000 cells per sample) to answer specific questions about the cell population (e.g., fraction of mitotic cells, dead cells) (35). However, the sample must be in a single-cell suspension, and tissue samples, particularly fixed pathological specimens, are not easily dissociated into single cells (36).

Apart from mitotic index, another major cell cycle metric that researchers frequently wish to quantify is cancer cell ***proliferation rate***. A variety of proliferation assays are available to quantify growth rate under experimental conditions, for instance, assessing the effect of a tumor suppressor knockout or the effect of a mitogen on a cell line. Different metrics can be used to measure proliferation rates. The simplest measurement of proliferation is cell counting, but this can be tedious or inaccurate. For in vitro experiments, the amount of ATP in a well is proportional to the number of live cells, and by measuring ATP at different time points, the proliferation rate can be measured (37). A number of assays are available to quantify ATP and typically use an ATP-dependent enzyme to convert a substrate into a fluorescent, luminescent, or colored product. Relative ATP concentrations can be compared between a control and experimental condition (e.g., drug treatment), or a standard curve of known cell numbers per well can be generated to determine absolute cell number per well.

The rate of incorporation of a tracer (3H-thymidine or BrdU) into newly synthesized DNA is a direct measure of the rate of DNA synthesis and, thus, of cell division rate. ***3H-thymidine*** (tritiated thymidine) is a radioactive analog of the nucleoside thymidine and can be added to cells in culture for a period of time followed by washing (38). The remaining thymidine has presumably been incorporated into DNA and can be measured using a scintillation counter. ***BrdU***, another thymidine analog, is a nonradioactive alternative that can be detected with an anti-BrdU antibody for immunostaining applications (39). Both 3H-thymidine and BrdU can also be used in animal models with intraperitoneal injections of the tracer or addition of tracer to the water supply. A major advantage of using 3H-thymidine or BrdU is the ability to perform ***pulse chase experiments***, allowing the researcher to study proliferation over a defined period of time (29). The amount of BrdU tracer used should be titrated for the cell line, as too great a concentration can actually inhibit cell proliferation (40).

Proliferation rate can also be measured using the dilution rate of a stable fluorescent dye in a population of cells. For instance, carboxyfluorescein succinimidyl ester (CFSE) is a fluorescent dye that covalently binds cytoplasmic proteins (Figure 4.2). In CFSE-labeled cells, each cell division results in halving of the CFSE fluorescence intensity in the two daughter cells, which can be quantified by flow cytometry (41). CFSE labeling can be combined with use of other stains and antibodies for flow cytometry to answer questions about the differences between a highly proliferative population of cells and a slower growing population.

Example: Flow cytometry on cancer cells treated with an antimicrotubule agent—staining with PI, Hoescht 33342, and anti-histone H3 phospho-ser-10 for cell cycle analysis

Antimicrotubule drugs, a commonly used class of antineoplastic agents, interfere with the segregation of chromosomes during mitosis. In characterizing a new antimitotic agent, one would want to perform a variety of cell cycle studies to determine the effect of the drug on cell cycle progression, namely, halting mitotic division. In this example, we demonstrate how cell cycle analysis dyes and flow cytometry can be used to answer this question.

A breast cancer cell line is plated at low confluency in tissue culture wells and incubated at 37°C. At set time points (8 and 16 hours) after plating, the antimitotic agent is added at a specified concentration to different wells, and cells are harvested at the 26-hour time point, such that different wells have been exposed to the agent for different time periods (18 and 10 hours, respectively). An untreated well is used as a baseline of cell cycle activity. Cells are harvested, fixed with paraformaldehyde, permeabilized with Triton X-100, treated with RNAse (to degrade RNA, which

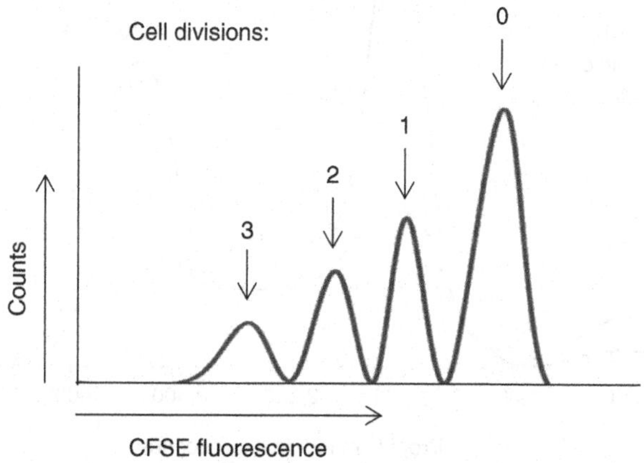

FIGURE 4.2 Number of mitotic cycles measured with CFSE staining.
CFSE, carboxyfluorescein succinimidyl ester.

can cause background), and stained with PI. Flow cytometry analysis in the red channel shows PI staining, with the level of PI staining proportional to the DNA present (Figure 4.3). On analysis, the 10-hour treatment results in a larger fraction of cells in G2/M phase, but by 18 hours, a significant fraction of cells have undergone apoptosis, distinguished by sub-G0/G1 levels of DNA. By disrupting normal microtubule–centromere attachment, this drug induces apoptosis via the spindle assembly checkpoint.

Alternatively, to evaluate cell cycle status of live cells only, cells can be harvested and simultaneously stained with PI and Hoescht 33342 without fixation and permeabilization (Figure 4.4). Live cells can be gated on the basis of low PI staining because live cell membranes are relatively impermeable to PI, unlike dying cells (more details in the next section). The Hoescht dye staining profile (measured in the UV channel) resembles that of the fixed, PI-stained cells, except now apoptotic cells are excluded.

Finally, one may wish to distinguish G2 phase cells from mitotic cells to confirm that indeed the antimicrotubule agent halts cells in mitosis by staining for a mitosis-specific marker. Phosphorylation of serine 10 on histone H3 is specific to mitosis and can be detected using an antibody. Cells are harvested, fixed, and permeabilized, followed by staining with a fluorophore-labeled anti-histone H3 Ser10 antibody and PI. On a scatterplot of PI staining versus anti-histone H3 staining, now the G2 phase and M phase populations can be distinguished (Figure 4.5).

MECHANISMS OF CELL DEATH

Neoplasia is the result of inappropriate cell growth resulting from the imbalance between exaggerated cell survival signals and lack of normal cell death. Thus, an understanding of the basic types, mechanisms, and regulation of cell death is critical to answering questions in many areas of cancer research. For example, knowledge of the specific pathways that particular cancers use to evade cell death can facilitate identification of druggable targets in those pathways (42). Furthermore, researchers frequently characterize antineoplastic agents based on the mechanism by which they

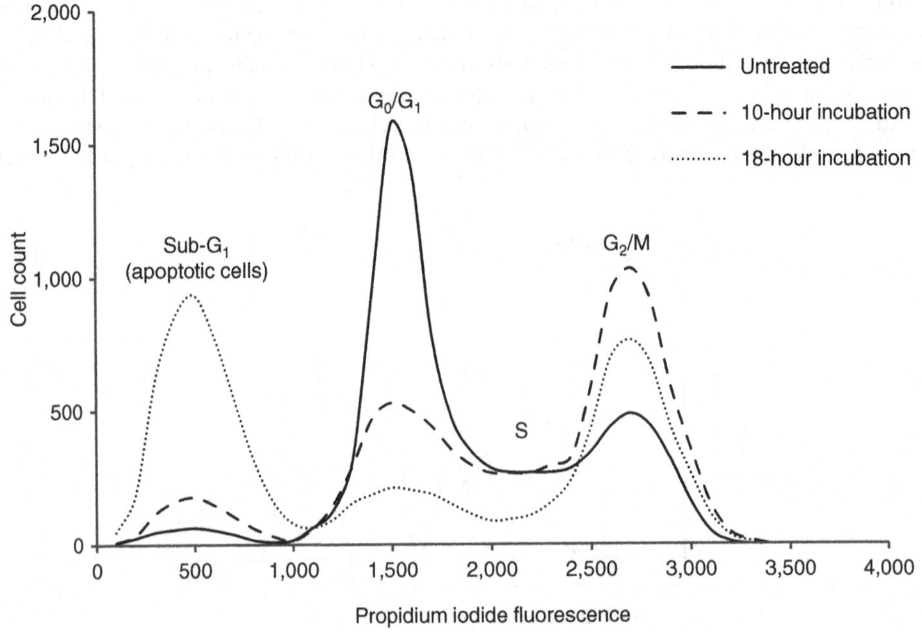

FIGURE 4.3 Histogram comparing propidium iodide (PI) staining of cells treated with antimicrotubule agent for 0, 10, and 18 hours.

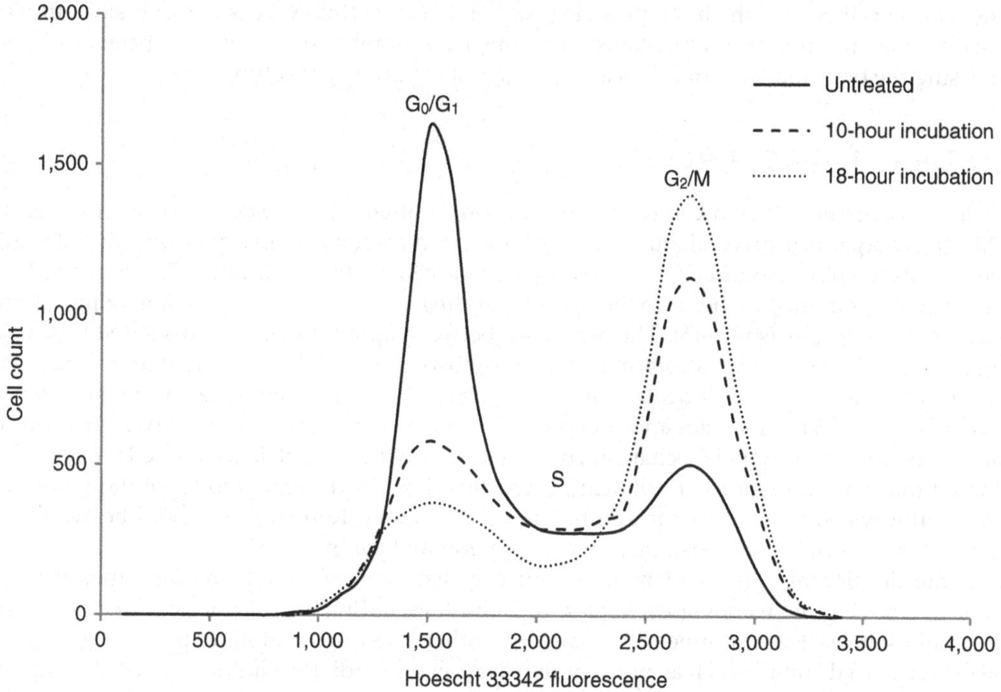

FIGURE 4.4 Histogram comparing Hoescht 33342 staining of cells treated with antimicrotubule agent for 0, 10, and 18 hours. Dead cells excluded with propidium iodide (PI).

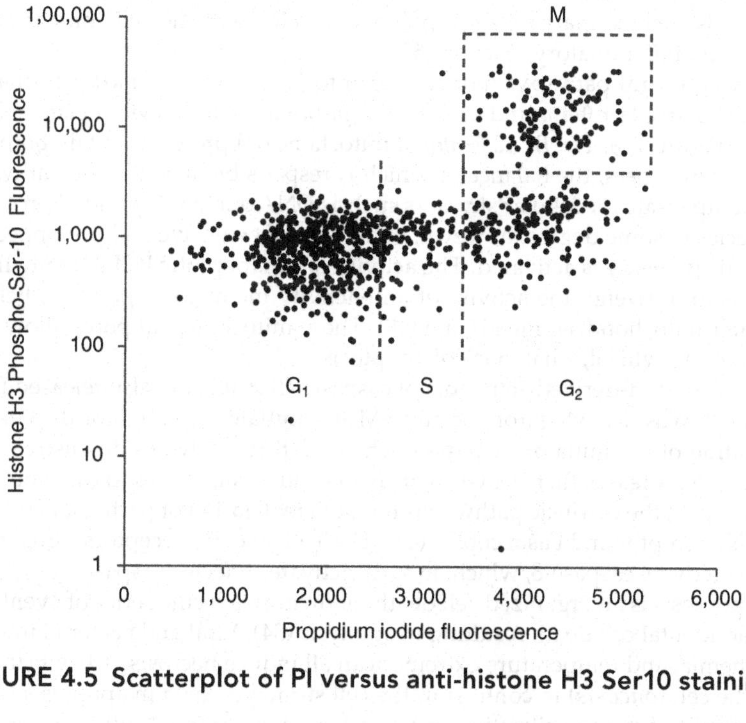

FIGURE 4.5 Scatterplot of PI versus anti-histone H3 Ser10 staining.

induce cancer cell death, which can provide insight into drug efficacy, possible toxic side effects to normal tissues, and tumor cell resistance mechanisms. A number of assays have been developed to measure the type and level of cell death in different experimental settings.

CELL DEATH—BACKGROUND

Cell death, occurring when a cell ceases to function, is often a physiologic process required for multicellular organism survival, but can be pathologic in response to injury or infection. The distinction between physiologic cell death and pathologic cell death is typically whether the cell was genetically programmed to die, as in the case of ***apoptosis***, or dies as a result of damaging external conditions, as in ***necrosis*** (43–45). The difference between apoptosis and necrosis is subtle, however, as external stressors can also bring about apoptosis, if the cell has sufficient time to respond. A third broad category of cell death is *autophagy associated* and results when a nutrient-starved cell consumes its own organelles and proteins to generate energy (46). Autophagy-associated cell death is a temporary survival mechanism, but eventually, without nutrients, the cell will die. Each of these three main categories of cell death is characterized by different modes of induction, signaling pathways, and morphologic and biochemical changes. Researchers should be aware that alternate forms of cell death exist, including *necroptosis* and *pyroptosis* (47).

In the developing fetus and in the adult organism, specific cells undergo apoptosis, for instance, removing the webbing between finger and toes, aiding in maturation of the brain, and eliminating self-reactive immune cells that could otherwise cause autoimmune disease (48–50). However, external stimuli such as nutrient deprivation and radiation-induced DNA damage can also bring about apoptosis via specific pathways that are activated by these stimuli. Apoptosis is an organized series of events in the cell, resulting in key morphologic features such as cell shrinkage, membrane blebbing, chromatin condensation (*pyknosis*), DNA fragmentation (*karyorrhexis*), and mRNA decay (48). In contrast to necrosis, the plasma membrane integrity is preserved, meaning that ion and adenosine 5′-triphosphate (ATP) levels are maintained in the cell to drive the specific series of steps to complete the process (51). Apoptosis is generally a nonimmunogenic form of cell death. Following the completion of the process, the resulting apoptotic bodies are consumed by phagocytic cells such as macrophages, preventing release of the cell contents, which would otherwise trigger an inflammatory reaction (52).

There are two general pathways inducing apoptosis, an ***intrinsic pathway*** that is mediated directly by mitochondrial proteins and an ***extrinsic pathway*** that acts via specific receptors on the cell surface (48) (Figure 4.6). The *BCL2 family* of mitochondrial proteins contain both proapoptotic and antiapoptotic members, the balance of which is responsible for intrinsic pathway activation (53). Cells can compensate for cellular stressors such as DNA damage, unfolded proteins, and reactive oxygen species to some degree; however, in the case of extensive and prolonged damage, the intrinsic apoptotic pathway is activated. The activity of proapoptotic BCL2 family members (e.g., Bad, Bax) begins to outweigh the activity of anti-activity members (e.g., Bcl-2, Bcl-xL), forming pores in the outer mitochondrial membrane (48). These mitochondrial pores allow the release of cytochrome c into the cytosol, a hallmark of apoptosis.

Second mitochondria-derived activators of caspases (*SMACs*) are also released from the mitochondria. Both cytoplasmic cytochrome c and SMACs initiate activation of the ***caspase*** cascade, first with activation of the initiator caspase-9, which, in turn, activates downstream effector caspases. Caspases are proteases that cleave an array of cellular substrates to carry out the apoptotic process. Alternatively, the extrinsic pathway is initiated by ligation of particular cell surface receptors, namely, TNF receptor and Fas receptor (48). The TNF and Fas receptors signal through adaptor molecules to activate caspase-8, which, in turn, activates effector caspases.

Whereas apoptosis is an organized cell death following a specific series of events, necrosis is a disorganized, accidental cell death resulting in autolysis (54). Viral and bacterial infections, physical trauma, ischemia, and temperature extremes can all induce necrosis. A key feature of necrosis is swelling of the cell (***oncosis***) in contrast to the cell shrinkage seen in apoptosis (48) (Table 4.1). Oncosis is the result of permeabilization of the plasma membrane, leading to disruption of ion

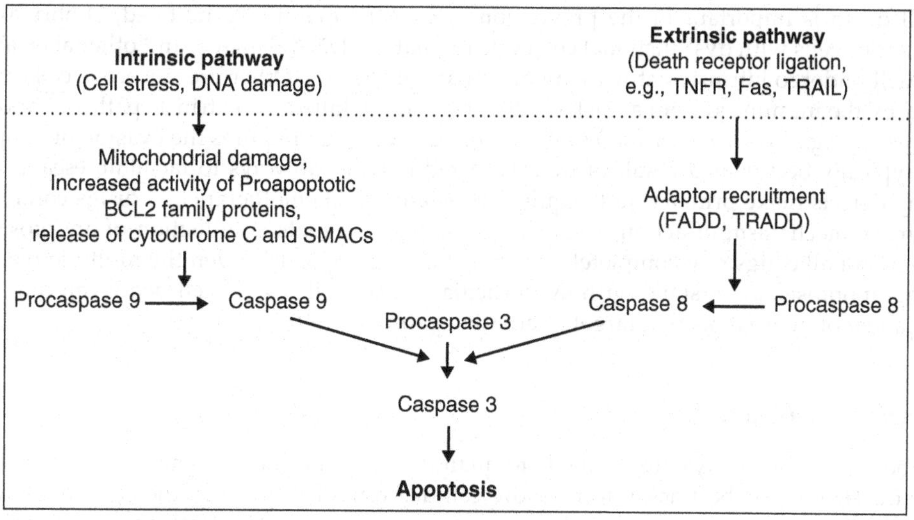

FIGURE 4.6 Extrinsic and intrinsic apoptotic pathways.
FADD, Fas-associated protein with death domain; SMAC, second mitochondria-derived activator of caspases; TNFR, tumor necrosis factor receptor; TRADD, tumor necrosis factor receptor type 1-associated DEATH domain protein; TRAIL, TNF-related apoptosis-inducing ligand.

gradients and loss of ATP. Organelle lysis results in release of destructive enzymes that degrade cellular proteins and DNA. Loss of plasma membrane integrity results in release of dying cell contents into the extracellular environment before phagocytic cells have a chance to consume the dying cells (55). These cellular contents trigger an inflammatory response, making necrosis generally an immunogenic form of cell death (56).

The third major form of cell death is ***autophagy***, which is an adaptive response to cellular stress, such as nutrient deprivation. Autophagy takes three main forms: macroautophagy, microautophagy, and chaperone-mediated autophagy. Macroautophagy typically serves to eliminate damaged organelles and involves the formation of an autophagosome around the target organelle. The double-membraned autophagosome ultimately fuses with a lysosome, where lysosomal hydrolases degrade the contents. In microautophagy, the lysosome forms an invagination around a segment of cytosolic contents, which are directly degraded. The third form of autophagy involves the chaperone protein hsc70 complexing with substrates, which are recognized by a lysosomal receptor and translocated into the lysosome for degradation.

TABLE 4.1 KEY DIFFERENCES BETWEEN APOPTOSIS AND NECROSIS

Apoptosis	Necrosis
Affects single cells or small clusters	Affects groups of neighboring cells
Cell shrinks	Cell swelling
Plasma membrane blebbing but intact	Plasma membrane integrity disrupted
Mitochondrial membrane permeability	Organelle swelling and damage
Pyknosis and karyorrhexis	Karyolysis, pyknosis, and karyorrhexis
No inflammation	Inflammation present

Cell death is important in the prevention of cancer to eliminate mutated, abnormal cells. Precancerous cells with dysfunctional cell cycle regulation, DNA damage, and other aberrant signaling will undergo intrinsic pathway-mediated apoptosis (57). Other precancerous cells are recognized by the immune system as sick or stressed and are killed via extrinsic pathway apoptotic mechanisms (e.g., *Fas-FasL signaling*) (58). Tumor cell evolution requires the evasion of apoptosis, which typically occurs as a result of defects in redundant pathways to facilitate escape. These pathway defects make primary and acquired resistance to chemotherapeutic drugs common, as the primary mechanism of action of many antineoplastic agents is induction of apoptosis (42). However, not all drugs rely completely on induction of apoptosis. Given the multiple pathways inducing apoptosis, understanding how particular cancer cells evade cell death can inform the development of new agents that target alternative pathways (59).

CELL DEATH ASSAYS

A number of in vitro assays are available to quantify general cell death and mechanism-specific cell death. There is no best assay to measure cell death in all situations; the optimal assay will depend on the particular experiment being performed. Compromised membrane integrity is a robust metric of cell death and even apoptotic cells in vitro will ultimately lose plasma membrane integrity in the absence of phagocytic cells (60,61). Dyes that are excluded by live cells but permeable to dead cells include trypan blue, PI, and 7-aminoactinomycin D (7-AAD) (60). Trypan blue is visualized with a bright-field microscope; PI and 7-AAD measurements use a fluorescent readout. Of note, only late-stage, and not early-stage, apoptotic cells will label with these dyes. Similarly, cell content release can be quantified to measure cell death, such as LDH, an enzyme present in all cells (62). Alternatively, live cells can be prelabeled with a substance (e.g., chromium-51 [Cr-51], calcein AM), and the release of that substance used as a metric for cell death. In the ***Cr-51 release assay***, cells are prelabeled with Cr-51, and afterward free Cr-51 is quantified with a gamma or scintillation counter (63). Use of calcein AM is a nonradioactive alternative to the Cr-51 release assay. Calcein AM is a nonfluorescent dye that can penetrate viable cells. Once in the cells, the calcein AM is hydrolyzed by cell esterases into calcein, which cannot penetrate the cell membrane. Calcein labeling can be used to identify viable cells via flow cytometry or fluorescence microscopy. However, upon cell death of labeled cells, the fluorescent calcein is released into the media and can be quantified via fluorometry (64).

Other assays are apoptosis specific, some of which work best at particular time points in the apoptotic process. Both early and late apoptotic cells can be identified by their caspase activity, which drives apoptosis. Caspase activity assays often consist of a membrane-penetrating peptide conjugated to a dye. The peptide in its native form prevents the dye from producing fluorescence; however, in the presence of active caspases, the peptide, which contains a caspase substrate amino acid sequence, is cleaved by the caspases, resulting in fluorescence (65). These caspase activity reporter peptides can also be used in vivo to study apoptosis in animal models. Other caspase activity dyes—for example, fluorescent inhibitors of caspases (FLICA™)—covalently bind to the active site of caspases (66). Unbound dye can be washed away, but bound dye remains and can be imaged via fluorescent microscopy. Alternatively, certain antibodies bind only the active, cleaved form of caspases or bind the cleaved form of canonical caspase substrates (e.g., the nuclear protein PARP) (67).

Mitochondrial permeability is another characteristic of early apoptosis that can be quantified. Enhanced membrane permeability is due in part to stabilization of the mitochondrial permeability transition pore (MPTP) that forms between the inner and outer membranes of the mitochondria and releases its contents into the cytosol (68). Fluorescent dyes such as tetramethylrhodamine methyl ester (TMRM) stain only permeabilized mitochondria, and other probes are available that produce a drop in fluorescence in the mitochondria when the mitochondrial membrane potential is disrupted (69).

The ***TUNEL assay*** is a classic assay of apoptosis, taking advantage of the enzyme terminal deoxynucleotidyl transferase (TdT)'s recognition of nicked DNA ends (70). TdT adds dUTP nucleotides to the ends of DNA. The use of labeled dUTPs, such as with fluorophores or haptens, allows detection either via direct fluorescence or via an anti-hapten antibody, respectively. Because DNA fragmentation occurs late in apoptosis, TUNEL only recognizes late-stage apoptotic cells (1.5–2 hours after induction of apoptosis) (71). DNA fragmentation can also be detected by performing gel electrophoresis on extracted DNA, with DNA from apoptotic cells showing a characteristic low-molecular-weight laddering pattern (72).

The ***comet assay***, also known as single-cell gel electrophoresis, also detects DNA fragmentation (73). In the comet assay, cells are imbedded and lysed in agarose. Application of an electric field results in DNA ends containing breaks to become free and migrate to a greater extent than the remainder of the supercoiled nuclear DNA, forming the "tail" of the comet. After electrophoresis, DNA is stained with a fluorescent dye and the ratio of the comet's tail to body can be quantified as a measure of DNA damage. Apart from detection of DNA fragmentation, chromatin condensation can be stained with certain fluorescent Hoechst dyes (74).

Certain dyes, such as ***annexin V***, selectively label plasma membrane changes in apoptotic cells. The protein annexin V recognizes phosphatidylserines on the outer cell membrane of apoptotic cells (75). In healthy cells, phosphatidylserine is present on the inner cell membrane. Apoptosis results in flipping of the phosphatidylserines, which are recognized by phagocytic cells as a signal to consume the dying cell. Annexin V can be conjugated to a fluorophore, enzyme, or other label for detection. Early-stage apoptotic cells will label with annexin V, but still have membrane integrity and so will not label with cell death dyes (e.g., PI, 7-AAD). Late-stage apoptotic cells will label both with the apoptotic-specific dyes and cell death dyes. Necrotic cells can be distinguished by exclusion of those cells staining with cell death dyes, but not with apoptosis indicator dyes.

Example: Flow cytometry analysis of cancer cells under hypoxic conditions—distinguishing early-apoptotic, late-apoptotic, and necrotic cells

Hypoxia is a common feature of many advanced solid tumors as the rapidly proliferating cancer cells outgrow their blood supply. One may want to characterize the effect of varying levels of oxygen deprivation on cancer cells in culture—specifically if and how cell death is induced. In this example, we expose colon cancer cells to different oxygen concentrations and evaluate the mechanism of resulting cell death. A colon cancer cell line is incubated in chambers with three oxygen concentrations chosen to mimic normoxia (8%), hypoxia (1%), and anoxia (0%; Figures 4.7, 4.8, and 4.9, respectively). After 8 hours, cells are harvested, stained with PI and annexin-V-FITC,

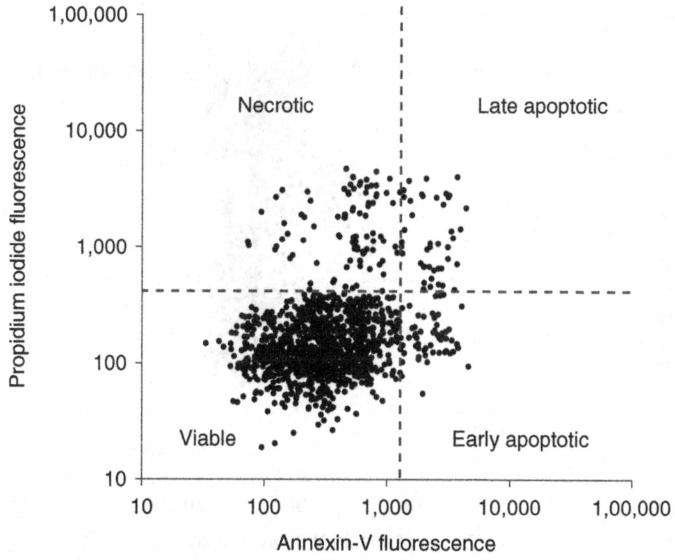

FIGURE 4.7 Propidium iodide (PI) and annexin V staining of colon cancer cells incubated under normoxic conditions.

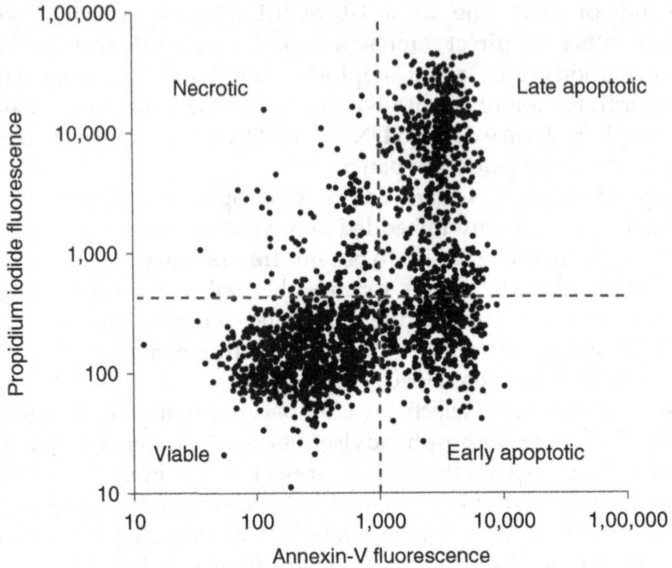

FIGURE 4.8 Propidium iodide (PI) and annexin V staining of colon cancer cells incubated under hypoxic conditions.

and analyzed by flow cytometry. In the normoxic conditions, the majority of the cells are viable, staining with neither PI nor annexin V. Under hypoxic conditions, some of the cells are undergoing apoptosis. Early apoptotic cells stain with annexin V but not PI because they still retain plasma integrity. Late apoptotic cells have loss of membrane integrity and stain with both dyes. Cells incubated under anoxic conditions are inviable, with a fraction staining with annexin V only (early apoptotic), a fraction staining with PI only (necrotic), and the majority staining with both PI and annexin V (late apoptotic).

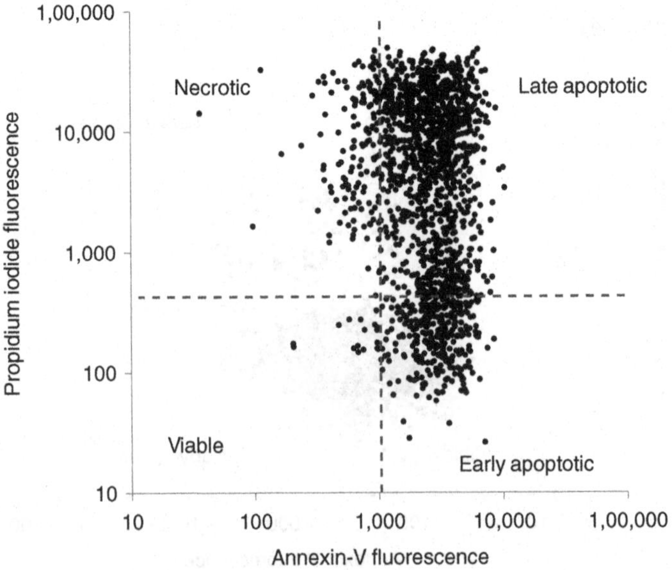

FIGURE 4.9 Propidium iodide (PI) and annexin V staining of colon cancer cells incubated under anoxic conditions.

CELL METABOLISM

Even for the experienced biochemist, metabolism is a complex field with an intricate web of pathways regulated by complicated mechanisms to carry out a vast array of biochemical processes in cells. However, even a basic understanding of metabolic pathways, their regulation, and experimental techniques to probe pathway activity can be critical for answering certain questions in biomedical research, particularly in the field of cancer biology. Cancer cells universally display aberrant regulation of basic metabolic pathways as a consequence of their increased metabolic demands for ATP and biochemical macromolecules to meet the need for rapid cell growth and division. Cancer researchers commonly use experimental techniques to elucidate the metabolic abnormalities in cancers to better understand drivers of malignant growth and identify possible therapeutic avenues.

BACKGROUND

Metabolism refers collectively to the enzyme-catalyzed reactions that produce useful forms of energy and synthesize biochemical compounds required for cellular function. Metabolic pathways can generally be divided into two categories. ***Catabolic pathways*** break down organic compounds into more basic components, freeing useful energy in the process. ***Anabolic pathways*** use energy and basic carbon building blocks to produce more complex biochemical substances such as proteins, carbohydrates, lipids, and nucleic acids.

All cells require energy, and two most important forms of energy in the cell are glucose and ATP, both of which contain high-energy bonds that can be broken to drive biochemical processes. Most cell types take up energy from the extracellular environment in the form of glucose via specific glucose transporters. Glucose then enters into the ***glycolysis pathway***, consisting of 10 cytosolic enzymatic steps to convert glucose into two molecules of pyruvate, producing ATP and reducing NAD+ (nicotinamide adenine dinucleotide) to NADH in the process (76). NADH and other forms of reducing equivalents (e.g., NADPH and QH2) are electron-donating cofactors critical for use in reductive biochemical reactions, such as the electron transport chain (77). Glycolysis is a highly controlled process with key regulated steps to tightly balance the levels of glycolysis substrates and products in the cell.

Glycolysis only produces two molecules of ATP per glucose entering the cycle, in contrast to the approximate 30 molecules of ATP produced from the use of pyruvate for downstream aerobic respiration (78). However, glycolysis is a quick source of ATP and does not require oxygen, important under hypoxic conditions. In animal cells suffering hypoxia, pyruvate is converted into lactic acid to regenerate NAD+ that is required to drive glycolysis to maintain ATP levels in the cell (79). Not all glucose entering glycolysis ends up as pyruvate. Some glycolysis intermediates are used as building blocks for other biochemical substances. For example, the intermediate dihydroxyacetone phosphate (DHAP) can be converted into glycerol, which combines with fatty acids to form triglycerides, an important form of energy storage (80). In addition, the intermediate glucose-5-phosphate can be shunted into the pentose phosphate pathway, which produces NADPH and carbon backbones for nucleotide and amino acid synthesis (81).

Following glycolysis, most pyruvate in the cell is used for aerobic respiration to maximize its full ATP-producing potential—a process also referred to as ***oxidative phosphorylation*** because of its dependence on oxygen. Pyruvate is first decarboxylated in the mitochondria, producing acetyl-CoA and carbon dioxide. The acetyl-CoA then enters the tricarboxylic acid (TCA) cycle (also known as the *Krebs cycle* or citric acid cycle), an eight-step enzymatic process occurring in the mitochondrial matrix (76). The TCA cycle results in full oxidation of acetyl-CoA to water and carbon dioxide, producing ATP and the reducing equivalents NADH and QH2 (a reduced form of coenzyme Q) in the process. Acetyl-CoA can also be derived from other carbohydrates, fats, and proteins, demonstrating how these complex biochemical macromolecules can be broken down into simpler forms to produce energy. The TCA cycle is important for anabolic pathways as well, with intermediates that can also be used to synthesize amino acids and nucleotides (76). As in glycolysis, key TCA enzymes are tightly regulated, predominantly via inhibition by its products and activation by its substrates.

The NADH and QH2 produced by the TCA cycle are used as reducing equivalents to drive the electron transport chain, located in the inner membrane of the mitochondria. The electron transport chain is a series of electron acceptors and donors that gradually transfers electrons from less to more electronegative acceptors, ending with oxygen, the most electronegative in the series (76). The reduction of electronegative acceptors releases energy, which is coupled to the pumping of hydrogens from the mitochondrial matrix into the inner membrane space. The ultimate goal of the electron transport chain is to harness the energy-releasing reduction of oxygen into water, to produce an electrochemical gradient of hydrogen ions across the inner mitochondrial membrane. This proton gradient drives ATP synthase, which acts as a molecular motor to produce ATP (82).

Cancers frequently display dramatic perturbations in metabolic pathways to support their abnormal growth. One of the most dramatic and longest known abnormalities of cancer metabolism is the ***Warburg effect***, also called ***aerobic glycolysis*** (83) (Figure 4.10). The Warburg effect is an observation that the majority of cancers predominantly depend on glycolysis followed by lactic acid fermentation for ATP generation, a completely anaerobic process, in contrast to normal cells that depend predominantly on aerobic respiration (TCA cycle and electron transport chain) for ATP generation. This dependence of anaerobic ATP production would be expected under hypoxic conditions; however, even in the presence of plentiful oxygen, cancer cells can display a glycolytic rate as much as 200 times that of normal cells (84).

The explanation for the high frequency with which the Warburg effect has been observed in a range of different cancer types has been a topic of uncertainty for decades. The effect could be the result of adaptation to hypoxic conditions during early tumor development, a consequence of mitochondrial damage (mitochondria being essential for aerobic respiration), an adaptive response by the cell to shut down the mitochondria to prevent the initiation of apoptosis, or simply a mechanism to generate extra building blocks for cell growth by shunting of glycolytic intermediates to biosynthetic pathways. Recently, an alternate form of ***pyruvate kinase*** (PKM2), a key glycolytic enzyme, has been implicated in driving the Warburg effect. PKM2 catalyzes the final step of glycolysis, producing pyruvate. The alternate form of the enzyme is

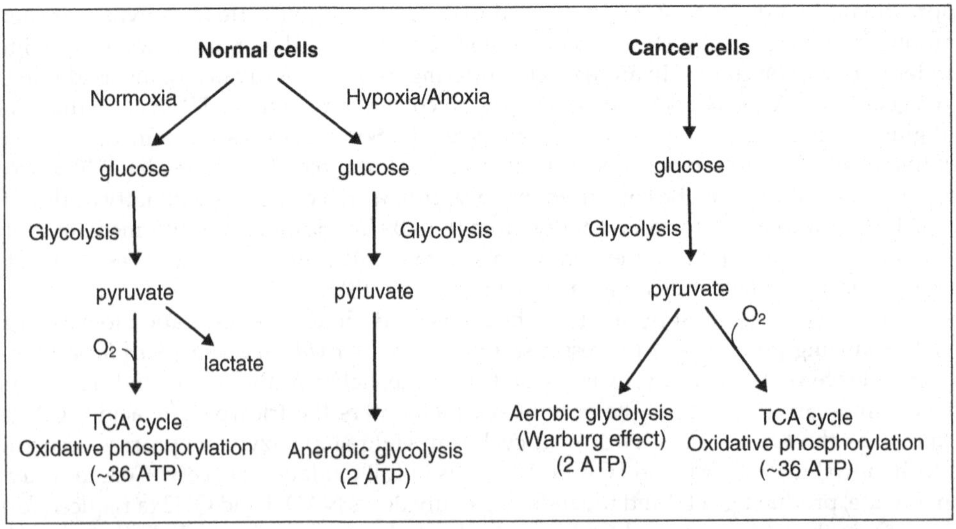

FIGURE 4.10 Glucose metabolism in normal cells versus cancer cells highlighting the Warburg effect found in cancer cells.

ATP, adenosine 5′-triphosphate; TCA, tricarboxylic acid.

less efficient than other isoforms, slowing down glycolysis and increasing shunting of intermediates to the pentose phosphate pathway, thereby producing NADPH and carbon backbones to support rapid cell growth. The Warburg effect has been used for diagnostic purposes. The high rate of glucose uptake by cancer cells underlies the use of ***^{18}F-fluorodeoxyglucose* (*^{18}F-FDG*)**, a radioactive glucose analog, for diagnostic PET imaging studies in cancer patients (83). Additionally, a number of glycolytic inhibitors are currently being investigated as anticancer agents (85).

Metabolic dysfunction in cancer is fundamentally the result of oncogene and tumor suppressor mutations. The summation of these mutations results in activation of pro-growth signaling pathways and transcription factors that alter metabolic enzyme regulation to support the increased growth demands (86). For example, mutations in the *PI3K pathway* (e.g., activation of PI3K, loss of function of *PTEN*) result in increased *AKT* activity. AKT has a number of downstream targets, resulting in an overall shift toward increased glycolysis and ATP generation. Importantly, one of AKT's substrates is *mTOR*, which normally integrates the cell's nutrient status and growth signals. Inappropriate activation of mTOR in cancer cells globally stimulates protein and lipid biosynthesis, thereby supporting growth and proliferation (86). Rapid tumor growth results in heterogeneous conditions for tumor cells, with variable access to oxygen, glucose, and other nutrients.

Tumor cells must be able to evade cellular checks that would initiate apoptosis in response to the metabolic stresses resulting from the abnormal tumor microenvironment. One such pathway is initiated by the kinase ***AMPK***, which acts as a metabolic checkpoint on the cell in the case of energetic stress, in part via inhibition of the pro-growth mTOR (86). AMPK is frequently downregulated in many cancer types, allowing those cells to continue to proliferate in response to oncogenic signaling even under abnormal metabolic conditions. While intrinsic genetic changes initiate and allow metabolic changes to occur, the heterogeneous conditions of the tumor microenvironment are thought to further contribute to metabolic abnormalities.

For example, hypoxia stabilizes the transcription factor ***HIF-1alpha***, resulting in expression of genes to help the cell compensate for the low-oxygen environment. HIF-1alpha signaling increases glycolytic activity and reduces citric acid cycle activity, further reinforcing the cell's dependence on glycolysis while diminishing its oxygen demand (79). Of note, HIF-1alpha can be inappropriately stabilized by oncogenic signaling even under normoxic conditions, an example of how a cancer cell can hijack existing pathways to meet the cell's metabolic needs (87).

METABOLISM ASSAYS

Many assays exist to investigate metabolic processes in the cell. The choice of particular assays will depend on the question being asked and the system studied. Such assays are useful for understanding the mechanisms driving malignant growth and discovering cancer-specific drugs. Given the strong dependence on glycolysis in many cancers, one may want to study glucose uptake, the rate of particular glycolytic steps, or levels of glycolytic intermediates.

Fluorescent glucose analogs, such as 2-NBDG, are available to monitor glucose uptake in cells (88). After a period of incubation with 2-NBDG, excess 2-NBDG is washed away and fluorescence evaluated using either microscopy or flow cytometry. A range of assays exists to quantify the activities of particular glycolytic enzymes, producing a fluorescent or colorimetric change proportional to the level of enzyme activity (88). Alternatively, to evaluate overall glycolytic activity, one can measure the ***extracellular acidification rate* (*ECAR*)** as cells relying primarily on glycolysis release more lactic acid into their environment (88). Fluorescent assays are available to measure the ECAR using fluorescent reagents sensitive to changes in pH.

Similarly, there are assays to assess the activities of specific TCA cycle enzymes and electron transport chain components, which may be important in demonstrating a particular cancer's reduced dependence on aerobic respiration (89,90). Alamar blue and tetrazolium salts (e.g., MTT, XTT) are compounds reduced by NAD(P)H-dependent enzymes in the cytosol, with the level of enzyme activity proportional to the overall metabolic activity of the cell (91). MTT is a positively charged yellow soluble compound that penetrates live cell membranes and is converted to the insoluble purple compound formazan upon reduction by mitochondrial enzymes, with the conversion rate proportional to the mitochondrial activity in the cell (37). Prior to measurement with a spectrometer, formazan should be solubilized using particular solvents or detergents, making this an endpoint assay.

The ***MTT assay*** was developed as a nonradioactive alternative to the 3H-thymidine incorporation assay; however, the two assays measure different cell processes: mitochondrial activity and DNA synthesis, respectively. Thus, while the MTT assay often correlates with proliferation, it is not, strictly speaking, an accurate measurement of proliferation (92). MTT has several limitations, including cytotoxicity, possibly altering measurements and requiring optimization for each cell line, and potential false signals due to reduction by chemicals tested in the assay (91,93).

The mechanism of the ***Alamar Blue assay*** is similar to that of MTT, but involves a fluorescent as well as colorimetric change. Alamar Blue has several advantages, such as being nontoxic to cells and having a reportedly higher sensitivity than MTT (91). Another metric of mitochondrial activity is the cellular oxygen consumption. Oxygen consumption is traditionally measured with a dissolved oxygen probe; however, more recently, compounds have been developed that undergo a fluorescent change in response to changes in oxygen concentration (94).

Assays are available to quantify redox cofactors such as NADH and NADPH, typically using a cofactor-specific enzyme to produce a colorimetric or fluorometric change proportional to the cofactor concentration (95). Other assays exist to study the synthesis or degradation of amino acids, lipids, carbohydrates, and nucleic acids. More recently, a number of "omics" technologies have been developed to evaluate global metabolic changes in cells. Metabolomics combines the use of nuclear magnetic resonance (NMR) spectroscopy and mass spectrometry to evaluate metabolite levels (96). Proteomic mass spectrometry and transcriptomics can assist in identifying the presence and expression patterns of enzymes and other proteins relevant to cell metabolism (97).

Example: Measuring ECAR, oxygen consumption rate (OCR), and ATP to compare relative rates of glycolysis and aerobic respiration upon treatment with metabolic pathway inhibitors

This example highlights the use of measuring the ECAR and ***oxygen consumption rate*** (***OCR***) as metrics of glycolytic and oxidative phosphorylation activities, respectively. A lung cancer cell line cultured in vivo is treated with agents that inhibit particular metabolic pathways, and the resulting inhibition of the target pathway and increased activity of compensatory pathways are quantified. The ECAR measures the conversion of pyruvate to lactic acid, proportional to glycolytic activity, using a pH-sensitive fluorescent probe. Fluorescence, as a function of time, is plotted, with the slope equal to the rate of extracellular acidification. Similarly, the oxygen consumption can be measured using an oxygen-sensitive fluorescent probe, with fluorescent change over time proportional to the OCR. ATP is measured by lysing cells and using a luciferase-based assay, with the level of luciferase activity proportional to ATP levels.

Oligomycin is used to probe the effect of oxidative phosphorylation inhibition on the lung cancer cell line. Oligomycin inhibits ATP synthase, the final component of the electron transport chain that uses the proton gradient between the mitochondrial matrix and inner membrane space to produce ATP. The cancer cells plated in three 96-well plates are treated with varying doses of oligomycin. One plate is used to measure ECAR and subjected to fluorescent monitoring after the addition of a pH-sensitive probe. A second plate is used to measure OCR, and the third plate is used to measure ATP concentrations. ECAR, OCR, and ATP levels are all plotted as a function of oligomycin dose (Figure 4.11). Increasing oligomycin results in a decrease in the OCR. Cells need less oxygen for electron acceptors, as inhibition of ATP synthase activity halts the electron transport chain. The cells compensate by increasing glycolytic rates, as measured by the ECAR. Because glycolysis activity is able to fully compensate for the drop in activity of the electron transport chain, ATP levels are maintained.

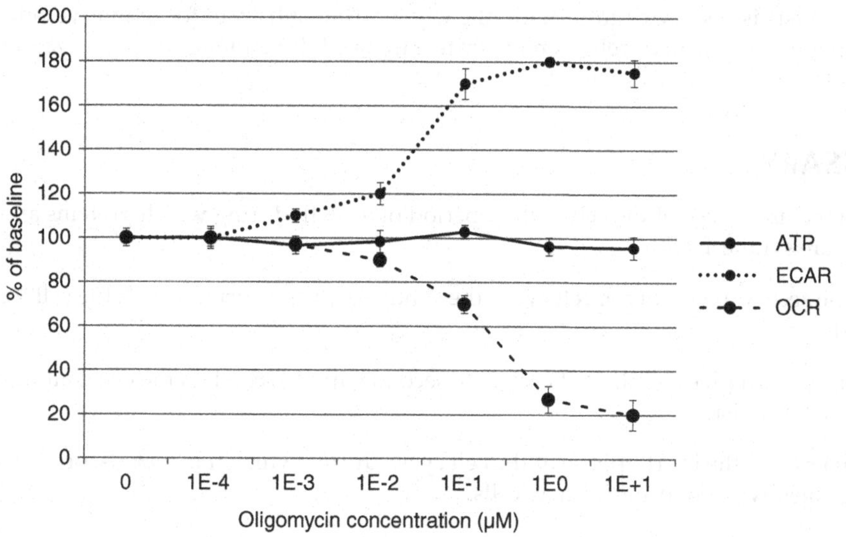

FIGURE 4.11 Effect of oligomycin concentration on ECAR, OCR, and ATP levels in a lung cancer cell line.

ATP, adenosine 5′-triphosphate; ECAR, extracellular acidification rate; OCR, oxygen consumption rate.

Next, the effect of glycolytic inhibition on the cancer cell line is investigated using *2-deoxy glucose (2-DG),* which blocks the first step of glycolysis. Increasing doses of 2-DG result in a decrease in the ECAR (Figure 4.12). To some degree, oxidative phosphorylation can compensate for decreased glycolytic activity, but ATP levels still drop compared to baseline levels.

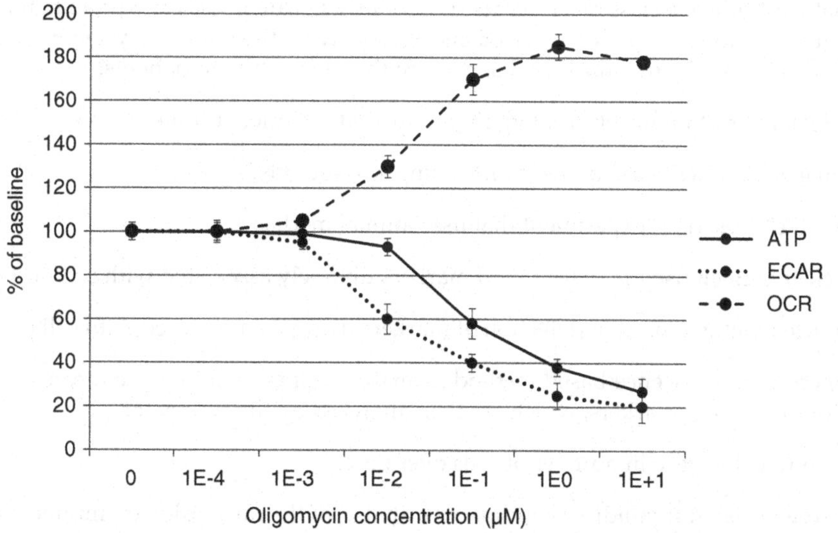

FIGURE 4.12 Effect of 2-DG concentration on ECAR, OCR, and ATP levels in a lung cancer cell line.

ATP, adenosine 5′-triphosphate; ECAR, extracellular acidification rate; OCR, oxygen consumption rate.

While glycolysis is necessary to provide the key starting substrate for oxidative phosphorylation (pyruvate), most cancer cells demonstrate enhanced dependence on glycolysis even in the presence of oxygen (Warburg effect).

GLOSSARY

G1 phase: the first phase of the cell cycle; a period of growth during which proteins and organelles are synthesized.

S phase: the second phase of the cell cycle; the synthesis phase during which the cell's genome is duplicated.

G2 phase: the third phase of the cell cycle; the second gap phase, when the cell continues to grow and prepare for division.

M (mitotic) phase: the fourth phase of the cell cycle, during which the nucleus, organelles, and cell membrane divide to form two new cells.

cytokinesis: separation of a cell into two daughter cells.

interphase: the G1, S, and G2 periods of the cell cycle.

quiescent: describes a cell in the resting G0 phase.

cyclins: One of the master regulators of the cell cycle.

cyclin-dependent kinases (CDKs): One of the master regulators of the cell cycle.

alkylating agents: drugs that damage DNA.

antimitotic: descriptor of chemotherapies that disrupt the microtubules that form the mitotic spindle, interrupting cell division.

monoclonal antibodies: a class of "Y" shaped proteins that can bind to any protein, not just to growth factor receptors. They are produced endogenously by the immune system to neutralize pathogens but can also be manufactured and given therapeutically to patients.

mitotic index: the fraction of cells undergoing mitosis at a particular time.

in vitro: "in glass"; describes experiment not using live subjects.

in vivo: "in live"; describes experiment that uses animal models.

Ki67: a nuclear antigen used in detection of markers uniquely associated with cell proliferation.

PCNA: a nuclear antigen used in detection of markers uniquely associated with cell proliferation.

flow cytometry: a fluorescence-based method to analyze cell populations. Cells can be stained with dyes or fluorescent markers, which are then analyzed by the cytometer.

proliferation rate: Increase in number of cells over time.

3H-thymidine: tritiated thymidine; a radioactive analog of the nucleoside thymidine used to measure the rate of DNA synthesis.

BrdU: a nonradioactive analog of the nucleoside thymidine used to measure the rate of DNA synthesis.

pulse chase experiment: a method of studying a process over time during which a tracer is introduced for a set amount of time (pulse), followed by a wash out period (chase). It can be used to study proliferation among many other cellular processes.

apoptosis: genetically programmed cell death.

necrosis: cell death occurring as a result of damaging external conditions.

intrinsic pathway: apoptosis-inducing pathway that is triggered by internal cellular signals and mediated by mitochondrial proteins.

extrinsic pathway: apoptosis-inducing pathway that is triggered by specific receptors on the cell surface.

caspase: a protease that cleaves an array of cellular substrates to carry out the apoptotic process.

oncosis: swelling of the cell; the result of permeabilization of the plasma membrane, leading to disruption of ion gradients and loss of ATP.

autophagy: when the cell degrades and recycles damaged or unused cell parts. It is often triggered when a cell is stressed. If recycling a few parts is not sufficient, the cell will die of "autophagy associated cell death."

Cr-51 release assay: an in vitro cell death assay.

TUNEL assay: a classic assay of apoptosis that uses the enzyme terminal deoxynucleotidyl transferase (TdT)'s recognition of nicked DNA ends.

comet assay: also known as *single-cell gel electrophoresis*; a means of detecting DNA fragmentation.

Annexin V: a dye that selectively labels plasma membrane changes in apoptotic cells.

hypoxia: lack of oxygen; a common feature of many advanced solid tumors as the rapidly proliferating cancer cells outgrow their blood supply.

catabolic pathways: metabolic pathways that break down organic compounds into more basic components, freeing useful energy in the process.

anabolic pathways: metabolic pathways that use energy and basic carbon building blocks to produce more complex biochemical substances.

glycolysis pathway: pathway for cellular energy derivation.

oxidative phosphorylation: process that uses pyruvate in the cell is used for aerobic respiration.

Warburg effect: also called **aerobic glycolysis**; an observation of an abnormality of cancer metabolism that the majority of cancers predominantly depend on glycolysis followed by lactic acid fermentation for ATP generation (a completely anaerobic process).

pyruvate kinase: (PKM2) a key glycolytic enzyme implicated in driving the Warburg effect.

^{18}F-fluorodeoxyglucose: (18F-FDG) a radioactive glucose analog used for diagnostic PET imaging studies in cancer patients.

AMPK: a kinase that acts as a metabolic checkpoint on the cell in the case of energetic stress.

HIF-1alpha: transcription factor that helps cells compensate for a low-oxygen environment.

extracellular acidification rate (ECAR): the rate at which a cell's extracellular environment is acidified, largely as a result of lactate production but in part due to CO_2 production.

MTT assay: a nonradioactive alternative to the 3H-thyimidine incorporation assay; measures mitochondrial activity.

Alamar Blue: (assay) assay method is similar to MTT, but involves a fluorescent as well as colorimetric change.

oxygen consumption rate (OCR): a measure of oxidative phosphorylation.

REFERENCES

1. Vermeulen K, Van Bockstaele DR, Berneman ZN. The cell cycle: A review of regulation, deregulation and therapeutic targets in cancer. *Cell Prolif.* 2003;36:131–149. doi:10.1046/j.1365-2184.2003.00266.x
2. Williams GH, Stoeber K. The cell cycle and cancer. *J Pathol.* 2012;226:352–364. doi:10.1002/path.3022.
3. Abraham E, Singer M. Mechanisms of sepsis-induced organ dysfunction. *Crit Care Med.* 2007;35:2408–2416. doi:10.1097/01.CCM.0000282072.56245.91
4. Potten CS, Loeffler M. Stem cells: attributes, cycles, spirals, pitfalls and uncertainties. Lessons for and from the crypt. *Development.* 1990;110:1001–1020. http://dev.biologists.org/content/develop/110/4/1001.full.pdf
5. Malumbres M, Barbacid M. Cell cycle, CDKs and cancer: a changing paradigm. *Nat Rev Cancer.* 2009;9:153–166. doi:10.1038/nrc2602
6. Nigg EA. Mitotic kinases as regulators of cell division and its checkpoints. *Nat Rev Mol Cell Biol.* 2001;2:21–32. doi:10.1038/35048096
7. Planas-Silva MD, Weinberg RA. The restriction point and control of cell proliferation. *Curr Opin Cell Biol.* 1997;9: 768–772. doi:10.1016/S0955-0674(97)80076-2
8. Bloom J, Cross FR. Multiple levels of cyclin specificity in cell-cycle control. *Nat Rev Mol Cell Biol.* 2007;8:149–160. doi:10.1038/nrm2105
9. Blagosklonny MV, Pardee AB. The restriction point of the cell cycle. *Cell Cycle.* 2002;1:103–110. doi:10.4161/cc.1.2.108
10. Di Leonardo A, Linke SP, Clarkin K, Wahl GM. DNA damage triggers a prolonged p53-dependent G1 arrest and long-term induction of Cip1 in normal human fibroblasts. *Genes Dev.* 1994;8:2540–2551. doi:10.1101/gad.8.21.2540
11. Cuddihy AR, O'Connell MJ. Cell-cycle responses to DNA damage in G2. *Int Rev Cytol.* 2003;222:99–140. doi:10.1016/S0074-7696(02)22013-6
12. Lara-Gonzalez P, Westhorpe FG, Taylor SS. The spindle assembly checkpoint. *Curr Biol.* 2012;22:R966–R980. doi:10.1016/j.cub.2012.10.006
13. Velasco-Velázquez MA, Li Z, Casimiro M, et al. Examining the role of cyclin D1 in breast cancer. *Future Oncol.* 2011;7: 753–765. doi:10.2217/fon.11.56
14. Yin Y, Shen WH. PTEN: a new guardian of the genome. *Oncogene.* 2008;27:5443–5453. doi:10.1038/onc.2008.241
15. Bachmann IM, Straume O, Akslen LA. Altered expression of cell cycle regulators Cyclin D1, p14, p16, CDK4 and Rb in nodular melanomas. *Int J Oncol.* 2004;25:1559–1565. doi:10.3892/ijo.25.6.1559
16. Vogelstein B, Papadopoulos N, Velculescu VE, et al. Cancer genome landscapes. *Science.* 2013;339:1546–1558. doi:10.1126/science.1235122
17. Jackson AL, Loeb LA. The mutation rate and cancer. *Genetics.* 1998;148:1483–1490. http://www.genetics.org/content/148/4/1483
18. Storchova Z, Pellman D. From polyploidy to aneuploidy, genome instability and cancer. *Nat Rev Mol Cell Biol.* 2004;5: 45–54. doi:10.1038/nrm1276
19. De Falco M, De Luca A. Cell cycle as a target of antineoplastic drugs. *Curr Pharm Des.* 2010;16:1417–1426. doi:10.2174/138161210791033914
20. Janssen A, Medema RH. Mitosis as an anti-cancer target. *Oncogene.* 2011;30:2799–2809. doi:10.1038/onc.2011.30
21. Fischer AH, Jacobson KA, Rose J, Zeller R. Hematoxylin and eosin (H & E) staining of tissue and cell sections. *CSH Protoc.* 2008;2008:pdb.prot4986. doi:10.1101/pdb.prot4986
22. Kim YJ, Ketter R, Steudel WI, Feiden W. Prognostic significance of the mitotic index using the mitosis marker anti-phosphohistone H3 in meningiomas. *Am J Clin Pathol.* 2007;128:118–125. doi:10.1309/HXUNAG34B3CEFDU8
23. Kadota K, Suzuki K, Kachala SS, et al. A grading system combining architectural features and mitotic count predicts recurrence in stage I lung adenocarcinoma. *Mod Pathol.* 2012;25:1117–1127. doi:10.1038/modpathol.2012.58
24. Lehr H-A, Rochat C, Schaper C, et al. Mitotic figure counts are significantly overestimated in resection specimens of invasive breast carcinomas. *Mod Pathol.* 2012;26(3):336–342. doi:10.1038/modpathol.2012.140
25. Keshgegian AA, Cnaan A. Proliferation markers in breast carcinoma: Mitotic figure count, S-phase fraction, proliferating cell nuclear antigen, Ki-67 and MIB-1. *Am J Clin Pathol.* 1995;104:42-49. doi:10.1093/ajcp/104.1.42
26. Ben-Izhak O, Bar-Chana M, Sussman L, et al. Ki67 antigen and PCNA proliferation markers predict survival in anorectal malignant melanoma. *Histopathology.* 2002;41:519–525. doi:10.1046/j.1365-2559.2002.01444.x
27. Stuart-Harris R, Caldas C, Pinder SE, Pharoah P. Proliferation markers and survival in early breast cancer: A systematic review and meta-analysis of 85 studies in 32,825 patients. *Breast.* 2008;17:323–334. doi:10.1016/j.breast.2008.02.002

28. Zink D, Sadoni N, Stelzer E. Visualizing chromatin and chromosomes in living cells. *Methods*. 2003;29:42–50. doi:10.1016/S1046-2023(02)00289-X
29. Henderson L, Bortone DS, Lim C, Zambon AC. Classic "broken cell" techniques and newer live cell methods for cell cycle assessment. *Am J Physiol Cell Physiol*. 2013;304:C927–C938. doi:10.1152/ajpcell.00006.2013
30. Martin RM, Leonhardt H, Cardoso MC. DNA labeling in living cells. *Cytom Part A*. 2005;67:45–52. doi:10.1002/cyto.a.20172
31. Pozarowski P, Darzynkiewicz Z. Analysis of cell cycle by flow cytometry. *Methods Mol Biol*. 2004;281:301–311. doi:10.1385/1-59259-811-0:301
32. Nunez R. DNA measurement and cell cycle analysis by flow cytometry. *Curr Issues Mol Biol*. 2001;3:67–70. doi:10.21775/cimb.003.067
33. Cecchini MJ, Amiri M, Dick FA. Analysis of cell cycle position in mammalian cells. *J Vis Exp*. 2012;7:1–7. doi:10.3791/3491
34. Crosio C, Fimia GM, Loury R, et al. Mitotic phosphorylation of histone H3: spatio-temporal regulation by mammalian Aurora kinases. *Mol Cell Biol*. 2002;22:874–885. doi:10.1128/MCB.22.3.874-885.2002
35. Rieseberg M, Kasper C, Reardon KF, Scheper T. Flow cytometry in biotechnology. *Appl Microbiol Biotechnol*. 2001;56:350–360. doi:10.1007/s002530100673
36. Chang Q, Hedley D. Emerging applications of flow cytometry in solid tumor biology. *Methods*. 2012;57:359–367. doi:10.1016/j.ymeth.2012.03.027
37. Riss T, Moravec R, Niles A, et al. Cell viability assays. In: Sittampalam GS, Coussens NP, Brimacombe K, et al., eds. *Assay Guidance Manual*. Bethesda, MD: Eli Lilly & Company and National Center for Advancing Translational Sciences; 2013. https://www.ncbi.nlm.nih.gov/books/NBK144065
38. Pollard PC, Moriarty DJW. Validity of the tritiated thymidine method for estimating bacterial growth rates: measurement of isotope dilution during DNA synthesis. *Appl Environ Microbiol*. 1984;48:1076–1083.
39. Taupin P. BrdU immunohistochemistry for studying adult neurogenesis: paradigms, pitfalls, limitations, and validation. *Brain Res Rev*. 2007;53:198–214. doi:10.1016/j.brainresrev.2006.08.002
40. Levkoff LH, Marshall GP, Ross HH, et al. Bromodeoxyuridine inhibits cancer cell proliferation in vitro and in vivo. *Neoplasia*. 2008;10:804–816. doi:10.1593/neo.08382
41. Lyons AB, Blake SJ, Doherty KV. Flow cytometric analysis of cell division by dilution of CFSE related dyes. *Curr Protoc Cytom*. 2013;64:9.11.1–9.11.12. doi:10.1002/0471142956.cy0911s64
42. Tan T-T, White E. Therapeutic targeting of death pathways in cancer: mechanisms for activating cell death in cancer cells. *Adv Exp Med Biol*. 2008;615:81–104. doi:10.1007/978-1-4020-6554-5_5
43. Lazar T. Histology and cell biology—An introduction to pathology. *Tissue Cell*. 2002;34:460. doi:10.1016/S0040816602000733
44. Kanduc D, Mittelman A, Serpico R, et al. Cell death: apoptosis versus necrosis (review). *Int J Oncol*. 2002;21:165–170. doi:10.3892/ijo.21.1.165
45. Nikoletopoulou V, Markaki M, Palikaras K, Tavernarakis N. Crosstalk between apoptosis, necrosis and autophagy. *Biochim Biophys Acta–Mol Cell Res*. 2013;1833:3448–3459. doi:10.1016/j.bbamcr.2013.06.001
46. Levine B, Yuan J. Autophagy in cell death: an innocent convict? *J Clin Invest*. 2005;115:2679–2688. doi:10.1172/jci26390
47. Inoue H, Tani K. Multimodal immunogenic cancer cell death as a consequence of anticancer cytotoxic treatments. *Cell Death Differ*. 2014;21:39–49. doi:10.1038/cdd.2013.84
48. Elmore S. Apoptosis: a review of programmed cell death. *Toxicol Pathol*. 2007;35:495–516. doi:10.1080/01926230701320337
49. Eguchi K. Apoptosis in autoimmune diseases. *Intern Med*. 2001;40:275–284. doi:10.2169/internalmedicine.40.275
50. Roth KA, D'Sa C. Apoptosis and brain development. *Ment Retard Dev Disabil Res Rev*. 2001;7:261–266. doi:10.1002/mrdd.1036
51. Eguchi Y, Shimizu S, Tsujimoto Y. Intracellular ATP levels determine cell death fate by apoptosis or necrosis. *Cancer Res*. 1997;57:1835–1840.
52. Fadok VA, Bratton DL, Henson PM. Phagocyte receptors for apoptotic cells: recognition, uptake, and consequences. *J Clin Invest*. 2001;108:957–962. doi:10.1172/JCI200114122
53. Ola MS, Nawaz M, Ahsan H. Role of Bcl-2 family proteins and caspases in the regulation of apoptosis. *Mol Cell Biochem*. 2011;351:41–58. doi:10.1007/s11010-010-0709-x
54. Proskuryakov SY, Konoplyannikov AG, Gabai VL. Necrosis: a specific form of programmed cell death? *Exp Cell Res*. 2003;283:1–16. doi:10.1016/S0014-4827(02)00027-7
55. Srikrishna G, Freeze HH. Endogenous damage-associated molecular pattern molecules at the crossroads of inflammation and cancer. *Neoplasia*. 2009;11:615–628. doi:10.1593/neo.09284
56. Green DR, Ferguson T, Zitvogel L, Kroemer G. Immunogenic and tolerogenic cell death. *Nat Rev Immunol*. 2009;9:353–363. doi:10.1038/nri2545
57. Kelly GL, Strasser A. The essential role of evasion from cell death in cancer. *Adv Cancer Res*. 2011;111:39–96. doi:10.1016/B978-0-12-385524-4.00002-7
58. Kim R. Cancer immunoediting: From immune surveillance to immune escape. *Immunology*. 2007:9–27. doi:10.1111/j.1365-2567.2007.02587.x
59. Ricci MS, Zong W-X. Chemotherapeutic approaches for targeting cell death pathways. *Oncologist*. 2006;11:342–357. doi:10.1634/theoncologist.11-4-342
60. Atale N, Gupta S, Yadav UCS, Rani V. Cell-death assessment by fluorescent and nonfluorescent cytosolic and nuclear staining techniques. *J Microsc*. 2014;255:7–19. doi:10.1111/jmi.12133
61. Wickman GR, Julian L, Mardilovich K, et al. Blebs produced by actin-myosin contraction during apoptosis release damage-associated molecular pattern proteins before secondary necrosis occurs. *Cell Death Differ*. 2013;20:1293–1305. doi:10.1038/cdd.2013.69

62. Chan FKM, Moriwaki K, De Rosa MJ. Detection of necrosis by release of lactate dehydrogenase activity. *Methods Mol Biol.* 2013;979:65–70. doi:10.1007/978-1-62703-290-2_7
63. Nelson DL, Kurman CC, Serbousek DE. 51Cr release assay of antibody-dependent cell-mediated cytotoxicity (ADCC). *Curr Protoc Immunol.* 2001;Chapter 7:Unit 7.27.
64. Neri S, Mariani E, Meneghetti A, et al. Calcein-acetyoxymethyl cytotoxicity assay: standardization of a method allowing additional analyses on recovered effector cells and supernatants. *Clin Diagn Lab Immunol.* 2001;8:1131–1135. doi:10.1128/CDLI.8.6.1131-1135.2001
65. He L, Wu X, Meylan F, et al. Monitoring caspase activity in living cells using fluorescent proteins and flow cytometry. *Am J Pathol.* 2004;164:1901–1913. doi:10.1016/S0002-9440(10)63751-0
66. Darzynkiewicz Z, Pozarowski P, Lee BW, Johnson GL. Fluorochrome-labeled inhibitors of caspases: convenient in vitro and in vivo markers of apoptotic cells for cytometric analysis. *Methods Mol Biol.* 2011;682:103–114. doi:10.1007/978-1-60327-409-8_9
67. Boulares AH, Yakovlev AG, Ivanova V, et al. Role of poly(ADP-ribose) polymerase (PARP) cleavage in apoptosis. Caspase 3-resistant PARP mutant increases rates of apoptosis in transfected cells. *J Biol Chem.* 1999;274:22932–22940. doi:10.1074/jbc.274.33.22932
68. Brenner C, Moulin M. Physiological roles of the permeability transition pore. *Circ Res.* 2012;111:1237–1247. doi:10.1161/CIRCRESAHA.112.265942
69. Hüser J, Rechenmacher CE, Blatter LA. Imaging the permeability pore transition in single mitochondria. *Biophys J.* 1998;74:2129–2137. doi:10.1016/S0006-3495(98)77920-2
70. Gavrieli Y, Sherman Y, Ben-Sasson SA. Identification of programmed cell death in situ via specific labeling of nuclear DNA fragmentation. *J Cell Biol.* 1992;119:493–501. doi:10.1083/jcb.119.3.493
71. Kyrylkova K, Kyryachenko S, Leid M, Kioussi C. Detection of apoptosis by TUNEL assay. *Methods Mol Biol.* 2012;887: 41–47. doi:10.1007/978-1-61779-860-3_5
72. Matassov D, Kagan T, Leblanc J, et al. Measurement of apoptosis by DNA fragmentation. *Methods Mol Biol.* 2004;282: 1–17. doi:10.1385/1-59259-812-9:001
73. Choucroun P, Gillet D, Dorange G, et al. Comet assay and early apoptosis. *Mutat Res–Fundam Mol Mech Mutagen.* 2001;478:89–96. doi:10.1016/S0027-5107(01)00123-3
74. Frey T. Nucleic acid dyes for detection of apoptosis in live cells. *Cytometry.* 1995;21:265–274. doi:10.1002/cyto.990210307
75. Vermes I, Haanen C, Steffens-Nakken H, Reutelingsperger C. A novel assay for apoptosis. Flow cytometric detection of phosphatidylserine expression on early apoptotic cells using fluorescein labelled Annexin V. *J Immunol Methods.* 1995;184:39–51. doi:10.1016/0022-1759(95)00072-I
76. Berg JM, Tymoczko JL, Stryer L. Biochemistry. In: *Biochemistry Textbook.* 5th ed. New York, NY: WH Freeman; 2006:1120.
77. Hou J, Lages NF, Oldiges M, Vemuri GN. Metabolic impact of redox cofactor perturbations in Saccharomyces cerevisiae. *Metab Eng.* 2009;11:253–261. doi:10.1016/j.ymben.2009.05.001
78. Rich PR. The molecular machinery of Keilin's respiratory chain. *Biochem Soc Trans.* 2003;31:1095–1105. doi:10.1042/bst0311095
79. Kim JW, Tchernyshyov I, Semenza GL, Dang CV. HIF-1-mediated expression of pyruvate dehydrogenase kinase: a metabolic switch required for cellular adaptation to hypoxia. *Cell Metab.* 2006;3:177–185. doi:10.1016/j.cmet.2006.02.002
80. Coleman RA, Bell RM. Selective changes in enzymes of the sn-glycerol 3-phosphate and dihydroxyacetone-phosphate pathways of triacylglycerol biosynthesis during differentiation of 3T3-L1 preadipocytes. *J Biol Chem.* 1980;255:7681–7687.
81. Kruger NJ, Von Schaewen A. The oxidative pentose phosphate pathway: structure and organisation. *Curr Opin Plant Biol.* 2003;6:236–246. doi:10.1016/S1369-5266(03)00039-6
82. Boyer PD. The ATP synthase--a splendid molecular machine. *Annu Rev Biochem.* 1997;66:717–749. doi:10.1146/annurev.biochem.66.1.717
83. Vander Heiden MG, Cantley LC, Thompson CB. Understanding the Warburg effect: the metabolic requirements of cell proliferation. *Science.* 2009;324:1029–1033. doi:10.1126/science.1160809
84. Pecqueur C, Oliver L, Oizel K, et al. Targeting metabolism to induce cell death in cancer cells and cancer stem cells. *Int J Cell Biol.* 2013;2013:1–13. doi:10.1155/2013/805975
85. Pelicano H, Martin DS, Xu R-H, Huang P. Glycolysis inhibition for anticancer treatment. *Oncogene.* 2006;25:4633–4646. doi:10.1038/sj.onc.1209597
86. Cairns RA, Harris IS, Mak TW. Regulation of cancer cell metabolism. *Nat Rev Cancer.* 2011;11:85–95. doi:10.1038/nrc2981
87. Doe MR, Ascano JM, Kaur M, Cole MD. Myc posttranscriptionally induces HIF1 protein and target gene expression in normal and cancer cells. *Cancer Res.* 2012;72:949–957. doi:10.1158/0008-5472.CAN-11-2371
88. Teslaa T, Teitell MA. Techniques to monitor glycolysis. *Methods Enzymol.* 2014;542:91–114. doi:10.1016/B978-0-12-416618-9.00005-4
89. Reisch AS, Elpeleg O. Biochemical assays for mitochondrial activity: Assays of TCA cycle enzymes and PDHc. *Methods Cell Biol.* 2007;80:199–222. doi:10.1016/S0091-679X(06)80010-5
90. Frazier AE, Thorburn DR. Biochemical analyses of the electron transport chain complexes by spectrophotometry. *Methods Mol Biol.* 2012;837:49–62. doi:10.1007/978-1-61779-504-6_4
91. Hamid R, Rotshteyn Y, Rabadi L, et al. Comparison of alamar blue and MTT assays for high through-put screening. *Toxicol Vitr.* 2004;18:703–710. doi:10.1016/j.tiv.2004.03.012
92. Quent VMC, Loessner D, Friis T, et al. Discrepancies between metabolic activity and DNA content as tool to assess cell proliferation in cancer research. *J Cell Mol Med.* 2010;14:1003–1013. doi:10.1111/j.1582-4934.2010.01013.x
93. Maioli E, Torricelli C, Fortino V, et al. Critical appraisal of the MTT assay in the presence of Rottlerin and uncouplers. *Biol Proced Online.* 2009;11:227–240. doi:10.1007/s12575-009-9020-1

94. Jonckheere AI, Huigsloot M, Janssen AJM, et al. High-throughput assay to measure oxygen consumption in digitonin-permeabilized cells of patients with mitochondrial disorders. *Clin Chem.* 2010;56:424–431. doi:10.1373/clinchem.2009.131441
95. Xie W, Xu A, Yeung ES. Determination of NAD + and NADH in a single cell under hydrogen peroxide stress by capillary electrophoresis. *Anal Chem.* 2009;81:1280–1284. doi:10.1021/ac802249m
96. Dieterle F, Riefke B, Schlotterbeck G, et al. NMR and MS methods for metabonomics. *Methods Mol Biol.* 2011;691:385–415. doi:10.1007/978-1-60761-849-2_24
97. Zhou W, Liotta LA, Petricoin EF. Cancer metabolism and mass spectrometry-based proteomics. *Cancer Lett.* 2015;356:176–183. doi:10.1016/j.canlet.2013.11.003

5

Metastasis and the Tumor Microenvironment

JACQUELINE DOUGLASS ■ ANDREW SHARABI ■ PHUOC T. TRAN

TUMOR MICROENVIRONMENT

The ***tumor microenvironment*** (***TME***), consisting of the ***extracellular matrix*** (***ECM***) and cells surrounding tumor cells, exhibits dramatic abnormalities over the microenvironment of normal tissues. These abnormalities, characterized by a state of chronic inflammation, support the growth and metastasis of tumor cells (Figure 5.1). Thus, it is advantageous for cancer researchers to consider cancer cells in the context of their surrounding environment rather than the isolation of a cell culture dish. This context is important for understanding how neoplastic lesions develop, proliferate, metastasize, and evade the immune system. Additionally, understanding the TME can inform the development of new anticancer drugs, particularly in the field of tumor immunology. A number of drugs are currently on the market or under evaluation that reverse or seek to overcome abnormalities of the TME. Furthermore, for any new drug under development, its access to, stability in, and impact on the TME should all be considered.

TUMOR MICROENVIRONMENT—BACKGROUND

Approximately 90% percent of human cancers are carcinomas (1), meaning they are derived from cells of ***epithelial*** origin, as opposed to cells of ***hematopoietic*** origin (leukemias and lymphomas), ***mesenchymal*** origin (sarcomas), or ***germ cell*** origin (germinomas). Epithelial cells line the inner and outer surfaces of the body atop the basement membrane, a thin fibrous layer serving as a mechanical barrier and an anchor for epithelial attachment.

Below the basement membrane is the ***stroma***. The stroma is the connective tissue of an organ that plays a supportive, structural role rather than an organ-specific function. Stroma consists of fibroblasts, immune cells, vasculature, and ECM, in a milieu of secreted signaling molecules (2). While normal tissue stroma is typically cancer suppressing, as the tumor cells grow and evolve, they manipulate their environment to support malignant growth. A carcinoma starts as in situ neoplasia, with an intact basement membrane and relatively normal microenvironment. As the tumor grows, it penetrates the basement membrane, growing into the underlying stroma. Extracellular

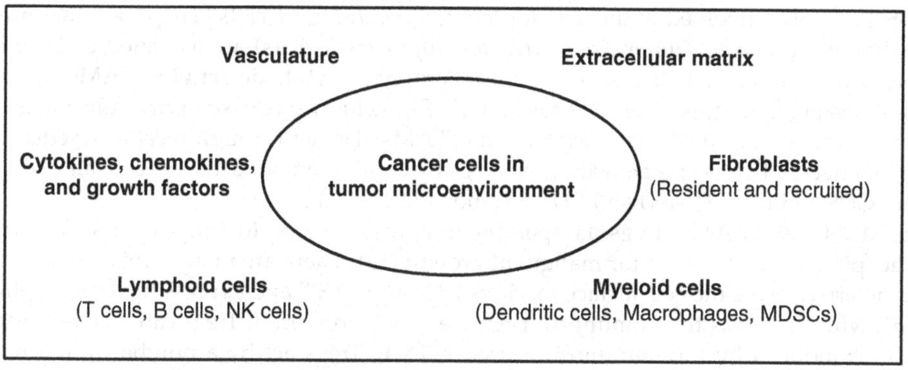

FIGURE 5.1 Key components of the tumor microenvironment.
MDSC, myeloid-derived suppressor cell; NK, natural killer.

proteases, released by either fibroblasts or the tumor itself, degrade the ECM and basement membrane, facilitating tumor invasion into the underlying stroma.

Fibroblasts, connective tissue cells responsible for producing the collagen and other components of the ECM, are one of the most prominent cell types of the TME, comprising up to 90% of total tumor mass (3). Tumors recruit fibroblasts via secretion of ***cytokines*** (such as *beta*), ***chemokines***, and ***growth factors***. The fibroblasts recruited by the tumor transform into myofibroblasts, a type of fibroblast involved in wound healing and chronic inflammation. Myofibroblasts are responsible for fibrosis associated with wounds and tumors (desmoplasia) (4). Other cell types such as myeloid-derived progenitors and other mesenchymal cells are recruited by the tumor and transdifferentiate into fibroblast-like cells (3). Collectively, this heterogeneous population is termed cancer-associated fibroblasts (CAFs).

Recruited CAFs, in turn, play a number of pro-tumorigenic roles to support cancer growth and aggression that parallel the roles they would play in normal wound healing (3,5,6). CAFs secrete a variety of factors not produced by normal fibroblasts, including cytokines, chemokines, and growth factors, that reinforce that CAF phenotype via paracrine signaling. Many of the secreted CAF factors encourage tumor cell proliferation, migration, and invasion, in part by altering tumor cell phenotype to express mesenchymal and stem cell–like features.

CAFs secrete ***metalloproteinases*** (***MMP***) and other enzymes that remodel and damage the normal ECM structure, facilitating tumor cell migration and metastasis. Metalloproteinase activity also releases TGF-beta, which is trapped in the ECM, driving the ***epithelial–mesenchymal transition*** (***EMT***) response. Other growth factors and cytokines also support tumor growth. Furthermore, CAFs aid in supplying nutrients to the tumor, by encouraging the formation of vasculature. Finally, CAFs dampen inflammation in the TME, by recruiting immunosuppressive immune cells and secreting immunosuppressive cytokines, both of which inhibit the activities of pro-inflammatory tumor-reactive immune cells (7).

Many solid tumors exhibit chronic inflammation, characterized by the infiltration of a variety of immune cells. ***Myeloid-derived suppressor cells*** (***MDSCs***) are a mixed population of immature cells of myeloid origin that strongly inhibit the activity of pro-inflammatory immune cells, including T cells and natural killer (NK) cells, which would otherwise act to eliminate the abnormal tumor cells (8). MDSCs normally play an important role in wound healing and infection response by tightly regulating the immune system to prevent autoimmunity against autoantigens and excessive immune response to infection. Cytokines (e.g., GM-CSF, G-CSF, IL-6, and IL-10) released by many tumors recruit MDSCs and maintain their immunosuppressive phenotype (9). MDSC-suppressive mechanisms include the metabolism of L-arginine, production of nitric oxide, release of *reactive oxygen species (ROS)*, and secretion of immunosuppressive cytokines (e.g., TGF-beta, IL-10), all of which suppress the function of effector cells.

MDSCs are also involved in the development of ***regulatory T cells (Tregs)***, another immunosuppressive immune cell. ***Tumor-associated macrophages (TAMs)*** are a related class of immunosuppressive myeloid cells that lack typical macrophage cytotoxic activity. TAMs act through many of the same mechanisms as MDSCs and CAFs, including release of pro-tumorigenic cytokines, chemokines, and MMPs (10). MDSCs and TAMs also act through receptor-mediated suppression of effector T cells and activation of Tregs by expression of particular cell surface ligands, including CD80 (binds CTLA-4) and PD-L1 (binds PD-1) (11,12).

Like MDSCs and TAMs, Tregs dampen the immune response to injury or infection, creating a more hospitable environment for malignant growth (13). There are many subtypes of Tregs; the best characterized have the cell surface markers CD4 and CD25 and express the transcription factor ***Foxp3***, which controls the immunosuppressive genetic program. Tregs can be either naturally occurring or induced by the immunosuppressive TME. Tregs act by a number of mechanisms, including secretion of immunosuppressive cytokines (e.g., TGF-beta and IL-10) and metabolites (e.g., adenosine), competition for IL-2 (a T cell pro-growth cytokine), and downregulation of dendritic cell activity via cell surface receptors (e.g., CD80, CD86) (13).

The TME frequently contains pro-inflammatory immune cells called ***tumor-infiltrating lymphocytes (TILs)***, collectively referring to CD4+ or CD8+ T cells, NK cells, and other effector immune cells (14). Tumors express a number of antigens, either mutated proteins or inappropriately expressed proteins, that are recognized as abnormal by TILs. TILs seek to kill cells expressing such tumor antigens, eliminating them via cytokine release (CD4+ T cells) or cytolytic activity (CD8+ T cells and NK cells) (15). To some degree, particularly in early neoplasia, TILs can eliminate dysfunctional or foreign-appearing cells (16). However, both via ***immunoediting*** (the process whereby the most immunogenic antigens are eliminated) and immunosuppression, cancers evade this immune response. TIL function is suppressed by both the tumor cells and other immune cells in the TME through a number of mechanisms, including suppressive cytokines, metabolite abnormalities (e.g., increased adenosine, reduced L-arginine), receptor-mediated inhibition, hypoxia, and poor presentation of antigens by resident antigen-presenting cells (17–19).

The TME is also characterized by abnormal and increased vascularization. Normal epithelial tissue lacks vasculature, which is below the basement membrane in the underlying stroma. Without the formation of new blood vessels, tumors would not grow larger than 1 to 2 mm (20). Thus, carcinomas induce the formation of new blood vessels from existing vessels (***angiogenesis***) or de novo (***vasculogenesis***) by recruiting endothelial precursor cells (EPCs) (21). EPCs recruited by fibroblasts transdifferentiate into endothelial cells in response to ***vascular endothelial growth factor (VEGF)*** signaling, forming new vessels (22). The high degree of vascularization in many cancers allows the delivery of nutrients to support high growth rates, carries away waste products, and facilitates the escape of individual tumor cells that form metastasis (23). Like other aspects of the TME, the tumor vasculature is a target of anticancer therapies. Typical tumor vasculature is dilated and abnormal in architecture, resulting in the enhanced permeability and retention (EPR) effect (24). The EPR effect results in increased accumulation of larger molecules (nanoparticles or large drugs) in the tumor, which may be co-opted for therapeutic purposes.

TUMOR MICROENVIRONMENT—ASSAYS

There is a vast array of experimental tools and techniques to study components of the TME. This chapter cannot exhaustively cover all assays, but instead highlights a select set of key assays. Cancer researchers should be aware that additional assays exist and that study of TME components in isolation does not fully recapitulate their interactions in a spontaneously arising tumor. As a result, many experiments studying the TME are done either in mouse models or on *ex vivo* samples.

Immunohistochemistry (IHC) is commonly performed on research and clinical tissue sections to study the cellular and ECM architecture. Antibodies to cell type–specific markers are used to simultaneously label different cell populations; differentiate between immune cell subtypes, tumor cells, and fibroblasts; and provide morphology and co-localization information. Cell localization staining can be combined with other staining types to better elucidate the processes occurring in the TME. For instance, IHC can also be used to evaluate in situ protein expression, such as the distribution of cytokines or cell surface receptors in different cell types using protein-specific antibodies.

Ribonucleic acid (RNA) ***in situ hybridization*** (*ISH*) expression uses a nucleic acid probe complementary to the sequence of interest, with either radio, hapten, or fluorophore labeling, to provide information on expression patterns on messenger RNA (mRNA) and other RNA types (25,26). However, given RNA's instability and possible low copy numbers, RNA ISH requires rapid sample processing and frequent protocol optimization to achieve sufficient sensitivity for the RNA of interest.

Other techniques can be used to detect fibrosis on tissue sections, using either stains that highlight connective tissue (e.g., trichrome stain) or antibodies specific to ECM proteins (e.g., collagen, fibronectin) (27). Although IHC and other tissue stains provide good qualitative information about localization, general expression patterns, and tissue architecture, the major disadvantage is the inability to easily quantify these characteristics. More recently, automated computer algorithms have been developed to quantify staining metrics, including fractions of particular cell types and protein expression levels (28). Alternatively, TME cells can be analyzed by flow cytometry following tissue dissociation, but cell localization and morphology information is lost.

To investigate functions of particular TME cell types, cells can be isolated and subjected to various assays. For instance, the release of cytokines (e.g., interferon gamma [IFNγ]) or other secreted factors from fibroblasts or infiltrating immune cells can be assessed using an ***enzyme-linked immunosorbent assay*** (***ELISA***) on conditioned culture media (29). ELISA is a highly sensitive method to detect protein (or other antigen) levels using an antibody specific to the antigen, followed by an enzyme-conjugated secondary (Figure 5.2). The enzyme catalyzes a colorimetric change in a substrate that is proportional to the amount of enzyme, and thus shows how much antigen is present. ELISAs, however, evaluate the phenotype of whole cell populations.

Intracellular cytokine staining and other immunofluorescence staining techniques followed by flow cytometry can differentiate different subtypes of cells in a population (30). Co-culturing different cell types, such as T cells with cancer cells, followed by many of the assays discussed here (e.g., ELISAs, flow cytometry, or cell death assays), can be used to assess cell–cell interaction, particularly immune responses (31). Additionally, invasion and migration assays can be used to mimic the invasion of cells into the tumor stroma. The ***transwell invasion assay*** quantifies cell penetration through an ECM-coated membrane toward a chemoattractant (32). Three-dimensional (3-D) organoid models allow the in vitro study of tumor cells, immune cells, fibroblasts, and other cell types in the context of an ECM scaffold particularly well suited for studying complex TME processes (33). Organoid models offer some of the advantages of in vitro culture, namely, a more controlled and observable assay in a more biologically relevant system.

Researchers use a number of assays to study angiogenesis with in vitro and in vivo models, but these assays have trade-offs, namely, how well controlled, reproduced, and quantified the results are versus how well they recapitulate angiogenesis in the native TME. Many of these in vitro assays assess the proliferation, migration, and differentiation of human endothelial cells in response to particular drugs, upon co-culturing with other cell types (e.g., CAFs, tumor cells), or in

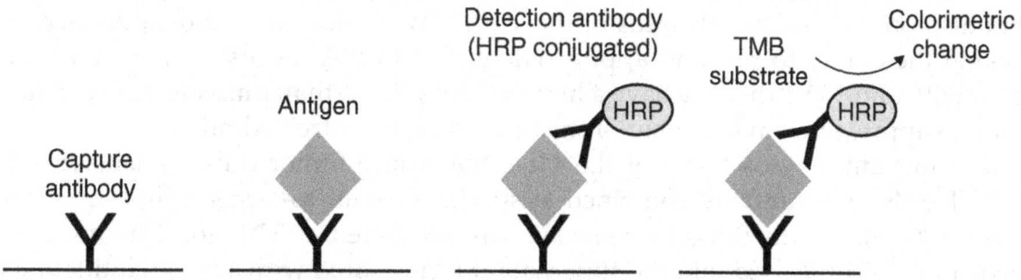

FIGURE 5.2 Capture (or sandwich) enzyme-linked immunosorbent assay (ELISA).
HRP, horseradish peroxidase; TMB, tetramethylbenzidine.

certain ECM environments (34). Traditionally, human umbilical cord endothelial cells (HUVECs) have been used for these assays; however, endothelial cells from the organ of interest have been shown to more accurately recapitulate in vivo activity. Researchers should also keep in mind that the length of time in culture affects endothelial cell phenotype, as is true for many primary cells, and could alter assay results (35).

Standard proliferation assays (e.g., cell number, tetrazolium MTT salt assay (3), H-thymidine incorporation) are used to study endothelial cell growth in response to stimuli. Tube formation assays are used to investigate endothelial cell differentiation into vessels and involve plating endothelial cells in different ECM environments and quantifying tube formation over time (36). While results are more easily quantified and reproduced, all of these in vitro endothelial cell assays are limited by their applicability to processes in an actual solid tumor. To overcome these limitations, harvested organ tissue can be cultured *ex vivo* to study angiogenesis. Quantification of vascularization in *ex vivo* organ culture is performed manually or digitally, but is challenging and frequently lacks standardization (35). A number of in vivo assays to study angiogenesis exist, but researchers should keep in mind that the choice of tumor environment (e.g., animal species, implantation location) and quantification technique (e.g., IHC on specimens, live imaging) can all influence results. As with any other area of research, scientists studying angiogenesis should use a variety of assays in different biological systems to confirm observed results.

Example: T cell–cancer cell co-culture assay—IFNγ ELISA and Cr-51 release

The study of tumor-infiltrating immune cells is a promising area of cancer research, as subpopulations of these cells have anti-cancer effects. A number of cancer immunotherapies specifically work by augmenting the function of these cells, thereby overcoming tolerance in the TME, for example, anti-CTLA-4 and anti-PD-1/L1 monoclonal antibodies (37). These antibodies work by blocking inhibitory receptors (or their ligands) found on effector cells—namely, T lymphocytes—resulting in a net increase in effector cell antitumor activity. In this example, we use a syngeneic mouse tumor model (mouse tumor models are discussed in more detail in the next section) to study the impact of PD-1 blockade on the function of TILs.

Immunocompetent mice are injected subcutaneously with syngeneic tumor cells. After 1 week, mice are treated with either an anti-PD-1 antibody or placebo. Two weeks later, mice are sacrificed and tumors are harvested. Tumors are cut into small pieces with a scalpel, digested in cell culture media containing collagenase and DNAse, and passed through a filter to achieve a single-cell suspension. Cells are incubated with anti-mouse CD3 antibody conjugated to magnetic microbeads to label all TILs. The cell suspension is passed through a magnetic column, and CD3+ cells are eluted. Alternatively, cytotoxic T cells (CD8+) and helper T cells (CD4+) can be individually isolated using anti-CD8 and anti-CD4 microbeads, respectively, to probe the functions of these separate populations.

An ELISA is performed to measure cytokine release from the isolated T lymphocytes upon co-culture with tumor cells (Figure 5.3). In this assay, T cells (from anti-PD-1- or placebo-treated mice) are cultured overnight with tumor cells from the syngeneic tumor cells at a 1:1 ratio. The next day, the supernatant is removed and used to perform an ELISA with an *interferon gamma capture antibody* (although other cytokines such as IL-2 are frequently quantified). IFNg is a commonly monitored cytokine released by T cells and NK cells to stimulate an immune response. The ability of T cells to release IFNg depends on the T cells recognizing their cognate antigen on the tumor cell surface but also on the functional status of the T cells, with more immunosuppressed "anergic" T cells lacking the ability to respond appropriately. The ELISA results show that TILs from the mice treated with anti-PD-1 therapy have a higher IFNg release than untreated mice, reflecting the more immunosuppressive environment of the tumors in the untreated mice.

To assess antitumor cytotoxicity of the TILs, the mouse tumor cells are labeled with Cr-51 (Figure 5.4). T cells (effectors) are combined at specific effector-to-target ratio (1:1, 3:1, 9:1, 27:1) with the labeled cancer cells (target cells). Cells are incubated at 37°C for 4 hours. The plate is centrifuged, and Cr-51 released into the supernatant is measured with a beta scintillation counter. Specific lysis is calculated by subtracting from the sample values the spontaneous Cr-51 release from intact cells and dividing this value by maximal lysis minus spontaneous Cr-51 release. Specific lysis as a function of effector-to-target ratio for each lymphocyte population is plotted. The plot shows that higher effector-to-target ratios result in greater target cell death and that the TILs isolated from mice treated with anti-PD-1 therapy have greater cytotoxic activity against tumor cells.

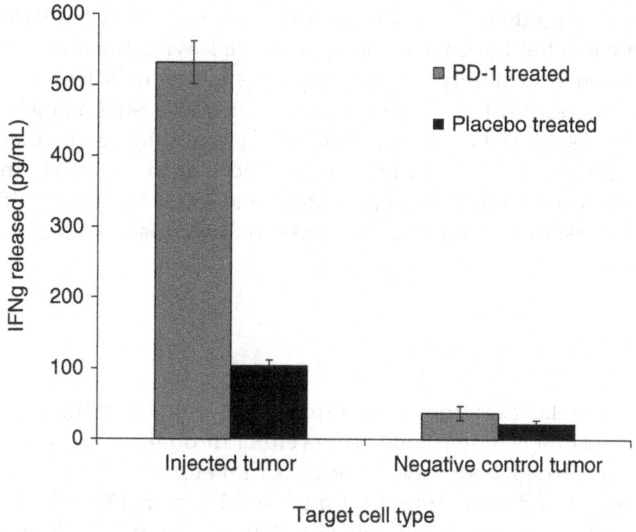

FIGURE 5.3 ELISA of IFNg released by T cells isolated from tumor-bearing mice treated with either PD-1 antibody or placebo. T cells are incubated at a 1:1 ratio with the same tumor cell line used for animal injections or a different murine tumor line.
ELISA, enzyme-linked immunosorbent assay; IFNg, interferon gamma.

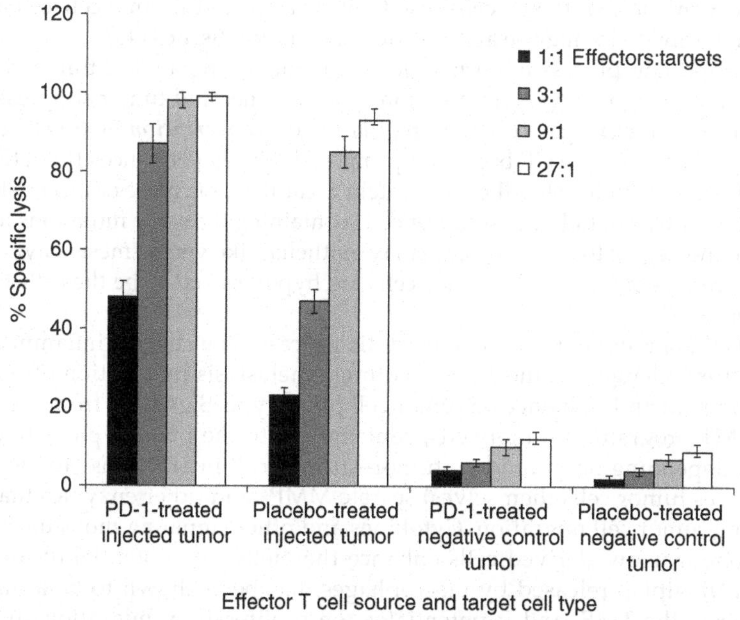

FIGURE 5.4 Specific lysis of target cells measured by a Cr-51 release assay. Target cells prelabeled with Cr51 are incubated with T cells isolated from anti-PD-1-treated or placebo-treated mice.

METASTASIS

The majority of cancer deaths are not due to the primary tumor but are instead the result of metastatic disease. As a result, understanding the biology of metastasis with hopes of blocking this process is a major goal in the field of cancer research. The formation of metastasis is a complex event requiring tumor cells to migrate into the vasculature, survive in the bloodstream, infiltrate other organs, and proliferate in a foreign environment, all while leaving the familiar microenvironment of the primary tumor. Such flexibility in phenotype has led many scientists to propose that the cells able to undergo this journey have acquired unique characteristics, namely, mesenchymal-like and stem cell–like features. Metastasis is a challenging field of study, given that so many cell types and tissue environments are involved in the process and that to accurately model it, one would need to follow the actions of single cells at an organismal level. Most assays focus on individual steps of metastasis, for instance, assessing the migration potential of cancer cells in the presence of a particular stimulus.

METASTASIS—BACKGROUND

For cancer cells to form metastases, they must break away from the primary tumor and spread to other sites in the body. Tumor cell migration occurs either through circulation, via the bloodstream or lymphatic system, or through body cavities (e.g., peritoneum). Hematogenous spread is the primary method of transport to distant organs for most solid tumors (38). However, the mechanism of spread varies depending on cancer cell type (39). This section primarily focuses on the mechanism of hematogenous dissemination in carcinomas, although many of the assays discussed can be applied to other cancer types and other routes of dissemination.

Early in the metastatic process, tumor cells must overcome the mechanical and biological boundaries of the stroma and invade (***intravasate***) into the vasculature. Normal epithelial cells maintain highly structured sheets and polarity mediated by cell–cell adhesion proteins. However, these characteristics are lost in carcinomas through a process called the EMT. During EMT, a hallmark of many carcinomas, epithelial cells lose their polarity and normal cell–cell adhesion molecules and gain the ability to migrate and invade surrounding tissues (40).

EMT is an important process in normal development and repair, but tumor cells co-opt this process to carry out malignant spread. Mutations in oncogenes and tumor suppressor genes help drive this transition. For example, certain upregulation of ***transcription factors*** (e.g., Twist, Snail, and Slug) and pathways (e.g., TGF-beta) that promote EMT also enhances the rate of metastasis (41–43), while loss of the cell–cell adhesion protein E-cadherin increases cancer cell motility and invasiveness (44). However, individual cancer cells containing the same mutations tend to display heterogeneity in the degree to which they display epithelial-like versus mesenchymal-like characteristics. The more mesenchymal-like tumor cells are hypothesized to be the cells that ultimately form metastases.

Tumor cells do not alone drive the metastatic process. The chronic inflammatory environment and structural changes of the TME encourage metastasis by creation of the appropriate physical environment and influence on tumor cell phenotype. Signaling from the tumor stroma activates the EMT program in tumor cells, contributing to the phenotypic heterogeneity seen in cancer cells, depending on individual tumor–stromal cell interactions (40). Recruited CAFs (and in some cases tumor cells themselves) secrete MMPs and other enzymes that degrade the ECM, permitting tumor cell migration. Cytokines and other signaling molecules released from stromal and bone marrow–derived cells enhance the metastatic potential of tumor cells (45). For example, TNF-alpha, released by macrophages, has been shown to be a major regulator of inflammation in the TME, and it potentiates the proliferation, migration, and invasion of tumor cells.

Angiogenesis further facilitates escape, increasing physical access of cancer cells to the vasculature. The newly formed vasculature lacks the tight endothelial junctions seen in most normal vessels, with the resulting "leakiness" permitting tumor cell intravasation. Similarly, lymph vessels, which are inherently leaky, promote tumor cell intravasation into the lymphatic system, with tumor cells lodging in nearby draining lymph nodes (46). Lymph node metastases are often the first site of metastatic spread. Sampling of lymph nodes for cancer cells (such as with *sentinel node* assays) is commonly used clinically as a prognostic marker and guide for aggressiveness of therapies.

While research has shown that macroscopic primary tumors shed a large number of cancer cells (estimated at several million tumor cells per gram of tumor tissue daily) (47), only a small fraction of these cells, typically fewer than 0.01%, ultimately form metastases (48). Cancer cells are subject to mechanical shearing in the bloodstream (49). Additionally, they are targets for potential destruction by the immune system, particularly NK cells that recognize tumor cells as diseased (49). However, many tumor cells express ***tissue factor***, a complement receptor and coagulation activator, resulting in aggregation of platelets around the tumor cell. Platelets act as a shield against mechanical shearing and immune recognition for tumor cells in circulation. This larger complex more easily lodges into capillaries.

Certain organs—namely, lungs, liver, brain, and bones—are the sites of the majority of metastases, although each cancer type tends to metastasize to characteristic locations. For instance, prostate cancers often metastasize to the bone, whereas melanoma frequently metastasizes to the brain. This stereotypical behavior of particular cancers was noted over a century ago by Stephen Paget, who posited the ***"seed and soil" theory***, stating that cancer cells ("seeds") have difficulty surviving outside their primary environment and thus tend to metastasize to tissues ("soils") with appropriate characteristics. Others disagree with this theory, arguing that the location of most metastases is determined by physical access, either via movement in body cavities (e.g., ovarian cancer tends to metastasize intraperitoneally to the liver surface) or through lymphatic or vascular routes (e.g., colon cancer tends to metastasize to the liver, through which blood from the colon directly drains).

A large body of research suggests that both active and passive mechanisms determine the location of metastases and that this balance is a function of the cancer type. Tumor cells, particularly tumor cell aggregates, can easily become trapped in capillaries, arguing in favor of the physical access hypothesis. Passive trapping of cancer cells in capillaries provides an immediate blood supply to the tumor cells, a critical source of nutrients for the growing ***micrometastasis***. The high frequency of intraperitoneal metastases in ovarian cancer and intrapleural metastases in mesothelioma further indicates the importance of physical routes to cancer spread.

However, research in animal models has demonstrated that of the tumor cells that lodge in particular tissues, only a fraction ultimately form ***macrometastases***. While this in part is due to the fitness of that individual tumor cell to form a metastasis, this phenomenon is also a function of the tissue type, independent of physical access (50). Although vascular supply is important for metastasis growth, tumor cells must also establish the appropriate TME, which the tumor cell accomplishes by invading the underlying tissue parenchyma (50).

Tumor cells can extravasate into select tissues by active recruitment, such as through the secretion of chemokines or expression of particular homing receptors or ligands in those tissues. For example, breast cancer cells that express the receptor CXCR4 often home to tissues that express the ligand CXCL12, specifically bone, brain, liver, lung, and lymph node, which are indeed the most common locations for breast cancer metastases (51,52). Other physical attributes of the target organ play a role in stereotypic metastatic patterns. For example, the bone microenvironment is thought to provide a good metastatic niche, not only because of the milieu of growth-promoting chemokines and cytokines found in bone but also because of the acidic pH, low oxygen concentration, and high extracellular calcium concentrations found in bone, which promote the growth of many cancers (53).

Of the tumor cells that translocate to new tissues, most ultimately die or remain dormant (54). Other cells may grow to some degree, but never become macrometastases because they are unable to establish a blood supply (55). As in the primary tumor, the establishment of the appropriate TME is important for metastasis growth. Recruitment of bone marrow–derived cells to promote immunosuppression, endothelial progenitor cells for angiogenesis, and fibroblasts for ECM remodeling all support tumor cell colonization. The primary tumor in many patients may facilitate this process, for instance, through systemic immunosuppression. In other patients, excision of the primary tumor may actually encourage metastatic growth (49,56). Therefore, while the tissue environment to which a cancer cell translocates plays a significant role in the ability to proliferate, typically only the most aggressive and fit cells ultimately form macroscopic metastases. This process selects for increasingly malignant tumor cell variants with the most appropriate mutations for disseminated, rapid growth (57).

The flexible phenotype required for cells to form metastases and the small fraction of cancer cells that actually have these characteristics give credence to the ***cancer stem cell (CSC) hypothesis***. Critical for normal fetal development and homeostasis in adults, stem cells are undifferentiated cells capable of indefinite divisions, producing progenitor cells that ultimately give rise to the mature, differentiated cell types in a particular tissue. The CSC theory states that cancers arise from tissue-specific stem cells or from cells that express a stem cell–like genetic program, resulting in a fraction of cells in the primary tumor with stem cell–like features, including the ability to self-renew and differentiate into different cell types (58), with the majority of the tumor composed of a heterogeneous population of daughter cells. First identified in leukemias, CSCs have now been identified in solid tumors, although in many other solid tumor types, the definition of such cells remains elusive (59). Not all cancer cells are tumorigenic (capable of forming tumors), but researchers have been able to isolate the subpopulations of cells using surface markers that were responsible for tumor formation in mice (60). Most chemotherapies readily kill differentiated cells, but CSCs are believed to be relatively immune to such treatments, thus becoming a principal driver of cancer relapse (60).

CSCs are likely the primary cells giving rise to metastases, which inherently require the initiating cell to have tumorigenic ability (60). Many of the EMT protein expression patterns conveying the capacity to invade and migrate are highly linked with a CSC-like state. As with normal stem cells, it is hypothesized that CSCs require a particular niche to maintain their stem cell–like state and that microenvironments in certain tissues may be more amenable to CSC colonization and, thus, metastasis formation (59). Finally, while mesenchymal-like cells initiate metastases, most carcinoma metastases contain epithelial-like cells, suggesting that the "seed" cell for metastases is highly plastic, capable of undergoing EMT and its reverse—***mesenchymal–epithelial transition*** (MET) (61).

METASTASIS ASSAYS

Metastasis is challenging to study in its entirety, given the necessity to monitor individual cancer cells at an organismal level and the complexity of the cellular and environmental interactions. A number of in vitro assays are available to parse out details of particular steps in the process. These assays have proven valuable for studying the biology driving metastasis and screening drugs that could inhibit steps in the process. These assays tend to be faster, more reproducible, and less costly than in vivo models. The development of 3-D cell culture and 3-D assays has significantly improved modeling in vivo interactions. Culturing cells in a 3-D setting versus traditional two-dimensional (2-D) culture more accurately mimics cellular behavior and drug sensitivity in vivo (62). However, researchers should keep in mind that these systems tend to be highly simplified and in many cases not biologically accurate or clinically relevant. As with many areas of biology, but especially in studying metastasis, hypotheses should ultimately be tested in animal models or with patient samples.

Given the strong connection between the abnormalities in the TME and the capacity of the TME to promote metastasis, many of the methods discussed in the previous section for studying angiogenesis, stromal recruitment, and bone marrow–derived cell phenotypes are relevant to studying the metastatic process. Principles of many of these assays can be applied to studying cancer cell functions. For instance, invasion assays using transwells with an ECM protein–coated membrane can be used to study cancer cell *chemotaxis* in response to a stimulus. Similarly, many of the in vitro assays (e.g., *migration assays*) discussed in this section can be applied to study other cell types of the TME.

Cancers display abnormalities in adhesion to particular ECM proteins and cell surface molecules, which allow them to carry out the metastatic cascade. ECM adhesive properties can be studied in vitro by coating a plate with a particular ECM protein (e.g., collagen), incubating the cells for a period of time, and then counting bound cells, typically with a fluorescent dye (63,64). The ECM protein used should reflect the specific step that is being studied. Shorter incubation periods and serum-free media are preferred for these assays, as some cancer cells secrete matrix proteins (64) and serums contain proteins that coat plates, acting as a surface for cell attachment (65). Alternatively, cancer cell adhesion to nonmalignant cells can be studied by growing a confluent layer of the nonmalignant cell, followed by a short incubation with cancer cells and assessing cancer cell binding. For instance, this assay can be used to model tumor cell adhesion to endothelial cells to mimic the early steps of vasculature extravasation (64). In this case, the organ source of endothelial cells can affect assay results, reflecting differential tumor cell organ tropism, so researchers should use nonmalignant cells that most closely mimic the process they wish to study.

Many in vitro assays have been developed to quantify cell motility. In the ***wound healing assay***, a linear scratch is made across the surface of a confluent plate of cells. Migration can be assessed by microscopy, making real-time kinetics studies possible (66). To inhibit proliferation, cells are typically serum starved and treated with a low-dose mitomycin C prior to the test (67). Because scratching may damage cells, electric impulses or a temporary physical barrier can create a cell-free area, referred to as a ***cell exclusion zone assay*** (68). A variety of microfluidic assays are available to quantify cell chemotaxis toward a chemokine or other stimulus (69,70).

The major advantage of microfluidic assays is tight control over stimulus gradients and lower cost due to smaller volumes of reagents. Automated cell-tracking software and single-cell tracking assays are available to study the movement of individual cells. All of these assays have the disadvantage of assessing cell behavior in two dimensions; however, other assays are available that measure cell motility in three dimensions. For example, in the ***microcarrier bead assay***, cells are grown to confluency on dextran beads, then incubated in cell culture dishes, following which the number of cells migrating to the plate is quantified (68). The ***spheroid migration assay*** is similar to the microcarrier bead assay, but uses multicellular tumor spheroids as the origin from which cells migrate. Because the cells form a 3-D structure, versus the 2-D structure of cells coating a bead, this assay far more accurately models the cell–cell interactions and nutrient and oxygen variability present in solid tumors (68). Furthermore, tumor cells can be labeled with ***green fluorescent protein*** (***GFP***) or a fluorescent dye and the assay carried out in the presence of another cell type (e.g., fibroblasts) to assess the influence of other cell types on tumor cell migration.

Migration refers to unobstructed cell movement on a substrate, whereas ***invasion*** refers to penetration into a tissue barrier (68). The most commonly used assay for cancer cell invasion is the transwell assay (Figure 5.5), with different ECM protein–coated membranes used to evaluate cancer cell invasion through different tissues (e.g., laminin to mimic basement membrane or certain collagens to mimic parenchyma) (64). These assays are relatively easy and fast to set up, but typically are endpoint assays with quantification of migrated cell number terminating the experiment. Furthermore, they only study movement of the cell in one direction (across the membrane) and do not provide information about cell path.

A variety of other assays that provide more information can be used to measure cell invasiveness. For instance, certain assays can quantify cell penetration into an ECM block that is either acellular or contains another cell type (e.g., fibroblasts) (71,72). Invasion can be assessed using microscopy, and the incorporation of 3-D cell-tracking software can track cell movement, given that the cell number is not too high. However, 3-D cell tracking generally requires specialized microscopy equipment and a higher level of data-processing expertise (73). Alternatively, the blocks can be fixed and sectioned as formalin-fixed paraffin-embedded (FFPE) samples, followed by IHC, giving the researcher the advantage of staining for protein expression.

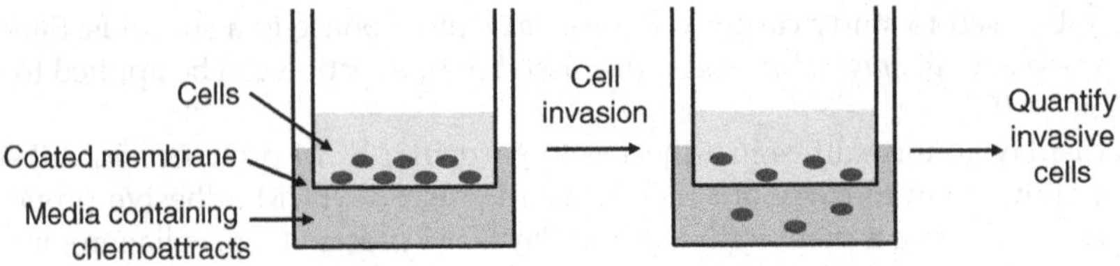

FIGURE 5.5 Transwell invasion assay.

Because cancer cells in vivo tend to invade tissue in cellular clusters, 3-D models to assess cluster invasion are more biologically relevant. In the spheroid gel invasion assay, multicellular spheroids are embedded into an ECM gel and invasion into the gel measured (74). To study the invasion of one cell type into another, a dispersed population of one cell type can be co-cultured with spheroids of another cell type, containing tight cell–cell junctions, similar to what an invading cell would encounter in tissue (75). This spheroid invasion assay can be used to study either the invasion of nonmalignant cells into a spheroid of malignant cells or the reverse. Invasion into the spheroid can be assessed using microscopy, *trypsinization* followed by flow cytometry, or IHC. While invasion through cell–cell junctions is a major advantage of this assay, it requires that the invaded cell type be capable of forming spheroids.

Animal models, most commonly using mice, are the standard to investigate multiple aspects of metastasis in a controlled setting simultaneously. Carcinogen-induced or spontaneously arising tumors derived from a particular mouse strain can be implanted back into that mouse strain, referred to as ***syngeneic models*** (76,77). Syngeneic models have the advantage of allowing researchers to study metastasis in an animal with a competent immune system, a genetically identical background, and with all cell types and microenvironments derived from the same species. However, syngeneic tumors may lack certain features of human tumors (78).

Alternatively, immunodeficient mice can be implanted with human-derived tumors, referred to as ***xenograft models*** (79). Xenograft models based on tumors derived from patients are termed ***patient-derived xenograft*** (***PDX***) models. Xenograft tumors may not accurately recapitulate cancer cell–stroma interactions, given the mixed species origins. Furthermore, because the mice lack a fully functional immune system, immune-mediated effects on metastasis cannot be studied (80). A third class of animal tumor models are tumors that arise spontaneously in the tissue of origin as they would in human patients, referred to as ***autochthonous models***. Autochthonous models are typically generated using carcinogens or genetically predisposed mice with somatic tumor suppressor or oncogene mutations (78). Autochthonous models do not always form metastases or may be slow to metastasize, but they allow the researcher to most closely mimic human disease.

In both syngeneic and xenograft models, the formation of metastases can occur by either implanting a primary tumor and waiting for distant spontaneous metastases to arise or by directly injecting tumor cells into systemic circulation, seeding multiple metastatic sites at once (78). The spontaneous metastatic model allows researchers to study the full process of metastasis in the presence of a primary tumor. However, not all tumors metastasize, and the location of the primary tumor transplant can have a significant impact on the tumor's metastatic potential. Tumors are frequently injected subcutaneously on the flank of the animal, referred to as ***heterotopic models***, but research has shown that ***orthotopic transplants***, where tumor cells are injected in the tissue of origin, more closely resemble patient tumor architecture and behavior, generally with higher rates of metastasis (81).

Direct tumor cell injection is the most common method to study metastasis in animal models. It has several advantages over spontaneously arising metastases (namely, rapidity and reproducibility), allowing the researcher to control the number of cells injected (82). However, along with the inherent tissue tropism of the cancer cells, the site of injection will influence the location of the metastases, depending on the first capillary bed encountered by the tumor cells. For instance, tail vein injections and portal vein injections frequently result in pulmonary metastases and liver metastases, respectively (78). One downside of injecting tumor cells into circulation is the inability to study early steps of the metastatic process, which selects for particular tumor cells having phenotypes conveying the highest metastatic potential. This important difference may influence downstream measurements of metastasis behavior.

A number of assays can be performed using animal models or, in some cases, patient samples. Metastases can be monitored using imaging techniques (PET or MRI), allowing the same metastasis to be followed over time. Tumor cells expressing luciferase or GFP can be tracked using bioluminescent and fluorescent imaging, respectively (83,84). Rare tumor cells in circulation can be isolated using methods to enrich for tumor-specific cell surface markers, and these cells used for downstream applications (85). Circulating tumor nucleic acids can be assessed using ***reverse transcriptase-polymerase chain reaction*** (***RT-PCR***) with tumor-specific RNA primers. Recently, improvements in sequencing technologies and sample preparation have made identification of rare tumor nucleic acids in circulation feasible (86). Presence of micrometastases in lymph nodes and organs can be assessed by surgical removal of the tissue followed by RT-PCR or IHC probing for tumor-specific markers (87).

Example: Cancer cell transwell invasion assay

Integrins are a broad class of plasma membrane receptors that are involved in cell–cell and cell–ECM interactions. Dysregulation of certain integrins has been implicated in metastasis. In this example, we evaluate the role of a hypothetical integrin, integrin a8b3, in the migration and invasion of a prostate cancer cell line in vitro. The hypothetical integrin has been found to be upregulated in a subset of patient prostate cancer bone metastases, although it is not typically found in normal prostate epithelium or in situ prostate carcinoma. Knockdown of the integrin in a prostate cancer cell line followed by adhesion and invasion assays sheds light on the possible role of the hypothetical integrin in the metastatic process.

The prostate cancer line is infected with lentivirus containing short hairpin RNA (shRNA) specific to integrin subunits a8 and b3. shRNA works via *RNA interference (RNAi)* to degrade mRNA transcripts complementary to the shRNA sequence. Transduction with lentiviral shRNA results in integration of the shRNA into the cellular genome and long-term silencing on the target gene. Individual prostate cancer cell clones are picked and screened for integrin knockdown. The knockdown clone is compared to the parental line in an adhesion assay (Figure 5.6). A 96-well plate is coated with either collagen I or fibronectin, both components of the ECM, or left uncoated

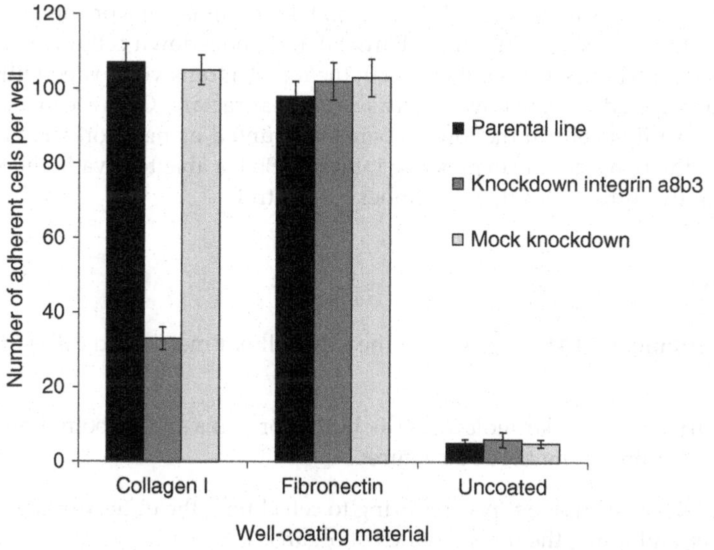

FIGURE 5.6 Adherence assay comparing adherence of the parental prostate cancer line, integrin a8b3 knockdown line, and a mock knockdown control line to various well coatings.

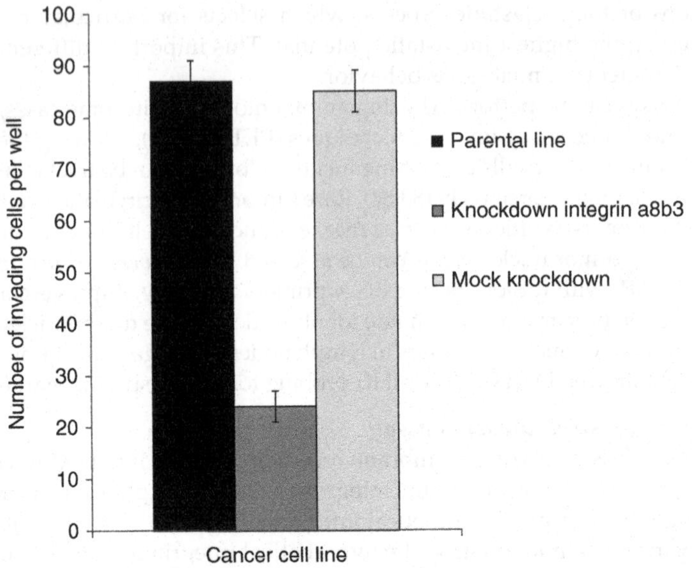

FIGURE 5.7 Transwell invasion assay comparing ability of parental line and knockdown lines to invade through a laminin-coated membrane.

as a control. The knockdown and parental cells are stained with carboxyfluorescein succinimidyl ester (CFSE) to allow fluorescent detection of live cells and then incubated in the coated wells for 30 minutes. Wells are gently washed with a multichannel pipette and adherent cells per well are manually counted using fluorescent microscopy. Alternatively, cell quantification can be performed using an MTT or ATP assay. The results show that loss of integrin results in lower adhesion to collagen I, but fibronectin adhesion is unchanged. Thus, in this example, enhanced ECM adhesion via upregulation of integrin a8b3 could facilitate prostate cancer cell migration.

To assess the role of integrin a8b3 in basement membrane invasion, an invasion assay with laminin-coated membranes is performed (Figure 5.7). Laminin is a major component of the basal lamina, a layer of the basement membrane. Parental and knockdown cells are stained with CFSE and serum starved for 8 hours. Cells are placed in the top of a transwell coated with laminin, using 2% serum-containing media in the lower well as a chemoattractant. Cells are incubated for several hours, and then invading cells in the lower assay are counted using fluorescent microscopy. The results show that the parental line expressing integrin a8b3 is able to invade the basement membrane at significantly higher rates than the knockout control.

GLOSSARY

tumor microenvironment (TME): consists of the extracellular matrix and cells surrounding tumor cells.

extracellular matrix: non-cellular molecules (including proteins and carbohydrates) supporting cell maintenance and providing tissue structure.

epithelial: one of the basic tissue types, referring to cells lining the outer surfaces of skin, organs, and blood vessels, and lining the inner cavities of organs.

hematopoietic: blood-related.

germ cell: cell giving rise to gametes.

stroma: the connective tissue of an organ that plays a supportive, structural role.

proteases: an enzyme that degrades other proteins or peptides.

fibroblasts: connective tissue cells responsible for producing collagen and other components of the ECM.

cytokine: small proteins secreted by certain cells to signal to other cells.

chemokine: a type of cytokine that functions to attract particular cell types, typically immune cells.

growth factor: substance encouraging the growth of certain cell types.

metalloproteinase: metal-dependent protease, often involved in hydrolysis of ECM proteins.

epithelial–mesenchymal transition (EMT): Process by which cells lose their epithelial-like characteristics (polarity, cell–cell, and basement membrane adhesion) and become mesenchymal-like (with migratory and invasive abilities).

myeloid-derived suppressor cells (MDSCs): a mixed population of immature cells of myeloid origin that strongly inhibit the activity of pro-inflammatory immune cells.

regulatory T cells (Tregs): a subpopulation of T cells (T lymphocytes) with immunosuppressive functions.

tumor-associated macrophages (TAMs): a class of immunosuppressive monocyte derived cells involved in cancer-related inflammation.

Foxp3: a transcription factor that controls the regulatory T cell phenotype.

tumor-infiltrating lymphocytes (TILs): general term for pro-inflammatory lymphocytes, such as T cells and NK cells, found in the tumor microenvironment.

immunoediting: the process whereby the most immunogenic antigens are eliminated.

angiogenesis: formation of new blood vessels from existing vessels.

vasculogenesis: de novo formation of new blood vessels.

vascular endothelial growth factor (VEGF): substance that signals EPCs recruited by fibroblasts to transdifferentiate into endothelial cells.

immunohistochemistry: antibody staining procedure commonly performed on research and clinical tissue sections to study the cellular and ECM architecture.

in situ hybridization (ISH): procedure that uses a nucleic acid probe complementary to the sequence of interest, with either radio, hapten, or fluorophore labeling, to provide information on a nucleic acid's expression patterns.

enzyme-linked immunosorbent assay (ELISA): highly sensitive, plate-based assay to quantify the amount of an antigen in a liquid.

transwell invasion assay: quantifies cell penetration through an ECM-coated membrane toward a chemoattractant.

intravasate: invade into the vasculature.

transcription factors: protein controlling the rate of DNA expression (transcription) into RNA.

tissue factor: a complement receptor and coagulation activator.

"seed and soil" theory: proposed by Stephen Paget based on stereotypical metastasis behavior of particular cancers, stating that cancer cells ("seeds") have difficulty surviving outside their primary environment and thus tend to metastasize to tissues ("soils") with appropriate characteristics.

micrometastasis: small collection of tumor cells that has spread (metastasized) from the primary tumor.

macrometastases: population of cells metastasized from a primary tumor that has formed a large metastatic mass.

cancer stem cell (CSC) hypothesis: theory stating that cancers arise from tissue-specific stem cells or from cells that express a stem cell–like genetic program, resulting in a fraction of cells in the primary tumor with stem cell–like features, including the ability to self-renew and differentiate into different cell types.

mesenchymal–epithelial transition (MET): reverse of EMT.

wound healing assay: an in vitro assay used to study cell migration and cell–cell adhesion. It is performed by making a scratch across a surface and studying cell migration across the gap.

cell exclusion zone assay: A method similar to the wound healing assay, but instead in which electric impulses or temporary physical barriers create a cell-free area.

microcarrier bead assay: method in which cells are grown to confluency on dextran beads, then incubated in cell culture dishes, after which the number of cells migrating to the plate is quantified.

spheroid migration assay: method similar to the microcarrier bead assay that uses multicellular tumor spheroids as the origin from which cells migrate.

green fluorescent protein (GFP): fluorescent protein that can be made to be expressed by cells to label them.

migration: unobstructed cell movement on a substrate.

invasion: penetration into a tissue barrier.

syngeneic model: animal model that implants carcinogen-induced or spontaneously arising tumors derived from a particular mouse strain back into that mouse strain.

xenograft model: animal model in which immunodeficient mice are implanted with human-derived tumors.

patient-derived xenograft (PDX): [model] xenograft model based on tumors derived from patients.

autochthonous model: class of animal tumor model that uses tumors arising spontaneously in the tissue of origin.

heterotopic model: animal model is which tumor is introduced to a non-physiological site, such as subcutaneously on the animal's flank.

orthotopic transplant: animal model in which tumor cells are injected in the tissue of origin.

reverse transcriptase-polymerase chain reaction (RT-PCR): a technique similar to PCR, but used to amplify RNA instead of DNA.

integrins: a broad class of plasma membrane receptors that are involved in cell–cell and cell–ECM interactions.

REFERENCES

1. Wodarz D. Dynamics of cancer: incidence, inheritance, and evolution. *Q Rev Biol.* 2009;84:117–118. doi:10.1086/598317
2. Pietras K, Östman A. Hallmarks of cancer: interactions with the tumor stroma. *Exp Cell Res.* 2010;316:1324–1331. doi:10.1016/j.yexcr.2010.02.045
3. Karagiannis GS, Poutahidis T, Erdman SE, et al. Cancer-associated fibroblasts drive the progression of metastasis through both paracrine and mechanical pressure on cancer tissue. *Mol Cancer Res.* 2012;10:1403–1418. doi:10.1158/1541-7786.MCR-12-0307
4. De Wever O, Demetter P, Mareel M, Bracke M. Stromal myofibroblasts are drivers of invasive cancer growth. *Int J Cancer.* 2008;123:2229–2238. doi:10.1002/ijc.23925
5. Augsten M. Cancer-associated fibroblasts as another polarized cell type of the tumor microenvironment. *Front Oncol.* 2014;4:62. doi:10.3389/fonc.2014.00062
6. Madar S, Goldstein I, Rotter V. "Cancer associated fibroblasts"—more than meets the eye. *Trends Mol Med.* 2013;19:447–453. doi:10.1016/j.molmed.2013.05.004
7. Fearon DT. The carcinoma-associated fibroblast expressing fibroblast activation protein and escape from immune surveillance. *Cancer Immunol Res.* 2014;2:187–193. doi:10.1158/2326-6066.CIR-14-0002
8. Talmadge JE, Gabrilovich DI. History of myeloid-derived suppressor cells. *Nat Rev Cancer.* 2013;13:739–752. doi:10.1038/nrc3581
9. Gabrilovich DI, Nagaraj S. Myeloid-derived suppressor cells as regulators of the immune system. *Nat Rev Immunol.* 2009;9:162–174. doi:10.1038/nri2506
10. Quatromoni JG, Eruslanov E. Tumor-associated macrophages: function, phenotype, and link to prognosis in human lung cancer. *Am J Transl Res.* 2012;4:376–389.
11. Youn J-I, Nagaraj S, Collazo M, Gabrilovich DI. Subsets of myeloid-derived suppressor cells in tumor-bearing mice. *J Immunol.* 2008;181:5791–5802. doi:10.4049/jimmunol.181.8.5791
12. Francisco LM, Salinas VH, Brown KE, et al. PD-L1 regulates the development, maintenance, and function of induced regulatory T cells. *J Exp Med.* 2009;206:3015–3029. doi:10.1084/jem.20090847
13. Vignali DA, Collison LW, Workman CJ. How regulatory T cells work. *Nat Rev Immunol.* 2008;8:523–532. doi:10.1038/nri2343
14. Man YG, Stojadinovic A, Mason J, et al. Tumor-infiltrating immune cells promoting tumor invasion and metastasis: existing theories. *J Cancer.* 2013;4:84–95. doi:10.7150/jca.5482
15. Alderton GK, Bordon Y. Tumour immunotherapy—leukocytes take up the fight. *Nat Rev Immunol.* 2012;12:237–237. doi:10.1038/nri3197
16. Mittal D, Gubin MM, Schreiber RD, Smyth MJ. New insights into cancer immunoediting and its three component phases: elimination, equilibrium and escape. *Curr Opin Immunol.* 2014;27:16–25. doi:10.1016/j.coi.2014.01.004
17. Bellone M, Calcinotto A. Ways to enhance lymphocyte trafficking into tumors and fitness of tumor infiltrating lymphocytes. *Front Oncol.* 2013;3:231. doi:10.3389/fonc.2013.00231
18. Mellman I, Coukos G, Dranoff G. Cancer immunotherapy comes of age. *Nature.* 2011;480:480–489. doi:10.1038/nature10673
19. Schreiber RD, Old LJ, Smyth MJ. Cancer immunoediting: integrating immunity's roles in cancer suppression and promotion. *Science.* 2011;331:1565–1570. doi:10.1126/science.1203486
20. Nishida N, Yano H, Nishida T, et al. Angiogenesis in cancer. *Vasc Health Risk Manag.* 2006;2:213–219. doi:10.2147/vhrm.2006.2.3.213
21. Tang HS, Feng YJ, Yao LQ. Angiogenesis, vasculogenesis, and vasculogenic mimicry in ovarian cancer. *Int J Gynecol Cancer.* 2009;19:605–610. doi:10.1111/IGC.0b013e3181a389e6
22. Clarke JM, Hurwitz HI. Understanding and targeting resistance to anti-angiogenic therapies. *J Gastrointest Oncol.* 2013;4:253–263. doi:10.3978/j.issn.2078-6891.2013.036
23. Fang J, Nakamura H, Maeda H. The EPR effect: unique features of tumor blood vessels for drug delivery, factors involved, and limitations and augmentation of the effect. *Adv Drug Deliv Rev.* 2011;63:136–151. doi:10.1016/j.addr.2010.04.009
24. Greish K. Enhanced permeability and retention (EPR) effect for anticancer nanomedicine drug targeting. *Methods Mol Biol.* 2010;624:25–37. doi:10.1007/978-1-60761-609-2_3
25. Jensen E. Technical review: in situ hybridization. *Anat Rec (Hoboken).* 2014;297:1349–1353. doi:10.1002/ar.22944
26. Woodruff TK. Cellular localization of mRNA and protein: in situ hybridization histochemistry and in situ ligand binding. *Methods Cell Biol.* 1998;57:333–351. doi:10.1016/S0091-679X(08)61589-7
27. Ayala G, Tuxhorn JA, Wheeler TM, et al. Reactive stroma as a predictor of biochemical-free recurrence in prostate cancer. *Clin Cancer Res.* 2003;9:4792–4801.
28. Moeder CB, Giltnane JM, Moulis SP, Rimm DL. Quantitative, fluorescence-based in-situ assessment of protein expression. *Methods Mol Biol.* 2009;520:163–175. doi:10.1007/978-1-60327-811-9_12
29. Leng SX, McElhaney JE, Walston JD, et al. ELISA and multiplex technologies for cytokine measurement in inflammation and aging research. *J Gerontol A Biol Sci Med Sci.* 2008;63:879–884. doi:10.1093/gerona/63.8.879
30. Lovelace P, Maecker HT. Multiparameter intracellular cytokine staining. *Methods Mol Biol.* 2011;699:165–178. doi:10.1007/978-1-61737-950-5_8
31. Gros A, Robbins PF, Yao X, et al. PD-1 identifies the patient-specific $CD8^+$ tumor-reactive repertoire infiltrating human tumors. *J Clin Invest.* 2014;124:2246–2259. doi:10.1172/JCI73639
32. Tolboom TCA, Huizinga TWJ. In vitro matrigel fibroblast invasion assay. *Methods Mol Med.* 2007;135:413–421. doi:10.1007/978-1-59745-401-8_27

33. Infanger DW, Lynch ME, Fischbach C. Engineered culture models for studies of tumor-microenvironment interactions. *Annu Rev Biomed Eng*. 2013;15:29–53. doi:10.1146/annurev-bioeng-071811-150028
34. Auerbach R, Lewis R, Shinners B, et al. Angiogenesis assays: a critical overview. *Clin Chem*. 2003;49:32–40. doi:10.1373/49.1.32
35. Staton C, Reed MWR, Brown NJ. A critical analysis of current in vitro and in vivo angiogenesis assays. *Int J Exp Pathol*. 2009;90:195–221. doi:10.1111/j.1365-2613.2008.00633.x
36. Arnaoutova I, George J, Kleinman HK, Benton G. The endothelial cell tube formation assay on basement membrane turns 20: State of the science and the art. *Angiogenesis*. 2009;12:267–274. doi:10.1007/s10456-009-9146-4
37. Pardoll DM. The blockade of immune checkpoints in cancer immunotherapy. *Nat Rev Cancer*. 2012;12:252–264. doi:10.1038/nrc3239
38. Bacac M, Stamenkovic I. Metastatic cancer cell. *Annu Rev Pathol*. 2008;3:221–247. doi:10.1146/annurev.pathmechdis.3.121806.151523
39. Gerhardt H, Semb H. Pericytes: gatekeepers in tumour cell metastasis? *J Mol Med*. 2008;86:135–144. doi:10.1007/s00109-007-0258-2
40. Kalluri R, Weinberg RA. The basics of epithelial-mesenchymal transition. *J Clin Invest*. 2009;119:1420–1428. doi:10.1172/JCI39104
41. Yang J, Mani SA, Donaher JL, et al. Twist, a master regulator of morphogenesis, plays an essential role in tumor metastasis. *Cell*. 2004;117(7):927–939. doi:10.1016/j.cell.2004.06.006
42. Kurrey NK, Amit K, Bapat SA. Snail and Slug are major determinants of ovarian cancer invasiveness at the transcription level. *Gynecol Oncol*. 2005;97(1):155–165. doi:10.1016/j.ygyno.2004.12.043
43. Siegel PM, Shu W, Cardiff RD, et al. Transforming growth factor beta signaling impairs Neu-induced mammary tumorigenesis while promoting pulmonary metastasis. *Proc Natl Acad Sci U S A*. 2003;100(14):8430–8435. doi:10.1073/pnas.0932636100
44. Jeanes A, Gottardi CJ, Yap AS. Cadherins and cancer: how does cadherin dysfunction promote tumor progression? *Oncogene*. 2008;27(55):6920–6929. doi:10.1038/onc.2008.343
45. Wu Y, Zhou BP. TNF-alpha/NF-kappaB/Snail pathway in cancer cell migration and invasion. *Br J Cancer*. 2010;102:639–644. doi:10.1038/sj.bjc.6605530
46. Wong SY, Hynes RO. Lymphatic or hematogenous dissemination: how does a metastatic tumor cell decide? *Cell Cycle*. 2006;5:812–817. doi:10.4161/cc.5.8.2646
47. Butler TP, Gullino PM. Quantitation of cell shedding into efferent blood of mammary adenocarcinoma. *Cancer Res*. 1975;35:512–516.
48. Zhe X, Cher ML, Bonfil RD. Circulating tumor cells: finding the needle in the haystack. *Am J Cancer Res*. 2011;1:740–751.
49. Joyce JA, Pollard JW. Microenvironmental regulation of metastasis. *Nat Rev Cancer*. 2009;9:239–252. doi:10.1038/nrc2618
50. Langley RR, Fidler IJ. The seed and soil hypothesis revisited: The role of tumor-stroma interactions in metastasis to different organs. *Int J Cancer*. 2011;128:2527–2535. doi:10.1002/ijc.26031
51. Müller A, Homey B, Soto H, et al. Involvement of chemokine receptors in breast cancer metastasis. *Nature*. 2001;410(6824):50–56. doi:10.1038/35065016
52. Kang Y, Siegel PM, Shu W, et al. A multigenic program mediating breast cancer metastasis to bone. *Cancer Cell*. 2003;3(6):537–549. doi:10.1016/S1535-6108(03)00132-6
53. Guise T. Examining the metastatic niche: targeting the microenvironment. *Semin Oncol*. 2010;37 Suppl 2:S2–S14. doi:10.1053/j.seminoncol.2010.10.007
54. Barkan D, Green JE, Chambers AF. Extracellular matrix: a gatekeeper in the transition from dormancy to metastatic growth. *Eur J Cancer*. 2010;46:1181–1188. doi:10.1016/j.ejca.2010.02.027
55. Hedley BD, Chambers AF. Tumor dormancy and metastasis. *Adv Cancer Res*. 2009;102:67–101. doi:10.1016/S0065-230X(09)02003-X
56. Demicheli R, Retsky MW, Hrushesky WJM, et al. The effects of surgery on tumor growth: a century of investigations. *Ann Oncol*. 2008;19:1821–1828. doi:10.1093/annonc/mdn386
57. Klein C. Selection and adaptation during metastatic cancer progression. *Nature*. 2013;501:365–372. doi:10.1038/nature12628
58. Tan BT, Park CY, Ailles LE, Weissman IL. The cancer stem cell hypothesis: a work in progress. *Lab Invest*. 2006;86:1203–1207. doi:10.1038/labinvest.3700488
59. Shiozawa Y, Nie B, Pienta KJ, et al. Cancer stem cells and their role in metastasis. *Pharmacol Ther*. 2013;138:285–293. doi:10.1016/j.pharmthera.2013.01.014
60. Kreso A, Dick JE. Evolution of the cancer stem cell model. *Cell Stem Cell*. 2014;14:275–291. doi:10.1016/j.stem.2014.02.006
61. Yao D, Dai C, Peng S. Mechanism of the mesenchymal-epithelial transition and its relationship with metastatic tumor formation. *Mol Cancer Res*. 2011;9:1608–1620. doi:10.1158/1541-7786.MCR-10-0568
62. Lovitt C, Shelper T, Avery V. Advanced cell culture techniques for cancer drug discovery. *Biology (Basel)*. 2014;3:345–367. doi:10.3390/biology3020345
63. Bartsch JE, Staren ED, Appert HE. Adhesion and migration of extracellular matrix-stimulated breast cancer. *J Surg Res*. 2003;110:287–294. doi:10.1016/S0022-4804(03)00004-0
64. Pouliot N, Connolly LM, Moritz RL, et al. Colon cancer cells adhesion and spreading on autocrine laminin-10 is mediated by multiple integrin receptors and modulated by EGF receptor stimulation. *Exp Cell Res*. 2000;261:360–371. doi:10.1006/excr.2000.5065
65. Underwood PA, Bennett F. A comparison of the biological activities of the cell-adhesive proteins vitronectin and fibronectin. *J Cell Sci*. 1989;93(Pt 4):641–649.
66. Jonkman JEN, Cathcart J., Xu F, et al. An introduction to the wound healing assay using live-cell microscopy. *Cell Adh Migr*. 2015;8:440–451. doi:10.4161/cam.36224

67. Li W, Fan J, Chen M, et al. Mechanism of human dermal fibroblast migration driven by type I collagen and platelet derived growth factor-BB. *Mol Biol Cell*. 2004;15:294–309. doi:10.1091/mbc.e03-05-0352
68. Kramer N, Walzl A, Unger C, et al. In vitro cell migration and invasion assays. *Mutat Res*. 2013;752:10–24. doi:10.1016/j.mrrev.2012.08.001
69. Nie F-Q, Yamada M, Kobayashi J, et al. On-chip cell migration assay using microfluidic channels. *Biomaterials*. 2007;28:4017–4022. doi:10.1016/j.biomaterials.2007.05.037
70. Zhang M, Li H, Ma H, Qin J. A simple microfluidic strategy for cell migration assay in an in vitro wound-healing model. *Wound Repair Regen*. 2013;21:897–903. doi:10.1111/wrr.12106
71. Lim SO, Kim H, Jung G. P53 inhibits tumor cell invasion via the degradation of snail protein in hepatocellular carcinoma. *FEBS Lett*. 2010;584:2231–2236. doi:10.1016/j.febslet.2010.04.006
72. Schor SL, Allen TD, Winn B. Lymphocyte migration into three-dimensional collagen matrices: a quantitative study. *J Cell Biol*. 1983;96:1089–1096. doi:10.1083/jcb.96.4.1089
73. Meijering E, Dzyubachyk O, Smal I. Methods for cell and particle tracking. *Methods Enzymol*. 2012;504:183–200. doi:10.1016/B978-0-12-391857-4.00009-4
74. Dolznig H, Rupp C, Puri C, et al. Modeling colon adenocarcinomas in vitro: A 3D co-culture system induces cancer-relevant pathways upon tumor cell and stromal fibroblast interaction. *Am J Pathol*. 2011;179:487–501. doi:10.1016/j.ajpath.2011.03.015
75. Kunz-Schughart LA, Heyder P, Schroeder J, Knuechel R. A heterologous 3-D coculture model of breast tumor cells and fibroblasts to study tumor-associated fibroblast differentiation. *Exp Cell Res*. 2001;266:74–86. doi:10.1006/excr.2001.5210
76. Double JA, Ball CR, Cowen PN. Transplantation of adenocarcinomas of the colon in mice. *J Natl Cancer Inst*. 1975;54:271–275. doi:10.1093/jnci/54.1.271
77. Bobek V, Kolostova K, Pinterova D, et al. A clinically relevant, syngeneic model of spontaneous, highly metastatic B16 mouse melanoma. *Anticancer Res*. 2010;30:4799–4804.
78. Khanna C, Hunter K. Modeling metastasis in vivo. *Carcinogenesis*. 2005;26:513–523. doi:10.1093/carcin/bgh261
79. Aparicio S, Hidalgo M, Kung AL. Examining the utility of patient-derived xenograft mouse models. *Nat Rev Cancer*. 2015;15:311–316. doi:10.1038/nrc3944
80. Morgan R. Human tumor xenografts: the good, the bad, and the ugly. *Mol Ther*. 2012;20:882–884. doi:10.1038/mt.2012.73
81. Bobek V, Kolostova K, Pinterova D, et al. Tail spontaneous metastatic mouse model: comparison of metastatic potential of orthotopic and heterotopic models imaged by GFP and RFP protein. *In Vivo*. 2011;25:849–852.
82. Elkin M, Vlodavsky I. Tail vein assay of cancer metastasis. *Curr Protoc Cell Biol*. 2001;Chapter 19:Unit 19.2. doi:10.1002/0471143030.cb1902s12
83. Hoffman RM. Imaging cancer dynamics in vivo at the tumor and cellular level with fluorescent proteins. *Clin Exp Metastasis*. 2009;26:345–355. doi:10.1007/s10585-008-9205-z
84. Kocher B, Piwnica-Worms D. Illuminating cancer systems with genetically engineered mouse models and coupled luciferase reporters in vivo. *Cancer Discov*. 2013;3:616–629. doi:10.1158/2159-8290.CD-12-0503
85. Alix-Panabières C, Pantel K. Challenges in circulating tumour cell research. *Nat Rev Cancer*. 2014;14:623. doi:10.1038/nrc3820
86. Kinde I, Wu J, Papadopoulos N, et al. Detection and quantification of rare mutations with massively parallel sequencing. *Proc Natl Acad Sci U S A*. 2011;108:9530–9535. doi:10.1073/pnas.1105422108
87. Leong SPL, Tseng WW. Micrometastatic cancer cells in lymph nodes, bone marrow, and blood: clinical significance and biologic implications. *CA Cancer J Clin*. 2014;64:195–206. doi:10.3322/caac.21217

Preclinical Methods

HAILUN WANG ■ PHUOC T. TRAN

Preclinical studies, including in vitro studies with cells and in vivo studies with animal models, comprise a critical facet of cancer research. These preclinical studies are a critical starting point for elucidating mechanisms of diseases and discovery of novel molecularly targeted agents. Through biomarker discovery and establishing proof-of-concept principles, preclinical studies also lay the framework for incorporation of translational endpoints into trial design. Usually, preclinical studies are not very large. However, these studies must provide detailed information on dosing and toxicity levels. After preclinical testing, researchers review their findings and decide whether the treatment regiments and drugs should be tested in patients and whether they should move forward with large-scale clinical trials in which patients may be exposed to potentially toxic therapy.

RATIONAL TARGET SELECTION

Cancer is a class of diseases characterized in the broadest terms by dysregulated cell growth. There are more than 100 types of cancer (www.cancer.gov/types). Conventional cancer therapies are based on the inhibition of the division of rapidly growing cells, which is a characteristic of the cancerous cells. Most of the traditional chemotherapeutic agents function by directly interfering with cell division or DNA synthesis. Based on their targets and mechanisms of action, traditional chemotherapeutic agents can be categorized as **alkylating** (and alkylating-like) agents, **antimetabolites**, **anthracyclines**, and plant **alkaloids** (see Chapter 7 for additional detail).

Alkylating and alkylating-like agents are among the most commonly used chemotherapeutics. These compounds add alkyl groups on DNA and lead to breaks or point mutations in DNA strands and can interfere with DNA replication through cross-linking. The damaged DNA will eventually result in the death of cancer cells. Examples of alkylating/alkylating-like agents include cyclophosphamide, cisplatin, carboplatin, and oxaliplatin (1,2).

Antimetabolites are analogs of nucleic acid precursors or nucleic acids. They mimic a purine and can be incorporated into the DNA or ribonucleic acid (RNA) and interfere with DNA replication and cell division. Methotrexate is a commonly used antimetabolite that is related structurally to folate and inhibits the enzyme dihydrofolate reductase, which is required for DNA synthesis. Three other commonly used antimetabolites are mercaptopurine, 5-fluorouracil (5-FU), and gemcitabine, which also function by blocking replication of DNA (3,4).

Anthracyclines are aromatic polyketide-based chemotherapeutic agents. They were originally derived from *Streptomyces* and their antitumor activities are due to their ability to intercalate into base pairs, effectively inhibit topoisomerase II enzyme activity, and block DNA and RNA synthesis. Therefore, they can prevent the replication of cancer cells. The first anthracycline discovered was daunorubicin; shortly thereafter, doxorubicin, a derivative of daunorubicin, was developed. Many others have followed, including idarubicin, epirubicin, and mitoxantrone (5,6).

Plant alkaloids are compounds derived from plants. Vinblastine (Velbe) and vincristine (Oncovin) are representative plant alkaloids obtained from the periwinkle plant. Another class of microtubule inhibitors, taxanes (e.g., paclitaxel, docetaxel), was originally isolated from the bark of the Pacific yew tree, *Taxus brevifolia*. These compounds specifically target the M phase of the cell cycle and act by blocking tubulin assembly into microtubules in the mitotic spindle during cell division (7,8).

All of the traditional cancer treatments already described have significant side effects, in part due to their lack of selectivity for tumor cells over normal cells with fast proliferation rates, such as the hair follicles, bone marrow, and gastrointestinal tract cells, generating the characteristic systemic toxicity observed with traditional cytotoxic chemotherapies. Recent advances in cancer genomics and novel insight into the complex biology of cancer have revealed numerous cancer-specific mutations and abnormalities. Novel approaches are being developed to specifically target the biologic transduction pathways and inhibit the activities of **oncoproteins**, such as kinases, transcriptional factors, and cell surface receptors, and preventing activation of pathways that are dysregulated in cancer.

Two types that are currently being developed are small molecule inhibitors and monoclonal antibodies (mAbs) (9–14). Many small molecule inhibitors have been successfully developed so far. Imatinib (Gleevec) was one of the first cancer therapies to show the potential for such targeted action and it ushered in the concept of ***precision medicine***. Imatinib is used to treat chronic myeloid leukemia (CML). The disease arises because of a translocation of chromosomes to generate an abnormal protein, BCR-ABL (breakpoint cluster region-Abelson proto-oncogene), and imatinib can target this aberrant protein (15,16). The **epidermal growth factor receptor** (**EGFR**) is a transmembrane receptor involved in many cell processes, including cell growth, proliferation, survival, migration, and tissue invasion (17). In a wide range of epithelial cells, including breast, colon, head, neck, kidney, lung, pancreas, and prostate, the mutations and constitutive activation of the EGFR family members, particularly EGFR and HER2, have been reported to trigger cancer initiation, metastasis, and tumor progression (18).

Several small molecules that directly bind to the tyrosine kinase domain of ErbB receptors have been developed and act as **tyrosine kinase inhibitors (TKIs)**. The first representatives of this class, gefitinib, erlotinib, and lapatinib, are reversible EGFR or EGFR/HER2 selective TKIs, which effectively bind to the EGFR with the common sensitizing mutations (exon 19 deletions and L858R point mutations) (19,20). However, acquisition of resistance invariably occurs in cancers due to additional second site EGFR mutations (T790M). Therefore, several next-generation TKIs have been developed, such as osimertinib (target T790M) and afatinib (irreversible EGFR TKI) (21–23). Monoclonal antibodies have also been successfully used in inhibiting signaling from ErbB family members by interacting with the extracellular domains. These include cetuximab (20), which targets EGFR, and trastuzumab, which targets HER2 (24).

Several other pathways that often show abnormal activities in cancer and can serve as therapeutic targets include the **PI3K/Akt/mTOR** pathway (25) (promotes tumor metabolism, growth, and survival); the **vascular endothelial growth factor** (**VEGF**) pathway (26) (promotes tumor angiogenesis); the **hypoxia inducible factor** (**HIF-1**) pathway (27) (promotes tumor metastasis, angiogenesis, and survival); the **Myc** pathway (28,29) (promotes tumor metabolism, growth, and survival); the **epithelial-to-mesenchymal transition** (**EMT**) pathway (9,30–33) (promotes tumor onset, tumor metastasis, and therapeutic resistance); and the **DNA damage repair** pathway (34–39) (promotes tumor formation and growth, but sensitive to radiation treatment). Unfortunately, there are still many molecular targets that are not tractable targets to current medicinal chemistry approaches. **KRAS** is the most frequently mutated oncogene in human cancer. However, in the 30 years since its discovery, only minimal strides have been made to specifically target KRAS. Today, patients with KRAS-mutated cancer are largely treated with standard chemotherapy and radiation (40–43).

Recently, immunologic checkpoint blockade with antibodies that target **cytotoxic T lymphocyte–associated antigen 4** (**CTLA-4**) and the **programmed cell death protein 1** (**PD-1/PD-L1**) pathway has emerged as a potent new class of anticancer therapy (see Chapter 7 for additional detail). These antibodies have changed the treatment landscape for a range of tumors. Tumors with high mutational rates resulting in more tumor-associated neoantigens are thought to be particularly susceptible to immunotherapy (44–46).

Given the number of candidate-targeted agents and treatment approaches that are available, it is nearly impossible to test every combination in a preclinical study. However, many agents have mechanisms of action that are well positioned to inhibit specific biological pathways and treat particular disease conditions. Preclinical testing should focus research efforts only on those agents with established biomarkers predictive of clinical benefit and focus on confirming activity when combined with their studied treatment and identifying mechanisms of resistance.

IN VITRO METHODS

Although in vitro studies often do not address all the complexities and nuances of cancer biology in patients, such as differences in immune system, metabolism, and tumor microenvironment, they are a necessary starting point in preclinical development. In vitro studies typically include cell lines in standard tissue culture or in three-dimensional (3-D) culture. They are conducted to elucidate mechanisms of action and resistance pathways and to demonstrate agent activity as well as potential tumor selectivity. The selection of cell lines and assays should be based on knowledge of expression of the target with consideration of what types of tumors will be studied in clinical trials. Several classical in vitro and in vivo methods used in preclinical studies are summarized in the following text.

2-D/3-D CELL CULTURE

Most of our current knowledge of signaling pathway and disease mechanisms is derived from cell lines cultured in vitro. These studies provide us an efficient, easy, and invaluable way to understand the molecular basis of many human diseases. In 1885, Wilhelm Roux demonstrated 2-D methodology using glass plates and warm saline solution (47). Ever since then, there has been considerable progress in 2-D culture techniques, with improved understanding of tissue-specific requirements for culture medium. In a 2-D culture, culture plates are precoated with collagen, fibronectin, or a mixture of different components to simulate an optimal **extracellular matrix** (**ECM**) for primary tumor cells to attach and grow. Meanwhile, the tumor tissues are minced with scissors or sharp blades and dissociated into single-cell suspensions with enzymatic digestion. Enzymes used for tumor dissociation include trypsin, papain, elastase, hyaluronidase, collagenase, pronase, and deoxyribonuclease (48–51). These enzymes have distinct target specificity; specific tissues require the use of different combinations of enzymes to achieve efficient dissociation (52). The resulting single-cell suspension from tumors is then seeded in Petri dishes that have been precoated with the ECM materials mentioned earlier. Every 2 days, the mixture is serially subcultured until a specific cell line is generated.

Creating cell lines from tumor tissues has always been a challenge due to low success rate. For decades, a limited number of immortal cancer cell lines have been used as biological models to investigate cancer biology and explore the potential efficacy of anticancer drugs. However, with the advances of genome sequencing technology, numerous studies have revealed the molecular heterogeneity of cancers, even within the same bulk of tumors. Furthermore, there is a wide range of variability in patients' response to the same drugs treating the same type of cancer. Therefore, it is difficult to comprehend the genetic and epigenetic diversities of millions of patients from a small number of cancer cell lines. The need to tailor medical treatment to individual patients provides the impetus to develop methods of efficiently generating and culturing primary tumor cells from patients.

Several additional cell culture techniques have been developed. Each one has its own advantages, but few methods have been found to be universally promising. For example, in the **explant cell culture** system, explants of human normal and tumor tissues are cut into small pieces (2 mm^3) or very thin slices (160 um) and plated into plates that have been coated with gelatin/ collagen and fetal bovine serum. It is then supplemented with essential nutrients for optimal growth. The amount of media needs to be adjusted to ensure the explants stay attached to the plate surface and do not float. The explants with fibroblast outgrowth are discarded. When the outgrowth of epithelial layer forms a halo, the explants need to be taken out and transferred into a new plate for subculturing. The explant cell culture system has a relatively high success rate in generating primary tumor cell lines (50% efficiency). It largely retains the native tissue structure and microenvironment at early passages, which provide us a better representation of molecular interactions in vivo. However, the method cannot be used in soft tissues (melanoma), and it requires serial subculturing to enrich tumor cells. Also, the primary cells in long-term culture are prone to genetic and phenotypic drift (53–56).

Another example is the **sandwich culture** system, which cultures tumor cells between two glass slides. It provides a nutritionally deprived environment, like the hypoxic conditions present in some tumors, in which a set of tumor cells can survive but normal cells do not. However, the success rate in generating heterogeneous primary tumor cells is limited (57).

Recently, **conditionally reprogrammed cells** (**CRC**) technology has been developed by Drs. Richard Schlegel and Xuefeng Liu, which can be used to generate primary epithelial cell lines from a wide variety of normal or tumor tissues with high success rates (58). Generally, primary epithelial cells derived from human tissue have limited ability to proliferate in standard tissue culture conditions. The limit of proliferation, often referred to as the **Hayflick limit** (59), consists of two restrictive phases of growth referred to as **senescence** (60,61) and **agonescence** (62). Previously, normal cells could not divide indefinitely unless these restriction points were inactivated by cellular or viral oncogenes, such as the two viral oncogenes E6 and E7 from human papillomavirus (HPV), to create immortalized cells (63). However, such genetic manipulation disrupts critical cell regulatory pathways and induces altered growth and differentiation phenotypes.

CRC technology uses a combination of feeder cells and a Rho kinase inhibitor (Y-27632) to induce normal and tumor epithelial cells to proliferate indefinitely in vitro without modification of phenotypes and genetic drifts (58). In this method, minced tumor tissues are suspended in a complete medium containing collagenase type I and hyaluronidase at 37°C in a tube rotator for about 1 hour or until the suspension medium becomes turbid. The digested tissue is then filtered through a cell strainer to get single-cell suspension. The cells are centrifuged and cell pellet resuspension is seeded in the culture plates precoated with lethally irradiated NIH3T3-J2 murine fibroblast feeder cells. The Rho kinase inhibitor (Y-27632) is added in appropriate cell culture media. After reaching subconfluency, cells are periodically split and subcultured to grow definite cell lines. Continued cell proliferation is dependent upon the continued presence of both feeder cells and Y-27632. The CRCs generated from normal tissues are reprogrammed toward a stemlike state and remain non-tumorigenic. More importantly, these CRCs retain their lineage commitment and establish normal epithelial architecture when returned to appropriate environmental stimuli. Thus, the induction of CRCs is reversible and the removal of Y-27632 and feeders allows the cells to differentiate normally (63).

One limitation of characterizing tumor samples from individual patients has been the lack of appropriate genetic matched cell lines and cell culture system. The CRCs generated from tumor tissues are the result of reprogramming of the entire cell population, rather than the selection of a minor subpopulation, largely maintaining the heterogeneity of the original tumor tissues. Therefore, any favorable treatment results from in vitro studies on CRCs can be readily used in clinical therapies on the same patient. Several recent successful applications of CRCs for evaluating human lung cancers and developing appropriate therapeutic drug screens have demonstrated the potential and efficiency of CRCs in personalized medicine (64,65).

Because 2-D culture is easy to carry out, it is still the predominant cell culture technique. However, in 2-D cultures, cells are grown as a **monolayer** and lack architectural diversity because of the flat environmental surface. Also, cell cultures in a 2-D system lack the metabolic and proliferative gradients that are present in the body, and cells do not have the physiologically relevant microenvironment and ECM that has been found to be critical for mechanical signaling, growth, migration, invasion, and differentiation. Therefore, 2-D cultures cannot accurately reproduce tissue-specific characters such as topology, differentiation, and gene expression.

Three-dimensional (3-D) cell cultures have great potential for overcoming the challenges inherent in 2-D cell cultures (66). To mirror the environment experienced by cells in the body, 3-D cultures grow cells in a 3-D environment, matrix, or on a scaffold with 3-D architecture, as opposed to the flat surface of a conventional 2-D culture vessel. For example, tumor-dissociated cells can be seeded as a monolayer within two layers of ECM or on some other scaffolds that simulate the in vivo microenvironment. The natural environment or ECM is a complex mixture of glycoproteins, proteoglycans, and collagens that make up the structural scaffold to support cell attachment and survival (48,67,68).

In recent years, researchers have discovered numerous **biomimetic scaffolds** such as hydrogel (69), Matrigel (70), collagen (71), and even decellularized organs (72). These biocompatible materials show great promise as a means to mimic natural environmental conditions (73). Several recent studies have demonstrated that 3-D culture system can be used to generate **organoids** efficiently from human tumor tissues (74–76). The genetic mutations in the organoid cultures closely match those in the corresponding tumor biopsies. In contrast to cell lines, these organoids display the hallmarks of the original tissue in terms of its 3-D architecture, the cell types present, and their proliferating properties. Orthotopically transplanted neoplastic organoids recapitulate the full spectrum of tumor development. Furthermore, these organoid cultures are amenable to large-scale drug screens for the detection of genetic changes associated with drug sensitivity. With these advances in culturing technologies, 3-D cell cultures will redefine our conventional in vitro model and provide us powerful tools for cancer biology research and clinical practice.

TARGET INHIBITION

Recent advances in cancer genomics and insight into the complex biology of cancer have revealed numerous cancer-specific gene mutations and abnormalities. Understanding the role of these mutated genes in tumor development will provide us novel targets for cancer treatment. Currently, several genetic and pharmacological approaches are available to inhibit individual genes and their cognate gene products in tumor cells, which include siRNA/shRNA, CRISPR-Cas9, small molecular inhibitors, and monoclonal antibodies.

Small interfering RNA (**siRNA**) is the most commonly used RNA interference (RNAi) tool for inducing short-term silencing of protein coding genes. siRNA is a single-stranded RNA molecule (usually from 21 to 25 nucleotides in length) produced by the cleavage and processing of double-stranded RNA. It binds to complementary sequences in mRNA and forms the **RNA-induced silencing complex** (**RISC**), inducing cleavage and degradation of the mRNA (77,78). Delivery of siRNA intracellularly is usually done by transfecting cells with siRNA-containing cationic liposomes (79). For cells that are difficult to transfect, such as floating cultured cells and primary cells, electrical pulses (electroporation) are used to intracellularly deliver siRNA into cells (80). To achieve long-term silencing effects, siRNA containing a **short hairpin RNA vector** (**shRNA**) can be used to silence target gene expression. The shRNA vector can be delivered intracellularly using adenovirus and lentivirus. The latter is the most efficient virus that transduces both dividing and nondividing cells, as well as directly inserting the shRNA unit into the genome of the recipient cell and stably expressing siRNA in target cells (81). However, significant barriers to successful siRNA therapies remain, the most significant of which is off-target effects (82).

CRISPR-Cas9 is a recently developed powerful new genome-editing technology. It was adapted from a naturally occurring system in bacteria. The CRISPR-Cas9 system is faster, cheaper, more accurate, and more efficient than other existing genome-editing methods (83). The CRISPR-Cas9 system consists of two key components: a small piece of short guide RNA (sgRNA) that can bind to a specific target sequence of DNA in a genome; and a nuclease, such as Cas9, Cas9n, or Cpf1, that can cut a single or both strands of DNA.

When we transfect plasmids containing sequences of both sgRNA and an expression construct encoding the Cas9 protein into a cell, the complex directed by the sgRNA will bind to the DNA sequence of a gene of interest, and Cas9 will incise the DNA target. The incised DNA is then repaired using endogenous DNA repair machinery. Depending on the repair process, genetic material may be randomly added or deleted during the repair process, resulting in mutations that give rise to functional deficiency of the target coding sequence. Therefore, no protein product will be generated from the mutated genes. We can also make defined changes on the DNA by replacing an existing segment of the gene with a co-transfected customized DNA sequence during the repair process (84). CRISPR-Cas9 is of great interest in the prevention and treatment of human diseases. Currently, most research is done to understand diseases using cells and animal models. It is being explored in the treatment of a wide variety of diseases in animals, including age-related macular degeneration, virus infection, cystic fibrosis, hemophilia, and sickle cell disease (84–89). Clinical trials in humans also are emerging for the treatment and prevention of more complex diseases, such as cancer and HPV infection (90,91).

Other than targeting DNA and mRNA, proteins represent a vast class of therapeutic targets both inside and outside the cell. Extensive biological and clinical investigations have led to the identification of protein interaction hubs and nodes that are critical for cancer development. With the increased knowledge of the structural information of binding sites on the target proteins and improved chemical compound library design, many small molecule inhibitors have been successfully developed (92). For example, ganetespib competitively binds the N-terminal ATP binding site of HSP90 and inhibits its function in cancer (39,93). Several small molecules (gefitinib, erlotinib, lapatinib, osimertinib) directly bind to the tyrosine kinase domain of ErbB receptors and act as TKIs (20–22).

mAbs can also be used to target abnormal proteins outside the tumor cells. These bind specifically to certain cells or proteins and may result in cancer cell death through direct and indirect means (see Chapter 7 for additional detail). Many mAbs have been approved by the U.S. Food and Drug Administration (FDA) for therapeutic use. For example, bevacizumab is a mAb that targets VEGF, inhibiting tumor blood vessel growth (94,95). Cetuximab is an antibody that targets EGFR, which is overexpressed in many cancers (96,97). Immunologic checkpoint blockade with mAbs targeting CTLA-4 (ipilimumab) and PD-1/PD-L1 (nivolumab, pembrolizumab, durvalumab, etc.) is a powerful new and complementary pillar of cancer therapy (44–46).

CELL VIABILITY ASSAYS

Assays to measure the number and viability of cultured cells are commonly used to monitor the response and health of cells in culture after various treatments. Cell viability, proliferation, and cell death assays are generally grouped together, despite the fact that they measure different parameters. The proper choice of an assay method depends on the number and type of cells used as well as the expected outcome (98).

Trypan Blue Exclusion Assay

This method is based on the principle that live (viable) cells do not take up certain dyes, whereas dead (nonviable) cells do. **Trypan blue** is one of several dyes recommended for use in dye exclusion procedures for viable cell counting. Staining facilitates the visualization of cell morphology. Cell counting using viability dyes can provide both the rate of proliferation and the percentage of viable cells (99).

DNA Synthesis Proliferation Assays

Cell proliferation may be studied by monitoring the incorporation of a nucleoside analog, such as the radioisotope [3H]-thymidine, into cellular DNA, followed by autoradiography. Alternatively, bromodeoxyuridine (BrdU) assays may be used instead of thymidine. Actively proliferating cells that have incorporated BrdU into DNA are easily detected using a monoclonal antibody against BrdU and an enzyme- or fluorochrome-conjugated second antibody (100).

Metabolic Proliferation Assays

Assays that measure metabolic activity are also suitable for analyzing proliferation, viability, and cytotoxicity. The reduction of tetrazolium salts such as MTT, XTT, and WST-1 to colored formazan compounds or the bioreduction of resazurin only occurs in the mitochondria of metabolically active cells. Actively proliferating cells have high metabolic activity, whereas dying cells will have decreased activity. The water-insoluble colored compounds generated from this assay can be solubilized using isopropanol or other solvents. The dissolved material is measured spectrophotometrically, yielding absorbance as a function of concentration of converted dye (101–103).

Cell Death Assays

Apoptosis assays are among the most commonly used methods to study cell death. **Apoptosis** is a process of programmed cell death that occurs in multicellular organisms. It is ATP dependent and is characterized by cell shrinkage, maintenance of plasma membrane integrity, chromatin condensation, nuclear fragmentation, and activation of a family of cysteine-containing, aspartate-directed proteases called caspases. During early apoptosis, the phosphatidylserines flip onto the outer leaflet of the plasma membrane where they can be easily stained by fluorescently labeled **annexin V**. This feature, in combination with DNA binding dyes, such as propidium iodide (PI) and 7-amino-actinomycin D (7-AAD), which are impenetrable to intact membranes, can be used to determine the apoptotic state of a cell (104,105).

During apoptosis, caspases are activated and cleave a number of cell proteins as part of the programmed cell death pathway. This activity can be detected in a **Western blot** and immunofluorescent staining of cells using antibodies that specifically recognize total or cleaved caspase 3 to determine the level of apoptosis present within a sample (106). Alternatively, the **terminal transferase-mediated dUTP nick end labeling (TUNEL)** assay can be used to determine apoptosis in cells and in whole-tissue sections. It is based on the fact that apoptosis leads to a controlled digestion of the nuclear DNA, which can be identified by terminal deoxynucleotidyl transferase, an enzyme that catalyzes the addition of dUTPs that are secondarily labeled with a fluorochrome or another marker (107).

CLONOGENIC ASSAY

A **clonogenic assay** or **colony formation assay** serves as a useful tool to test whether a given cancer therapy can reduce the clonogenic survival of tumor cells after treatment with ionizing radiation. It can also be used to determine the effectiveness of other cytotoxic agents. It was first developed by T.T. Puck and Philip I. Marcus at the University of Colorado in 1955 (108). The assay detects all cells that have retained the capacity for producing a large number of progeny after treatments that can cause cell reproductive death, including mitotic catastrophe, apoptosis, senescence, necrosis, and so forth (61,109–111). The assay involves three major steps:

1. A certain number of cells are plated in tissue culture dishes and allowed to attach overnight.
2. Treatment is applied to the cells, and the cells are allowed to grow for 2 to 3 weeks.
3. The colonies produced are fixed and stained.

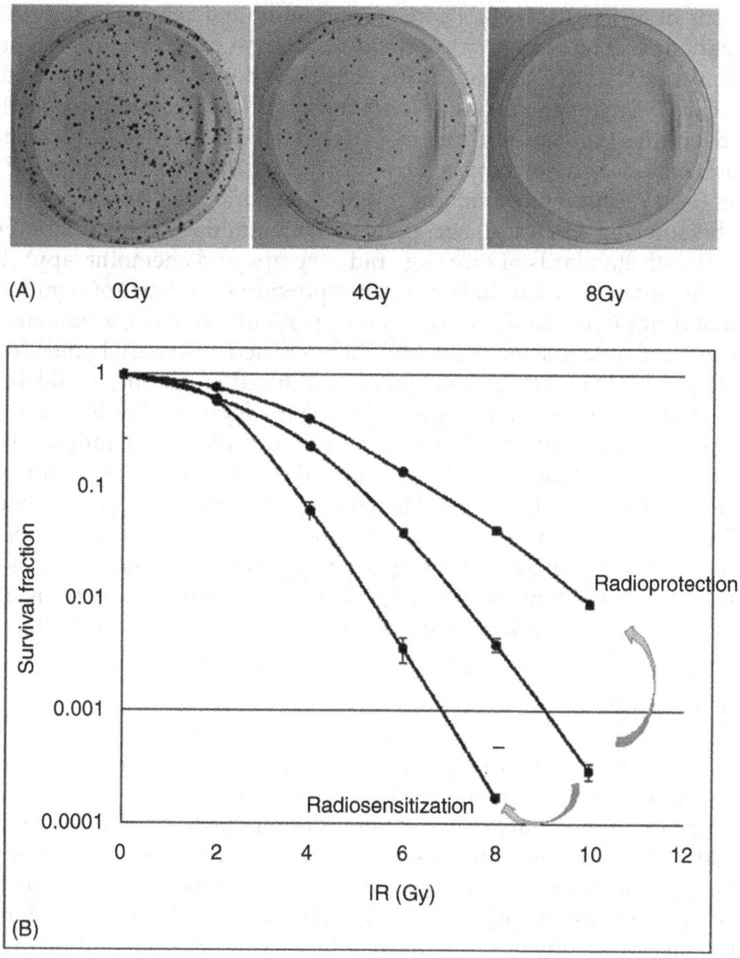

FIGURE 6.1 Clonogenic assay—a graphical representation of survival versus dose of ionizing radiation (or drug concentration) is plotted to compare treatment efficiency between several groups. (A) Representative images of number of colonies formed after radiation treatment. (B) Compounds that either protect cells or sensitize them to radiation treatment will shift the curves accordingly.

Colonies with more than 50 cells are counted. At the conclusion of the experiment, the percentage of cells that survived the treatment is calculated. A graphical representation of survival versus drug concentration or dose of ionizing radiation is plotted to compare treatment efficiency between several groups (112). The assay is easy to set up and can provide accurate results (Figure 6.1).

COMBINATION ANTICANCER DRUG STUDIES

Cancers usually harbor many mutations in multiple molecular pathways that limit the long-term benefit of single-agent therapies in patients. Even in cancers that depend on one major oncogene, responses to single agents can be short-lived, as resistance is common (see Chapters 4 and 5). For example, the median duration of response to erlotinib, a highly selective mutant EGFR (L858R) inhibitor for lung cancer, is approximately 13.1 months, despite an initial response rate of 83% (113). Analyses of tissues from relapsed patients and laboratory studies with cell lines identified several mechanisms of resistance (114). These studies and other reports support the hypothesis that drug combinations will be necessary to provide long-term tumor control for most patients.

Complementary agents or treatments are selected based on scientific and medical rationale. The aims are to achieve a synergistic (or additive) therapeutic effect with acceptable toxicity and to minimize or delay the induction of treatment resistance. Examples of combination therapy in cancer include combinations of molecularly targeted agents, combinations of two or more immunotherapies (e.g., vaccines plus immune modulating antibodies or two immunomodulatory antibodies), combinations of DNA damage agents with immunotherapy, or combinations of an experimental agent with standards of care (e.g., radiotherapy and chemotherapy) (115,116).

In order to evaluate combination studies, or when providing evidence of significant superiority of a combination of drugs over the single agents is of particular interest, a standard definition for additive, synergistic, and antagonistic effects should be created (also see Chapter 7) (117–119). One popular and widely accepted method was jointly introduced by Chou and Talalay in the 1980s (120,121). This approach views **synergy** as a reaction, operating on physiochemical mass action laws rather than a statistical consideration. The resulting **combination index (CI)** of the Chou-Talalay method offers a quantitative definition of an additive effect (CI = 1), synergism (CI < 1), and antagonism (CI > 1) in drug combinations. Therefore, they proposed that one should determine synergy with CI values, not p values. The CI provides a quantitative measure of the degree of interaction between two or more agents. A slight modification of this method was optimized for combination studies with radiation therapy (RT) where experiments are performed using a range of doses in a nonconstant ratio checkerboard design in order to derive a CI (122).

METASTASIS ASSAYS

Given that metastasis is the leading cause of death in cancer patients, the molecular and cellular processes underlying metastasis continue to be a major focus of cancer research. Cell migration and invasion are integral parts of metastasis. Many pro-migratory factors, including chemokines and growth factors, have now been identified and shown to contribute to tumor dissemination (123). These factors and their downstream signaling pathways constitute attractive therapeutic targets to prevent or delay metastatic progression (33,124). Accordingly, several in vitro assays have been developed to investigate the mechanisms regulating cancer cell migration or invasion, or to test the efficacy of potential therapeutic drugs. These include scratch or wound healing assays, trans-membrane migration assays (Transwell/Boyden chamber), and migration assays using microfluidic devices (MFDs).

Wound Healing Assays

The **wound healing assay** refers to the measurement of cell migration into a wound (cell-free area) that is created by a linear scratch across the surface of a tissue culture well containing a confluent monolayer of cells (125,126). To avoid cell growth influencing the rate of wound closure, cells are often serum starved 10 to 24 hours prior to wounding, and the post-scratch medium is typically supplemented with nontoxic doses of mitomycin C to inhibit proliferation (125). Migration may be quantitated manually by standard microscope or by using quantitation software such as ImageJ (www.le.ac.uk/biochem/microscopy/pdf/Wound%20healing%20assay.pdf). Scratch assays are cheap and straightforward, and allow the assessment of cell migration kinetics in real time by time-lapse microscopy. However, this approach is not suitable for chemotaxis measurement or for nonadherent cells.

Transwell/Boyden Chamber Assays

Cell migration assays in **Transwell chambers** involve seeding cells into an upper chamber and monitoring the movement of cells to a lower well separated by a microporous membrane. The chemotactic gradient is created by addition of serum or specific chemotactic factors in the lower well. The ECM may also be coated on the upside of the porous membrane to measure tumor cell invasion. The cells can be visualized after migration using fluorescent dyes. The advantage of this approach is that different chemotactic gradients can be applied and the migratory response of both adherent and nonadherent cells can be measured.

Microfluidic Assays

Microfluidic assays involve seeding cells into a chamber that is bridged to a second chamber by an internal microchannel (127). Microfluidic assays require very small volumes, which facilitates establishing a stable and linear concentration gradient that can last for more than 48 hours. The small volume makes them more suitable for drug testing against rare primary cell populations, such as biopsies, and decreases the amount of chemoattractant or therapeutic agent needed, reducing the cost of reagents. These represent clear advantages over the other 2-D cell migration assays described earlier. Moreover, this approach allows live cell tracking of single cell migration and quantitative measurements of cell migration. The limitations of microfluidic assays are that they are relatively expensive and unsuitable for high throughput applications.

IN VIVO METHODS

In order to understand cancer as a biological process that has effects on a whole organism, it is necessary to study cancer cells in a physiologically relevant setting. The question that a research biologist or a clinical oncologist wishes to address will determine the system chosen for study. The quality and significance of the findings are heavily affected by the model system chosen.

NONMAMMALIAN MODEL SYSTEMS

When studying gene functions or screening small molecular inhibitors, nonmammalian models can offer a variety of advantages. These include genetic simplicity and experimental accessibility in early development. Given the frequent conservation of gene function along evolution, the results gathered using nonmammalian models often lead us to new realizations about gene activities in mammals. The three most commonly used nonmammalian animal models are flies (***Drosophila***), nematodes (***Caenorhabditis elegans***), and **zebrafish**.

Drosophila has been used for over a century to study gene function and perform genetic screens. It has been an instrumental model organism in the identification of cancer-related genes (128). Some of the highly implicated pathways in human tumorigenesis, including Notch (N), Hedgehog (Hh), and Salvador/Warts/Hippo (SWH), were first identified in the fly (129). A number of cancer-related drug screenings have been run in *Drosophila* models. For example, Tin Su et al. ran a screen for radiation sensitizers using wild-type and cell cycle checkpoint mutants in *Drosophila* (130).

The *C. elegans* worm has also been used as a model system for several decades. Several characteristics of the worm make it highly amenable for cancer research (131). Many human genes and pathways involved in cancer are highly conserved in *C. elegans*. For example, many hyperproliferation-inducing cell cycle genes have **orthologs*** in *C. elegans*, and their functions have generally been shown to be well conserved (*orthologs are genes from different species that evolve from a common ancestral gene by speciation) (132). In addition, *C. elegans* has a completely characterized somatic cell lineage, thereby facilitating the analysis of phenotypes that disrupt normal proliferation and patterning (133).

Zebrafish has become a very popular model for studying developmental processes and human disorders. Zebrafish shares a high level of genetic and physiologic homology with humans, including brain, digestive tract, musculature, vasculature, and an innate immune system (134–138). In addition, zebrafish has a transparent body and rapid development, which allow easy disease evaluation. Therefore, it has been widely employed in the study of developmental processes, angiogenesis, wound healing, microbe–host interactions, and drug screening. Moreover, approximately 70% of all human disease genes have functional **homologs*** with this species (139), which greatly widened its use as a model for studying tumor development in vivo (*homologs are genes related by descent from a common ancestral DNA sequence) (140,141). To date, several models of cancer have been generated in zebrafish, such as pancreatic adenocarcinoma (142), sarcomas (143), intestinal hyperplasia (144), melanoma (145–147), and leukemia (148–150).

In addition to the advantages already mentioned, a major limitation of nonmammalian models are that genes of interest and target inhibitors identified in such models may not function in exactly the same way as in mammalian species, due to species differences.

MICE

The mouse is the most frequently used animal model for cancer research, owing to its relative physiologic similarity to humans and the relative efficiency in breeding and housing. In addition, the mouse genome can be easily manipulated with greater speed, scale, and sophistication than that of other mammals. In the past decade, the number and diversity of murine models available for preclinical evaluation have increased exponentially. These models have played a vital role in understanding the mechanisms of tumor development and identifying better diagnostic and therapeutic strategies (151,152). Currently, animal models of cancer biology are becoming more sophisticated by application of new technology, and they play ever-increasingly important roles in mechanistic studies and preclinical research.

Xenograft Models

In this model, human tumor cells are transplanted, either under the skin or **orthotopically*** in the organ type in which the tumor originated, into immunocompromised mice that do not reject human cells (*orthotopic means in the same [*ortho*] place [*topos*]). Immunodeficiency is a prerequisite for preventing human tumor cell rejection. Several mouse strains exhibiting various types of immune deficiency are now available, such as **athymic nude mice** and **severely compromised immunodeficient** (**SCID**) mice (153–156).

Implanted tumor cells normally engraft, and in few weeks, a solid tumor mass is palpable. This method is simple and fast. The tumor growth can be easily followed by measuring tumor volume change, and the results are fairly reproducible. It provides a simple testing format for genetic and pharmacodynamic studies prior to analysis in more complex models. However, the most commonly used tumor cell lines used in xenograft experiments have been grown in vitro for a *long* time (e.g., the HeLa cell line was generated in 1951, PC3 in 1979), and carry additional genomic mutations and aberrations. This has sometimes led to complicated interpretations of positive as well as negative results (157,158). In addition, because of the clonal selection process during tumor cells' adaptation to growth on plastic culture plates, many of these cell lines do not fully recapitulate the genetic diversity observed across human tumors, nor do they properly mimic intratumoral heterogeneity.

To overcome this, **patient-derived xenograft** (**PDX**) mouse models have been developed, which are generated by implanting chunks of cancerous tissue from a patient biopsy directly into an immunodeficient mouse. The PDX tumors maintain the genetic and histological heterogeneity as observed in cancer patients, even after serial passaging in mice (159). In recent years, implementing new technology, such as using more immunodeficient mice—like SCID mice and **nonobese diabetic** (**NOD**)/**SCID** mice—has significantly increased the tumor engraftment rate in mice (160), resulting in a large rise in the use of PDX mice in personalized cancer medicine. Many studies demonstrating the successful translation from PDX mouse to clinical drug response have been published, underlining the current status of the PDX as a highly useful model (159,161–163).

Tumors arise from a range of anatomical sites in humans, but PDX xenografts are almost always implanted subcutaneously in the mouse, not at the orthotopic site. This results in the lack of relevant tissue-specific microenvironment to support the implanted tumor and contributes to different responses in mouse and human. Additionally, a notable limitation of the immune-compromised systems required for xenograft transplantation is that they cannot readily be used for evaluating immune-targeting therapies for oncology (164). One new solution is to generate **humanized mice** by engrafting immunodeficient mice with human CD34+ hematopoietic stem cells or precursor cells. This appears promising as another model to use in preclinical cancer research, particularly for immunotherapy-related studies (165,166).

Genetically Engineered Mouse Models

In the early 1980s, the first cloned cancer genes were introduced into the genome of transgenic mice, which were termed **oncomice** (167). The first oncomouse was a **genetically engineered mouse model (GEMM)** with transgenic expression of an oncogene (v-HRas) under control of a mammary-specific promoter (MMTV), making the mouse prone to developing mammary tumors (168). Recent technological developments enable more sophisticated manipulation of the mouse genome and fast generation of GEMMs that harbor mutations that mimic the somatic alterations observed in human tumors. GEMMs can now be designed that more closely mimic human cancer in terms of genetic composition, tumor microenvironment, multistep tumor development process, drug response, and resistance (169).

There are three basic technical approaches to produce GEMMs. The first involves pronuclear injection of a gene construct into the pronuclei of fertilized mouse eggs, which are subsequently implanted in the oviduct of pseudopregnant recipient mice. The injected gene constructs will randomly integrate into the mouse genome, and the offspring will be screened for transgene expression. Where positive, these are used to develop transgenic lines with stable integration and expression of the transgene (170).

To achieve spatially and temporally controlled gene expression in specific tissues, an inducible system will often be included in the injected gene construct. The most commonly used system is the **tetracycline-controlled transcriptional activation (Tet-On)** system developed in 1992 by Hermann Bujard and Manfred Gossen at the University of Heidelberg (171). The Tet-On system contains two elements: a **transactivator protein (rtTA)** and its consensus binding sequence—a **tetracycline response element (TRE)**. The expression of the rtTA is usually driven by a tissue-specific promoter. In the presence of tetracycline or its derivatives (such as doxycycline), rtTA can bind to the TRE sequence upstream of the gene of interest and increase the transcription of the gene. The Tet-On system allows for rapid and reversible gene expression control and has demonstrated its utility in many mouse model studies (9,32) (Figure 6.2).

The second approach to generate GEMMs, pioneered by Oliver Smithies and Mario Capecchi, involves injecting a DNA construct into mouse embryonic stem cells. The DNA construct contains DNA sequences homologous to the target gene, and recombination with the genomic DNA results in the replacement of the endogenous wild-type gene with the injected mutant DNA, which will modify the activity of the gene product or totally silence the target gene (**knockout**). Embryonic stem cells that possess the recombinant DNA are selected for and they are then injected into mouse blastocysts (172).

With a conventional knockout, loss of a vital gene can often lead to embryonic lethality or severe developmental abnormalities, making it impossible to study the gene functions in cancer. To circumvent conventional knockout limitations, sophisticated conditional genetic engineering technology has been developed to enable genetic events to be tightly controlled spatially and temporally. For example, **Cre enzyme** is a site-specific recombinase that catalyzes specific recombination between two defined loxP sites. By temporally and spatially controlling expression of the Cre recombinase, recombination is induced between loxP sites that flank the gene of interest, resulting in deletion (173).

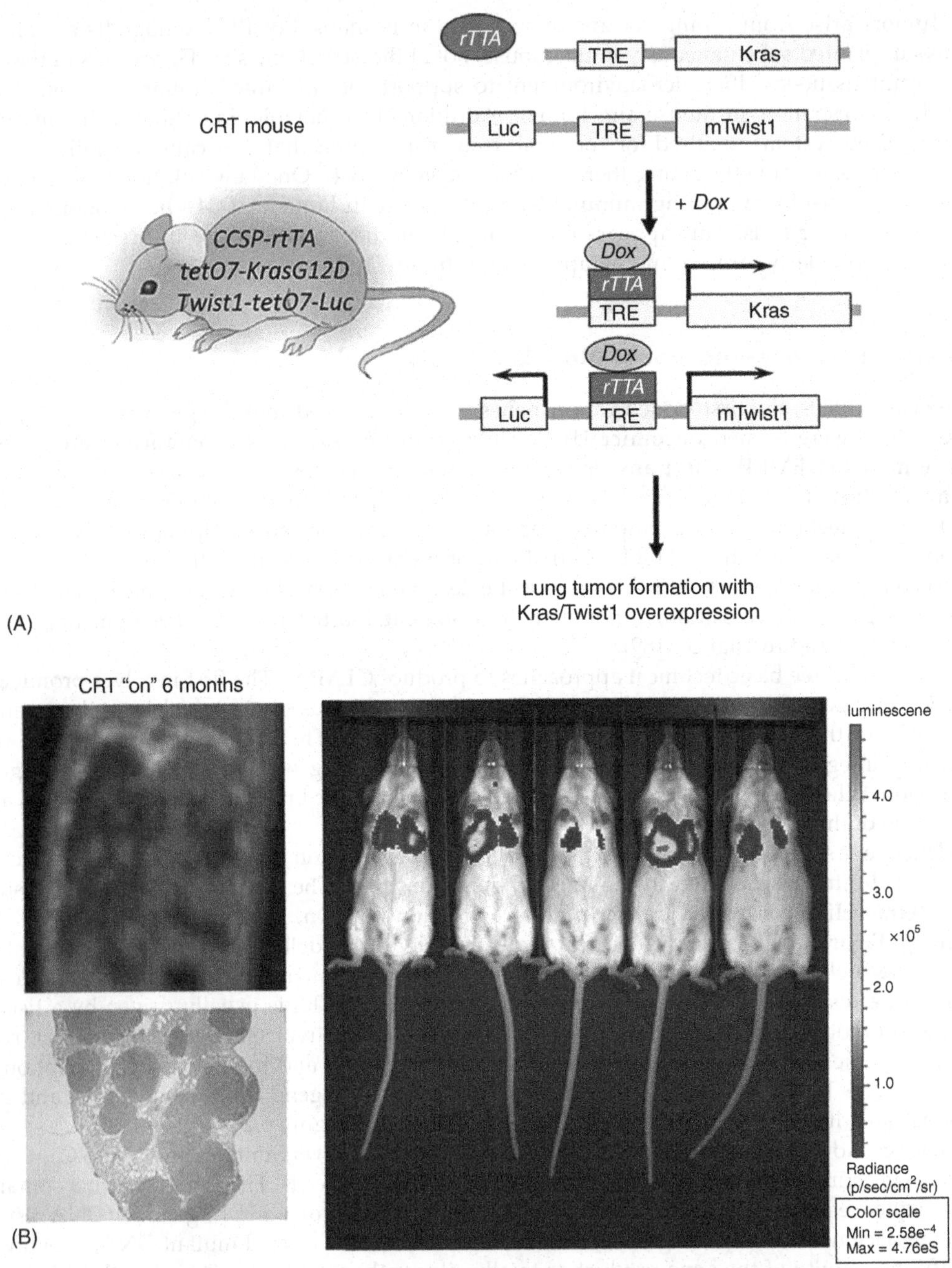

FIGURE 6.2 Inducible lung tumor models for studying the role of Twist1 on tumor formation. (A) Schematic diagram of an inducible transgenic mouse model of lung cancer. Tet-On system is used to express KrasG12D and Twist1 in mouse lung. (B) Representative CT scan, bioluminescent imaging, and hematoxylin and eosin (H&E) stain to demonstrate the tumor formation.

Source: Tran PT, Shroff EH, Burns TF, et al. Twist1 suppresses senescence programs and thereby accelerates and maintains mutant Kras-induced lung tumorigenesis. *PLoS Genet.* 2012;8:e1002650. doi:10.1371/journal.pgen.1002650

Cre expression can be controlled by multiple types of delivery/induction systems. These include tissue-specific promoters, viral delivery, and temporally inducible systems. For the promoter-driven system, mice carrying the Cre recombinase under control of a tissue-specific promoter plus an inducible system (such as Tet-On) are crossed with mice carrying the gene of interest flanked by loxP sites to conditionally knock out the gene in a specific tissue or cell type, such as progenitor cells, or at specific times during development. For viral delivery, the Cre gene is packaged into viral particles, such as adenovirus or lentivirus and the virus can be locally delivered topically, in any accessible tissue lumen, or by direct injection into tissues, creating a regional or clonal knockout of cells within a given area (174,175). Although the recombination approach can achieve precise knockout or knock-in in a gene's natural locus, homologous recombination of a targeting DNA into a genomic locus of interest occurs at a very low frequency (at a frequency of 10^{-3} to 10^{-4}) (176). To circumvent this limitation, novel and more efficient genome-editing technologies are now available.

The recent development of CRISPR-Cas9 systems for genome editing has revolutionized biological research (84,177). CRISPR stands for **clustered regularly interspaced short palindromic repeats**. It was first discovered as a component of a prokaryotic immune system that confers resistance to foreign genetic elements, but soon thereafter was exploited to achieve gene editing in many diverse organisms (178,179).

The CRISPR-Cas9 system consists of two key components that introduce a change into the genomic DNA. One of them is an enzyme called Cas9, which is an RNA-guided DNA endonuclease enzyme. It acts as a pair of "molecular scissors" that can cut the two strands of DNA at a specific location in the genome so that parts of DNA can then be added or removed during DNA repair, resulting in functional gene knockouts. The other component is a small piece of RNA called a guide RNA (gRNA). The gRNA is designed to find and bind to a specific sequence in the DNA. Then the Cas9 follows the gRNA to the same location in the DNA sequence and makes a cut across both strands of the DNA. By using appropriate gRNA, the Cas9 nuclease can be directed to any genomic locus. The CRISPR-Cas9 system can also be used to introduce defined mutations or loxP recombination sites, by simply co-introducing oligonucleotides that contain desired sequences and serve as a template for repair of the Cas9-induced DNA damage (84,180,181).

Because CRISPR-Cas9 technology is faster, cheaper, and more accurate than previous techniques of editing DNA, it is expected to significantly facilitate rapid cancer modeling in mice. Indeed, it has already proven to be an efficient gene-targeting strategy with the potential for multiplexed genome editing (182–186). Virtually all genetic alterations found in human tumors can now be rapidly introduced in the mouse germline, including gene deletions (183,184), point mutations (187), and translocations (188–190). CRISPR-Cas9 technology can also be used for direct somatic editing of oncogenes or tumor suppressor genes in mice, such as generation of non-germline mouse models of lung cancer (191,192), hepatocellular carcinoma (187,193), pancreatic cancer (194,195), brain cancer (196), and breast cancer (197). Recently, the development of a catalytically inactive form of Cas9 fused to a transcriptional activation or suppression domain has repurposed the CRISPR-Cas9 system as a platform for RNA-guided transcriptional regulation. These modified systems may be used to generate mice with inducible and reversible activation of oncogenes or tumor suppressor genes (186,198–200).

GEMMs of human cancer have provided us a unique tool for understanding the mechanisms of cancer initiation, progression, and metastasis. They offer us the most advanced preclinical opportunity for validating candidate drug targets, assessing therapy efficacy like radiotherapy (Figure 6.3), and evaluating mechanisms of drug resistance. Because GEMMs develop de novo tumors in the context of an intact immune system, they are uniquely suited for investigating the potential of cancer immunotherapy. Taken together, the xenograft models and these next-generation GEMMs are of great importance to improve our understanding of the complex mechanisms underlying cancer biology, and they are anticipated to improve translation of new therapeutic strategies into the clinic and improve personalized cancer treatment efficiency.

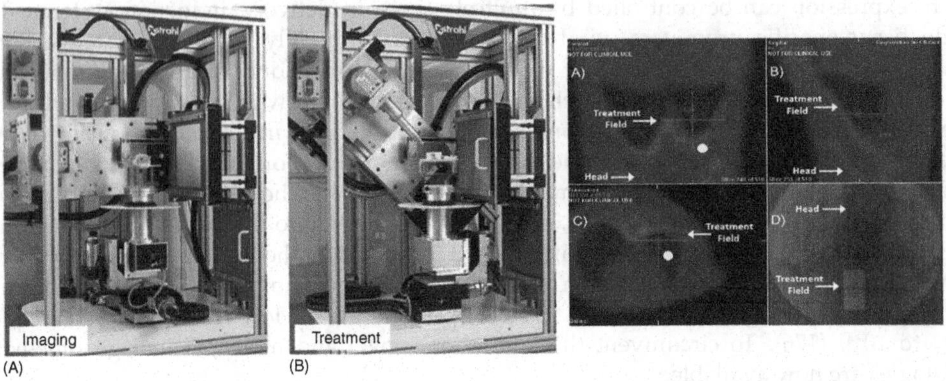

(A) (B)

FIGURE 6.3 A small animal radiation research platform (SARRP) can deliver focused radiation to lung tumors in mice (left figure). Picture of SARRP at imaging or treatment (right figure). (A–C) Representative images of a cone beam computed tomography (CBCT) scan of a mouse thorax in orthogonal planes. The hemi-thorax treatment region is designated by the red crosshairs. (D) Double exposure using the treatment beam showing the hemi-thorax treatment field.

Source: Courtesy of Xstrahl Ltd.

RATS AND LARGER MAMMALS

Similar to mice, rats are widely used in medical research. In the past 10 years, considerable progress has been made in rat genetic studies, which significantly facilitates the modeling of human cancer in rats (201,202). Recent advances in genome-editing technology have led to the generation of genetically modified rats, such as the immunodeficient rats, which provide another platform for modeling human cancer and PDX tissues (203–210). The rat offers a number of advantages over the mouse, including easier surgical manipulation, larger tumor size, and greater blood volume for downstream analyses, as well as being the preferred model for drug efficacy and toxicology studies. However, the low engraftment rate of human tumors in rat limits its application. Further genetic modification may be necessary to create a rat that phenotypically more closely mimics the NOD/SCID mouse to be able to humanize the immune system and engraft the widest range of human cancer cell lines and PDX tissues.

Other than rodent models, swine have been widely used in many areas of biomedical research due to the high anatomical, physiological, and genetic similarities between swine and humans (211). For example, the similarity in size and anatomy of the swine cardiovascular system allows design and testing of stents and tissue engineering of blood vessels (212,213). Imaging modalities such as CT, MRI, and PET can be easily applied to pigs. Furthermore, the size of the pig allows for refinement of surgical techniques, chemotherapies, radiation therapies, and studies of local tumor recurrence, which are otherwise difficult or impossible to perform in rodents. Pigs have also been widely used in preclinical drug toxicology and are standard large animal models for preclinical toxicology prior to human studies (214,215).

In cancer modeling, the advances in genome-editing technologies also facilitate the development of swine models of cancers with targeted mutations in a single generation. Recently, a basal cell carcinoma model was created by making a transgenic pig in which Gli2 was expressed under control of a keratinocyte-specific promoter (216). Similarly, a dominant-negative missense mutation, R167H, was introduced in TP53 in swine fetal fibroblasts, which later developed lymphomas, osteogenic tumors, and renal tumors at varying rates (217,218). Most recently, a transgenic "oncopig" was developed in which a Cre-inducible transgene expressing $KRAS^{G12D}$ and $TP53^{R167H}$ was engineered, in which rapid and reproducible tumor development of mesenchymal origin was observed (219). Although pigs may be better models to investigate cancer and potential therapeutics, one obvious downside of this model is the considerable expense and labor associated with large animals over their extended lifetimes, which may impede their widespread adoption into mainstream science.

CONCLUSION

In summary, decisions on initiating clinical trials have relied and will rely heavily on the results of preclinical studies. The breakthrough in technologies and our increased understanding of cancer biology will enable the development of more sophisticated preclinical disease models to help drive improvements to accurately recapitulate human cancer in the laboratory. These improvements in preclinical cancer disease modeling will in turn increase the success rates of future clinical trials.

GLOSSARY

alkylating agents: compounds that add alkyl groups on DNA and lead to breaks or point mutations in DNA strands and can interfere with DNA replication through cross-linking.

antimetabolites: analogs of nucleic acid precursors or nucleic acids that mimic a purine and can be incorporated into the DNA or RNA and interfere with DNA replication and cell division.

anthracyclines: aromatic polyketide-based chemotherapeutic agents originally derived from *Streptomyces*; antitumor activities are due to their ability to intercalate into base pairs, effectively inhibit topoisomerase II enzyme activity, and block DNA and RNA synthesis.

alkaloids: compounds derived from plants; specifically target the M phase of the cell cycle and act by blocking tubulin assembly into microtubules in the mitotic spindle during cell division.

oncoproteins: substance grouping that includes kinases, transcriptional factors, and cell surface receptors.

precision medicine: treatment that uses small molecule inhibitors to achieve specifically targeted action.

epidermal growth factor receptor (EGFR): a transmembrane receptor involved in many cell processes.

tyrosine kinase inhibitors (TKIs): small molecules that directly bind to the tyrosine kinase domain of ErbB receptors.

PI3K/Akt/mTOR pathway: pathway that often shows abnormal activities in cancer and can serve as a therapeutic target.

vascular endothelial growth factor (VEGF) pathway: pathway that often shows abnormal activities in cancer and can serve as a therapeutic target.

hypoxia inducible factor (HIF-1) pathway: pathway that often shows abnormal activities in cancer and can serve as a therapeutic target.

Myc pathway: pathway that often shows abnormal activities in cancer and can serve as a therapeutic target.

epithelial-to-mesenchymal transition (EMT) pathway: pathway that often shows abnormal activities in cancer and can serve as a therapeutic target.

DNA damage repair pathway: pathway that often shows abnormal activities in cancer and can serve as a therapeutic target.

KRAS: the most frequently mutated oncogene in human cancer.

cytotoxic T lymphocyte–associated antigen 4 (CTLA-4) pathway: pathway that often shows abnormal activities in cancer and can serve as a therapeutic target for immunologic checkpoint blockade.

programmed cell death protein 1 (PD-1/PD-L1) pathway: pathway that often shows abnormal activities in cancer and can serve as a therapeutic target for immunologic checkpoint blockade.

extracellular matrix (ECM): culture-plate medium for growing primary tumor cells.

explant cell culture: cell culture system that consists of explants of human normal and tumor tissues plated into coated plates and supplemented with essential nutrients for optimal growth.

sandwich culture: system that cultures tumor cells between two glass slides to provide a nutritionally deprived/hypoxic environment.

Hayflick limit: a limit of primary epithelial cell proliferation consisting of two restrictive phases of growth, senescence and agonescence.

agonescence: a restrictive phase of primary epithelial cell-culture growth.

monolayer: 2-D culture technique; lacks architectural diversity.

biomimetic scaffolds: biocompatible culture materials that mimic natural environmental conditions.

organoids: 3-D cultures that closely match the corresponding tumor biopsies.

small interfering RNA (siRNA): the most commonly used RNA interference tool for inducing short-term silencing of protein coding genes.

RNA-induced silencing complex (RISC): complex formed by use of siRNA that induces cleavage and degradation of the mRNA.

short hairpin RNA vector (shRNA): component of siRNA that can be used to silence target gene expression.

CRISPR-Cas9: a genome-editing technology adapted from a naturally occurring system in bacteria.

Trypan blue: one of several dyes recommended for use in dye exclusion procedures for viable cell counting.

apoptosis: process of programmed cell death.

Annexin V: type of stain used for cell-death assays.

Western blot: type of cell-death assay.

terminal transferase-mediated dUTP nick end labeling (TUNEL) assay: procedure used to determine apoptosis in cells and whole-tissue sections.

clonogenic assay or **colony formation assay:** a tool for testing whether a given cancer therapy can reduce the clonogenic survival of tumor cells after treatment with ionizing radiation.

combination index (CI): part of the Chou-Talalay method that offers a quantitative definition of an additive effect (CI = 1), synergism (CI < 1), and antagonism (CI > 1) in drug combinations.

synergy: a reaction operating on physiochemical mass action laws.

wound healing assay: test that permits the measurement of cell migration into a wound (cell-free area) created by a linear scratch across the surface of a tissue culture well containing a confluent monolayer of cells.

transwell chambers: apparatus consisting of an upper chamber and a lower well separated by a microporous membrane; used in cell migration assays.

microfluidic assay: test done by seeding cells into a chamber that is bridged to a second chamber by an internal microchannel.

Drosophila: flies commonly used as a nonmammalian animal model.

nematodes: *Caenorhabditis elegans*; commonly used as a nonmammalian animal model.

zebrafish: species commonly used as a nonmammalian animal model.

orthologs: genes from different species that evolve from a common ancestral gene by speciation

homologs: genes related by descent from a common ancestral DNA sequence.

orthotopic: in the same (*ortho*) place (*topos*).

athymic nude mice: mouse strain exhibiting various types of immune deficiency.

severely compromised immunodeficient (SCID) mice: mouse strain exhibiting various types of immune deficiency.

patient-derived xenograft (PDX): model developed by implanting chunks of cancerous tissue from a patient biopsy directly into an immunodeficient mouse.

nonobese diabetic (NOD)/SCID: type of immunodeficient mouse.

humanized mice: immunodeficient mice engrafted with human CD34+ hematopoietic stem cells or precursor cells; used for evaluating immune-targeting therapies for oncology.

oncomice: transgenic mice with cloned cancer cells.

genetically engineered mouse model (GEMM): oncomice.

tetracycline-controlled transcriptional activation (Tet-On): inducible system to achieve spatially and temporally controlled gene expression in specific tissues.

transactivator protein (rtTA): element of the Tet-On system.

tetracycline response element (TRE): element of the Tet-On system.

knockout: DNA construct that totally silences the target gene.

Cre enzyme: a site-specific recombinase that catalyzes specific recombination between two defined loxP sites.

clustered regularly interspaced short palindromic repeats (CRISPR): a component of a prokaryotic immune system that confers resistance to foreign genetic elements; used for gene editing.

CRISPR: *see clustered regularly interspaced short palindromic repeats.*

REFERENCES

1. Alkylating Agents. *United States Natioal Library of Medicine* (2017). https://livertox.nih.gov/AlkylatingAgents.htm
2. Kondo N, Takahashi A, Ono K, Ohnishi T. DNA damage induced by alkylating agents and repair pathways. *J Nucleic Acids*. 2010;2010:1–7. doi:10.4061/2010/543531
3. Peters GJ, van der Wilt CL, van Moorsel CJA, et al. Basis for effective combination cancer chemotherapy with antimetabolites. *Pharmacol Ther*. 2000;87:227–253. doi:10.1016/S0163-7258(00)00086-3
4. Antineoplastic Antimetabolites. *US National Library of Medicine Medical Subject Headings (MeSH)* (2017). https://www.ncbi.nlm.nih.gov/mesh?term=Antimetabolites,+Antineoplastic
5. Weiss RB. The anthracyclines: will we ever find a better doxorubicin? *Semin Oncol*. 1992;19:670–686.
6. Rabbani A, Finn RM, Ausio J. The anthracycline antibiotics: antitumor drugs that alter chromatin structure. *Bioessays*. 2004;27:50–56. doi:10.1002/bies.20160
7. Kittakoop P, Mahidol C, Ruchirawat S. Alkaloids as important scaffolds in therapeutic drugs for the treatments of cancer, tuberculosis, and smoking cessation. *Curr Top Med Chem*. 2014;14:239–252. doi:10.2174/1568026613666131216105049
8. Qiu S, Sun H, Zhang A-H, et al. Natural alkaloids: basic aspects, biological roles, and future perspectives. *Chin J Nat Med*. 2014;12:401–406. doi:10.1016/S1875-5364(14)60063-7
9. Yochum ZA, Cades J, Mazzacurati L, et al. A first-in-class TWIST1 inhibitor with activity in oncogene-driven lung cancer. *Mol Cancer Res*. 2017;15:1764–1776. doi:10.1158/1541-7786.MCR-17-0298
10. Singh M, Jadhav HR. Targeting non-small cell lung cancer with small-molecule EGFR tyrosine kinase inhibitors. *Drug Discov Today*. 2018;23:745–753. doi:10.1016/j.drudis.2017.10.004
11. Zhang J, Yang PL, Gray NS. Targeting cancer with small molecule kinase inhibitors. *Nat Rev Cancer*. 2009;9:28–39. doi:10.1038/nrc2559
12. Breedveld FC. Therapeutic monoclonal antibodies. *Lancet*. 2000;355:735–740. doi:10.1016/S0140-6736(00)01034-5
13. Stern M, Herrmann R. Overview of monoclonal antibodies in cancer therapy: present and promise. *Crit Rev Oncol Hematol*. 2005;54;11–29. doi:10.1016/j.critrevonc.2004.10.011
14. Sharma P, Allison JP. The future of immune checkpoint therapy. *Science*. 2015;348:56–61. doi:10.1126/science.aaa8172
15. Druker BJ, Tamura S, Buchdunger E, et al. Effects of a selective inhibitor of the Abl tyrosine kinase on the growth of Bcr-Abl positive cells. *Nat Med*. 1996;2:561–566. doi:10.1038/nm0596-561
16. Druker BJ, Talpaz M, Resta DJ, et al. Efficacy and safety of a specific inhibitor of the BCR-ABL tyrosine kinase in chronic myeloid leukemia. *N Engl J Med*. 2001;344:1031–1037. doi:10.1056/NEJM200104053441401
17. Holbro T, Hynes NE. ErbB receptors: directing key signaling networks throughout life. *Annu Rev Pharmacol Toxicol*. 2004;44:195–217. doi:10.1146/annurev.pharmtox.44.101802.121440
18. Gullick WJ. Prevalence of aberrant expression of the epidermal growth factor receptor in human cancers. *Br Med Bull*. 1991;47:87–98. doi:10.1093/oxfordjournals.bmb.a072464
19. Cohen MH, Williams GA, Sridhara R, et al. United States Food and Drug Administration Drug Approval summary: Gefitinib (ZD1839; Iressa) tablets. *Clin Cancer Res*. 2004;10:1212–1218. doi:10.1158/1078-0432.CCR-03-0564
20. Horn L, Sandler A. Epidermal growth factor receptor inhibitors and antiangiogenic agents for the treatment of non-small cell lung cancer. *Clin Cancer Res*. 2009;15:5040–5048. doi:10.1158/1078-0432.CCR-09-0520
21. Modjtahedi H, Cho BC, Michel MC, Solca F. A comprehensive review of the preclinical efficacy profile of the ErbB family blocker afatinib in cancer. *Naunyn Schmiedebergs Arch Pharmacol*. 2014;387:505–521. doi:10.1007/s00210-014-0967-3
22. Soejima K, Yasuda H, Hirano T. Osimertinib for EGFR T790M mutation-positive non-small cell lung cancer. *Expert Rev Clin Pharmacol*. 2017;10:31–38. doi:10.1080/17512433.2017.1265446
23. Gao X, Le X, Costa DB. The safety and efficacy of osimertinib for the treatment of EGFR T790M mutation positive non-small-cell lung cancer. *Expert Rev Anticancer Ther*. 2016;16:383–390. doi:10.1586/14737140.2016.1162103
24. Wong AL, Lee SC. Mechanisms of resistance to trastuzumab and novel therapeutic strategies in HER2-positive breast cancer. *Int J Breast Cancer*. 2012;2012:415170. doi:10.1155/2012/415170
25. Porta C, Paglino C, Mosca A. Targeting PI3K/Akt/mTOR signaling in cancer. *Front Oncol*. 2014;4:64. doi:10.3389/fonc.2014.00064
26. Kieran MW, Kalluri R, Cho YJ. The VEGF pathway in cancer and disease: responses, resistance, and the path forward. *Cold Spring Harb Perspect Med*. 2012;2:a006593. doi:10.1101/cshperspect.a006593
27. Semenza GL. Hypoxia-inducible factors: mediators of cancer progression and targets for cancer therapy. *Trends Pharmacol Sci*. 2012;33:207–214, doi:10.1016/j.tips.2012.01.005
28. Hsieh AL, Walton ZE, Altman BJ, et al. MYC and metabolism on the path to cancer. *Semin Cell Dev Biol*. 2015;43:11–21. doi:10.1016/j.semcdb.2015.08.003
29. Dang CV. MYC on the path to cancer. *Cell*. 2012;149:22–35. doi:10.1016/j.cell.2012.03.003
30. Ye X, Weinberg RA. Epithelial-mesenchymal plasticity: A central regulator of cancer progression. *Trends Cell Biol*. 2015;25:675–686. doi:10.1016/j.tcb.2015.07.012
31. Burns TF, Dobromilskaya I, Murphy SC, et al. Inhibition of TWIST1 leads to activation of oncogene-induced senescence in oncogene-driven non-small cell lung cancer. *Mol Cancer Res*. 2013;11:329–338. doi:10.1158/1541-7786.MCR-12-0456
32. Tran PT, Shroff EH, Burns TF, et al. Twist1 suppresses senescence programs and thereby accelerates and maintains mutant Kras-induced lung tumorigenesis. *PLoS Genet*. 2012;8:e1002650. doi:10.1371/journal.pgen.1002650
33. Malek R, Wang H, Taparra K, Tran PT. Therapeutic targeting of epithelial plasticity programs: focus on the epithelial-mesenchymal transition. *Cells Tissues Organs*. 2017;203:114–127. doi:10.1159/000447238
34. O'Connor MJ. Targeting the DNA damage response in cancer. *Mol Cell*. 2015;60:547–560. doi:10.1016/j.molcel.2015.10.040
35. Dietlein F, Thelen L, Reinhardt HC. Cancer-specific defects in DNA repair pathways as targets for personalized therapeutic approaches. *Trends Genet*. 2014;30;326–339. doi:10.1016/j.tig.2014.06.003
36. Han Z, Fu A, Wang H, et al. Noninvasive assessment of cancer response to therapy. *Nat Med*. 2008;14:343–349. doi:10.1038/nm1691

37. Wang H, Yan H, Fu A, et al. TIP-1 translocation onto the cell plasma membrane is a molecular biomarker of tumor response to ionizing radiation. *PLoS One*. 2010;5:e12051. doi:10.1371/journal.pone.0012051
38. Hariri G, Yan H, Wang H, et al. Radiation-guided drug delivery to mouse models of lung cancer. *Clin Cancer Res*. 2010;16:4968–4977. doi:10.1158/1078-0432.CCR-10-0969
39. Chettiar ST, Malek R, Annadanam A, et al. Ganetespib radiosensitization for liver cancer therapy. *Cancer Biol Ther*. 2016;17:457–466, doi:10.1080/15384047.2016.1156258
40. Ostrem JM, Shokat KM. Direct small-molecule inhibitors of KRAS: from structural insights to mechanism-based design. *Nat Rev Drug Discov*. 2016;15:771–785. doi:10.1038/nrd.2016.139
41. Cully M. Cancer: closing the door on KRAS-mutant lung cancer. *Nat Rev Drug Discov*. 2016;15:747. doi:10.1038/nrd.2016.216
42. Stephen AG, Esposito D, Bagni RK, McCormick F. Dragging ras back in the ring. *Cancer Cell*. 2014;25:272–281. doi:10.1016/j.ccr.2014.02.017
43. Cox AD, Fesik SW, Kimmelman AC, et al. Drugging the undruggable RAS: mission possible? *Nat Rev Drug Discov*. 2014;13:828–851. doi:10.1038/nrd4389
44. Topalian SL, Taube JM, Anders RA, Pardoll DM. Mechanism-driven biomarkers to guide immune checkpoint blockade in cancer therapy. *Nat Rev Cancer*. 2016;16:275–287. doi:10.1038/nrc.2016.36
45. Topalian SL, Drake CG, Pardoll DM. Immune checkpoint blockade: a common denominator approach to cancer therapy. *Cancer Cell*. 2015;27:450–461 doi:10.1016/j.ccell.2015.03.001
46. Postow MA, Callahan MK, Wolchok JD. Immune checkpoint blockade in cancer therapy. *J Clin Oncol*. 2015;33:1974–1982. doi:10.1200/JCO.2014.59.4358
47. Kurz H, Sandau K, Christ B. On the bifurcation of blood vessels–Wilhelm Roux's doctoral thesis (Jena 1878)–a seminal work for biophysical modelling in developmental biology. *Ann Anat*. 1997;179:33–36. doi:10.1016/S0940-9602(97)80132-X
48. Li WC, Ralphs KL, Tosh D. Isolation and culture of adult mouse hepatocytes. *Methods Mol Biol*. 2010;633:185–196. doi:10.1007/978-1-59745-019-5_13
49. Ljung BM, Mayall B, Lottich C, et al. Cell dissociation techniques in human breast cancer--variations in tumor cell viability and DNA ploidy. *Breast Cancer Res Treat*. 1989;13:153–159. doi:10.1007/BF01806527
50. Mitaka T. The current status of primary hepatocyte culture. *Int J Exp Pathol*. 1998;79:393–409. doi:10.1046/j.1365-2613.1998.00083.x
51. Mitra R, Morad M. A uniform enzymatic method for dissociation of myocytes from hearts and stomachs of vertebrates. *Am J Physiol*. 1985;249:H1056–H1060. doi:10.1152/ajpheart.1985.249.5.H1056
52. *Introduction to Enzymes*. Lakewood, NJ: WB Corporation. http://www.worthington-biochem.com/introbiochem/introEnzymes.html
53. Torsvik A, Stieber D, Enger PO, et al. U-251 revisited: genetic drift and phenotypic consequences of long-term cultures of glioblastoma cells. *Cancer Med*. 2014;3:812–824. doi:10.1002/cam4.219
54. Pei XF, Noble MS, Davoli MA, et al. Explant-cell culture of primary mammary tumors from MMTV-c-Myc transgenic mice. *In Vitro Cell Dev Biol Anim*. 2004;40:14–21. doi:10.1290/1543-706X(2004)40<14:ECOPMT>2.0.CO;2
55. Johnson TV, Martin KR. Development and characterization of an adult retinal explant organotypic tissue culture system as an in vitro intraocular stem cell transplantation model. *Invest Ophthalmol Vis Sci*. 2008;49:3503–3512. doi:10.1167/iovs.07-1601
56. Natalie Bull TJ, Martin K. Organotypic explant culture of adult rat retina for in vitro investigations of neurodegeneration, neuroprotection and cell transplantation. *Protoc Exch*. 2011. doi:10.1038/protex.2011.215
57. Dairkee SH, Deng G, Stampfer MR, et al. Selective cell culture of primary breast carcinoma. *Cancer Res*. 1995;55:2516–2519.
58. Liu X, Ory V, Chapman S, et al. ROCK inhibitor and feeder cells induce the conditional reprogramming of epithelial cells. *Am J Pathol*. 2012;180:599–607. doi:10.1016/j.ajpath.2011.10.036
59. Hayflick L, Moorhead PS. The serial cultivation of human diploid cell strains. *Exp Cell Res*. 1961;25:585–621. doi:10.1016/0014-4827(61)90192-6
60. Shay JW, Wright WE, Werbin H. Defining the molecular mechanisms of human cell immortalization. *Biochimica Et Biophysica Acta*. 1991;1072:1–7. doi:10.1016/0304-419x(91)90003-4
61. Campisi J, d'Adda di Fagagna F. Cellular senescence: when bad things happen to good cells. *Nat Rev Mol Cell Biol*. 2007;8:729–740. doi:10.1038/nrm2233
62. Romanov SR, Kozakiewicz BK, Holst CR, et al. Normal human mammary epithelial cells spontaneously escape senescence and acquire genomic changes. *Nature*. 2001;409:633–637. doi:10.1038/35054579
63. Hawley-Nelson P, Vousden KH, Hubbert NL, et al. HPV16 E6 and E7 proteins cooperate to immortalize human foreskin keratinocytes. *EMBO J*. 1989;8:3905–3910.
64. Yuan H, Myers S, Wang J, et al. Use of reprogrammed cells to identify therapy for respiratory papillomatosis. *N Engl J Med*. 2012;367:1220–1227. doi:10.1056/NEJMoa1203055
65. Crystal AS, Shaw AT, Sequist LV, et al. Patient-derived models of acquired resistance can identify effective drug combinations for cancer. *Science*. 2014;346:1480–1486. doi:10.1126/science.1254721
66. Sterneckert JL, Reinhardt P, Scholer HR. Investigating human disease using stem cell models. *Nat Rev Genet*. 2014;15:625–639. doi:10.1038/nrg3764
67. Kim JB, Stein R, O'Hare MJ. Three-dimensional in vitro tissue culture models of breast cancer—a review. *Breast Cancer Res Treat*. 2004;85:281–291. doi:10.1023/B:BREA.0000025418.88785.2b
68. Jechlinger M, Podsypanina K, Varmus H. Regulation of transgenes in three-dimensional cultures of primary mouse mammary cells demonstrates oncogene dependence and identifies cells that survive deinduction. *Genes Dev*. 2009;23:1677–1688. doi:10.1101/gad.1801809
69. Malinen MM, Palokangas H, Yliperttula M, Urtti A. Peptide nanofiber hydrogel induces formation of bile canaliculi structures in three-dimensional hepatic cell culture. *Tissue Eng*. 2012;18:2418–2425. doi:10.1089/ten.TEA.2012.0046

70. Fischbach C, Chen R, Matsumoto T, et al. Engineering tumors with 3D scaffolds. *Nat Methods*. 2007;4:855–860. doi:10.1038/nmeth1085
71. Berdichevsky F, Alford D, D'Souza B, Taylor-Papadimitriou J. Branching morphogenesis of human mammary epithelial cells in collagen gels. *J Cell Sci*. 1994;107(Pt 12):3557–3568.
72. Andree B, Bar A, Haverich A, Hilfiker A. Small intestinal submucosa segments as matrix for tissue engineering: review. *Tissue Eng*. 2013;19:279–291. doi:10.1089/ten.TEB.2012.0583
73. Fridman R, Benton G, Aranoutova I, et al. Increased initiation and growth of tumor cell lines, cancer stem cells and biopsy material in mice using basement membrane matrix protein (Cultrex or Matrigel) co-injection. *Nature Protoc*. 2012;7:1138–1144. doi:10.1038/nprot.2012.053
74. van de Wetering M, Francies HE, Francis JM, et al. Prospective derivation of a living organoid biobank of colorectal cancer patients. *Cell*. 2015;161:933–945. doi:10.1016/j.cell.2015.03.053
75. Boj SF, Hwang C-I, Baker LA, et al. Organoid models of human and mouse ductal pancreatic cancer. *Cell*. 2015;160:324–338. doi:10.1016/j.cell.2014.12.021
76. Gao D, Vela I, Sboner A, et al. Organoid cultures derived from patients with advanced prostate cancer. *Cell*. 2014;159:176–187. doi:10.1016/j.cell.2014.08.016
77. Hamilton AJ, Baulcombe DC. A species of small antisense RNA in posttranscriptional gene silencing in plants. *Science*. 1999;286:950–952.
78. Elbashir SM, Harborth J, Lendeckel W, et al. Duplexes of 21-nucleotide RNAs mediate RNA interference in cultured mammalian cells. *Nature*. 2001;411:494–498. doi:10.1038/35078107
79. Brazas RM, Hagstrom JE. Delivery of small interfering RNA to mammalian cells in culture by using cationic lipid/polymer-based transfection reagents. *Methods Enzymol*. 2005;392:112–124. doi:10.1016/S0076-6879(04)92007-1
80. siRNA Delivery Methods into Mammalian Cells. *QIAGEN*. https://www.qiagen.com/kr/resources/molecular-biology-methods/transfection/#Guidelines%20for%20transfection%20of%20siRNA
81. Morris KV, Rossi JJ. Lentiviral-mediated delivery of siRNAs for antiviral therapy. *Gene Ther*. 2006;13:553–558. doi:10.1038/sj.gt.3302688
82. Shen H, Sun T, Ferrari M. Nanovector delivery of siRNA for cancer therapy. *Cancer Gene Ther*. 2012;19:367–373. doi:10.1038/cgt.2012.22
83. Doudna JA, Charpentier E. Genome editing. The new frontier of genome engineering with CRISPR-Cas9. *Science*. 2014;346:1258096. doi:10.1126/science.1258096
84. Hsu PD, Lander ES, Zhang F. Development and applications of CRISPR-Cas9 for genome engineering. *Cell*. 2014;157:1262–1278. doi:10.1016/j.cell.2014.05.010
85. Kim K, Park SW, Kim JH, et al. Genome surgery using Cas9 ribonucleoproteins for the treatment of age-related macular degeneration. *Genome Res*. 2017;27:419–426. doi:10.1101/gr.219089.116
86. Yang L, Guell M, Niu D, et al. Genome-wide inactivation of porcine endogenous retroviruses (PERVs). *Science*. 2015;350:1101–1104. doi:10.1126/science.aad1191
87. DeWitt MA, Magis W, Bray NL, et al. Selection-free genome editing of the sickle mutation in human adult hematopoietic stem/progenitor cells. *Science Trans Med*. 2016;8:360ra134. doi:10.1126/scitranslmed.aaf9336
88. Schwank G, Koo B-K, Sasselli V, et al. Functional repair of CFTR by CRISPR/Cas9 in intestinal stem cell organoids of cystic fibrosis patients. *Cell Stem Cell*. 2013;13:653–658. doi:10.1016/j.stem.2013.11.002
89. Nguyen TH, Anegon I. Successful correction of hemophilia by CRISPR/Cas9 genome editing in vivo: delivery vector and immune responses are the key to success. *EMBO Mol Med*. 2016;8:439–441. doi:10.15252/emmm.201606325
90. Cyranoski D. CRISPR gene-editing tested in a person for the first time. *Nature*. 2-16;539:479. doi:10.1038/nature.2016.20988
91. Le Page M. Boom in human gene editing as 20 CRISPR trials gear up. *New Scientist*. 2017.
92. Ivanov AA, Khuri FR, Fu H. Targeting protein-protein interactions as an anticancer strategy. *Trends Pharmacol Sci*. 2013;34:393–400. doi:10.1016/j.tips.2013.04.007
93. Jhaveri K, Modi S. Ganetespib: research and clinical development. *OncoTargets Ther*. 2015;8:1849–1858. doi:10.2147/OTT.S65804
94. Ellis LM. Bevacizumab. *Nat Rev Drug Discov*. 2005;4:S8–S9. doi:10.1038/nrd1727
95. Muhsin M, Graham J, Kirkpatrick P. Bevacizumab. *Nat Rev Drug Discov*. 2004;3:995–996. doi:10.1038/nrd1601
96. Goldberg RM. Cetuximab. *Nat Rev Drug Discov*. 2005;4:S10–S11. doi:10.1038/nrd1728
97. Graham J, Muhsin M, Kirkpatrick P. Cetuximab. *Nat Rev Drug Discov*. 2004;3:549–550. doi:10.1038/nrd1445
98. Stoddart MJ. Cell viability assays: introduction. *Methods Mol Biol*. 2011;740:1–6. doi:10.1007/978-1-61779-108-6_1
99. Strober W. Trypan blue exclusion test of cell viability. *Curr Protoc Immunol*. 2001;Appendix 3:Appendix 3B. doi:10.1002/0471142735.ima03bs21
100. Miller MW, Nowakowski RS. Use of bromodeoxyuridine-immunohistochemistry to examine the proliferation, migration and time of origin of cells in the central nervous system. *Brain Res*. 1988;457:44–52.
101. Mosmann T. Rapid colorimetric assay for cellular growth and survival: application to proliferation and cytotoxicity assays. *J Immunol Methods*. 1983;65:55–63. doi:10.1016/0022-1759(83)90303-4
102. Liu Y, Peterson DA, Kimura H, Schubert D. Mechanism of cellular 3-(4,5-dimethylthiazol-2-yl)-2,5-diphenyltetrazolium bromide (MTT) reduction. *J Neurochem*. 2002;69:581–593. doi:10.1046/j.1471-4159.1997.69020581.x
103. Scudiero DA, Shoemaker RH, Paull KD, et al. Evaluation of a soluble tetrazolium/formazan assay for cell growth and drug sensitivity in culture using human and other tumor cell lines. *Cancer Res*. 1988;48:4827–4833.
104. Schmid I, Krall WJ, Uittenbogaart CH, et al. Dead cell discrimination with 7-amino-actinomycin D in combination with dual color immunofluorescence in single laser flow cytometry. *Cytometry*. 1992;13:204–208. doi:10.1002/cyto.990130216
105. Koopman G, Reutelingsperger CP, Kuijten GA, et al. Annexin V for flow cytometric detection of phosphatidylserine expression on B cells undergoing apoptosis. *Blood*. 1994;84:1415–1420.
106. Kurokawa M, Kornbluth S. Caspases and kinases in a death grip. *Cell*. 2009;138:838–854. doi:10.1016/j.cell.2009.08.021

107. Gavrieli Y, Sherman Y, Ben-Sasson SA. Identification of programmed cell death in situ via specific labeling of nuclear DNA fragmentation. *J Cell Biol.* 1992;119:493–501. doi:10.1083/jcb.119.3.493
108. Kudriashov Iu B, Parkhomenko IM. Molecular-cellular mechanisms of the biological action of low x-ray doses on isolated mammalian cells. *Radiobiologiia.* 1987;27:297–302.
109. Castedo M, Perfettini J-L, Roumier T, et al. Cell death by mitotic catastrophe: a molecular definition. *Oncogene.* 2004;23:2825–2837. doi:10.1038/sj.onc.1207528
110. Brown JM, Attardi LD. The role of apoptosis in cancer development and treatment response. *Nat Rev Cancer.* 2005;5:231–237. doi:10.1038/nrc1560
111. Proskuryakov SY, Konoplyannikov AG, Gabai VL. Necrosis: a specific form of programmed cell death? *Exp Cell Res.* 2003;283:1–16. doi:10.1016/S0014-4827(02)00027-7
112. Franken NA, Rodermond HM, Stap J, et al. Clonogenic assay of cells in vitro. *Nat Protoc.* 2006;1:2315–2319. doi:10.1038/nprot.2006.339
113. Zhou C, Wu, Y-L, Chen G, et al. Erlotinib versus chemotherapy as first-line treatment for patients with advanced EGFR mutation-positive non-small-cell lung cancer (OPTIMAL, CTONG-0802): a multicentre, open-label, randomised, phase 3 study. *Lancet Oncol.* 2011;12:735–742. doi:10.1016/S1470-2045(11)70184-X
114. Rotow J, Bivona TG. Understanding and targeting resistance mechanisms in NSCLC. *Nat Rev Cancer.* 2017;17:637–658. doi:10.1038/nrc.2017.84
115. Palmer AC, Sorger PK. Combination cancer therapy can confer benefit via patient-to-patient variability without drug additivity or synergy. *Cell.* 2017;171:1678–1691. doi:10.1016/j.cell.2017.11.009
116. Humphrey RW, Brockway-Lunardi LM, Bonk DT, et al. Opportunities and challenges in the development of experimental drug combinations for cancer. *J Natl Cancer Inst.* 2011;103:1222–1226. doi:10.1093/jnci/djr246
117. Greco WR, Bravo G, Parsons JC. The search for synergy: a critical review from a response surface perspective. *Pharmacol Rev.* 1995;47:331–385.
118. Chou TC. Theoretical basis, experimental design, and computerized simulation of synergism and antagonism in drug combination studies. *Pharmacol Rev.* 2006;58:621–681. doi:10.1124/pr.58.3.10
119. Geary N. Understanding synergy. *Am J Physiol Endocrinol Metab.* 2013;304:E237–E253. doi:10.1152/ajpendo.00308.2012
120. Chou TC, Talalay P. Quantitative analysis of dose-effect relationships: the combined effects of multiple drugs or enzyme inhibitors. *Adv Enzyme Regul.* 1984;22:27–55.
121. Chou TC. Drug combination studies and their synergy quantification using the Chou-Talalay method. *Cancer Res.* 2010;70:440–446. doi:10.1158/0008-5472.CAN-09-1947
122. Twigger K, Vidal L, White CL, et al. Enhanced in vitro and in vivo cytotoxicity of combined reovirus and radiotherapy. *Clin Cancer Res.* 2008;14:912–923. doi:10.1158/1078-0432.CCR-07-1400
123. Roussos ET, Condeelis JS, Patsialou A. Chemotaxis in cancer. *Nat Rev Cancer.* 2011;11:573–587. doi:10.1038/nrc3078
124. Palmer TD, Ashby WJ, Lewis JD, Zijlstra A. Targeting tumor cell motility to prevent metastasis. *Adv Drug Deliv Rev.* 2011;63:568–581. doi:10.1016/j.addr.2011.04.008
125. Cory G. Scratch-wound assay. *Methods Mol Biol.* 2011;769:25–30. doi:10.1007/978-1-61779-207-6_2
126. Liang CC, Park AY, Guan JL. In vitro scratch assay: a convenient and inexpensive method for analysis of cell migration in vitro. *Nat Protoc.* 2007;2:329–333. doi:10.1038/nprot.2007.30
127. Nie FQ, Yamada M, Kobayashi J, et al. On-chip cell migration assay using microfluidic channels. *Biomaterials.* 2007;28:4017–4022. doi:10.1016/j.biomaterials.2007.05.037
128. Tipping M, Perrimon N. Drosophila as a model for context-dependent tumorigenesis. *J Cell Physiol.* 2014;229:27–33. doi:10.1002/jcp.24427
129. Perrimon N, Pitsouli C, Shilo BZ. Signaling mechanisms controlling cell fate and embryonic patterning. *Cold Spring Harb Perspect Biol.* 2012;4:a005975. doi:10.1101/cshperspect.a005975
130. Jaklevic B, Uyetake L, Lemstra W, et al. Contribution of growth and cell cycle checkpoints to radiation survival in Drosophila. *Genetics.* 2006;174:1963–1972. doi:10.1534/genetics.106.064477
131. Kirienko NV, Mani K, Fay DS. Cancer models in Caenorhabditis elegans. *Dev Dyn.* 2010;239:1413–1448. doi:10.1002/dvdy.22247
132. van den Heuvel S. The C. elegans cell cycle: overview of molecules and mechanisms. *Methods Mol Biol.* 2005;296:51–67.
133. Sulston JE, Schierenberg E, White JG, Thomson JN. The embryonic cell lineage of the nematode Caenorhabditis elegans. *Dev Biol.* 1983;100:64–119. doi:10.1016/0012-1606(83)90201-4
134. Gore AV, Monzo K, Cha YR, et al. Vascular development in the zebrafish. *Cold Spring Harb Perspect Med.* 2012;2:a006684. doi:10.1101/cshperspect.a006684
135. Kanungo J, Cuevas E, Ali SF, Paule MG. Zebrafish model in drug safety assessment. *Curr Pharm Des.* 2014;20:5416–5429.
136. Kalueff AV, Stewart AM, Gerlai R. Zebrafish as an emerging model for studying complex brain disorders. *Trends Pharmacol Sci.* 2014;35:63–75. doi:10.1016/j.tips.2013.12.002
137. Guyon JR, Steffen LS, Howell MH, et al. Modeling human muscle disease in zebrafish. *Biochim Biophys Acta.* 2007;1772:205–215. doi:10.1016/j.bbadis.2006.07.003
138. Lieschke GJ, Oates AC, Crowhurst MO, et al. Morphologic and functional characterization of granulocytes and macrophages in embryonic and adult zebrafish. *Blood.* 2001;98:3087–3096. doi:10.1182/blood.V98.10.3087
139. Santoriello C, Zon LI. Hooked! Modeling human disease in zebrafish. *J Clin Invest.* 2012;122:2337–2343. doi:10.1172/JCI60434
140. Blackburn JS, Langenau DM. Zebrafish as a model to assess cancer heterogeneity, progression and relapse. *Dis Model Mech.* 2014;7:755–762. doi:10.1242/dmm.015842
141. Mione MC, Trede NS. The zebrafish as a model for cancer. *Dis Model Mech.* 2010;3:517–523. doi:10.1242/dmm.004747
142. Park SW, Davison JM, Rhee J, et al. Oncogenic KRAS induces progenitor cell expansion and malignant transformation in zebrafish exocrine pancreas. *Gastroenterol.* 2008;134:2080–2090. doi:10.1053/j.gastro.2008.02.084

143. Ju B, Spitsbergen J, Eden CJ, et al. Co-activation of hedgehog and AKT pathways promote tumorigenesis in zebrafish. *Mol Cancer*. 2009;8:40. doi:10.1186/1476-4598-8-40
144. Phelps RA, Chidester S, Dehghanizadeh S, et al. A two-step model for colon adenoma initiation and progression caused by APC loss. *Cell*. 2009;137:623–634. doi:10.1016/j.cell.2009.02.037
145. Schartl M, Wilde B, Laisney JAGC, et al. A mutated EGFR is sufficient to induce malignant melanoma with genetic background-dependent histopathologies. *J Invest Dermatol*. 2010;130:249–258. doi:10.1038/jid.2009.213
146. Dovey M, White RM, Zon LI. Oncogenic NRAS cooperates with p53 loss to generate melanoma in zebrafish. *Zebrafish*. 2009;6:397–404. doi:10.1089/zeb.2009.0606
147. Patton EE, Widlund HR, Kutok JL, et al. BRAF mutations are sufficient to promote nevi formation and cooperate with p53 in the genesis of melanoma. *Curr Biol*. 2005;15:249–254. doi:10.1016/j.cub.2005.01.031
148. Langenau DM, Traver D, Ferrando AA, et al. Myc-induced T cell leukemia in transgenic zebrafish. *Science*. 2003;299:887–890. doi:10.1126/science.1080280
149. Sabaawy HE, Azuma M, Embree LJ, et al. TEL-AML1 transgenic zebrafish model of precursor B cell acute lymphoblastic leukemia. *Proc Natl Acad Sci U S A*. 2006;103:15166–15171. doi:10.1073/pnas.0603349103
150. Chen J, Jette C, Kanki JP, et al. NOTCH1-induced T-cell leukemia in transgenic zebrafish. *Leukemia*. 2007;21:462–471. doi:10.1038/sj.leu.2404546
151. Lunardi A, Nardella C, Clohessy JG, Pandolfi PP. Of model pets and cancer models: an introduction to mouse models of cancer. *Cold Spring Harb Protoc*. 2014;2014:17–31. doi:10.1101/pdb.top069757
152. Bock BC, Stein U, Schmitt CA, Augustin HG. Mouse models of human cancer. *Cancer Res*. 2014;74:4671–4675. doi:10.1158/0008-5472.CAN-14-1424
153. Morton CL, Houghton PJ. Establishment of human tumor xenografts in immunodeficient mice. *Nat Protoc*. 2007;2:247–250. doi:10.1038/nprot.2007.25
154. Pantelouris EM. Absence of thymus in a mouse mutant. *Nature*. 1986;217:370–371.
155. Bosma MJ, Carroll AM. The SCID mouse mutant: definition, characterization, and potential uses. *Annu Rev Immunol*. 1991;9:323–350. doi:10.1146/annurev.iy.09.040191.001543
156. Rygaard J, Povlsen CO. Heterotransplantation of a human malignant tumour to "Nude" mice. *Acta Pathol Microbiol Scand*. 1969;77:758–760. doi:10.1111/j.1699-0463.1969.tb04520.x
157. Masters JR. HeLa cells 50 years on: the good, the bad and the ugly. *Nat Rev Cancer*. 2002;2:315–319. doi:10.1038/nrc775
158. Frattini A, Fabbri M, Valli R, et al. High variability of genomic instability and gene expression profiling in different HeLa clones. *Sci Rep*. 2015;5:15377. doi:10.1038/srep15377
159. Hidalgo M, et al. Patient-derived xenograft models: an emerging platform for translational cancer research. *Cancer Disc*. 2014;4:998–1013. doi:10.1158/2159-8290.CD-14-0001
160. Siolas D, Hannon GJ. Patient-derived tumor xenografts: transforming clinical samples into mouse models. *Cancer Res*. 2013;73:5315–5319. doi:10.1158/0008-5472.CAN-13-1069
161. Julien S, Merino-Trigo A, Lacroix L, et al. Characterization of a large panel of patient-derived tumor xenografts representing the clinical heterogeneity of human colorectal cancer. *Clin Cancer Res*. 2012;18:5314–5328. doi:10.1158/1078-0432.CCR-12-0372
162. Weroha SJ, Becker MA, Enderica-Gonzalez S, et al. Tumorgrafts as in vivo surrogates for women with ovarian cancer. *Clin Cancer Res*. 2014;20:1288–1297. doi:10.1158/1078-0432.CCR-13-2611
163. Zhao X, Liu Z, Yu L, et al. Global gene expression profiling confirms the molecular fidelity of primary tumor-based orthotopic xenograft mouse models of medulloblastoma. *Neurooncol*. 2012;14:574–583. doi:10.1093/neuonc/nos061
164. Aparicio S, Hidalgo M, Kung AL. Examining the utility of patient-derived xenograft mouse models. *Nat Rev Cancer*. 2015;15:311–316. doi:10.1038/nrc3944
165. Drake AC, Chen Q, Chen J. Engineering humanized mice for improved hematopoietic reconstitution. *Cell Mol Immunol*. 2012;9:215–224. doi:10.1038/cmi.2012.6
166. Holzapfel BM, Wagner F, Thibaudeau L, et al. Concise review: humanized models of tumor immunology in the 21st century: convergence of cancer research and tissue engineering. *Stem Cells*. 2015;33:1696–1704. doi:10.1002/stem.1978
167. Hanahan D, Wagner EF, Palmiter RD. The origins of oncomice: a history of the first transgenic mice genetically engineered to develop cancer. *Genes Dev*. 2007;21:2258–2270. doi:10.1101/gad.1583307
168. Sinn E, Muller W, Pattengale P, et al. Coexpression of MMTV/v-Ha-ras and MMTV/c-myc genes in transgenic mice: synergistic action of oncogenes in vivo. *Cell*. 1987;49:465–475. doi:10.1016/0092-8674(87)90449-1
169. Singh M, Murriel CL, Johnson L. Genetically engineered mouse models: closing the gap between preclinical data and trial outcomes. *Cancer Res*. 2012;72:2695–2700. doi:10.1158/0008-5472.CAN-11-2786
170. Gordon JW, Scangos GA, Plotkin DJ, et al. Genetic transformation of mouse embryos by microinjection of purified DNA. *Proc Nat Acad Sci U S A*. 1980;77:7380–7384. doi:10.1073/pnas.77.12.7380
171. Gossen M, Bujard H. Tight control of gene expression in mammalian cells by tetracycline-responsive promoters. *Proc Nat Acad Sci U S A*. 1992;89:5547–5551. doi:10.1073/pnas.89.12.5547
172. Thomas KR, Capecchi MR. Site-directed mutagenesis by gene targeting in mouse embryo-derived stem cells. *Cell*. 1987;51:503–512. doi:10.1016/0092-8674(87)90646-5
173. Branda CS, Dymecki SM. Talking about a revolution: the impact of site-specific recombinases on genetic analyses in mice. *Dev Cell*. 2004;6:7–28. doi:10.1016/S1534-5807(03)00399-X
174. Jackson EL, Wills N, Mercer K, et al. Analysis of lung tumor initiation and progression using conditional expression of oncogenic K-ras. *Genes Dev*. 2001;15:3243–3248. doi:10.1101/gad.943001
175. Marumoto T, Tashiro A, Friedmann-Morvinski D, et al. Development of a novel mouse glioma model using lentiviral vectors. *Nature Med*. 2009;15:110–116. doi:10.1038/nm.1863
176. Jasin M, Berg P. Homologous integration in mammalian cells without target gene selection. *Genes Dev*. 1988;2:1353–1363. doi:10.1101/gad.2.11.1353

177. Cong L, Ran FA, Cox D, et al. Multiplex genome engineering using CRISPR/Cas systems. *Science*. 2013;339:819–823. doi:10.1126/science.1231143
178. Mojica FJ, Diez-Villasenor C, Soria E, Juez, G. Biological significance of a family of regularly spaced repeats in the genomes of Archaea, Bacteria and mitochondria. *Mol Microbiol*. 2000;36:244–246. doi:10.1046/j.1365-2958.2000.01838.x
179. Jansen R, Embden JD, Gaastra W, Schouls LM. Identification of genes that are associated with DNA repeats in prokaryotes. *Mol Microbiol*. 2002;43:1565–1575. doi:10.1046/j.1365-2958.2002.02839.x
180. Yang H, Wang H, Jaenisch R. Generating genetically modified mice using CRISPR/Cas-mediated genome engineering. *Nat Protoc*. 2014;9:1956–1968. doi:10.1038/nprot.2014.134
181. Cong L, Zhang F. Genome engineering using CRISPR-Cas9 system. *Methods Mol Biol*. 2015;1239:197–217. doi:10.1007/978-1-4939-1862-1_10
182. Sanchez-Rivera FJ, Jacks, T. Applications of the CRISPR-Cas9 system in cancer biology. *Nat Rev Cancer*. 2015;15:387–395. doi:10.1038/nrc3950
183. Yang H, Wang H, Shivalila CS, et al. One-step generation of mice carrying reporter and conditional alleles by CRISPR/Cas-mediated genome engineering. *Cell*. 2013;154:1370–1379. doi:10.1016/j.cell.2013.08.022
184. Wang H, Yang H, Shivalila CS, et al. One-step generation of mice carrying mutations in multiple genes by CRISPR/Cas-mediated genome engineering. *Cell*. 2013;153:910–918. doi:10.1016/j.cell.2013.04.025
185. Zetsche B, Heidenreich M, Mohanraju P, et al. Multiplex gene editing by CRISPR-Cpf1 using a single crRNA array. *Nat Biotechnol*. 2017;35:31–34. doi:10.1038/nbt.3737
186. Konermann S, Brigham MD, Trevino AE, et al. Genome-scale transcriptional activation by an engineered CRISPR-Cas9 complex. *Nature*. 2015;517:583–588. doi:10.1038/nature14136
187. Xue W, Chen S, Yin H, et al. CRISPR-mediated direct mutation of cancer genes in the mouse liver. *Nature*. 2014;514:380–384. doi:10.1038/nature13589
188. Blasco RB, Karaca E, Ambrogio C, et al. Simple and rapid in vivo generation of chromosomal rearrangements using CRISPR/Cas9 technology. *Cell Rep*. 2014;9:1219–1227. doi:10.1016/j.celrep.2014.10.051
189. Choi PS, Meyerson M. Targeted genomic rearrangements using CRISPR/Cas technology. *Nature Commun*. 2014;5:3728. doi:10.1038/ncomms4728
190. Torres R, Martin MC, Garcia A, et al. Engineering human tumour-associated chromosomal translocations with the RNA-guided CRISPR-Cas9 system. *Nature Commun*. 2014;5:3964. doi:10.1038/ncomms4964
191. Sanchez-Rivera FJ, Papagiannakopoulos T, Romero R, et al. Rapid modelling of cooperating genetic events in cancer through somatic genome editing. *Nature*. 2014;516:428–431. doi:10.1038/nature13906
192. Platt RJ, Chen S, Zhou Y, et al. CRISPR-Cas9 knockin mice for genome editing and cancer modeling. *Cell*. 2014;159:440–455. doi:10.1016/j.cell.2014.09.014
193. Weber J, Öllinger R, Friedrich M, et al. CRISPR/Cas9 somatic multiplex-mutagenesis for high-throughput functional cancer genomics in mice. *Proc Natl Acad Sci U S A*. 2015;112:13982–13987. doi:10.1073/pnas.1512392112
194. Chiou SH, Winters IP, Wang J, et al. Pancreatic cancer modeling using retrograde viral vector delivery and in vivo CRISPR/Cas9-mediated somatic genome editing. *Genes Dev*. 2015;29:1576–1585. doi:10.1101/gad.264861.115
195. Maresch R, Mueller S, Veltkamp C, et al. Multiplexed pancreatic genome engineering and cancer induction by transfection-based CRISPR/Cas9 delivery in mice. *Nature Commun*. 2016;7:10770. doi:10.1038/ncomms10770
196. Zuckermann M, Hovestadt V, Knobbe-Thomsen CB, et al. Somatic CRISPR/Cas9-mediated tumour suppressor disruption enables versatile brain tumour modelling. *Nature Commun*. 2015;6:7391. doi:10.1038/ncomms8391
197. Annunziato S, Kas SM, Nethe M, et al. Modeling invasive lobular breast carcinoma by CRISPR/Cas9-mediated somatic genome editing of the mammary gland. *Genes Dev*. 2016;30:1470–1480. doi:10.1101/gad.279190.116
198. Zetsche B, Volz SE, Zhang F. A split-Cas9 architecture for inducible genome editing and transcription modulation. *Nat Biotechnol*. 2015;33:139–142. doi:10.1038/nbt.3149
199. Joung J, Konermann S, Gootenberg JS, et al. Genome-scale CRISPR-Cas9 knockout and transcriptional activation screening. *Nat Protoc*. 2017;12:828–863. doi:10.1038/nprot.2017.016
200. Gilbert LA, Larson MH, Morsut L, et al. CRISPR-mediated modular RNA-guided regulation of transcription in eukaryotes. *Cell*. 2013;154:442–451. doi:10.1016/j.cell.2013.06.044
201. Aitman TJ, Critser JK, Cuppen E, et al. Progress and prospects in rat genetics: a community view. *Nat Genet*. 2008;40:516–522. doi:10.1038/ng.147
202. Szpirer C, Szpirer J. Mammary cancer susceptibility: human genes and rodent models. *Mamm Genome*. 2007;18:817–831. doi:10.1007/s00335-007-9073-x
203. Hougen HP, Klausen B. Effects of homozygosity of the nude (rnu) gene in an inbred strain of rats: studies of lymphoid and non--lymphoid organs in different age groups of nude rats of LEW background at a stage in the gene transfer. *Lab Anim*. 1984;18:7–14. doi:10.1258/002367784780865018
204. Chapman KM, Medrano GA, Jaichander P, et al. Targeted germline modifications in rats using CRISPR/Cas9 and spermatogonial stem cells. *Cell Rep*. 2015;10:1828–1835. doi:10.1016/j.celrep.2015.02.040
205. Tsuchida T, Zheng YW, Zhang RR, et al. The development of humanized liver with Rag1 knockout rats. *Transplant Proc*. 2014;46:1191–1193. doi:10.1016/j.transproceed.2013.12.026
206. Mashimo T, Takizawa A, Kobayashi J, et al. Generation and characterization of severe combined immunodeficiency rats. *Cell Rep*. 2012;2:685–694. doi:10.1016/j.celrep.2012.08.009
207. Mashimo T, Takizawa A, Voigt B, et al. Generation of knockout rats with X-linked severe combined immunodeficiency (X-SCID) using zinc-finger nucleases. *PloS One*. 2010;5:e8870. doi:10.1371/journal.pone.0008870
208. Colston MJ, Fieldsteel AH, Dawson PJ. Growth and regression of human tumor cell lines in congenitally athymic (rnu/rnu) rats. *J Natl Canc Inst*. 1981;66:843-848.
209. Maruo K, Ueyama Y, Kuwahara Y, et al. Human tumour xenografts in athymic rats and their age dependence. *Br J Cancer*. 1982;45:786–789. doi:10.1038/bjc.1982.122

210. Takenaka K, Prasolava TK, Wang JCY, et al. Polymorphism in Sirpa modulates engraftment of human hematopoietic stem cells. *Nat Immunol.* 2007;8:1313–1323. doi:10.1038/ni1527
211. Swindle MM, Makin A, Herron AJ, et al. Swine as models in biomedical research and toxicology testing. *Vet Pathol.* 2012;49:344–356. doi:10.1177/0300985811402846
212. Bedoya J, Meyer CA, Timmins LH, et al. Effects of stent design parameters on normal artery wall mechanics. *J Biomech Eng.* 2006;128:757–765. doi:10.1115/1.2246236
213. Gyongyosi M, Strehblow C, Sperker W, et al. Platelet activation and high tissue factor level predict acute stent thrombosis in pig coronary arteries: prothrombogenic response of drug-eluting or bare stent implantation within the first 24 hours. *Thromb Haemost.* 2006;96:202–209. doi:10.1160/TH06-03-0178
214. Earl FL, Tegeris AS, Whitmore GE, et al. The use of swine in drug toxicity studies. *Ann N Y Acad Sci.* 1964;111:671–688. doi:10.1111/j.1749-6632.1964.tb53136.x
215. Helke KL, Swindle MM. Animal models of toxicology testing: the role of pigs. *Expert Opin Drug Metab Toxicol.* 2013;9:127–139. doi:10.1517/17425255.2013.739607
216. McCalla-Martin AC, Chen X, Linder KE, et al. Varying phenotypes in swine versus murine transgenic models constitutively expressing the same human Sonic hedgehog transcriptional activator, K5-HGLI2 Delta N. *Transgenic Res.* 2010;19:869–887. doi:10.1007/s11248-010-9362-0
217. Sieren JC, Meyerholz DK, Wang XJ, et al. Development and translational imaging of a TP53 porcine tumorigenesis model. *J Clin Invest.* 2014;124:4052–4066. doi:10.1172/JCI75447
218. Leuchs S, Saalfrank A, Merkl C, et al. Inactivation and inducible oncogenic mutation of p53 in gene targeted pigs. *PloS One.* 2012;7:e43323. doi:10.1371/journal.pone.0043323
219. Schook LB, Collares TV, Hu W, et al. A genetic porcine model of cancer. *PloS One.* 2015;10:e0128864. doi:10.1371/journal.pone.0128864

7

Cancer Therapeutic Strategies and Treatment Resistance

KEKOA TAPARRA ■ PHUOC T. TRAN

Knowledge of molecular and cellular biology has inspired clinical cancer therapies for more than a century. Modern standard-of-care cancer treatment options consist of surgery, chemotherapy, radiation therapy, and more recently immunotherapy. At the end of the 19th century, William Halsted pioneered the field of surgical oncology, which continues to be the major curative cancer treatment option. This is particularly true for patients who present with localized disease that can be encompassed by a surgical field. Despite the continued success of surgery, experience from the operating room reveals that surgery has limitations for cancer patients, particularly when the disease is advanced. Due to difficult resections of tumors embedded within vital tissues (e.g., brain and liver), new approaches emerged out of necessity in the field of cancer therapy. Thus, pioneers of cancer research shifted from physical resection to chemical cytotoxicity. In this chapter, we discuss the progress and experimental basis of cancer therapies (e.g., chemotherapy, radiation, biological, and immunotherapies) followed by mechanisms of resistance and strategies for overcoming treatment resistance.

TRADITIONAL CHEMOTHERAPY AND EARLY CANCER MODELS

To address the limitations of surgery, the earliest concepts of chemotherapies aimed to treat metastatic cancer systemically. The birth of cancer chemotherapy is attributed to Louis Goodman and Alfred Gilman in 1942 for their work on nitrogen mustard in the treatment of non-Hodgkin lymphoma (1). As pharmacologists, Goodman and Gilman were intrigued by the myelosuppression observed in autopsies of World War II soldiers. They had the insight to recognize the cytotoxic potential of sulfur mustard to kill cancer cells in patients with lymphoma. This initiated the decades of research identifying nitrogen mustard as an alkylating agent, which covalently binds to DNA, resulting in apoptosis. Like nitrogen mustard, most chemotherapies today fall under five broad categories:

1. Alkylating and alkylating-like agents (e.g., nitrogen mustard, cisplatin)
2. Antimetabolites (e.g., methotrexate and gemcitabine)

3. Antimicrotubule agents (e.g., alkaloids and taxols)
4. Topoisomerase inhibitors (e.g., camptothecin and etoposide)
5. Cytotoxic antibiotics (e.g., doxorubicin and bleomycin)

In their initial studies on the first alkylating chemotherapies, Goodman and Gilman transplanted lymphoid tumors into mice to study the cytotoxic effects of nitrogen mustard (2). To their surprise they observed tumor regression, which led to the first clinical trials of nitrogen mustard in patients (2). This work demonstrated for the first time that a chemical compound had the capacity to induce tumor regression in a controlled study. Despite frequent cancer relapse following this treatment, their work showed proof of principle and was emblematic of the now classic bench-to-bedside approach to targeting cancer with systemic treatments.

The approach of tumor engraftment in mice remains a useful tool to evaluate potential efficacy of chemical therapies. In combination with in vitro tissue culture experiments, experiments using in vivo models are a necessary preclinical step that helps justify clinical trials. In vivo models demonstrate the physiological relevance of in vitro studies. This is due to the limitations of two-dimensional (2-D) cell culture, including cell growth in three-dimensional space, tissue signaling interactions, and the **tumor microenvironment** (**TME**).

Tumor graft material is referred to as **xenogeneic** or **syngeneic** depending on whether the animal model is immunodeficient or immunocompetent, respectively. Two common tumor graft models are the T-cell–deficient athymic nude (nu/nu) mice and the B-cell– and T-cell–deficient severe combined immunodeficient (scid/scid) mice (3). Selecting the correct mouse model depends on the capacity for successful engraftment. For example, certain leukemias are difficult to grow in athymic nude mice; however, they are more successful in a type of scid mouse called the non-obese diabetic (NOD)-scid mouse. Thus, when planning an experiment to assess preclinical efficacy of a new cancer chemotherapy, it is essential to consider the proper mouse model of choice.

In general, the procedure for tumor grafting in mouse models follows the same principle and is outlined by Morton and Houghton (4). Briefly, patient-derived tumor cells or cells from tissue culture are collected and treated under sterile conditions. Approximately $0.5–5 \times 10^6$ cells are needed per engraftment depending on the growth rates and tumorigenicity of the specific cell line. Cells should be free from contamination as they may infect the immunocompromised mice. The medium that the cells are suspended in will depend on the cell type; however, examples include phosphate buffered saline (PBS), cell culture media (e.g., RPMI/DMEM), or a gelatinous protein mixture called Matrigel™. After sterilizing the hind limbs with an alcohol swab, cancer cells are injected into the flanks of an anesthetized immunocompetent mouse. The site of injection will form a visible prominence that is a product of the tumor engraftment and will disappear within the first week. The actual tumor may take approximately 1 to 3 months to establish and grow depending on the proliferative capacity of the cell line. For aggressive cancer cells, however, this process may occur in as little as 1 to 2 weeks. The site of injection should be monitored for growth and eventually measured multiple times a week once a tumor forms. Typical experiments will assess growth response of tumors after they reach a threshold volume (e.g., typically ~100 mm^3).

The use of tumor engraftment to test the toxicity and efficacy of drugs paved a path for chemotherapeutic strategies starting with nitrogen mustard. Following the alkylating chemotherapies was an era of antimetabolites. In the 1940s, initial studies on folic acid therapy were conducted by a pathologist named Sydney Farber at the Harvard Medical School and the Children's Hospital in Boston (5). Farber and his collaborators identified synthetic compounds structurally similar to metabolites that promoted cellular proliferation in cancer. Despite modest remissions, these molecules could inhibit key metabolic enzymes and the viability of cancer cells. This chemical approach exploited biological vulnerabilities of cancer to induce cytotoxicity. While antimetabolites and subsequent cancer therapeutics in this era made progress by targeting rapidly dividing cells, there were significant associated short- and long-term toxicities that posed a major challenge. At this time, it was apparent that cancer researchers were making progress toward treating cancer, but there was still work to be done.

HORMONAL THERAPY AND MOLECULARLY TARGETED THERAPY

The next era of pharmacotherapy arose from a greater understanding of underlying molecular mechanisms of cancer. Improvements in treatment strategies aimed to directly treat the patient's malignancy while limiting toxicity. Advances in genetics and biotechnology identified novel signaling networks orchestrated by cancer. One treatment strategy still widely used in the clinic is **hormone therapy**, also called hormonal or endocrine therapy. These therapies are particularly effective against certain types of hormone-driven breast and prostate cancers (6).

This treatment strategy works by one of two mechanisms: (a) by blocking the body's ability to produce the hormone that promotes tumor growth and (b) by interfering with the interaction between the hormone and cancer cell. Hormone therapies generally work by blocking the activity of **estrogen receptor** (**ER**) in breast cancer and **androgen receptor** (**AR**) in prostate cancer. These hormone receptors function as transcription factors upon ligand binding, receptor dimerization, and translocation to the nucleus. Inhibition by hormone therapy prevents transcriptional activity in cancers, thus inhibiting cellular proliferation and survival.

Tamoxifen is the prototypical hormonal therapy for ER+ breast cancer. Due to a number of notable side effects, however, including irregular menses, infertility, hot flashes, secondary cancers, and drug resistance, tamoxifen is no longer the gold standard for breast cancer therapy. **Aromatase inhibitors** (**AIs**) have recently gained traction as an efficacious alternative. AIs inhibit the synthesis of estrogen, rather than blocking ER protein function. Both strategies target the underlying growth mechanism of the cancer, varying primarily in the side effect profile.

Beyond hormonal therapies, progress in cancer biology has led to a plethora of agents that specifically target unique characteristics of cancer cells not seen in normal cells, thus limiting drug-associated toxicity. The **molecularly targeted therapy** that revolutionized modern cancer therapy and ushered in the era of what is known as *precision medicine* is imatinib mesylate (Gleevec), a treatment for chronic myeloid leukemia (CML) (7). A team of chemists at Novartis led by physicians Brian Druker and Charles Sawyers developed this small molecule to target the aberrant protein product of the Philadelphia chromosome. The Philadelphia chromosome gives rise to a fusion protein of the Breakpoint Cluster Region (*BCR*) gene on chromosome 22 and the Abelson (*ABL*) tyrosine kinase gene on chromosome 9. The BCR–ABL fusion protein forms an oncogenic tyrosine kinase that activates numerous downstream effectors of cancer-like cell cycle proteins. Over 90% of CML cases are Philadelphia chromosome positive, making imatinib an excellent option for these patients.

Since the discovery of imatinib, the scientific and medical communities have made great progress in targeted therapy discovery with the advent of new technologies. Due to this targeted approach to treating cancer, recent developments in clinical trial design assess efficacy of new therapeutic options in patients based on specific genetic mutation profile rather than the tumor site. These so-called **"basket" trials** have the advantage of accelerating the Food and Drug Administration (FDA) approval process with the aim of more precisely treating cancer patients (8). For example, the drug vemurafenib has been approved for the treatment of melanoma patients harboring the $BRAF^{V600E}$ mutation. In a recent basket trial study, patients with various tumor types—including lung, breast, colorectal, blood, ovarian, and other rare cancers—were treated with vemurafenib. The results showed that the treatment worked best in the setting of lung malignancies and two rare cancers. The study demonstrated the importance of focusing on drug mechanism of action and matching this with the mutation driving the patient's tumor. These clinical trials, among others, are currently being designed in an era of medical progress and patient-centered precision medicine.

Although genetic sequencing is becoming exponentially more affordable, basket trials are still very costly and require each tumor to be sequenced before placing the patient on a trial. Even when the patient tumors are sequenced, it may ultimately reveal a genetic mutation that is too rare to be placed in a basket. Furthermore, unlike the traditional experimental setup, there are no patient controls. Rather than receiving a placebo, patients are placed into baskets with hopes of observing a significant difference. This inadvertently highlights only the success of each drug with each gene mutation. Thus, without proper controls it is challenging to determine cause and effect pertaining to observed side effects. Despite the setbacks, this up-and-coming approach puts into action our knowledge of targeted therapies and has resulted in significant discoveries.

RADIATION THERAPY

While systemic chemotherapies may have significant toxicities due to drug distribution, radiation therapy aims to manage or cure localized tumors. Physicians have tried to use low-powered x-rays to treat cancer since the discovery of radioactive elements well over a century ago. Modern-day radiation therapy is said to have been founded by Kaplan and Ginzton with their coinvention of the first medical **linear accelerator** (**LINAC**) in the Western hemisphere (9). A LINAC works by using microwaves to accelerate electrons that will then collide with a heavy metal target to produce high-energy x-rays. Their technology first demonstrated efficacy in the setting of Hodgkin lymphoma and retinoblastoma (9). Today, LINACs are used in hospitals around the world by radiation oncologists to deliver high-energy x-rays directly to the tumor while sparing the surrounding normal tissue. Radiation therapy can be used for cancer management or may even be curative due to the physiological effects radiation has on cancer cells.

The approach of radiation therapy is incredibly patient-specific, as treatment plans are personalized on the anatomical level. Treatment plans involve contouring anatomical features of each patient to ensure the x-rays are delivered to the tumor and not the surrounding normal tissues. There are three phases to the radiation therapy process: (a) simulation, (b) planning, and (c) treatment. Simulation typically involves positioning and immobilizing the patient for future treatments. This step maximizes the possibility of specifically delivering the radiation to the tumor. Planning involves locating the anatomical position of the tumor so that it can be targeted relative to other body structures. The key medical imaging used for planning and calculating the appropriate dose comes from CT, although additional imaging may help delineate the tumor. Treatment is the final step in which the radiation is directly delivered internally or externally.

The techniques used by radiation oncologists have greatly improved over the decades since Kaplan and Ginzton. Two major classes of radiation therapy include **external beam radiation therapy** (**EBRT** or XRT) and **brachytherapy** or internal source radiotherapy. Both techniques require highly technical treatment planning with careful consideration of radiation energy loss, scatter, range, dose/isodose, stopping power, and relative biological effect.

Clinically, the effects of radiation therapy are delayed for both tumor response and side effects. This is due to the mechanism of action of radiation therapy. Cancer cells treated with radiation are damaged either by direct or indirect means of DNA damage. The impact of DNA damage on cellular death takes time, as mutations and genomic alterations need to accumulate. The latent effects occur when cells approach cell cycle checkpoints and respond to DNA damage by arresting cell cycle progression or initiating programmed cell death. Direct DNA damage occurs when ionized radiation from a photon or charged particle directly damages the DNA of the cancer cell. Indirect DNA damage occurs with the ionization of water, which forms free radicals (e.g., hydroxyl radicals) that damage DNA and other cellular components.

A limitation to radiation therapy also reflects the mechanism of cellular damage. Oxygen is known to be a potent radiosensitizer due to radical formation (10). However, solid tumors can have areas of hypoxia if the growth outpaces the supporting vasculature, thus depleting the available oxygen for the ionizing radiation to react with to form free radicals. This results in an increased radioresistant phenotype for hypoxic tumors, which translates to a reduced response to radiation therapy. To combat this challenge, some strategies have been proposed, including the administration of drugs or methods to physically or functionally increase intratumoral oxygenation.

With the limitation of hypoxia in radiation therapy, a common preclinical question that may be considered is whether a novel therapeutic agent acts as a **radiosensitizer**. That is to say, can a drug increase the toxicity of radiation in a cancer cell line relative to a noncancer control cell line? This question can be addressed experimentally both in vitro and in vivo. The equipment required for delivering radiation to cancer cells or mouse models of cancer can be purchased through industries specializing in preclinical x-ray irradiators (e.g., Xstrahl Life Sciences). Radiation delivered for in vitro experiments can be performed using the Xstrahl CIXD device, whereas in vivo experiments can be performed using Xstrahl Small Animal Radiation Research Platform (SARRP). Both research platforms provide safe irradiation administration to experimental samples of interest to answer questions, such as whether a drug acts as a radiosensitizer.

To illustrate these experimental designs, we will use a recent example by Hastak et al. examining whether the **poly(adenosine diphosphate [ADP]-ribose) polymerase inhibitor (PARPi) LT626** acts as a radiosensitizer (11). Their research highlights key concepts in preclinical in vitro experiments of radiation therapy and many anticancer agents. Various cancer cell lines, including pancreatic (Miapaca2, PDA) and lung (H1299, H460) cell lines, were treated with varying concentrations of the PARPi, LT626. After 5 days, cell viability was measured using the metabolism-based colorimetric MTT assay. A dose–response curve was constructed and half maximal inhibitory concentration (IC_{50}) or concentration of the agent needed for 50% growth inhibition was determined. For radiosensitization, cell lines are treated with various dose levels of radiation (0–10 Gy) and the sensitivity of the cell lines to radiation alone assessed first, using the gold standard long-term anticancer in vitro assay, the **colony formation assay**. Radiosensitization by LT626 is next addressed by treating cells first with the 1 or 10 μM concentration of drug followed by 0 to 6 Gy of radiation. To assess for radiosensitization, calculation of a numeric **combination index (CI)** can be used to determine synergism ($CI < 1$), additivity ($CI = 1$), or antagonism ($CI > 1$).

Although slightly different, drug–drug combinations can be approached in essentially the same fashion to examine for combination anticancer effects. In vivo experiments (typically in a murine model) are then useful to follow up in vitro data to determine if the anticancer effects can be validated. Most studies utilize nude mice in an experimental xenograft setup similar to one described earlier in this chapter. Tumor volumes and overall survival (OS) are measured over time. Results are compared between the groups with drug alone, radiation alone, and in combination. As an alternative to nude mice, **genetically engineered mouse models (GEMMs)** may be used to better recapitulate tumor biology in an autochthonous model (12) (Figure 7.1).

Researchers typically then interrogate the underlying molecular mechanisms of the anticancer if not already known. In the example provided by Hastak et al., key players important in

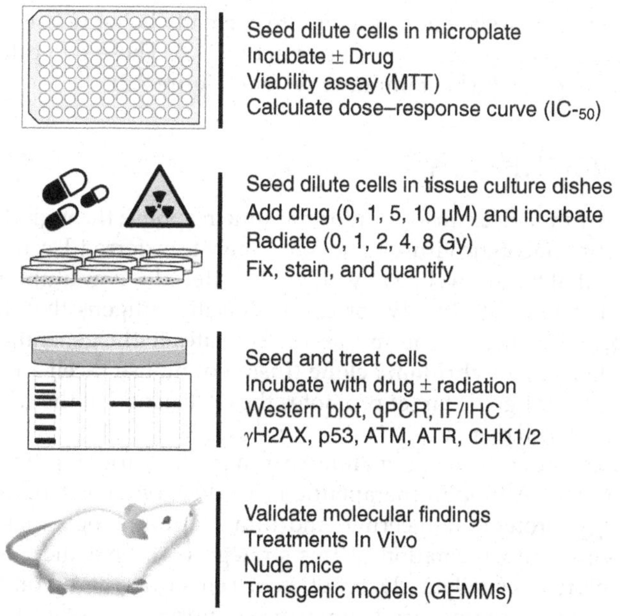

FIGURE 7.1 Experimental design for validating drug radiosensitization.
GEMM, genetically engineered mouse model.

the assessment of radiosensitization are the DNA double strand break associated histone protein (γH2AX) and the DNA damage checkpoint protein (p53). Significant increases in levels of γH2AX and p53 are associated with cellular stress and can suggest whether a chemotherapeutic agent is capable of radiosensitization compared to radiation alone. These proteins are easily assessed using immunofluorescence (IF), as the antibodies are well optimized for such experiments. To evaluate the immunofluorescence, cells are counted either manually from individual images or automatically using programs such as the ImageJ cell counter feature. These markers serve as surrogates for direct measurement of DNA damage from radiation. Additional DNA damage response (DDR) proteins implicated in radiosensitization—ATR, ATM, Chk1, and Chk2—are also phosphorylated (activated) and can be evaluated similarly. These phosphorylated proteins can also be interrogated via Western blotting using cell extracts from radiation and drug–radiation combination treated cell lines. Collectively, these proteins are a part of the DNA repair process and offer a molecular perspective of radiosensitization in preclinical experiments.

IMMUNOTHERAPY AND OTHER BIOLOGICAL THERAPIES

One of the most active areas of preclinical and clinical cancer research is the field of biological therapies. The goal of biological therapies is to use living organisms, their derivatives, or synthetic versions of these organismal products to treat disease. There are many examples of biological therapies, which include:

- Adoptive cell transfer
- Angiogenesis inhibitors
- Cytokine therapy
- Gene therapy
- Immunoconjugates (e.g., antibody drug conjugates [ADCs])
- Monoclonal antibodies
- Oncolytic virus therapy
- Vaccinations (e.g., cancer neoantigens or bacillus Calmette–Guérin [BCG])

Perhaps the most promising area of cancer therapy research in the past decade is cancer **immunotherapy**. Although classification systems are currently being reassessed, immunotherapy has historically been classified as either passive or active (13). These two categories are based on the therapy's ability to engage the host immune system (Figure 7.2).

PASSIVE IMMUNOTHERAPY

Passive immunotherapy enhances an antitumor immune response through tumor-specific monoclonal antibodies (mAbs), oncolytic viruses, and adoptively transferred T-cells. One passive immunotherapeutic strategy that has been clinically utilized for decades is antitumor mAbs. Monoclonal antibodies are used that have an affinity for cancer-specific antigens that are expressed in low levels or absent in normal tissues. The term *monoclonal* relates to the generation of the therapeutic mAbs, which are made from a **hybridoma clone** (fusion of mouse B-cell and myeloma cell). The binding of the mAb to its antigenic target promotes the destruction of the cancer cell by inducing direct or indirect forms of cell death.

Researchers may consider developing an mAb as a strategy for targeting a cancer antigen of interest to kill cancer cells. Although therapeutic mAb development requires extensive knowledge of cancer serology, protein engineering, and tumor immunology, there are key themes in approaches to successful implementation of this strategy (14). First there is the need to determine the antigen of interest, usually a glycoprotein or cell surface receptor. These targets can be identified using serological, genomic, proteomic, or bioinformatic methods. Antigens capable of developing mAbs are then isolated and a hybridoma clone is produced in the lab. Once the mAb is acquired, a series of preclinical and clinical evaluations is necessary prior to the consideration

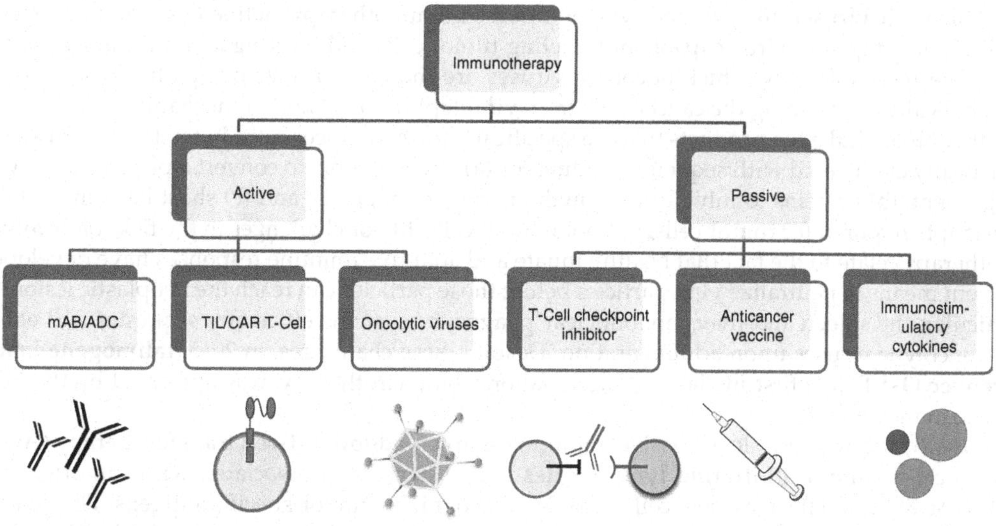

FIGURE 7.2 The big picture of immunotherapy strategies in cancer treatment.
ADC, antibody drug conjugate; CAR, chimeric antigen receptor; mAB, ; TIL, tumor-infiltrating lymphocytes.

as a potential therapeutic agent. The antibody is first administered in preclinical models of cancer to assess in vivo antibody localization, biodistribution, therapeutic activity, immune effector functions, and effects on the tumor vasculature or stroma. The mechanism of any antitumor properties would also have to be identified as either direct (receptor blockade and inhibition of cell signaling) or indirect (immune-mediated killing via antibody-dependent cell-mediated cytotoxicity, complement-dependent cytotoxicity, and antibody-dependent cellular phagocytosis) effects. Clinical evaluation of the developed mAb should evaluate toxicity and therapeutic efficacy, particularly focusing on the ratio of antibody uptake in the tumor versus normal tissues. Deposition of the antibody nonspecifically into nontumor tissues is a major concern and is associated with adverse events for this therapeutic strategy. Exemplar cancer antigen specific mAb agents target such receptors as CD20 (rituximab for non-Hodgkin lymphoma), CD52 (alemtuzumab for chronic lymphocytic leukemia), or epidermal growth factor receptor (EGFR; cetuximab and panitumumab for head and neck or colon cancers).

In addition to the direct antitumor application of mAbs, **ADCs** or mAbs covalently bound to a linker that carries a cytotoxic agent or radioisotope are other strategies. The antigen specificity of the mAb allows the cytotoxic drug complex to home in on the cancer cell and deliver the therapy upon endocytosis. Upon entry into the cell, endosomal or lysosomal enzymes aid in the cleavage of the labile linker to ensure the conjugated drug is only deployed within the cancer cell. Examples of ADCs include brentuximab vedotin (relapsed or refractory Hodgkin lymphoma) and trastuzumab emtansine (HER2-positive metastatic breast cancer).

In addition to directly targeting the tumor, mAbs serve as a biological therapeutic strategy for targeting the TME and angiogenesis. **Angiogenesis** is a biological phenomenon by which blood vasculature is generated de novo through a process of migration, growth, and differentiation of endothelial cells that line blood vessel walls. In the context of cancer, it is an appreciated hallmark of cancer that enables the delivery of oxygen and nutrients to the developing tumor. Antiangiogenic agents have been utilized in the clinic that prevent tumors from forming new blood vessels and thus effectively deprive the tumor of essential growth factors. The major mechanism of this class of drugs targets the vascular endothelial growth factor (VEGF). The agent bevacizumab is an mAb that binds to VEGF, inhibiting the proangiogenic signaling. Other small molecules have been developed as nonspecific tyrosine kinases with some affinity for VEGF receptor (VEGFR), namely sorafenib and sunitinib. While antiangiogenic agents have showed some promise, a major caveat is that off-target effects can lead to patient toxicity.

Oncolytic viruses are a second type of passive immunotherapy, defined as a nonpathogenic replication-competent virus capable of targeting tumor cells and eliciting an antitumor response (15). One mechanism by which oncolytic viruses are thought to have cytopathic activity is by metabolically overloading the cancer cells from viral replication. Another mechanism includes the production of viral gene products that are specifically toxic to cancer cells. In the latter, viruses are genetically engineered with sequences coding for (a) enzymes able to convert a prodrug to a cytotoxic agent, (b) proteins to inhibit the growth or trigger apoptosis, and (c) short hairpins to bind transcripts required for tumor cells, but not normal cells. Major challenges in the field of oncolytic virotherapy relate to the fact that healthy innate and adaptive immune responses have developed efficient means to neutralize viral particles before those particles can reach the neoplastic lesion. In particular, the spleen and liver mononuclear phagocytic systems efficiently sequester and eliminate oncolytic viruses upon administration. Despite these challenges, in 2015, **talimogene laherparepvec (T-VEC)**, a first-in-class intralesional oncolytic virotherapy, was approved by the FDA for use in melanoma.

Finally, a third example of passive immunotherapy is **adoptive T-cell transfer therapy** (ACT). The so-called **tumor-infiltrating lymphocytes (TILs)** have been associated with tumorigenesis and some of these TILs may be T-cells capable of recognizing tumor-specific antigens. The general principle of ACT involves the collection of lymphocytes (circulating or tumor-infiltrating), biomarker selection, ex vivo modification, clonal expansion, and patient readministration. Prior to readministration of the lymphocytes, patients are usually lymphodepleted. When TILs are modified ex vivo, they may be genetically engineered with a tumor associated antigen (TAA) specific T-cell receptor (TCR). These TCRs can be further modulated with intracellular TCR immunostimulatory domains, generating what is known as a **chimeric antigen receptor (CAR) T-cell**. The end result of ACT is the generation of a tumor-specific cell-based therapy that harnesses the biological function of the immune system. Limitations of this strategy relate to the feasibility of ACT and high financial cost, but these can be overcome, as signaled by the success and FDA approval of CAR T-cell therapies for B-cell malignancies in 2017.

ACTIVE IMMUNOTHERAPY

Active immunotherapy mounts a potentially durable immune response through immunomodulatory mAbs, anticancer vaccines, and immunostimulatory cytokines. The class of mAbs that target so-called T-cell checkpoint inhibitors holds incredible promise for the future of cancer treatment. Immune checkpoint inhibitors are immunomodulators that serve to augment an antitumor immune response. The current era of immunomodulatory mAb checkpoint inhibitors derives from an inherent property of T-cell biology. Early researchers realized that despite an abundance of immunogenic antigens and neoantigens expressed by cancer cells, it was perplexing that the immune system was ignoring these antigenic signals. This led to the realization that there are immune "checkpoints" that prevent TILs from recognizing and destroying the tumor cells, which are normally present in normal physiology likely to prevent autoimmunity (16).

Normally, a CD8+ cytotoxic T-cell requires two signals presented by an antigen presenting cell (APC) upon its activation. In Signal 1, the TCR recognizes a peptide-bound major histocompatibility complex I (MHC I) molecule on the APC. In Signal II, the T-cell receives a costimulatory signal by the CD28 molecule activated by either CD80 (B7-1) or CD86 (B7-2) on an APC. Without both signals, the CD8+ T-cell is unable to deploy its cytotoxic granules. Immune checkpoints were discovered that act upon Signal II in an "immune-inhibitory" fashion to dampen the effector function of the CD8+ T-cells. Cancer cells are able to inhibit Signal II via interactions using PD-1 and CTLA-4 to block the T-cell PD-L1/PD-L2 and CD80/CD86, respectively.

PD-1 and CTLA-4 are absent on resting naïve and memory T-cells and only expressed upon TCR engagement. Expression of the checkpoint inhibitor molecules on tumor cells is thought to be a result of chronic exposure of T-cells to TAAs. The inhibitory signal promotes a state of immune unresponsiveness called *anergy*. Although PD-1 and CTLA-4 are functionally similar, there are also notable differences, including downstream effectors, chronological expression, subset of cells expressing the molecules, and interactions with the TME. The discovery of natural immune checkpoint blockade by immune-evading cancer cells gave rise to the generation of multiple FDA-approved mAbs targeting PD-1 (nivolumab and pembrolizumab), PD-L1 (atezolizumab, durvalumab), and CTLA-4 (ipilimumab) (17). These drugs inhibit the immune checkpoint, thus releasing the breaks of cytotoxic T-cells and enabling the immune system to better kill tumor cells.

Despite the incredible clinical promise of these drugs, we are currently learning there are a number of restrictions to the success of immune checkpoint inhibitors in the clinic. There seems to be some tissue selectivity regarding the effectiveness of these agents. Current results suggest that not all tumor sites demonstrate the same clinical efficacy. Melanoma and non-small cell lung cancer (NSCLC) seem to be two tumor types with the most benefit. A pooled meta-analysis of 1,861 melanoma patients receiving ipilimumab in phase II and III clinical trials revealed that approximately 20% of melanoma patients demonstrate durable survival, in some cases extending beyond 10 years (18). Melanoma in particular demonstrates a cancer that responds well to this type of therapy due to the significant prevalence of TILs present. Despite the success, ipilimumab has shown only modest antitumor effects outside of melanoma patients. Moreover, not all patients with the same tumor type ultimately respond to these drugs. There are a number of proposed explanations for this. If the tumor lacks TILs, then these drugs will be ineffective, as there are no immune cells to mount a response irrespective of the immune checkpoints. Furthermore, we are only beginning to understand the existence of tumor biomarkers that need to be present for checkpoint inhibitors to be efficacious.

The development of biomarker analyses is a useful strategy to overcome the challenges of therapeutic failure. Biomarker development enables the identification of likely responders and nonresponders to immune checkpoint inhibitor therapy and is an active area of research (16). Biomarker development provides advantages to physicians because it allows for the selection of patients who will best respond to treatment while preventing a subset of patients from experiencing significant adverse events. In the case of melanoma, while biomarkers exist to identify candidates for the treatment of the common *BRAF*^{V600E} mutation with the tyrosine kinase vemurafenib, this biomarker would be uninformative in the context of immune checkpoint inhibitors. The first assay developed to correlate with response to anti-PD-1 treatment was the measurement of intratumoral lymphoid infiltrates via CD8+ T-cell density. The most mechanistically relevant biomarker for anti-PD-1 and anti-PD-L1 checkpoint blockade has been the **immunohistochemical analysis** of the tumor for PD-L1 positivity. In a recent analysis of 15 PD-1 inhibitor studies of varying tumor types, patients with PD-L1$^+$ tumors showed a response rate of 48% compared to 15% in PD-L1$^-$ tumors (19).

Beyond immunological biomarkers, large-scale genomic studies on patients receiving a given therapeutic constitute another excellent strategy to identify patients likely to respond to immunotherapy. A landmark paper published in 2015 integrated genomic analyses to identify **mutational load** as a potential biomarker for predicting tumor response to immune checkpoint inhibitors (20). The researchers understood that colorectal cancer (CRC) has a relatively low response rate to immune checkpoint inhibitors. They looked closely at one clinical trial that had a single patient of 33 enrolled who responded to anti-PD-1 therapy. They discovered that the one quality of responders in the pembrolizumab clinical trial was the high microsatellite instability (MSI) phenotype.

MSI tumors result from deficiencies in mismatch repair (MMR) that lead to genomic instability. The researchers rationalized that MSI tumors would have a significant mutational burden that may fuel the development of non-self-neoantigens that have potential for mounting an immune response. To test their hypothesis, they conducted a phase II clinical trial to evaluate the effects of pembrolizumab in patients specifically with MMR-deficient versus -proficient tumors. Recruited patients were previously treated and had progressive metastatic carcinoma with or without MMR deficiency. MMR deficiency was defined as one of two mechanisms: (a) hereditary nonpolyposis colorectal cancer (HNPCC or Lynch syndrome) with a germline defect and (b) sporadically occurring MMR deficiency due to a somatic mutation or epigenetic silencing of MMR genes. Both types of MMR-deficient patients harbor tumors with hundreds if not thousands of mutations. In the trial, three groups were evaluated: MMR-deficient CRC (n = 13), MMR-proficient CRC (n = 25), and MMR-deficient non-CRCs (n=10).

The clinical trial results demonstrated an improvement in objective response rate (ORR), progression-free survival (PFS), and OS in a variety of MMR-deficient tumor types, but not in MMR-proficient cancers. The immune-related ORR and PFS were 40% (4/10 patients) and 78% (7/9 patients), respectively, for MMR-deficient CRC and 0% (0/18 patients) and 11% (2/18 patients), respectively, for MMR-proficient CRC. Moreover, the responsiveness of MSI CRC to pembrolizumab was recapitulated in patients with non-CRC MSI tumors, with an immune-related ORR of 71% (5/7 patients) and PFS of 67% (4/6 patients). Although this study focused on CRC patients with MMR deficiencies, this hypothesis may also explain why melanoma and lung cancer are susceptible to immune checkpoint blockade. High mutational load can be found in melanoma due to ultraviolet-induced mutations and lung cancer due to carcinogenic cigarette smoke. Overall, this clinical trial highlights a pivotal link between basic scientific concepts, cancer genetics, and immunotherapy that led to the discovery of a clinically relevant biomarker.

Although much of the spotlight has focused on immune checkpoint inhibitors, two additional types of active immunotherapy are **anticancer vaccines** and **immunostimulatory cytokines**. Preclinical cancer vaccines are either peptide- or DNA-based anticancer vaccines. In this approach, TAA-derived epitopes are acquired by resident dendritic cells or other APCs during maturation and promote an antitumor specific immune response. Two major considerations when designing peptide-based vaccine therapies are (a) cancer specificity to avoid unwanted adverse events and (b) the length of the peptide to be administered. The length of the peptide is particularly important to consider because of the steps involved with antigen processing and presentation. Short peptides of about 8 to 12 amino acids are capable of directly binding to MHC molecules expressed on the surface of APCs, whereas longer peptides (25–30 amino acids) will have to undergo full antigen processing. Preliminary data support long synthetic peptides as superior to their shorter counterparts (21). The promise of cancer vaccination resonates with the need for precision medicine. Though still in preclinical development, autologous tumor lysates may be the future of cancer vaccination when complexed with immunostimulatory chaperones (e.g., heat shock proteins). While this strategy is desirable because it does not rely on a single TAA to mount the immune response and it is specific to each patient's tumor, the major challenge is that the cost of development is not currently justifiable.

The third type of active immunotherapy is immunostimulatory cytokines, namely IL-2, IFN-α2a, and IFN-α2b. Although these cytokines are immunostimulatory, they have been observed to have little, if any, clinical benefit to patients as single agents (13). Thus, cytokines are often implemented as an adjuvant to other immune stimulatory strategies. IL-2 is approved as a single-agent cancer treatment to treat melanoma and renal cell carcinoma. IFN-α therapies have been approved for nearly as long and are used in the high-dose adjuvant setting of multiple hematological and solid tumors, including CML, melanoma, and hairy cell leukemia. Overall, cytokines have been a known strategy for cancer therapy for decades, although the precise mechanism of action still remains poorly understood. With low response rates and significant, even lethal, toxicities, their implementation in the clinic has been limited.

Finally, in addition to passive and active immunotherapies, the third type of biological therapy is **gene therapy**. With advances in gene editing resulting in technology like CRISPR/Cas9, the goal is to introduce or modify DNA or RNA of living cells to treat cancer (22). Some broad applications of gene editing would be to administer gene therapy to specifically destroy cancer cells or to prevent the cells from proliferating. Alternatively, genetic alterations can be made in healthy cells (e.g., immune cells) to help combat cancer, as described throughout this section. Another example of implementing gene therapy would be to replace an altered tumor suppressor with the normal version of the gene to promote cancer cell cycle arrest. Another strategy is to insert and disrupt DNA sequences coding for protumorigenic genes to inhibit cell progression and induce treatment sensitization. While these ideas seemed grandiose just a few decades ago, due to our advancement in gene editing tools this is quickly becoming more of a reality. However, there are still many challenges with gene therapy that are currently being addressed, which primarily relate to the administration and specificity of targeting the cells of interest. Despite these challenges, gene therapy holds great promise in combination with many of the areas of cancer therapies discussed in this chapter.

THERAPEUTIC RESISTANCE MECHANISMS

Thus far we have covered a number of therapeutic strategies for cancer patients, including chemotherapy, radiation therapy, targeted precision medicine, and immunotherapy. As a disease based on evolutionary selection, a major clinical challenge that substantially limits the capacity and longevity of these treatment strategies is treatment resistance. From the very first chemotherapies and targeted agents, it became apparent that cancer possessed strategies to overcome clinical interventions, yielding even more aggressive and often lethal forms of cancer. Although clinical paradigms are currently shifting, patients with cancer relapse after an initial tumor response have historically been followed up with treatment agnostic to the molecular mechanism of resistance. However, cancer has been appreciated as a pathological state of multiple genetic and epigenetic mutations. Thus, drug resistance is due to genetic alterations and the ensuing activation of signaling pathways to drive cellular growth and evade cell death. In this current era of precision medicine, it is imperative to understand these mechanisms to counteract treatment resistance appropriately in patients with drug-resistant tumors. In this section, we cover the theories of drug resistance mechanisms and preclinical models that can be utilized to study this phenomenon in cancer.

Concepts of cancer therapy resistance have been present in every step of cancer drug discovery outlined in this chapter. Starting with the antimetabolites, nucleoside analogues, and alkyl agents discussed earlier, drug resistance mechanisms have been previously comprehensively reviewed in 1963 by Wallace Brockman (23). Brockman was the first to propose a biochemical and enzymatic perspective for drug resistance. He explained that drug-resistant cancer cells are a product of some deviation of a progenitor cancer cell. He proposed examples of drug resistance mechanisms including

> decreased conversion of the inhibitor to an active form, increased degradation of the inhibitor, increased synthesis of the inhibited enzyme, decreased sensitivity of an enzyme to an inhibitor (altered enzyme in the resistant cell), and decreased permeability of resistant cells to an inhibitor. (23)

This foresight set the foundation of cancer drug resistance mechanisms and the use of combinational therapies to combat this resistance.

Although Brockman's biochemical resistance mechanisms were incredibly insightful and showed preclinical integrity, there was little if any clinical evidence to support the theory at the time. Rather than focusing on a singular enzymatic target, another parallel mechanism of drug resistance is **multidrug resistance (MDR)**. This theory was founded by the identification of a P-glycoprotein associated with MDR followed by the discovery of the family of ABC transporter proteins. These transporters function as a cytoprotective means to bind nonspecifically to toxins for elimination out of the cell. Gene expression of *MDR1* correlated with multidrug-resistant cancers in the clinic (24). Consequently, multiple MDR inhibitors were developed, including verapamil, quinidine, and cyclosporine analogues. Clinical trials failed to show conclusive evidence demonstrating the link of MDR inhibition and chemoresistance and further exploration of these agents subsided. Despite the challenges of clinical application for these early drug resistance mechanisms, they highlighted the essential concepts of how cancers develop multiple routes of drug resistance.

With the development of more targeted therapies around the turn of the century, an alternative conceptualization of drug resistance was proposed. Rather than focusing on the biology of the drug itself, an integrative approach was developed that emphasized molecular signaling pathways with particular consideration of so-called "driver mutations." Rather than focusing on how the drug became ineffective, there was a shift in perspective in how the cancer cell was exploiting oncogenic dysregulation to refuel cellular proliferation. This change in perspective came at a time when the initial concepts of **oncogene addiction** and precision medicine were being formulated. This theory suggested that cancers required specific tumor-promoting signals and that without them cell cycle arrest and apoptosis would ensue (25). Thus, homing in on which oncogenes were required for the development and maintenance of cancer has helped shape the current paradigm of cancer drug resistance.

The current understanding of drug resistance is largely defined as one of two classifications with respect to when the drug resistance develops clinically: acquired resistance and innate resistance (26). Both mechanisms of resistance explain the two patient responses seen in the clinic. In acquired resistance a patient's tumor is initially responsive to the therapy for a period of time, followed by tumor progression. In this case, there is a genetic alteration that is positively selected from a subpopulation of cells in the tumor. This results in the expansion of the drug-resistant clones. Acquired resistance is due in part to the drug itself because it selects against cancer cells susceptible to the therapy, allowing the remaining resistant cancer cells to persist and repopulate the tumor. In contrast, innate (also called de novo or intrinsic) drug resistance is more straightforward. It is seen in the clinic when a patient's tumor is refractory at the outset to a therapy that should have been effective based on the histology or genetics of the tumor. The resistance is caused by a preexisting genetic alteration in the cancer that renders the therapy ineffective (Figure 7.3).

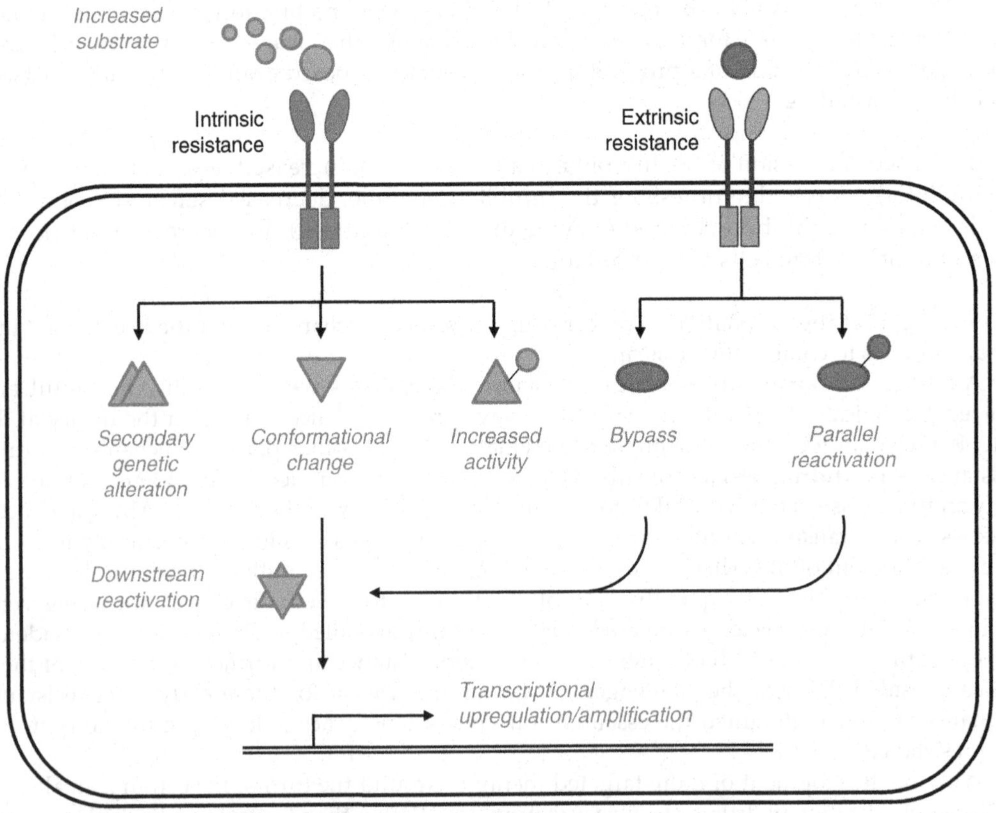

FIGURE 7.3 Common mechanisms of drug resistance.

Specifically related to acquired drug resistance, there are three main "pathway-dependent" categories that describe the precise molecular abnormality causing the refractory state. These hallmarks of drug resistance include (a) secondary reactivation of the target, (b) upstream/downstream pathway activation, and (c) parallel bypass effector pathway activation (26). A common theme is that some genetic alteration gives rise to a continual growth signal and/or evasion of cell death signals, rendering the administered drug futile, even in spite of inhibiting the intended target. These three categories of acquired resistance are particularly relevant to kinase inhibitor resistance. Kinase inhibitors are regularly utilized in the clinic and there has been a tremendous pharmaceutical investment in developing these drugs for cancer patients. While the illustrated examples primarily involve resistance to kinase inhibitors, the concepts may be applied to almost any treatment strategy where resistance is present.

First, the most common type of acquired drug resistance is **secondary reactivation** of the inhibited target. Secondary reactivation mutations were first described in CML patients treated with imatinib (27). In secondary reactivation, genetic alterations of the target kinase alter contact points for drug binding or confer an active conformational state of the protein itself. In general, tyrosine kinase inhibitors (TKIs) that target specific receptor tyrosine kinases (RTKs) are particularly problematic if there is a conserved amino acid residue, within the catalytic site, commonly mutated. These specific genetic alterations are known as a **gatekeeper mutation** and engender drug resistivity often found in cancer patient tumors. A classic example of a gatekeeper mutation is ABL^{T315I} in CML (imatinib, nilotinib, and dasatinib resistance). The mutation may also occur at the active site to increase adenosine triphosphate (ATP) affinity, thus creating a hyperactive form of the kinase. An example is $EGFR^{T790M}$ in NSCLC (gefitinib and erlotinib resistance). Moreover, the genetic alteration does not have to be a mutation. In the case of **genetic amplification** of BCR–ABL, the oncogene overcomes the targeted therapy by means of genetic duplication to put out more of the effector kinase.

A second category of acquired resistance commonly seen clinically is the activation of **upstream/downstream signaling pathway** targets. Drugs targeting the MAP kinase pathway best illustrate this scenario. This signaling cascade consists of a series of serine/threonine kinases (RAS–RAF–MEK–ERK) that drive proliferation. As mentioned previously, vemurafenib is a BRAF inhibitor used in the context of melanoma with the V600E mutation. While patients may initially respond to this drug, acquired resistance can promote a refractory state. In this case, activating mutations are often observed in the upstream *NRAS* or the downstream *MEK1* to overcome vemurafenib. In both cases, the secondary mutated oncoprotein is uncoupled from the targeted BRAF to reactivate the proliferation signal.

The third category of acquired resistance is activation of **bypass signaling** (26). While the first two categories address the pathway a drug was intended to inhibit, bypass signaling requires an alternative and parallel effector. Activation of parallel signaling is possible due to the redundancy of some proliferative intracellular signaling pathways. Again, a prime example of bypass signaling is seen in gefitinib-treated NSCLC. In this example, EGFR signaling through PI3K/AKT is thwarted by gefitinib. However, activation of the MET bypass oncogene reactivates EGFR signaling. This occurs via multiple routes, including gene amplification, elevation of the hepatocyte growth factor (HGF) ligand, or insulin growth factor-1 receptor (IGF-1R) signaling (28). In each situation, EGFR inhibition is unable to control proliferation because of the reactivation by a parallel RTK.

Beyond the three classic pathway-dependent mechanisms of acquired resistance, there are additional pathway-independent resistance mechanisms. Recent reports have suggested that resistance may arise from other cancer programs, including the **epithelial–mesenchymal transition (EMT)** and alterations in the TME. Perhaps the most studied of these mechanisms is EMT-induced drug resistance. Several studies have demonstrated that EMT promotes drug resistance and is thus a potential novel therapeutic strategy (29). As a transcriptional program, the key players (e.g., SNAIL, TWIST, and ZEB) are associated with a cancer stem cell (CSC) phenotype as well as expression of various transporters that are both chemo- and radioresistant. As for the

TME, studies have found that there is a complex relationship with cancer. The TME is capable of secreting a number of stromal cytokines and HGF to "feed" EGFR-driven cancer cells, thereby promoting TKI resistance. Put together, these pathway-independent mechanisms of drug resistance add a layer of complexity to the drug resistance story, contributing to the challenges of drug resistance.

THERAPY RESISTANCE MODELS

To address the challenges of overcoming treatment resistance, it is useful to establish preclinical models to study this phenomenon. Creating cancer models to study drug resistance aids in the development of novel strategies to overcome this barrier. While the gold standard of interrogating drug resistance would be to collect and analyze tumor samples pre- and posttreatment relapse in actual patients, it may take several months if not years to obtain these samples. Fortunately, there are both useful in vitro and in vivo treatment resistance preclinical models, but, as in the case for primary anticancer studies, critical questions to be evaluated regarding resistance mechanism include requirement and sufficiency of effectors and validation in clinical specimens and ultimately in patients (26).

A widely used experimental model to assess drug resistance involves culturing cancer cells. Both acquired and innate resistance can be investigated using cell culture. For example, a given cancer cell line can be cultured at first with low doses of an anticancer drug. Over weeks or months at a time, the drug dose is steadily increased. This process allows drug-sensitive cells to be selected against, while any drug-resistant clones may persist. The process is analogous to what is seen in patients, as there is an initial tumor response with reduction of tumor size, followed by an expansion of drug-resistant clones defining the recurrence. Additionally, with each increase of drug concentration, an aliquot of cells should be properly stored in liquid nitrogen to retain the cell population resistant at that concentration. After an extended period of time of dose escalation (e.g., 6 months with log-fold increase relative to starting drug dose), isogenic cell lines will have been established that differ primarily in their ability to tolerate different concentrations of drug.

As an example of this process and the subsequent analysis, after 6 months of erlotinib treatment, a given parental erlotinib-sensitive NSCLC cell line could result in low-, medium-, and high-dose resistant sublines. To investigate potential mechanisms of drug resistance, each of the resistant cell lines can be compared to the erlotinib-sensitive parental line. Candidates that should be assessed first are ones that relate to the drug mechanism of action. In this case, it is logical to hypothesize that there may be EGFR mutations and downstream/upstream activating mutations of the PI3K/AKT pathway. The use of genomics and/or proteomics may be useful in this analysis to determine the key gateway mutations driving erlotinib resistance. When using high-throughput bioinformatics-intensive methods, there may be a number of differences between the parental lines and the drug-resistant lines. Thus, it may be of interest to interrogate candidate genes that are sequentially mutated or amplified as the cell line transitions from parental, to low-, to medium-, to high-resistant isogenic cell lines. Taken together, this serves as a framework demonstrating the generation and assessment of a treatment-resistant in vitro cell-line–based model.

With the advent of large-scale RNAi and CRISPR-Cas9 targeting libraries, a more recent strategy for uncovering novel drug resistance mechanisms involves **systematic unbiased screening experiments**. Comprehensive RNAi and CRISPR-Cas9 based libraries have been developed to selectively knock down or knock out every mammalian gene and can be titrated in a way such that only a particular gene is knocked down in each cell. This enables comprehensive loss-of-function screens that may be used to investigate multiple mechanisms of drug resistance. A prime example of the use of a large-scale RNAi screen is a report that determined the loss of PTEN as a major determinant of trastuzumab resistance in breast cancer (30). In this report, the researchers followed up with a clinical analysis of 55 breast cancer patients. They found that activation of the PI3K pathway via downregulation of PTEN was associated with poor prognosis after trastuzumab therapy.

Once the mechanism of acquired resistance has been identified, four follow-up experiments should be considered. The mutated gene may be introduced into the parental cell line to directly show sufficiency for drug resistance. The gene of interest can also be knocked down or out using small interfering RNA (siRNA) or CRISPR-Cas9 in the high-dose drug-resistant line to demonstrate necessity for drug resistance. The mutated gene can be introduced into the parental cell line to assess whether downstream effectors are directly activated. Finally, there should be some analysis using patient samples to interrogate if the genetic alteration is clinically relevant as a bona fide mechanism of drug resistance in cancer patients. There are multiple user-friendly tools to determine clinical relevance if patient samples are not readily available. Web-based analyses of The Cancer Genome Atlas (TCGA) data can be performed through cBioPortal, UCSC Cancer Genomics Browser, or the Stanford Cancer Genome Atlas Clinical Explorer (31).

In vivo models are useful because they offer insight on drug resistance in relationship to TME interactions, metastatic potential, and drug metabolism. Using the in vitro model discussed earlier, these isogenic cell lines may be implanted into nude mice for xenograft experiments. One strategy is to implant a tumor with a drug-sensitive cell line in one flank and a drug-resistant cell line on the contralateral side. After a minimum tumor threshold volume is established, the mouse is treated with the drug over a period of time. If the gene confers drug resistivity, then it would be expected that the tumor would grow more aggressively compared to the parental cell line during drug treatment. Molecular analyses using Western blotting and immunohistochemistry can be performed for apoptotic markers and cell proliferation markers to quantify differences in drug resistance.

In a more complex model, GEMMs may be established to conditionally express transgenes of interest in an organ-specific manner. The transgenes required for this experiment include the cell/organ specific promoter, an oncogenic driver, and the gene of interest. Mice expressing both the oncogenic driver and the drug-resistant gene of interest would be compared to mice expressing the oncogenic driver alone. Much like the xenograft model, the mice would be given time to develop tumors, followed by a period of drug administration. The advantage of this model is that the organ and immune system effects can be taken into account. A great example of breast cancer drug resistance is described using a mammary gland-specific tetracycline-inducible model expressing human mutant $PIK3CA^{H1047R}$ and treated with a PI3K inhibitor (32) making phosphatidylinositol 3-kinase (PI3K). Mutant PIK3CA induced mammary tumors with elevated proliferative capacity as well as elevated activation of downstream p-AKT and p-S6RP. Unexpectedly, there were some tumors capable of overcoming PIK3CA oncogene addiction and tumor growth persisted upon removal of doxycycline. The group showed that the tumors which persisted despite PI3K signal withdrawal were innately resistant to clinically relevant PI3K inhibitors when tested in follow-up experiments. They determined the mechanism of action was due to MYC amplifications or MET upregulation.

The mechanistic understanding gained from in vitro and in vivo models drives the discovery of novel therapeutic combinations to combat drug resistance. One strategy is to identify the cause of cancer patient primary resistance and then select a second agent to circumvent the resistance. For example, in the setting of imatinib-resistant CML, dasatinib is clinically used to target the active conformation of ABL (33). A second strategy is to develop inhibitors that address the resistance up front by targeting known gateway mutations. For example, the CML drug nilotinib has shown efficacy even in the setting of imatinib-resistant mutant driven tumors (33). While both of these strategies are useful in the context of target reactivation, a third strategy is critical for bypass oncoprotein-mediated resistance. In the treatment of the bypass resistance, combinational therapies are warranted. An example of this is the combination of MEK and BRAF inhibitors used to treat acquired resistance in melanoma (34). A major consideration for combinational therapies is treatment toxicity. Combinational candidates should individually demonstrate high potency to reduce off-target effects when used in combination. As our understanding of cancer drug resistance evolves, we will be able to precisely optimize our arsenal of therapies to combat drug resistance a priori by treating patients with the right drug at the right dose in the first-line setting.

CONCLUSION

In this chapter, we highlighted some of the major pillars of cancer treatment including chemotherapy, hormonal therapy, targeted therapy, and radiation therapy. We discussed examples of experimental methodology used to evaluate cancer therapeutics in both laboratory and clinical settings. We reviewed the emerging players in the modern era of cancer immunotherapy. Finally, we discussed the key concepts behind drug resistance and provided examples of experimental approaches to probe mechanisms of cancer drug resistance.

GLOSSARY

xenogeneic: description of tumor graft material into an immunodeficient animal model.

syngeneic: description of tumor graft material into an immunocompetent animal model.

hormone therapy (hormonal or endocrine therapy): therapies that are particularly effective against certain types of hormone-driven breast and prostate cancers, which works either by blocking the body's ability to produce the hormone that promotes tumor growth or (b) by interfering with the interaction between the hormone and cancer cell.

estrogen receptor (ER): hormone targeted in breast cancer hormone therapy.

androgen receptor (AR): hormone targeted in prostate cancer hormone therapy.

aromatase inhibitors (AIs): breast cancer hormone therapy that inhibits the synthesis of estrogen.

molecularly targeted therapy: therapy type that specifically targets unique characteristics of cancer cells not seen in normal cells, thus limiting drug-associated toxicity.

"basket" trials: clinical trials designed to assess the efficacy of new therapeutic options in patients based on specific genetic mutation profile rather than the tumor site.

linear accelerator (LINAC): radiation therapy apparatus that works by using microwaves to accelerate electrons that then collide with a heavy metal target to produce high-energy x-rays.

external beam radiation therapy (EBRT, XRT): a major class of radiation therapy.

brachytherapy: internal source radiotherapy; a major class of radiation therapy.

radiosensitizer: drug that increases the toxicity of radiation in a cancer cell line relative to a noncancer control cell line.

poly(adenosine diphosphate [ADP]-ribose) polymerase inhibitor (PARPi) LT626: substance being tested for action as a radiosensitizer.

colony formation assay: the gold standard long-term anticancer in vitro assay.

combination index (CI): radiosensitization assessment measure in which a numeric is calculated to determine synergism (CI < 1), additivity (CI = 1), or antagonism (CI > 1).

genetically engineered mouse models (GEMMs): animal models being used for improved recapitulation of tumor biology in an autochthonous model.

immunotherapy: promising area of recent cancer therapy research.

hybridoma clone: fusion of mouse B-cell and myeloma cell.

ADCs: mAbs covalently bound to a linker that carries a cytotoxic agent or radioisotope.

angiogenesis: a biological phenomenon by which blood vasculature is generated de novo through a process of migration, growth, and differentiation of endothelial cells that line blood vessel walls.

oncolytic virus: a type of passive immunotherapy; a nonpathogenic replication-competent virus capable of targeting tumor cells and eliciting an antitumor response.

talimogene laherparepvec (T-VEC): a first-in-class intralesional oncolytic virotherapy.

adoptive T-cell transfer therapy (ACT): passive immunotherapy that uses the tumor-infiltrating lymphocytes (TILs) associated with tumorigenesis as T-cells capable of recognizing tumor-specific antigens.

tumor-infiltrating lymphocytes (TILs): lymphocytes associated with tumorigenesis.

chimeric antigen receptor (CAR) T-cell: a T-cell receptor further modulated with intracellular TCR immunostimulatory domains.

immunohistochemical analysis: means of finding the most mechanistically relevant biomarker for anti-PD-1 and anti-PD-L1 checkpoint blockade.

mutational load: a potential biomarker for predicting tumor response to immune checkpoint inhibitors.

anticancer vaccines: type of active immunotherapy.

immunostimulatory cytokines: type of active immunotherapy.

gene therapy: type of biological therapy.

multidrug resistance (MDR): a parallel mechanism of drug resistance.

oncogene addiction: perspective as to how cancer cells exploit oncogenic dysregulation to refuel cellular proliferation.

secondary reactivation: most common type of acquired drug resistance, in which genetic alterations of the target kinase alter contact points for drug binding or confer an active conformational state of the protein itself.

gatekeeper mutation: specific genetic alteration, often found in cancer patient tumors, that engenders drug resistivity.

upstream/downstream signaling pathway: category of acquired resistance.

bypass signaling: a category of acquired resistance.

epithelial–mesenchymal transition (EMT): cancer program through which resistance may arise.

systematic unbiased screening experiments: strategy for uncovering novel drug resistance mechanisms.

REFERENCES

1. Gilman A, Philips FS. The biological actions and therapeutic applications of the b-chloroethyl amines and sulfides. *Science*. 1946;103:409–436. doi:10.1126/science.103.2675.409
2. Gilman A. The initial clinical trial of nitrogen mustard. *Am J Surg*. 1963;105:574–578. doi:10.1016/0002-9610(63)90232-0
3. Kelland LR. 'Of mice and men': values and liabilities of the athymic nude mouse model in anticancer drug development. *Eur J Cancer*. 2004;40:827–836. doi:10.1016/j.ejca.2003.11.028
4. Morton CL, Houghton PJ. Establishment of human tumor xenografts in immunodeficient mice. *Nat Protoc*. 2007;2:247–250. doi:10.1038/nprot.2007.25
5. Farber S, Diamond LK. Temporary remissions in acute leukemia in children produced by folic acid antagonist, 4-aminopteroyl-glutamic acid. *N Engl J Med*. 1948;238:787–793. doi:10.1016/S0002-9343(48)90432-X
6. Groner AC, Brown M. Role of steroid receptor and coregulator mutations in hormone-dependent cancers. *J Clin Invest*. 2017;127:1126–1135. doi:10.1172/JCI88885
7. Druker BJ, Talpaz M, Resta DJ, et al. Efficacy and safety of a specific inhibitor of the BCR-ABL tyrosine kinase in chronic myeloid leukemia. *N Engl J Med*. 2001;344:1031–1037. doi:10.1056/nejm200104053441401
8. Hyman DM, Taylor BS, Baselga J. Implementing genome-driven oncology. *Cell*. 2017;168(4):584–599. doi:10.1016/j.cell.2016.12.015
9. Ginzton EL, Mallory KB, Kaplan HS. The Stanford medical linear accelerator. I. Design and development. *Stanford Med Bull*. 1957;15:123–140.
10. Dewhirst MW, Cao Y, Moeller B. Cycling hypoxia and free radicals regulate angiogenesis and radiotherapy response. *Nat Rev Cancer*. 2008;8:425–437. doi:10.1038/nrc2397
11. Hastak K, Bhutra S, Parry R, Ford JM. Poly (ADP-ribose) polymerase inhibitor, an effective radiosensitizer in lung and pancreatic cancers. *Oncotarget*. 2017;8(16):26344–26355. doi:10.18632/oncotarget.15464
12. Gierut JJ, Jacks TE, Haigis KM. Strategies to achieve conditional gene mutation in mice. *Cold Spring Harb Protoc*. 2014;2014(4):pdb.top069807. doi:10.1101/pdb.top069807
13. Galluzzi L, Vacchelli E, Bravo-San Pedro J-M, et al. Classification of current anticancer immunotherapies. *Oncotarget*. 2014;5(24):12472–12508. doi:10.18632/oncotarget.2998
14. Scott AM, Wolchok JD, Old LJ. Antibody therapy of cancer. *Nat Rev Cancer*. 2012;12:278–287. doi:10.1038/nrc3236
15. Russell SJ, Peng K-W. Oncolytic virotherapy: a contest between apples and oranges. *Mol Ther*. 2017;25(5):1107–1116. doi:10.1016/j.ymthe.2017.03.026
16. Topalian SL, Drake CG, Pardoll DM. Immune checkpoint blockade: a common denominator approach to cancer therapy. *Cancer Cell*. 2015;27:450–461. doi:10.1016/j.ccell.2015.03.001
17. Martin-Liberal J, de Olza MO, Hierro C, et al. The expanding role of immunotherapy. *Cancer Treat Rev*. 2017;54:74–86. doi:10.1016/j.ctrv.2017.01.008
18. Schadendorf D, Stephen Hodi F, Robert C, et al. Pooled analysis of long-term survival data from phase II and phase III trials of ipilimumab in unresectable or metastatic melanoma. *J Clin Oncol*. 2015;33:1889–1894. doi:10.1200/jco.2014.56.2736
19. Sunshine J, Taube JM. PD-1/PD-L1 inhibitors. *Curr Opin Pharmacol*. 2015;23:32–38. doi:10.1016/j.coph.2015.05.011
20. Le DT, Uram JN, Wang H, et al. PD-1 blockade in tumors with mismatch-repair deficiency. *N Engl J Med*. 2015;372:2509–2520. doi:10.1056/nejmoa1500596
21. Melief CJM, van der Burg SH. Immunotherapy of established (pre)malignant disease by synthetic long peptide vaccines. *Nat Rev Cancer*. 2008;8(5):351–360. doi:10.1038/nrc2373
22. Fellmann C, Gowen BG, Lin P-C, et al. Cornerstones of CRISPR-Cas in drug discovery and therapy. *Nat Rev Drug Discov*. 2017;16:89–100. doi:10.1038/nrd.2016.238
23. Brockman RW. Mechanisms of resistance to anticancer agents. *Adv Cancer Res*. 1963;7:129–234. doi:10.1016/S0065-230X(08)60983-5
24. Pastan I, Gottesman M. Multiple-drug resistance in human cancer. *N Engl J Med*. 1987;316:1388–1393. doi:10.1056/NEJM198705283162207
25. Felsher DW, Bishop JM. Reversible tumorigenesis by MYC in hematopoietic lineages. *Mol Cell*. 1999;4:199–207. doi:10.1016/S1097-2765(00)80367-6
26. Garraway LA, Jänne PA. Circumventing cancer drug resistance in the era of personalized medicine. *Cancer Discov*. 2012;2(3):214–226. doi:10.1158/2159-8290.cd-12-0012
27. Gorre ME. Clinical resistance to STI-571 cancer therapy caused by BCR-ABL gene mutation or amplification. *Science*. 2001;293:876–880. doi:10.1126/science.1062538
28. Engelman JA, Jänne PA. Mechanisms of acquired resistance to epidermal growth factor receptor tyrosine kinase inhibitors in non-small cell lung cancer. *Clin Cancer Res*. 2008;14:2895–2899. doi:10.1158/1078-0432.CCR-07-2248
29. Malek R, Wang H, Taparra K, Tran, PT. Therapeutic targeting of epithelial plasticity programs: focus on the epithelial-mesenchymal transition. *Cells Tissues Organs*. 2017;203:114–127. doi:10.1159/000447238
30. Berns K, Horlings HM, Hennessy BT, et al. A functional genetic approach identifies the PI3K pathway as a major determinant of trastuzumab resistance in breast cancer. *Cancer Cell*. 2007;12:395–402. doi:10.1016/j.ccr.2007.08.030

31. Lee H, Palm J, Grimes SM, Ji HP. The cancer genome atlas clinical explorer: a web and mobile interface for identifying clinical-genomic driver associations. *Genome Med.* 2015;7:112. doi:10.1186/s13073-015-0226-3
32. Liu P, Cheng H, Santiago S, et al. Oncogenic PIK3CA-driven mammary tumors frequently recur via PI3K pathway-dependent and PI3K pathway-independent mechanisms. *Nat Med.* 2011;17:1116–1120. doi:10.1038/nm.2402
33. O'Hare T, Eide CA, Deininger MWN. Bcr-Abl kinase domain mutations, drug resistance, and the road to a cure for chronic myeloid leukemia. *Blood.* 2007;110:2242–2249. doi:10.1182/blood-2007-03-066936
34. Villanueva J, Vultur A, Lee JT, et al. Acquired resistance to BRAF inhibitors mediated by a RAF kinase switch in melanoma can be overcome by cotargeting MEK and IGF-1R/PI3K. *Cancer Cell.* 2010;18:683–695. doi:10.1016/j.ccr.2010.11.023

8

Prognostic and Predictive Biomarkers

ARIEL E. MARCISCANO ■ PHUOC T. TRAN

Despite tremendous progress in screening, diagnosis, and treatment, cancer continues to be a major public health problem and a significant cause of morbidity and mortality. Death due to cancer is the second most common cause of mortality and accounts for nearly 25% of all deaths in the United States. In 2015, 1,658,370 new cases of cancer and 589,430 cancer deaths are projected to occur in the United States alone. Cancer is anticipated to surpass heart disease as the leading cause of death in the coming years (1).

Given these facts, there has been growing emphasis on the prevention and early detection of cancer as well as novel cancer treatments. However, even with a focus on preventive strategies and the implementation of novel therapeutics, many cancers continue to be diagnosed at late stages when treatments are generally less effective. Given the scope of this problem, there is great interest in the development, validation, and use of cancer biomarkers as a means to help lessen the cancer burden. The emergence of several new technologies has created new platforms for the discovery of novel cancer biomarkers.

DEFINITION OF CANCER BIOMARKERS

Cancer biomarkers are objective measures that rely upon the ability to identify and/or evaluate the unique molecular signature of a specific cancer type or malignant process. Cancer biomarkers are represented by a broad and heterogeneous group of biochemical entities, which range from nucleic acids, proteins, and metabolites to whole tumor cells as well as cytogenetic, cytokinetic, and imaging parameters (2). Ultimately, measurable changes in genes or gene products that provide clinically meaningful information are potential candidate biomarkers. Biomarkers are measurable in various biological materials, including the actual malignant cell of interest, tissues within the surrounding tumor microenvironment, and/or bodily fluids such as serum, plasma, and urine. At present, cancer biomarkers are utilized in a variety of different clinical contexts. They can be applied for the purposes of population screening, diagnosis, tumor staging, prognostication, and detection of disease recurrence as well as prediction of therapeutic response and monitoring the effectiveness of therapy (3).

To understand the clinical application of biomarkers, it is a requisite to have a functional knowledge of basic epidemiology and biostatistics. Specificity and sensitivity are statistical measures that assess the performance of a binary test or assay. **Specificity** refers to the proportion of control (without disease) subjects that are accurately identified as negative by the test (biomarker assay) under evaluation; it can be conceptualized as the "true negative rate." The **sensitivity** of a test is the proportion of subjects with confirmed disease that are accurately identified as positive by the test (biomarker assay); it can be conceptualized as the "true positive rate." The relationship between specificity and sensitivity in regard to a specific biomarker assay is graphically represented in Figure 8.1. Additionally, the receiver operating characteristic (ROC) curve can be used to evaluate the efficacy of a biomarker across a spectrum of values. As the ratio of the true positive rate to false positive rate increases, the area under the curve (AUC) consequently increases, as does the utility of the biomarker. An ideal ROC curve has a maximum AUC of 1.00 (Figure 8.2). A more in-depth review of basic biostatistics in cancer research appears in Chapter 11.

The prototypical cancer biomarker must fulfill several criteria, including: (a) the existence of significant and measurable differences (e.g., within biological fluid levels, gene expression patterns) from healthy subjects in order to distinguish between malignant and nonmalignant states, (b) the use of a consistent and standardized assay with well-defined reference limits, (c) outstanding analytic capacity with high sensitivity and specificity (e.g., high positive and negative predictive value), (d) cost-effectiveness, (e) easy accessibility, and (f) prospective clinical validation in a large cohort of subjects (3,4). In reality, few biomarkers, if any, are able to meet all of these criteria and there is an inherent trade-off between sensitivity and specificity of an assay as well as difficulty in selecting the subjects that are most appropriate for a specific test. Nevertheless, cancer biomarker identification remains essential to the goal of personalized and precision medicine, as this will allow physicians to identify the appropriate subsets of patients for therapy, to predict and to evaluate therapeutic response, and ultimately to tailor therapeutic intervention to a patient based upon his or her unique biological profile (5).

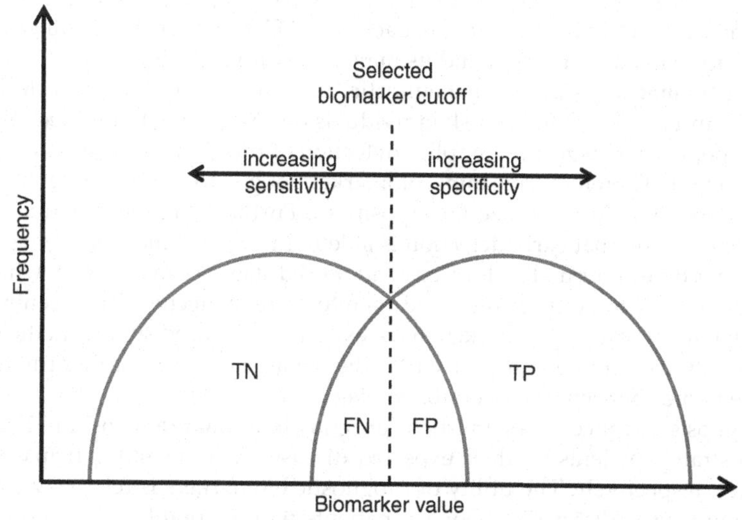

FIGURE 8.1 Graphical representation of the relationship between sensitivity and specificity.

FN, false negative; FP, false positive; TN, true negative; TP, true positive.

Source: Kulasingam V, Diamandis EP. Strategies for discovering novel cancer biomarkers through utilization of emerging technologies. *Nat Clin Pract Oncol.* 2008;5(10):588–599.

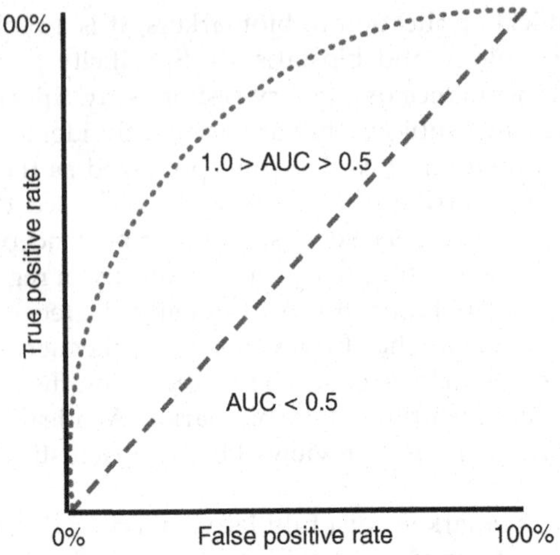

FIGURE 8.2 The receiver operating characteristic curve demonstrating the trade-off between true positive rate (sensitivity) and false positive rate (1 – specificity) for determining the optimal cutoff value for a biomarker test. A perfect biomarker test has a maximum AUC = 1.0. The dotted line represents a useful biomarker test with an AUC > 0.5 (albeit less than perfect, i.e., AUC < 1.0). The dashed line represents a nonuseful biomarker test with an AUC < 0.5.

AUC, area under the curve.

Source: Kulasingam V, Diamandis EP. Strategies for discovering novel cancer biomarkers through utilization of emerging technologies. *Nat Clin Pract Oncol*. 2008;5(10):588–599.

PROGNOSTIC AND PREDICTIVE BIOMARKERS

In general terms, there are three classes of biomarkers: screening/diagnostic biomarkers, prognostic biomarkers, and predictive biomarkers (6). Each class of biomarkers has distinct applications in relation to the natural history of cancer and its management (Figure 8.3).

A **screening biomarker** is used for diagnostic purposes on an individual level in order to detect a specific cancer type among at-risk individuals or on a population-based level for screening of an at-risk population. Screening implies detection of preclinical or early-stage disease in an asymptomatic subject. Therefore, screening biomarkers ought to possess exceptional specificity and high sensitivity so as to minimize false positives. Furthermore, an effective screening biomarker must demonstrate that early detection is able to improve clinical outcomes. Many cancer biomarkers only become abnormally elevated at advanced stages of malignancy when therapeutic intervention is less likely to be successful, and therefore are ineffective for screening. In practice, screening and diagnostic cancer biomarkers have experienced varied success in the clinical arena. They are commonly used in conjunction with other imaging or clinical information and often require invasive tissue confirmation to establish diagnosis.

Once a diagnosis of cancer is established, **prognostic biomarkers** and **predictive biomarkers** are used to stratify patients by their expected disease outcome and anticipated response to specific therapies, respectively. The utility of prognostic biomarkers is relatively straightforward in that they allow for the distinction between patients with favorable and unfavorable prognoses. Effective prognostic biomarkers correlate with the natural history of the cancer and provide meaningful information about a patient's clinical trajectory (e.g., overall survival, progression-free survival), which can help direct treatment selection, aggressiveness of therapy, and in some circumstances the need for adjuvant treatment versus postoperative surveillance (3). Classically, the definition of a prognostic biomarker applies to the expected clinical outcome among groups of

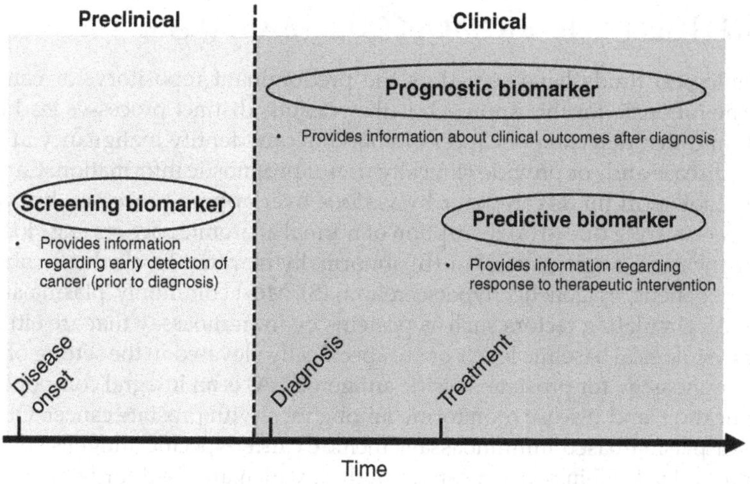

FIGURE 8.3 The application of screening, prognostic, and predictive biomarkers in the context of cancer progression from preclinical to clinical disease.

treatment-naïve patients. However, prognostic biomarkers are often used as a means to identify patients at risk for recurrence or metastasis following up-front therapy. Importantly, prognostic biomarkers explicitly do not provide information regarding response to a specific therapy (7).

In contrast to prognostic biomarkers, predictive biomarkers are objective measures that stratify patients based on their anticipated response to a specific therapeutic intervention. Indeed, for strictly predictive biomarkers, the use of a particular therapy is an independent predictor of outcome (8). The utility of predictive biomarkers lies in the ability to identify subgroups of patients who are likely or unlikely to respond to specific therapeutic interventions, thus guiding treatment selection in a more individualized fashion. Predictive biomarkers can be further subcategorized as (a) those that predict response prior to the therapeutic intervention and (b) those that provide information about early therapeutic response or treatment effect after intervention.

It is important to acknowledge that certain cancer biomarkers can serve as both prognostic and predictive factors, with the caveat that interpretation is dependent on the clinical context. An illustrative example is hormonal receptor status in breast cancer, which is both prognostic and predictive. Estrogen receptor/progesterone receptor (ER/PR) positivity is prognostic, in that it is independently associated with reduced mortality (9), and it is also a powerful predictive factor for the likelihood of benefit for adjuvant hormonal therapy (10).

METHODS FOR BIOMARKER DETECTION

Over the past two decades, there has been tremendous evolution in the field of cancer biomarker discovery given the emergence of several new technologies in conjunction with improved understanding of the biological underpinnings of cancer. Recent notable achievements include the completion of the Human Genome Project, next-generation sequencing (NGS) and various high-throughput technologies, and the complementary field of bioinformatics, which have laid foundation for the genomics, proteomics, and epigenomic revolutions. A veritable paradigm shift is occurring where single-biomarker analysis is being transitioned toward multiparametric analyses, which aim to identify unique molecular patterns and/or signatures that can better characterize the intrinsic complexity and heterogeneity of cancer (3,5). Often the methodologies used for candidate cancer biomarker detection have mirrored advances in knowledge and development of new technologies. Herein, we provide an overview of the various strategies employed for cancer biomarker evaluation and discovery.

CANCER-ANTIGEN AND BIOMOLECULE-BASED ASSAYS

Traditionally, biological fluids have served as the predominant repository for cancer biomarker identification. The rationale for this approach is that various distinct processes lead to elevation in biological fluids and that detection of cancer biomarkers can identify malignancy at early and preclinical stages of disease and/or provide clinically useful prognostic information. Cancer biomarker detection within biological fluids can occur by various overlapping processes, but can be broadly conceptualized as occurring due to (a) disruption of normal anatomic barriers (e.g., local destruction, lymphovascular invasion, angiogenesis) or (b) abnormally elevated levels due to aberrant biological processes (e.g., genetic, epigenetic, hypersecretion) (3). Most commonly, plasma and serum have been used to detect circulating factors such as proteins by immunoassay that are either abnormally elevated from physiological baseline levels or are specifically elevated in the setting of malignancy. A serum-based immunoassay for prostate-specific antigen (PSA) is an integral component in the diagnosis, risk stratification, and disease monitoring among men with prostate cancer. Other commonly utilized serum- or plasma-based immunoassays include cancer-specific antigens such as CA19-9 in pancreatic cancer and CA125 in ovarian cancer, both of which are used for the evaluation of treatment response, as well as oncofetal antigens such as alpha-fetoprotein (AFP), which is pathologically elevated in hepatocellular carcinoma and nonseminomatous germ cell tumors.

Tissue-based assays generally require invasive sampling of tumor or tissue of interest in order to qualitatively or quantitatively measure certain cancer biomarkers. Frequently, immunohistochemistry (IHC) is used to evaluate membrane-bound extracellular proteins and other intracellular or nuclear proteins (e.g., Ki-67, mitotic index). Examples include hormone receptor status in breast cancer in which the intensity of staining for ER and PR dictates receptor positivity or negativity, which is crucial for both prognostication and treatment selection. Recently, as immunotherapy, specifically immune checkpoint blockade, has rapidly become a mainstay in the anticancer armamentarium, there is great interest in the identification of biomarkers that will help predict treatment response and select patients who may benefit from this therapy. Programmed death-ligand 1 (PD-L1) expression has emerged as a potential predictive biomarker for both anti-programmed death-1 (anti-PD-1) and anti-PD-L1 therapies, as baseline intratumoral expression of PD-L1 has been correlated with clinical benefit in some cancer subtypes (11,12). However, variability between IHC-based assays, intrinsic difference in therapeutic antibodies, and arbitrary thresholds used to define positivity (based on percentage of tumor or immune cells expressing PD-L1) have complicated initial interpretation and early validation of this biomarker and are illustrative of the obstacles encountered by researchers and clinicians alike (13).

It deserves note that biological fluids and tissues also serve as the predominant medium for biomarker evaluation along with various newer technologies such as mass spectrometry or circulating tumor cell (CTC) analysis; these are reviewed later. Additionally, sampling of organ or tissue-specific biological compartments such as the cerebrospinal fluid, urine, or pleural fluid may help to identify biomarkers unique to certain cancer subtypes.

GENE-BASED ASSAYS (GENETIC, EPIGENETIC, AND GENOMIC)

The initial foray into the field of gene-based biomarkers is inextricably linked to the central dogma that genetic alterations are sentinel initiating events in carcinogenesis and that specific mutations, leading to either oncogene activation or tumor suppressor gene loss of function, are central to cancer development. This notion holds true in many circumstances, for instance, the translocation of chromosomes 9 and 22 and their oncogenic BCR–ABL gene fusion product, which is diagnostic in chronic myelogenous leukemia and predictive of response to targeted kinase inhibitors. However, it is generally accepted that this view underestimates the vast genetic complexity and intricacy of genetic and epigenetic changes that underlie malignant transformation and progression. Nevertheless, analysis of genetic mutations and mutation-based biomarkers has served important roles in diagnosis, prognostication, and prediction of therapeutic response in several cancer subtypes.

Modulation of gene expression occurs via multiple mechanisms and the wide array of genetic material alterations used as cancer biomarkers can be classified into three broad categories: (a) cytogenetic/chromosome based; (b) genetic/mutation based; and (c) epigenetic based (2). Structural alterations to chromosomes such as translocation of genetic elements or pathologic variants in ploidy can be used as cytogenetic markers of malignancy. In non-small cell lung cancer (NSCLC), genetic rearrangement of the anaplastic lymphoma kinase (*ALK*) gene and its fusion with various partner genes (e.g., echinoderm microtubule-associated protein-like 4 [*EML4*]) has been identified as an important predictive biomarker. Currently, fluorescence in situ hybridization (FISH) is the gold standard technique for the detection of *ALK*-rearranged lung adenocarcinomas, which identifies a subset of "*ALK*-positive" patients who are likely to have a favorable response to oral *ALK* inhibitors, such as crizotinib (14,15). The aforementioned BCR–ABL fusion product represents an additional example of a clinically integrated cytogenetic biomarker. In addition to FISH, other assays of cytogenetic biomarkers include conventional and spectral karyotyping as well as chromosome-based comparative genomic hybridization (CGH) (2).

With regard to gene-specific alterations, it has been well characterized that gain or loss of gene function can lead to oncogenic transformation (16). Deleterious mutations in tumor suppressor genes, *BRCA1* and *BRCA2*, are heavily associated with increased risk of developing breast and ovarian cancers as well as prostate, melanoma, and pancreatic cancers to a lesser extent (17–20). Furthermore, these mutations as well as other high-penetrance heritable mutations, such as *PTEN* and *TP53*, have been directly implicated in several hereditary cancer syndromes in addition to sporadic cancers.

Given this, identification of *BRCA1* and *BRCA2* mutations serves as a highly effective screening biomarker particularly when familial germline mutations or inherited cancer susceptibility syndromes are suspected. Indeed, they play an important role for both prevention and screening of at-risk individuals and their relatives by identifying asymptomatic individuals at preclinical states of disease, thus affording them the opportunity to pursue genetic counseling, preventive strategies, or risk reduction therapies when deemed appropriate (21). As such, well-defined screening recommendations and risk assessment criteria based on these genetic biomarkers exist to aid selection of the appropriate individuals for genetic testing.

At present, specific gene mutations are most commonly detected by basic DNA sequencing technologies such as polymerase chain reaction (PCR) using microsatellite probes. Intriguingly, the advent of NGS methods and other modern genomics tools has raised the possibility for population-wide screening for *BRCA1* and *BRCA2* mutations. However, various clinical, economic, and ethical considerations preclude this from being integrated in the immediate future (22). *BRCA1* and *BRCA2* mutations also carry prognostic implications, as *BRCA1* mutations have been linked with a higher incidence of triple-negative breast cancers, which traditionally carry a poorer prognosis than other molecular subtypes (23). Furthermore, among men with prostate cancer, BRCA mutation carriers have significantly poorer survival outcomes and more aggressive histologies as compared with noncarriers (24). Interestingly, a recent whole-exome sequencing observational study reported that *BRCA2* mutations among women with high-grade serous ovarian cancers are associated with improved survival and improved primary response to platinum chemotherapy in comparison to their wild-type counterparts, suggesting a putative role as a prognostic and potentially predictive biomarker (25).

The kinase-activating *BRAF V600E* mutation in metastatic melanoma is a prime example of a genetic biomarker and actionable mutation that has been actively targeted therapeutically. Patients harboring this mutation are sensitive to vemurafenib, a small molecular inhibitor of BRAF. The Food and Drug Administration (FDA) approval of vemurafenib was purposefully accompanied by the BRAF V600E mutation test to determine which patients would derive benefit from this therapy (26). Indeed, the notion of companion diagnostic markers for targeted agents represents a genuine step toward personalized medicine.

Gene overexpression is an additional genetic alteration that can serve as a biomarker and commonly results due to oncogene amplification (increased gene copy number) or increased transcriptional activity due to aberrant regulation (6). Finally, microsatellite instability (MSI), resulting from defects in mismatch repair (MMR) genes, can be detected via comparative PCR analysis or IHC.

This entity is best defined among patients with a predisposition for colorectal cancers, either with germline mutations leading to hereditary syndromes (Lynch syndrome) or with sporadic MSI-high (MSI-H) colon cancers, which generally manifest as a result of epigenetic silencing via MLH1 promoter hypermethylation (27,28). Another major advance in this field has been the FDA's first tissue/site-agnostic approval, which represents the first drug with an indication based on a tissue biomarker rather than a cancer subtype. As such, pembrolizumab (anti-PD-1) is now approved for patients with unresectable or metastatic MSI-H or mismatch repair deficient (dMMR) solid tumors, with progression on prior therapy and no satisfactory alternative treatment options (29).

Along these lines, it has become increasingly clear that epigenetic events are directly implicated in carcinogenesis and cancer progression. Genes and their functional products can be modified via epigenetic modifications to chromosomes that alter gene expression patterns. Epigenetic modification can occur directly through DNA methylation of genes or indirectly by methylation, acetylation, or phosphorylation of histones and other chromatin-associated proteins. Glioma biology has undergone a renaissance over the past decade, although prognosis remains quite poor among patients afflicted with glioblastoma and other high-grade gliomas. However, the addition of temozolomide to surgical resection and adjuvant radiotherapy resulted in survival benefit, which had been sorely missing for many years (30,31). Intriguingly, the benefit of temozolomide was mechanistically linked to epigenetic changes, which rendered tumors as either sensitive or resistant to alkylating therapies. Epigenetic silencing of a DNA repair enzyme, O-6-methylguanine-DNA-methyltransferase (MGMT), via promoter methylation results in reduced ability to repair DNA damage induced by alkylating agents, such as temozolomide, thus enhancing chemotherapeutic efficacy. As such, MGMT promoter methylation status has been shown to be a predictive biomarker of response to alkylating agents, although some clinicians view this as an imperfect biomarker because patients with MGMT promoter hypermethylation still derive some benefit from temozolomide (32).

Even more recently, comprehensive integrative genomic analyses have yielded tremendous progress in the arena of molecular characterization and stratification of glioma, as evidenced by several high-impact reports in 2015 (33,34). Whole-exome sequencing and rigorous evaluation of DNA methylation patterns, copy number, and RNA expression ultimately identified three key molecular aberrations (*IDH* mutation, *TERT* promoter mutation, and 1p/19q codeletion), which define five subsets of glioma patients with distinct molecular and clinical traits. Similar strides have been made in medulloblastoma via integrative genomic approaches (35,36). Comprehensive profiling using The Cancer Genome Atlas (TCGA) has also led to the identification of distinct molecular subtypes across a spectrum of non–central nervous system malignancies (e.g., urothelial bladder, invasive breast cancer, prostate), which has informed novel therapeutic targets and represents an important step toward the realization of precision medicine (37–41).While these advances demonstrate the evolving manner in which oncologists are beginning to stratify patients, much work is still needed to learn how to translate this prognostic information into clinical benefit.

As the sophistication of genomic assays increases, multigene expression signatures and gene expression pattern arrays have been able to improve the utility of prognostic and predictive biomarkers as compared to assays that rely on detection of solitary genetic aberrations. Perhaps the most well-integrated example is Oncotype DX, a 21-gene reverse transcriptase (RT) PCR-based panel that stratifies risk of recurrence among women with early-stage ER+ breast cancers and helps direct the decision for adjuvant chemohormonal therapies. Given that a low Oncotype DX recurrence score correlates with favorable prognosis and also indicates lack of benefit from adjuvant chemotherapy, it serves as both a prognostic and a predictive biomarker (42,43).

IMAGING-BASED ASSAYS

The field of quantitative imaging biomarkers has generated great optimism recently, as there have been considerable advances in the development of new applications for established technologies as well as the introduction of new imaging techniques. **Imaging biomarkers** are objective radiological (or molecular) measures that are able to assay in vivo anatomic and biologic processes in a noninvasive and quantitative manner. As such, imaging biomarkers are becoming a particularly appealing option for cancer biomarker discovery and are rapidly being integrated into clinical practice. Indeed, there has been success with the implementation of imaging biomarkers, particularly in the setting of assessment of therapeutic response, as predictive biomarkers. The Response Evaluation Criteria in Solid Tumors (RECIST) guidelines were introduced in 2000 and have been widely adopted as a clinical decision-making tool and standardized measure of tumor response in various solid malignancies (44,45). The RECIST criteria are a CT-based model that assesses all existing lesions characterized as either measurable or nonmeasurable and then further subcategorizes measurable lesions as either target or nontarget lesions. Evaluation of these lesions by standardized criteria is used to extrapolate the overall response to treatment as complete response, partial response, progressive disease, or stable disease. These guidelines have become key components in clinical trial design methodology as well as day-to-day clinical practice in the decision to continue or discontinue certain therapies.

Advances in molecular and functional imaging have also been promising and possess considerable advantages over other imaging techniques as they rely on the ability to assay biological processes in vivo rather than anatomic and/or structural-based changes. The noninvasive nature of quantitative imaging lends itself to serial measurements allowing for assessment of response over time or response to therapeutic intervention. Additionally, quantitative imaging biomarkers provide whole body information, thereby circumventing issues with sampling error or tissue heterogeneity that may arise with targeted tissue-based biomarker assays. A well-integrated molecular imaging tool is fluorine-18 2-fluoro-2-deoxyglucose PET (^{18}F-FDG PET), a marker of tumor metabolism by regional glucose uptake, which has become indispensable as a diagnostic modality and for evaluation of treatment response in various cancers.

Perhaps the most striking example is the modernization of the staging and response assessment criteria in both Hodgkin (HL) and non-Hodgkin lymphoma (NHL). The Lugano classification has recently been formally incorporated as the standard staging among all ^{18}F-FDG PET avid lymphomas, and response-adapted strategies based on the interim PET response to up-front therapy are rapidly gaining traction as a formalized criterion for treatment selection and the decision-making framework for treatment intensification or deintensification (46). Importantly, as with all cancer biomarkers, a standardized and reproducible assay with well-defined reference limits has been defined for ^{18}F-FDG PET based imaging in the form of the five-point Deauville scoring system (47). As molecular-based imaging techniques continue to mature and new targeted therapies continue to develop, an exciting convergence of imaging-based biomarkers to describe specific molecular phenotypes can be used to help identify appropriate subsets of patients for targeted approaches and monitor their response to such therapies. Cost considerations and development of standardized assessment criteria still pose considerable obstacles for many imaging-based biomarkers.

EMERGING TECHNOLOGIES

As previously mentioned, several recent technologies have granted opportunities for novel biomarker discovery. Warranting specific mention are CTCs and their detection in peripheral blood, which have steadily gained traction as clinical evidence matures demonstrating that CTCs can be of prognostic value and can potentially assist rational therapy selection. The noninvasive nature of CTC detection, which generally involves collection of peripheral blood and immunomagnetic capture and immunofluorescence of CTC-specific surface markers, makes this a very intriguing strategy. Indeed, elevated levels of CTCs were determined to be an independent predictor of progression-free survival and overall survival among patients with metastatic breast cancer in a prospective randomized study (48). Similar findings have been corroborated in the setting of metastatic prostate cancer (49) and advanced colorectal cancer (50). The detection or persistence of CTCs following therapy to evaluate treatment response is currently being evaluated; however, recent findings have tempered enthusiasm. SWOG S0500, a randomized phase III trial, ambitiously set out to use CTCs as a predictive metric of treatment response to cytotoxic therapy in metastatic breast cancer. Patients with persistently increased CTCs after 3 weeks of therapy were randomized to switch to an alternative regimen or continue with the initial therapeutic intervention. However, those patients who switched to alternative therapies did not show a survival benefit (51). Nevertheless, this approach still carries much promise and the ability to noninvasively assess which patients have complete responses to neoadjuvant therapy and can be spared potentially unnecessary surgery and the associated morbidities. Additionally, patients with persistent CTCs or rising CTCs following definitive treatment may be candidates for intensification of adjuvant therapy or consideration of early salvage therapy.

Unlike CTCs, circulating tumor DNA (ctDNA) profiling is a cell-free assay and an emerging plasma-based biomarker that uses high-resolution sequencing technologies to identify DNA fragments extruded from cancer cells, thus enabling noninvasive disease monitoring or treatment response assessment. Applications are similar to CTCs and quantification of ctDNA in the peripheral blood may be used to help personalize therapy and guide treatment or even potentially screen high-risk patients with a predisposition to develop cancer (52–53).

On a final note, the burgeoning field of functional proteomics and tools such as mass spectrometry or mass cytometry (CyTOF) pose an exciting challenge for scientists and clinicians as they learn how to apply newer technologies in order to discover and clinically validate cancer biomarkers and eventually integrate them with the current standards of care.

CANCER BIOMARKERS BY SITE

Several validated and emerging biomarkers have been integrated into clinical practice ranging from use in initial diagnostic workup through disease monitoring in advanced cancer (54,55). An introduction of established and emerging clinical biomarkers in the five most common noncutaneous solid tumors is provided as follows.

BREAST CANCER

Hormone receptor and HER2 status are critical prognostic and predictive biomarkers for the initial workup of any newly diagnosed breast cancer of any stage. Further, ER/PR-positive tumors help predict responsiveness to endocrine-based therapies, and therapies that target HER2 are now available (trastuzumab, pertuzumab), making the identification of ERBB2 gene amplification important both prognostically and as a predictive biomarker. The benefit of adjuvant chemotherapy in localized, node-negative ER/PR-positive disease that is >5 mm is heterogeneous. The 21-gene expression recurrence score based on the Oncotype DX assay helps address this issue and estimates the likelihood of recurrence and relative benefit from chemotherapy (56). Several other gene signature assays are in development for breast cancer. A 70-gene expression profiling (GEP) test (MammaPrint) is FDA approved and helps stratify patients with either ER-positive or -negative disease into those with high or low risk for recurrence. However, this assay does not predict response to adjuvant systemic therapy (57). Other GEP tests are being developed and integrated for noninvasive breast cancer (e.g., Oncotype DX Breast DCIS) to help understand which patients can undergo surveillance versus those who may benefit from definitive therapy. Finally, DNA microarray GEP has helped identify five distinct molecular subtypes: luminal A, luminal B, triple-negative/basal-like, HER2-enriched, and normal-like. Each subtype carries a distinct clinical outcome and these classifications are being integrated into clinical trial design (58).

NON-SMALL CELL LUNG CANCER

A number of predictive biomarkers have been integrated for NSCLC to help guide management, predominantly in the metastatic setting. Although rare, ALK fusions (2%–7% of all NSCLC) and ROS1 rearrangements (1%–2% of all NSCLC) identify a subset of patients who are sensitive to oral ALK inhibitors, such as crizotinib. Patients harboring ALK or ROS1 rearrangements are generally not sensitive to EGFR inhibitors and often these genetic aberrations are mutually exclusive. A host of sensitizing EGFR mutations have been identified that predict response to EGFR-targeting tyrosine kinase inhibitors (TKIs). Alternatively, KRAS mutations or EGFR exon 20 insertion predicts resistance to EGFR TKI therapy. Of note, presence of a KRAS mutation also serves as a prognostic biomarker, as these patients experience shorter survival relative to their wild-type counterparts (59). Recently, it has been recognized that acquired resistance to EGFR TKIs arises from the development of a second site EGFR T790M mutation that confers resistance. Furthermore, osimertinib, a third-generation EGFR inhibitor that is selective for EGFR TKI sensitizing and T790M resistance mutations, has demonstrated superior efficacy relative to cytotoxic chemotherapy among T790M-positive NSCLC patients that progressed following first-line EGFR TKIs (60). As such, the T790M mutation has rapidly become an important predictive biomarker and a therapeutic target, given the FDA approval of osimertinib. Similarly, PD-L1 expression is now being used as a predictive biomarker to identify patients more likely to respond to pembrolizumab in both the first- and second-line metastatic setting. As previously discussed, PD-L1 is an imperfect biomarker, and other FDA-approved anti-PD-1/PD-L1 agents (durvalumab, nivolumab) for NSCLC do not select patients based on PD-L1 status. Finally, there are a cadre of emerging biomarkers, such as MET amplification/mutations, which may have a more important role in the near future as therapeutics targeting MET begin to enter the clinic.

PROSTATE CANCER

PSA continues to be an integral biomarker in all stages of prostate cancer, from initial diagnostic workup to risk stratification and treatment/disease monitoring, and this serum test is used in conjunction with clinical exam and pathologic information. Recently, there has been great emphasis on the development of better tools for prognostication of patients to inform clinical decision making. The Decipher prostate biopsy and radical prostatectomy tests utilize whole-transcriptome expression profiling to stratify patients into low- or high-risk categories. The Decipher biopsy test is intended to help guide treatment selection among men with localized disease who have undergone biopsy. Those with high-risk Decipher biopsy classification may not be suitable for active surveillance and may benefit from treatment intensification. Alternatively, those with low-risk classification may not require multimodal therapy or can potentially undergo active surveillance (61). Similarly, in the postprostatectomy setting the Decipher identifies genomic "low" or "high" risk to inform prognosis and to guide adjuvant/salvage treatment decisions (or observation) (62). The Oncotype DX Genomic Prostate Score is a 17-gene signature score that helps refine risk stratification for men with clinically low-risk or low–intermediate risk prostate cancer to help individualize the decision to pursue active surveillance or definitive therapy (63). The Prolaris Score employs a similar concept using a 46-gene RNA expression signature to estimate 10-year risk of prostate cancer specific mortality (PCSM) for men with localized cancer who have undergone biopsy that helps determine the aggressiveness of disease and therefore guides treatment selection. This tool has also been applied in the postprostatectomy setting to estimate the 10-year risk of biochemical recurrence to identify patients with aggressive variants of prostate cancer who might benefit from treatment intensification (64,65). The ProMark system follows a slightly different approach with an 8-protein expression signature using a multiplex immunofluorescence platform, which is undergoing clinical validation for its use in the prediction of PCSM for men with National Comprehensive Cancer Network (NCCN) low-risk or very low-risk localized prostate (66). The development and availability of a myriad of clinically validated prognostic tests marks a new era in prostate cancer management; the next challenge will be to define their cost-effectiveness and suitability for large-scale application in addition to meeting regulatory requirements of the FDA and other governing agencies.

The FDA approval of six new agents since 2011 for metastatic castration-resistant prostate cancer has led to the discovery of several potential predictive biomarkers. One emerging target of interest is the androgen receptor splice variant 8 (AR-V7), which appears to predict resistance to enzalutamide and abiraterone (67). Further, AR-V7 has been validated as a treatment-specific biomarker that is associated with superior clinical outcomes with taxane-based therapy compared to enzalutamide or abiraterone (68). Interestingly, AR-V7 status can be detected through collection of CTCs and is being explored as a metric of treatment response. Another interesting development has been the appreciation that approximately 25% of metastatic castration-resistant prostate cancer patients harbor aberrations in the DNA repair pathways (69). This discovery has opened new therapeutic avenues, including DNA-damaging agents (e.g., poly(ADP-ribose) polymerase [PARP] inhibitors, platinum-based chemotherapy, ionizing radiation) and the tissue-agnostic indication of pembrolizumab for dMMR and MSI-H solid tumors.

COLORECTAL CANCER

Colorectal cancer biomarker development has largely been driven by the identification of genetic susceptibility syndromes, including hereditary nonpolyposis colorectal cancer (HNPCC) or Lynch syndrome. As mentioned, IHC testing for MMR protein expression (or absence in dMMR) or PCR-based assays for MSI are biomarker tools that have prognostic and/or predictive roles. Patients with stage II MSI-H tumors generally carry a more favorable prognosis relative to microsatellite-stable counterparts and therefore derive less benefit from adjuvant chemotherapy (70). More recently, the predictive utility of these biomarkers has gained traction with the approval of pembrolizumab (tissue/site agnostic) and nivolumab (colorectal only) for dMMR and MSI-H patients. Genotyping for KRAS, NRAS, and BRAF V600E mutations also has a role in the metastatic setting. KRAS exon 2 mutations often predict resistance and/or lack of response to EGFR-targeting monoclonal antibodies, panitumumab and cetuximab. Similarly, patients with non-exon 2 mutations of NRAS mutation also appear to derive minimal benefit from EGFR inhibition. Of note, EGFR status has not demonstrated predictive value (71). Trending of serum CEA levels is a long-standing and valuable disease status monitoring tool that functions as a surrogate for disease burden and can be used to assess treatment response longitudinally.

Finally, using a similar RT-PCR based platform, the Oncotype DX Colon Recurrence Score uses a 12-gene signature platform. This is a prognostic biomarker test that estimates the risk of recurrence following surgery for patients with stage II, mismatch repair proficient tumors and stage IIIA/IIIB disease. Patients who are stratified into the high recurrence score group are at increased risk of recurrence and thus may derive greater benefit from adjuvant chemotherapy (70). Other multigene signature assays for risk stratification are also in developmental or validation stages, including ColoPrint and ColDx. In line with other disease sites, recent investigation has defined four distinct molecular subtypes of colorectal cancer: (a) CMS1 (MSI immune)—MSI-H with strong immune activation; (b) CMS2 (canonical)—epithelial, WNT and MYC activated; (c) CMS3 (metabolic)—epithelial, metabolic dysregulation; and (d) CMS4 (mesenchymal)—TGFβ activated, stromal invasion, proangiogenic (72). These molecular stratifications are encouraging for future personalized therapies but have yet to be integrated into the clinic.

BLADDER CARCINOMA

The notion of developing urinary biomarkers for clinical use in bladder cancer is intriguing. Although many putative biomarkers have been identified and several assays have been granted FDA approval, their adoption into clinical practice has been limited given ongoing concerns about the added utility beyond the current standard of care. At present, the majority of urinary biomarker assays are designed to function as an adjunct to cystoscopy and urine cytology to aid initial diagnosis for high-risk or symptomatic individuals, as well as to detect early recurrence following resection. Broadly, the nuclear matrix protein (NMP22) BladderChek and bladder tumor–associated antigen (BTA) tests are urine-based immunoassays that qualitatively or quantitatively evaluate protein expression levels of targets that are produced by tumor cells (BTA) or released upon tumor cell apoptosis (NMP22) (73–75). The ImmunoCyt assay relies upon urine cytology with fluorescent labeling of cancer-associated proteins/antigens and may further assist detection of recurrent disease in conjunction with standard urine cytology (76). A FISH-based assay to detect common chromosomal alteration (chromosomes 3, 7, and 17) and a deletion of 9p12 is the foundation of the UroVysion biomarker test (77).

The recent emergence of immune checkpoint blockade in urothelial carcinoma has also introduced several candidate predictive biomarkers. The role and appropriate use of PD-L1 expression (on tumor cells or immune cells) to stratify or select patients for therapy remains unclear in bladder cancer. However, both high tumor mutational burden and a T-cell "inflamed" gene expression profile signature (e.g., IFNγ-gene signature) have been associated with improved response to different PD-1/PD-L1 blocking agents (78–80). There have also been attempts to understand if TCGA molecular subtypes for urothelial carcinoma can identify subsets of patients who may benefit from immunotherapy. However, there have been mixed results with different agents and across different studies. The cluster II luminal TCGA subtype has been demonstrated to have a high response rate to atezolizumab in the cisplatin-ineligible and second-line setting, whereas patients with cluster III basal 1 TCGA subtype have the highest response rate with nivolumab (78,79).

PITFALLS IN THE DEVELOPMENT AND VALIDATION OF BIOMARKERS

Despite tremendous advances in scientific research, biomarkers for precision cancer therapy remain an unmet clinical need. Following candidate biomarker discovery, multiple levels of validation are required before a biomarker becomes a useful tool that is integrated into clinical practice (81). A substantial proportion of candidate biomarkers fail because they lack the requisite specificity/sensitivity needed. For the subset of biomarkers with sufficient analytical capacity, the next step is clinical validation, which often involves retrospective analysis of biospecimens followed by evaluation in prospective trials across multiple cohorts. Issues pertaining to study bias and design may limit interpretation, such as small sample size, lack of appropriate control/comparison arms, or improper treatment of biospecimens (e.g., collection and storage) (82). Once clinically validated, approval from the FDA and other regulatory agencies for quality assurance and accreditation represents an additional hurdle to overcome. Ultimately, a biomarker must demonstrate clinical utility (81). A candidate biomarker must not only perform its intended prognostic or predictive role, but also must either surpass or complement the current standard of care.

CONCLUSIONS/FUTURE DIRECTIONS

Progress in cancer therapy and precision medicine necessitates that the pipeline for biomarker development be accelerated. Recent emphasis on biomarker-driven prospective clinical trials and the adaptation of novel trial design (e.g., adaptive, biomarker-enriched, hybrid) is a crucial step toward this goal. Further, to facilitate a patient-tailored approach, new therapies should increasingly be developed in tandem with companion diagnostics/validated biomarkers to identify the patients most likely to benefit from certain therapies. Finally, the recent tissue/site-agnostic FDA approval, "when the biomarker defines the indication," represents an important advance for biomarker development and a pathway forward for this field (29).

GLOSSARY

cancer biomarkers: objective measures that rely upon the ability to identify and/or evaluate the unique molecular signature of a specific cancer type or malignant process.

specificity: a statistical measure that assesses the performance of a binary test or assay; refers to the proportion of control (without disease) subjects that are accurately identified as negative by the test under evaluation; it can be conceptualized as the true negative rate.

sensitivity: a statistical measure that assesses the performance of a binary test or assay; refers to the proportion of subjects with confirmed disease that are accurately identified as positive by the test; it can be conceptualized as the true positive rate.

screening biomarker: an objective measure used for diagnostic purposes on an individual level to detect a specific cancer type among at-risk individuals or on a population-based level for screening of an at-risk population.

prognostic biomarkers: objective measures used to stratify patients by their expected disease outcome; allow for the distinction between patients with favorable and unfavorable prognoses.

predictive biomarkers: objective measures used to stratify patients by their anticipated response to specific therapies.

imaging biomarkers: objective radiological (or molecular) measures that are able to assay in vivo anatomic and biologic processes in a noninvasive and quantitative manner.

REFERENCES

1. Siegel RL, Miller KD, Jemal A. Cancer statistics, 2015. *CA Cancer J Clin.* 2015;65:5–29. doi:10.3322/caac.21254
2. Bhatt AN, Mathur R, Farooque A, et al. Cancer biomarkers—current perspectives. *Indian J Med Res.* 2010;132:129–149.
3. Kulasingam V, Diamandis EP. Strategies for discovering novel cancer biomarkers through utilization of emerging technologies. *Nat Clin Pract Oncol.* 2008;5(10):588–599. doi:10.1038/ncponc1187
4. Duffy MJ. Tumor markers in clinical practice: a review focusing on common solid cancers. *Med Princ Pract.* 2013;22(1):4–11. doi:10.1159/000338393
5. Mäbert K, Cojoc M, Peitzsch C, et al. Cancer biomarker discovery: current status and future perspective. *Int J Radiat Biol.* 2014;90(8):659–677. doi:10.3109/09553002.2014.892229
6. Srinivas PR, Kramer BS, Srivastava S. Trends in biomarker research for cancer detection. *Lancet Oncol.* 2001;2(11):698–704. doi:10.1016/S1470-2045(01)00560-5
7. Oldenhius CN, Oosting SF, Gietema JA, de Vries EG. Prognostic versus predictive value of biomarkers in oncology. *Eur J Cancer.* 2008;44(7):946–953. doi:10.1016/j.ejca.2008.03.006
8. Conley BA, Taube SE. Prognostic and predictive markers in cancer. *Dis Markers.* 2004;20(2):35–43. doi:10.1155/2004/202031
9. Early Breast Cancer Trialists' Collaborative Group. Tamoxifen for early breast cancer: an overview of the randomised trials. *Lancet.* 1998;351(9114):1451–1467. doi:10.1016/S0140-6736(97)11423-4
10. Fisher B, Redmond C, Fisher ER, Caplan R. Relative worth of estrogen or progesterone receptor and pathologic characteristics of differentiation as indicators of prognosis in node negative breast cancer patients: findings from National Surgical Adjuvant Breast and Bowel Project Protocol B-06. *J Clin Oncol.* 1988;6(7):1076–1087. doi:10.1200/JCO.1988.6.7.1076
11. Taube JM. Unleasing the immune system: PD-1 and PD-Ls in the pre-treatment tumor miroenvironment and correlation with response to PD-1/PD-L1 blockade. *Oncoimmunology.* 2014;3(11):e963413. doi:10.4161/21624011.2014.963413
12. Taube JM, Klein A, Brahmer JR, et al. Association of PD-1, PD-1 ligands, and other features of the tumor immune microenvironment with response to anti-PD-1 therapy. *Clin Cancer Res.* 2014;20(19):5064–5074. doi:10.1158/1078-0432.CCR-13-3271
13. Mahoney KM, Atkins MB. Prognostic and predictive markers for the new immunotherapies. *Oncology.* 2014; 28(Suppl 3):39–48.
14. Shaw AT, Yeap BY, Mino-Kenudson M, et al. Clinical features and outcome of patients with non-small-cell lung cancer who harbor EML4-ALK. *J Clin Oncol.* 2009;27(26):4247–4253. doi:10.1200/JCO.2009.22.6993
15. Kwak EL, Bang YJ, Camidge DR, et al. Anaplastic lymphoma kinase inhibition in non-small cell lung cancer. *N Engl J Med.* 2010;363(18):1693–1703. doi:10.1056/NEJMoa1006448
16. Hanahan D, Weinberg RA. Hallmarks of cancer: the next generation. *Cell.* 2011;144(5):646–674. doi:10.1016/j.cell.2011.02.013
17. Mavaddat N, Peock S, Frost D, et al. Cancer risks for BRCA1 and BRCA2 mutation carriers: results from prospective analysis of EMBRACE. *J Natl Cancer Inst.* 2013;105(11):812–822. doi:10.1093/jnci/djt095
18. Jazaeri AA, Lu K, Schmandt R, et al. Molecular determinants of tumor differentiation in papillary serous ovarian carcinoma. *Mol Carcinog.* 2003;36(2):53–59. doi:10.1002/mc.10098
19. Liede A, Karlan BY, Narod SA. Cancer risks for male carriers of germline mutations in BRCA1 or BRCA2: a review of the literature. *J Clin Oncol.* 2004;22:735–742. doi:10.1200/JCO.2004.05.055
20. Mersch J, Jackson MA, Park M, et al. Cancers associated with BRCA1 and BRCA2 mutations other than breast and ovarian. *Cancer.* 2014;121:269–275. doi:10.1002/cncr.29041
21. Weitzel JN, Blazer KR, MacDonald DJ, et al. Genetics, genomics, and cancer risk assessment: State of the art and future directions in the era of personalized medicine. *CA Cancer J Clin.* 2011;61(5):327–359. doi:10.3322/caac.20128
22. Levy-Lahad E, Lahad A, King MC. Precision medicine meets public health: population screening for BRCA1 and BRCA2. *J Natl Cancer Inst.* 2014;107(1):420. doi:10.1093/jnci/dju420
23. Tun NM, Villani G, Ong K, et al. Risk of having BRCA1 mutation in high-risk women with triple-negative breast cancer: a meta-analysis. *Clin Genet.* 2014;85(1):43–48. doi:10.1111/cge.12270
24. Castro E, Goh C, Olmos D, et al. Germline BRCA mutations are associated with higher risk of nodal involvement, distant metastasis, and poor survival outcomes in prostate cancer. *J Clin Oncol.* 2013;31(14):1748–1757. doi:10.1200/JCO.2012.43.1882

25. Yang D, Khan S, Sun Y, et al. Association of BRCA1 and BRCA2 mutations with survival, chemotherapy sensitivity, and gene mutator phenotype in patients with ovarian cancer. *JAMA*. 2011;306(14):1557–1565. doi:10.1001/jama.2011.1456
26. Chapman PB, Hauschild A, Robert C, et al. Improved survival with vemurafenib in melanoma with BRAF V600E mutation. *N Engl J Med*. 2011;364:2507–2516. doi:10.1056/NEJMoa1103782
27. Hampel H, Frankel WL, Martin E, et al. Screening for the Lynch syndrome (hereditary nonpolyposis colorectal cancer). *N Engl J Med*. 2005;352:1851–1860. doi:10.1056/NEJMoa043146
28. Weisenberger DJ, Siegmund KD, Campan M, et al. CpG island methylator phenotype underlies sporadic microsatellite instability and is tightly associated with BRAF mutation in colorectal cancer. *Nat Genet*. 2006;38:787–793. doi:10.1038/ng1834
29. Lemery S, Keegan P, Pazdur R. First FDA approval agnostic of cancer site—when a biomarker defines the indication. *N Engl J Med*. 2017;377(15):1409–1412. doi:10.1056/NEJMp1709968
30. Stupp R, Mason WP, van den Bent MJ, et al. Radiotherapy plus concomitant and adjuvant temozolomide for glioblastoma. *N Engl J Med*. 2005;352:987–996. doi:10.1056/NEJMoa043330
31. Stupp R, Hegi ME, Mason WP, et al. Effects of radiotherapy with concomitant and adjuvant temozolomide versus radiotherapy alone on survival in glioblastoma in a randomised phase III study: 5-year analysis of the EORTC-NCIC trial. *Lancet Oncol*. 2009;10:459–466. doi:10.1016/S1470-2045(09)70025-7
32. Hegi ME, Diserens AC, Gorlia T, et al. MGMT gene silencing and benefit from temozolomide in glioblastoma. *N Engl J Med*. 2005;352:997–1003. doi:10.1056/NEJMoa043331
33. Cancer Genome Atlas Research Network. Comprehensive, integrative genomic analysis of diffuse lower-grade gliomas. *N Engl J Med*. 2015;372:2481–2498. doi:10.1056/NEJMoa1402121
34. Eckel-Passow JE, Lachance DH, Molinaro AM, et al. Glioma groups based on 1p/19q, IDH, and TERT promoter mutations in tumors. *N Engl J Med*. 2015:372(26):2499–2508. doi:10.1056/NEJMoa1407279
35. Northcott PA, Korshunov A, Witt H, et al. Medulloblastoma comprises four distinct molecular variants. *J Clin Oncol*. 2011:29(11):1408–1414. doi:10.1200/JCO.2009.27.4324
36. Shih DJ, Northcott PA, Remke M, et al. Cytogenetic prognostication within medulloblastoma subgroups. *J Clin Oncol*. 2014;32(9):886–896. doi:10.1200/JCO.2013.50.9539
37. Robertson AG, Kim J, Al-Ahmadie H, et al. Comprehensive molecular characterization of muscle-invasive bladder cancer. *Cell*. 2017;171(3):556.e25. doi:10.1016/j.cell.2017.09.007
38. Ciriello G, Gatza ML, Beck AH, et al. Comprehensive molecular portraits of invasive lobular breast cancer. *Cell*. 2015;163(2):506–519. doi:10.1016/j.cell.2015.09.033
39. Cancer Genome Atlas Research Network. The molecular taxonomy of primary prostate cancer. *Cell*. 2015;163(4):1011–1025. doi:10.1016/j.cell.2015.10.025
40. Fishbein L, Leshchiner I, Walter V, et al. Comprehensive molecular characterization of pheochromocytoma and paraganglioma. *Cancer Cell*. 2017;31(2):181–193. doi:10.1016/j.ccell.2017.01.001
41. Robertson AG, Shih J, Yau C, et al. Integrative analysis identifies four molecular and clinical subsets in uveal melanoma. *Cancer Cell*. 2017;32(2):220.e15. doi:10.1016/j.ccell.2017.12.013
42. Paik S, Shak S, Tang G, et al. A multigene assay to predict recurrence of tamoxifen-treated, node-negative breast cancer. *N Engl J Med*. 2004;351:2817–2826. doi:10.1056/NEJMoa041588
43. Paik S, Tang G, Shak S, et al. Gene expression and benefit of chemotherapy in women with node-negative, estrogen receptor positive breast cancer. *J Clin Oncol*. 2006;24:3726–3734. doi:10.1200/JCO.2005.04.7985
44. Therasse P, Arbuck SG, Eisenhauer EA, et al. New guidelines to evaluate the response to treatment in solid tumors. European Organization for Research and Treatment of Cancer, National Cancer Institute of the United States, National Cancer Institute of Canada. *J Natl Cancer Inst*. 2000;92(3):205–216. doi:10.1093/jnci/92.3.205
45. Eisenhauer EA, Therasse P, Bogaerts J, et al. New response evaluation criteria in solid tumours: revised RECIST guideline (version 1.1). *Eur J Cancer*. 2009;45(2):228–247.doi:10.1016/j.ejca.2008.10.026
46. Cheson BD, Fisher RI, Barrington SF, et al. Recommendations for initial evaluation, staging, and response assessment of Hodgkin and non-Hodgkin lymphoma: the Lugano classification. *J Clin Oncol*.2014;32(27):3059–3069. doi:10.1200/JCO.2013.54.8800
47. Meignan M, Gallamini A, Haioun C. Report on the First International Workshop on interim-PET-scan. *Leuk Lymphoma*. 2009;50(8):1257–1260. doi:10.1080/10428190903040048
48. Cristofanilli M, Budd GT, Ellis MJ, et al. Circulating tumor cells, disease progression, and survival in metastatic breast cancer. *N Engl J Med*. 2004;351:781–791. doi:10.1056/NEJMoa040766
49. Scher HI, Heller G, Molina A, et al. Circulating tumor cell biomarker panel as an individual-level surrogate for survival in metastatic castration-resistant prostate cancer. *J Clin Oncol*. 2015;33(12):1348–1355. doi:10.1200/JCO.2014.55.3487
50. Cohen SJ, Punt CJ, Iannotti N, et al. Relationship of circulating tumor cells to tumor response, progression-free survival, and overall survival in patients with metastatic colorectal cancer. *J Clin Oncol*. 2008;26(19):3213–3221. doi:10.1200/JCO.2007.15.8923
51. Smerage JB, Barlow WE, Hortobagyi GN, et al. Circulating tumor cells and response to chemotherapy in metastatic breast cancer: SWOG S0500. *J Clin Oncol*. 2014;32(31):3483–3489. doi:10.1200/JCO.2014.56.2561
52. Chaudhuri AA, Binkley MS, Osmundson EC, et al. Predicting radiotherapy responses and treatment outcomes through analysis of circulating tumor DNA. *Semin Radiat Oncol*. 2015;25(4):305–312. doi:10.1016/j.semradonc.2015.05.001
53. Newman AM, Bratman SV, To J, et al. An ultrasensitive method for quantitating circulating tumor DNA with broad patient coverage. *Nat Med*. 2014;20(5):548–554. doi:10.1038/nm.3519
54. Sturgeon CM, Duffy MJ, Stenman UH, et al. National Academy of Clinical Biochemistry laboratory medicine practice guidelines for use of tumor markers in testicular, prostate, colorectal, breast, and ovarian cancers. *Clin Chem*. 2008;54(12):e11–e79. doi:10.1373/clinchem.2008.105601

55. Sturgeon CM, Duffy MJ, Hoffman BR, et al. National Academy of Clinical Biochemistry laboratory medicine practice guidelines for use of tumor markers in liver, bladder, cervical and gastric cancers. *Clin Chem*. 2010;56(6):e1–e48. doi:10.1373/clinchem.2009.133124
56. Sparano JA, Gray RJ, Makower DF, et al. Prospective validation of a 21-gene expression assay in breast cancer. *N Engl J Med*. 2015;373(21):2005–2014. doi:10.1056/NEJMoa1510764
57. Drukker CA, Bueno-de-Mesquita JM, Retel VP, et al. A prospective evaluation of a breast cancer prognosis signature in the observational RASTER study. *Int J Cancer*. 2013;133(4):929–936. doi:10.1002/ijc.28082
58. Sorlie T, Perou CM, Tibshirani R, et al. Gene expression patterns of breast carcinomas distinguish tumor subclasses with clinical implications. *Proc Natl Acad Sci U S A*. 2001;98(19):10869–10874. doi:10.1073/pnas.191367098
59. Mitsudomi T, Steinberg SM, Oie HK, et al. RAS gene mutations in non-small cell lung cancers are associated with shortened survival irrespective of treatment intent. *Cancer Res*. 1991;51(18):4999–5002.
60. Mok TS, Wu Y, Ahn M, et al. Osimertinib or platinum-pemetrexed in EGFR T790M-positive lung cancer. *N Engl J Med*. 2017;376(7):629–640. doi:10.1056/NEJMoa1612674
61. Klein EA, Santiago-Jimenez M, Yousefi K, et al. Molecular analysis of low grade prostate cancer using a genomic classifier of metastatic potential. *J Urol*. 2017;197(1):122–128. doi:10.1016/j.juro.2016.08.091
62. Erho N, Crisan A, Vergara IA, et al. Discovery and validation of a prostate cancer genomic classifier that predicts early metastasis following radical prostatectomy. *PLoS One*. 2013;8(6):e66855. doi:10.1371/journal.pone.0066855
63. Cullen J, Rosner IL, Brand TC, et al. A biopsy-based 17-gene genomic prostate score predicts recurrence after radical prostatectomy and adverse surgical pathology in a racially diverse population of men with clinically low- and intermediate-risk prostate cancer. *Eur Urol*. 2015;68(1):123–131. doi:10.1016/j.eururo.2014.11.030
64. Cooperberg MR, Simko JP, Cowan JE, et al. Validation of a cell-cycle progression gene panel to improve risk stratification in a contemporary prostatectomy cohort. *J Clin Oncol*. 2013;31(11):1428–1434. doi:10.1200/JCO.2012.46.4396
65. Cuzick J, Stone S, Fisher G, et al. Validation of an RNA cell cycle progression score for predicting death from prostate cancer in a conservatively managed needle biopsy cohort. *Br J Cancer*. 2015;113(3):382–389. doi:10.1038/bjc.2015.223
66. Blume-Jensen P, Berman DM, Rimm DL, et al. Development and clinical validation of an in situ biopsy-based multimarker assay for risk stratification in prostate cancer. *Clin Cancer Res*. 2015;21(11):2591–2600. doi:10.1158/1078-0432.CCR-14-2603
67. Antonarakis ES, Lu C, Wang H, et al. AR-V7 and resistance to enzalutamide and abiraterone in prostate cancer. *N Engl J Med*. 2014;371(11):1028–1038. doi:10.1056/NEJMoa1315815
68. Scher HI, Lu D, Schreiber NA, et al. Association of AR-V7 on circulating tumor cells as a treatment-specific biomarker with outcomes and survival in castration-resistant prostate cancer. *JAMA Oncol*. 2016;2(11):1441–1449. doi: 10.1001/jamaoncol.2016.1828
69. Robinson D, Van Allen EM, Wu YM, et al. Integrative clinical genomics of advanced prostate cancer. *Cell*. 2015;161(5):1215–1228. doi:10.1016/j.cell.2015.06.053
70. Saltz LB, Meropol NJ, Loehrer PJS, et al. Phase II trial of cetuximab in patients with refractory colorectal cancer that expresses the epidermal growth factor receptor. *J Clin Oncol*. 2004;22(7):1201–1208. doi:10.1200/JCO.2004.10.182
71. Gray RG, Quirke P, Handley K, et al. Validation study of a quantitative multigene reverse transcriptase-polymerase chain reaction assay for assessment of recurrence risk in patients with stage II colon cancer. *J Clin Oncol*. 2011;29(35):4611–4619. doi:10.1200/JCO.2010.32.8732
72. Guinney J, Dienstmann R, Wang X, et al. The consensus molecular subtypes of colorectal cancer. *Nat Med*. 2015;21(11):1350–1356. doi:10.1038/nm.3967
73. Grossman HB, Messing E, Soloway M, et al. Detection of bladder cancer using a point-of-care proteomic assay. *JAMA*. 2005;293(7):810–816. doi:10.1001/jama.293.7.810
74. Grossman HB, Soloway M, Messing E, et al. Surveillance for recurrent bladder cancer using a point-of-care proteomic assay. *JAMA*. 2006;295(3):299–305. doi:10.1001/jama.295.3.299
75. Babjuk M, Soukup V, Pesl M, et al. Urinary cytology and quantitative BTA and UBC tests in surveillance of patients with pTapT1 bladder urothelial carcinoma. *Urology*. 2008;71(4):718–722. doi:10.1016/j.urology.2007.12.021
76. Pfister C, Chautard D, Devonec M, et al. Immunocyt test improves the diagnostic accuracy of urinary cytology: results of a French multicenter study. *J Urol*. 2003;169(3):921–924. doi:10.1097/01.ju.0000048983.83079.4c
77. Liem, EIML, Baard J, Cauberg ECC, et al. Fluorescence in situ hybridization as prognostic predictor of tumor recurrence during treatment with Bacillus Calmette-Guerin therapy for intermediate- and high-risk non-muscle-invasive bladder cancer. *Med Oncol*. 2017;34(10):z. doi:10.1007/s12032-017-1033-z
78. Rosenberg JE, Hoffman-Censits J, Powles T, et al. Atezolizumab in patients with locally advanced and metastatic urothelial carcinoma who have progressed following treatment with platinum-based chemotherapy: a single-arm, multicentre, phase 2 trial. *Lancet*. 2016;387(10031):1909–1920. doi:10.1016/S0140-6736(16)00561-4
79. Sharma P, Retz M, Siefker-Radtke A, et al. Nivolumab in metastatic urothelial carcinoma after platinum therapy (CheckMate 275): a multicentre, single-arm, phase 2 trial. *Lancet Oncol*. 2017;18(3):312–322. doi:10.1016/S1470-2045(16)30496-X
80. Balar AV, Galsky MD, Rosenberg JE, et al. Atezolizumab as first-line treatment in cisplatin-ineligible patients with locally advanced and metastatic urothelial carcinoma: A single-arm, multicentre, phase 2 trial. *Lancet*. 2017;389(10064):67–76. doi:10.1016/S0140-6736(16)32455-2
81. Duffy MJ, Crown J. Precision treatment for cancer: Role of prognostic and predictive markers. *Crit Rev Clin Lab Sci*. 2014;51(1):30–45. doi:10.3109/10408363.2013.865700
82. Diamandis EP. Towards identification of true cancer biomarkers. *BMC Med*. 2014;12:156. doi:10.1186/s12916-014-0156-8

9

Working With Industry

SWAN LIN ■ YAZDI K. PITHAVALA ■ SANDIP PRAVIN PATEL

Historically, academic researchers have been major drivers of basic science research in molecular pathways and targets and have contributed to a better understanding of cancer biology. Conversely, discovery efforts and testing of candidate compounds in preclinical and clinical studies have largely been carried out by pharmaceutical industry scientists. The intersection of academia and industry research generally occurred at the clinical development stage of phase 1 through phase 3 trials. Over the past few decades, innovations for molecularly targeted therapies and cancer immunotherapy driven by collaboration between researchers from public and private sectors have blurred the traditional roles of academia and industry. This chapter highlights examples of successful collaborative efforts, discusses the evolving roles of academia and industry in discovery and development particularly with translational research, and provides insight into the training programs for future collaborative opportunities in oncology research and drug development.

TRADITIONAL ROLES OF ACADEMIA AND INDUSTRY

The ultimate goal of cancer research is to find treatments and cures; however, the driving forces and approach by which academia and industry scientists conduct cancer research differ. Academic research seeks to gain an understanding of the basic science of the pathophysiological mechanisms that drive tumor growth through deductive experimentation. Research is generally motivated by intellectual curiosity and there is often more freedom for exploration of theoretical ideas without the constraints of strict timelines. Although there is often more flexibility in selecting the work, obtaining resources is usually a major hurdle in academia.

In contrast, industry scientists are able to efficiently and effectively move a drug candidate into clinic through conducting more structured and well-defined experiments and trials. Product development and profit are the main drivers of private sector research. Particularly in large pharmaceutical companies, the financial resources and personnel expertise are comparatively more plentiful, which allows for more strategically planned research with the caveat of needing to meet tight timelines to ensure competitive advantage.

Not only do the drivers for research in academia and industry differ, the collaboration approach within these sectors is often different as well. In an academic laboratory, the team is generally limited to the principal investigator (PI) and those who work with the PI. In some instances, the collaborative effort may extend to other colleagues in the department. In industry, each drug candidate has an extensive team of experts who help guide the candidate from discovery to the market. The interdisciplinary work often extends beyond the research itself with involvement of team members with regulatory, supply chain, or even commercial marketing expertise. Thus, academic researchers often need to wear many hats, whereas industry researchers can hone in and become specialists in their own functional lines.

DRUG DISCOVERY AND DEVELOPMENT

The process from first understanding a pathway or target for cancer drug development to marketing of a drug is long and complicated. Figure 9.1 illustrates the chronological processes and

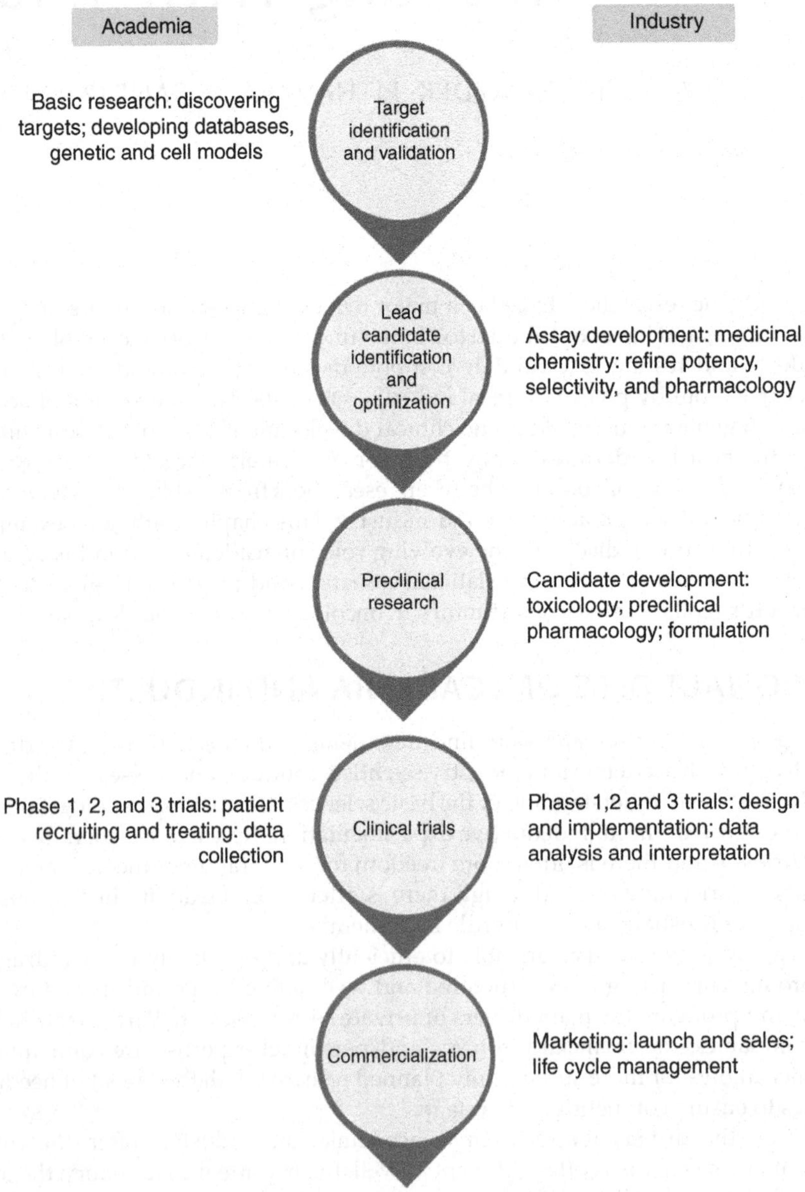

FIGURE 9.1 Relationship between academia and industry.

activities of drug discovery and development and summarizes the traditional roles that academic and industry researchers play at each step.

Academic researchers play a critical role in target identification and validation through their early discovery, basic science research efforts. Discovery research often leads to important publications about the target and creation of large databases that house this information. The lead drug candidate identification and optimization step often occurs in industry. The activities involved in this step are often part of a well-defined and regimented process, including assay development to optimize the medicinal chemistry, potency, selectivity of the candidate to the target, and pharmacology. Preclinical proof-of-concept, toxicology, and pharmacology studies are also often carried out in industry subsequent to the identification of a lead candidate. Simultaneously, efforts to develop a formulation of the lead candidate into drug form occur at this step. The crossroads for collaboration between academia and industry occurs in the clinical trial step of the process, where the industry partner often provides the funding and design for the studies and the academic partner helps with the recruiting of patients and data collection. Data analysis and interpretation are often done by the industry partner to support regulatory filing. With regulatory approval, commercialization of the drug is generally done in the private sector, along with conducting postmarketing trials and other life cycle management studies for the drug.

TRADITIONAL ROLES OF RESEARCHERS IN ACADEMIA AND INDUSTRY

"Translational research" and "personalized medicine" are hot phrases in the world of oncology. The idea of applying the progress in basic science research to development of new drugs or procedures that can readily benefit patients is the essence of translational research. Therefore, rather than taking the traditional, stepwise approach as outlined in Figure 9.1, it is necessary for academic and industry researchers to collaborate earlier on in the discovery and development timeline. *Translational research* can also refer to utilization of patient tissues or specimens collected from clinical research to then drive more basic science research in an effort to further the understanding of the nature of the disease. Thus, the paradigm for collaboration between academia and industry partners is ever evolving to allow for the fluid dialogue and in-parallel research from both sectors.

CLASSIC SUCCESSFUL COLLABORATIONS

The ever growing knowledge of molecular pathways and genetic alterations driving cancer cell proliferation and survival has generated a plethora of potential antitumor targets. The need to further evaluate and validate these targets to ultimately develop new therapeutic strategies in historically unassailable tumors is too great for academia, government, or industry to meet alone. In order to move novel targeted small-molecule inhibitors and biologics from bench to bedside more quickly and efficiently, collaborations between public and private sector researchers in complementary areas of expertise have grown. Case studies 1 and 2 describe the unique collaboration of researchers and clinicians from academic and industry sectors leading to the development of targeted therapies: trastuzumab and axitinib.

CASE STUDY 1

DEVELOPMENT OF TRASTUZUMAB (HERCEPTIN)

One of the classic academia and industry collaboration stories is the development of trastuzumab (Herceptin) for the treatment of breast cancer (1). This collaborative effort followed some aspects

(continued)

CASE STUDY 1 (*continued*)

of the traditional roles of academia and industry, in that target identification and discovery were first characterized by academic researchers and subsequent clinical development of a candidate compound was carried forward by the pharmaceutical industry. This case study describes the story of Herceptin, the evolving relationships and roles between academic researcher-oncologists and Genentech, and the challenges in development that eventually led to the approval of the first monoclonal antibody targeted against human epidermal growth factor receptor 2 (HER2) for breast cancer.

The breast cancer target discovery of *neu* gene in rats was first described by the laboratory of academic researcher Robert Weinberg from the Massachusetts Institute of Technology (2). The subsequent discovery that the human homolog of *neu*, HER2, could oncogenically transform normal cells was led by Dennis Slamon (University of California, Los Angeles [UCLA]) and Bill McGuire (University of Texas at San Antonio) and was instrumental in characterizing the clinical relevance of HER2 in breast cancer (3). At the time, Slamon was a junior faculty member at UCLA and divided his time between patient care and academic research. He collected excised tumors of a variety of cancers from surgeons and pathologists with the hope of finding oncogenes from these tumors.

The industry counterpart was Genentech, which in the late 1970s was a small biotechnology company in the Bay Area. Axel Ullrich was a postdoctoral fellow at the University of California, San Francisco (UCSF), before being recruited to join Genentech for his highly regarded work with isolating the gene for insulin from rats and producing the protein in bacteria. At Genentech, Ullrich's research was first focused on epidermal growth factors (EGFs) and he was part of the effort that discovered the oncogene called erb-b that leads to unrestrained cell growth and division (4). From there, Ullrich successfully isolated the gene for HER2 and purified the protein.

Dennis Slamon and Axel Ullrich first met at an airport in 1986 following a scientific conference. A few months after this chance meeting, Ullrich was in UCLA giving a seminar when Slamon approached him with the suggestion to collaborate: Ullrich had a rich collection of cloned growth factor genes and Slamon had his human tumor samples from a variety of different cancers. It naturally made sense to investigate whether there were any links between growth factor genes and specific cancer types. This collaboration yielded the important finding that the HER2 mutation in breast and ovarian cells produced normal HER2 proteins, but in abnormally high amounts. In order to characterize the type of breast cancer with this HER2 mutation, Slamon reached out to McGuire, who had a sizable collection of frozen breast tumors with detailed medical histories. In evaluating the number of cancerous lymph nodes before mastectomy in McGuire's breast tumors, Slamon discovered that HER2 breast cancers were generally faster spreading, more apt to recur, and deadlier than other breast cancers (5). In subsequent studies and exploration of the basic science, Slamon and Ullrich demonstrated that using a monoclonal antibody to block breast cancer cells that overexpress HER2 resulted in stopping the growth and division of the cancer

(*continued*)

CASE STUDY 1 (*continued*)

cells in vitro. This was further corroborated with remarkable tumor shrinkage in mouse xenograft models of human breast cells treated with monoclonal antibodies against HER2. Although these initial collaborative efforts on HER2 in breast cancer were instrumental in understanding the fundamental biology of breast cancer and revolutionizing oncogene research, a series of challenges in developing a therapy for HER2 breast cancers followed.

Genentech, being a small company, depended on Activase for its profits; additionally, Roche's acquisition of Genentech lent some uncertainty to the HER2 program. Having had unsuccessful trials in the development of alpha interferons in a broad range of cancers, there was hesitation within the upper management about investing in oncology programs. Moreover, developing antibody therapeutics at the time was novel and risky, as all monoclonal antibodies in the 1970s to 1980s were developed from genes in mice or other animals and could result in severe immunologic responses when administered to humans. The turning point came in late 1989, when the HER2 project found its champion in the vice president for manufacturing at Genentech, Bill Young, whose mother was coincidentally diagnosed with breast cancer. With the backing of senior management, the HER2 program had new life. To tackle the potential problem of severe immunologic responses with antibodies from mice or other animal species, Genentech hired Paul Carter to "humanize" monoclonal antibodies. In a short 10 months, the humanized HER2 antibody was developed and ready for evaluation in phase 1 studies, which were done at UCLA with Slamon, Sloan Kettering, and UCSF. At UCLA, Slamon tested the humanized HER2 antibody in combination with cisplatin and at Sloan Kettering and UCSF, HER2 antibody was given as monotherapy in breast cancer.

The development of a HER2 antibody seemed finally to be gaining steam. This was helped along by a large endowment to UCLA and Slamon from Revlon, the cosmetic company. Between 1989 and the end of 1997, the total contribution from Revlon to UCLA's work on women's cancer totaled $13 million. This money helped to set up phase 1 and phase 2 trials at UCLA. Throughout the years, Slamon continued to advocate for and champion the development of the HER2 antibody, trastuzumab, even in the volatile landscape of his industry partner at Genentech.

The initial trials of the humanized HER2 monoclonal antibody enrolled patients who had advanced, relapsed breast cancer. Even with the first phase 1 study of trastuzumab, Slamon saw remarkable response in some of his patients and the phase 2 trials had promising results as well; not only did trastuzumab shrink tumors, some patients even experienced cancer remissions (6). Soon, the promise of trastuzumab in treating women with breast cancer who otherwise had limited options was spreading publicly and widely. It was at this time that patient advocate groups Breast Cancer Action and the National Breast Cancer Coalition took to the media and government agencies to advocate for a compassionate use program for trastuzumab. It was apparent that collaborating with patient advocate groups in drug development would be important and soon these groups were involved in providing feedback on the inclusion/exclusion criteria of the

(*continued*)

CASE STUDY 1 (*continued*)

phase 3 protocols and in participating on Data Safety and Monitoring Boards. The data from women treated through the compassionate use program, along with its pivotal phase 3 studies (trials 648, 649, and 650) would later support the approval of trastuzumab.

The pivotal phase 3 study, trial 648, was initially designed as a double-blind, placebo controlled study of trastuzumab plus Cytoxan and Adriamycin (CA) in 450 women with newly diagnosed metastatic breast cancer. The selection of CA chemotherapy to be combined with trastuzumab had not previously been studied in earlier phases and went against many of the treating oncologists' preferences—Slamon had advocated for cisplatin, while other key opinion leaders had advocated for Taxol. The two other trials were smaller and conducted in 200 women each. Trial 649 evaluated trastuzumab monotherapy in women whose metastatic disease had failed to respond to one or more rounds of chemotherapy. Trial 650 evaluated trastuzumab monotherapy in newly diagnosed metastatic disease without prior chemotherapy treatment.

With 99 sites in the United States, 7 in Canada, and 33 in Europe, the phase 3 trials got under way in 1995. Even with 150 oncologists ready to enroll the 450 patients required for trial 648, enrollment ticked along slowly, although trial 649 accrued more rapidly. In trial 649, patients had few other alternatives for treatment, whereas trial 648 was in newly diagnosed patients. The biggest hurdles for enrollment in the key 648 trial were the placebo arm and the selection of the chemotherapy. With a placebo arm, physicians were concerned about withholding a possibly effective treatment from their patients. The selection of CA limited enrollment for physicians who would have otherwise chosen that regimen for their patients. About a year later, as the enrollment in trial 648 continued to lag, the protocol was amended to an open-label study of trastuzumab and added Taxol as an alternative to CA. With this change and the help of the patient advocate groups to advertise the revised protocol, enrollment in trial 648 was completed less than a year later. In September 1998, Herceptin received approval from the Food and Drug Administration (FDA) for use in women with metastatic breast cancer that overexpresses HER2 as first line in combination with chemotherapy or as monotherapy in patients who had failed one or more lines of chemotherapy.

The story of Herceptin is unique and highlights the importance of the partnership between academia, industry, and even patient advocate communities. Though the rationale for HER2 as a target for breast cancer stemmed from early academic researcher efforts, industry backing of Genentech in the development of humanized monoclonal antibodies and clinical development program proved to be crucial. However, given the many players in Genentech over the development course of trastuzumab, there were many setbacks along the way. With the persistence of researcher-oncologists, including Slamon and his UCLA–Revlon financial backing, the stalemate and near-failure of the pivotal phase 3 trial was averted, paving the way for Herceptin's approval in the treatment of breast cancer.

(*continued*)

CASE STUDY 1 (*continued*)

The development of Herceptin extends beyond breast cancer. Since its first indication in breast cancer, there have been other studies evaluating the use of Herceptin in patients with HER2-driven cancers arising from other anatomical sites. One such example is the *Trastuzumab for GAstric cancer* (ToGA) study, which was an open-label, international, phase 3, randomized controlled trial in patients with gastric or gastroesophageal cancer whose cancers expressed HER2 (7). In total, 594 patients were randomized in the study with $n = 298$ treated with trastuzumab plus chemotherapy and $n = 296$ in the control chemotherapy alone arm. The median overall survival was 13.8 months compared to 11.1 months in the chemotherapy group (hazard ratio 0.74, $p = .0046$), leading to its approval in this population in 2010. More recently, Roche/Genentech has an ongoing nonrandomized phase 2 open-label study, *My Pathway*, consisting of six treatment arms for patients with advanced solid tumors and expression of one of six targets for any cancer (trastuzumab and pertuzumab, erlotinib, vemurafenib plus cobimetinib, vismodegib, alectinib, and atezolizumab) (8). The approach to enroll patients based on biomarker expression and without regard to anatomic location of the primary tumor is revolutionizing the treatment approach and expanding options to oncology patients. This certainly will continue to drive increased collaborative efforts between academia and industry to coordinate such studies.

CASE STUDY 2

DEVELOPMENT OF AXITINIB (INLYTA)

The clinical development of axitinib (AG-013736, Inlyta) began in May 2002 with the First In Human study initiated in patients with solid tumors (9). Three clinical sites, University of Wisconsin Comprehensive Cancer Center, University of Texas MD Anderson Cancer Center, and UCSF, enrolled patients on this trial sponsored by Pfizer (9). Axitinib is a substituted indazole derivative that was developed using structure-based drug design as a potent small-molecule tyrosine kinase inhibitor of all known VEGF receptors (VEGFRs) at subnanomolar concentrations (9). Using the standard 3+3 design for safety-based dose finding, and based on real-time evaluation of patient tolerability by the three PIs and Pfizer, the 5 mg twice daily (BID) dose was identified as the maximum tolerated dose for axitinib and also the recommended dose for further clinical development (9).

Increase in blood pressure and proteinuria were two of the major class effects and it was important to characterize the drug exposure and side effect relationship in order to identify safe and efficacious doses. Results from dynamic contrast-enhanced MRI (DCE-MRI) employed in all patients on the study as a pharmacodynamic (PD) marker of antiangiogenic effect indicated

(*continued*)

CASE STUDY 2 (*continued*)

that near maximal reduction in permeability and blood flow was associated with axitinib mean steady-state plasma exposures (AUCtau) associated with the 5 mg BID dose (10). Hence, the dose identified based on intended mechanism of action dovetailed nicely with the dose suggested by safety criteria. From the first cohort of patients enrolled in the study, high intersubject variability in axitinib plasma exposure was noted, with coefficient of variation ranging from 30% to 98% in the doses evaluated in the trial (9). Flat dosing had been routinely applied for small-molecule, tyrosine kinase inhibitors until that point. Additional analysis with axitinib pharmacokinetic (PK) data that was subsequently published indicated that the intersubject variability in plasma exposures was not related to common demographic parameters such as age, body weight, body surface area, gender, or ethnicity (11). Hence, dosing based on body surface area or weight would not be helpful.

Subsequently, a phase 2 study was initiated in cytokine-refractory renal cell carcinoma patients, in which 44.2% objective response rate (ORR; 95% confidence interval [CI]: 30.5–58.7) was observed with the use of the flat 5 mg BID dose in the majority of patients (12). This demonstrated that a robust clinical response could be achieved with axitinib at a flat 5 mg BID dose. However, the high intersubject variability in pharmacokinetics suggested that a subset of patients with lower than typical drug concentrations at the 5 mg BID dose were likely getting subtherapeutic exposures. In order to maximize the likelihood of clinical response in the majority of patients, axitinib dose titration was proposed as a way of allowing patients who are able to tolerate the 5 mg BID starting dose to increase their dose. A specific dose algorithm was developed in collaboration between the industry sponsor and the key academic investigators participating in the axitinib clinical trials. If a patient was not already on hypertensive medications, did not have an increase in blood pressure, and did not have ≥ grade 2 drug-related toxicities after at least 2 weeks of dosing at the 5 mg BID starting dose, they were allowed to have their dose increased to 7 mg BID. After at least 2 weeks of dosing at the 7 mg BID, and applying the same criteria as before, the patient dose could be increased again to a final maximum dose of 10 mg BID. Investigator discretion was always to be applied prior to implanting this dose titration algorithm in individual patients (13).

With the agreement from investigators participating in axitinib trials at the time, this dose titration scheme was then implemented in a study in sorafenib-refractory renal cell carcinoma patients, and another study in Japanese cytokine-refractory patients with renal cell carcinoma (13,14). Additional guidance was provided to investigators participating in these trials regarding the logistics of the dose titration algorithm, and feedback was received on the challenges with implementing the individualized dosing strategy.

The proposed dose titration scheme was based entirely on individual patient tolerability; it did not take into account patient responses to treatment, nor did it involve therapeutic drug monitoring based on measured plasma concentrations of axitinib. Hence, in order to ascertain if the

(*continued*)

CASE STUDY 2 (*continued*)

implemented dose titration scheme did result in dose escalation in the right patients, a retrospective analysis was conducted using data from the three phase 2 studies in patients with renal cell carcinoma. The results from this analysis were presented by Dr. Brian Rini in an oral presentation at the American Society of Clinical Oncology Genitourinary (ASCO GU) Annual Meeting in 2012 (Table 9.1) (15).

TABLE 9.1 AXITINIB STEADY-STATE PLASMA EXPOSURES BEFORE AND AFTER TITRATION

Median AUC_{0-12} ng x h/mL (range)	**5 mg BID** N = 129	**7 mg BID** N = 30	**10 mg BID** N = 16
Before titration	**231** (42–931)	**160** (32.8–443)	**129** (31.9–304)
After titration		**225** (45.9–620)	**258** (63.9–608)

AUC, area under the curve.

In Figure 9.2, the individual steady-state plasma exposures are provided from the pooled data from the three clinical studies *prior to* dose titration. The data are divided into subgroups based on the highest dose that the patient dose was eventually increased to. It is evident that *prior to* dose titration, patients who eventually had their dose increased to 7 mg BID and particularly those whose dose increased to 10 mg BID had lower than typical plasma exposures, that is, 160 ng × h/mL mean area under the curve (AUC) for 7 mg BID group and 120 ng × h/mL compared to 231 ng.h/mL in patients not requiring dose escalation. Moreover, *after dose titration*, patients in all dose groups had normalized plasma exposures, as noted visually in Figure 9.2 and by similar mean AUC values of 231, 225, and 258 ng × h/mL in the three dose groups. This retrospective analysis therefore confirmed that dose titration implemented based on individual patient safety did in fact result in bringing all patients to similar plasma exposures. Also, this analysis confirmed that patients whose doses are increased from the 5 mg BID starting dose to the 10 mg BID maximal dose do not have higher than typical exposures; rather, this allows patients who had lower than typical exposures at the starting dose to catch up with the remaining patients at the 5 mg BID starting group.

Based on this analysis, the dose titration scheme was implemented for the phase 3 AXIS registrational study comparing axitinib with sorafenib in 723 patients enrolled from 175 sites in 22 countries (16). This large study, conducted collaboratively across academic and treatment centers around the world and in conjunction with the sponsor, led to the approval of axitinib in second-line renal cell carcinoma.

(*continued*)

CASE STUDY 2 (*continued*)

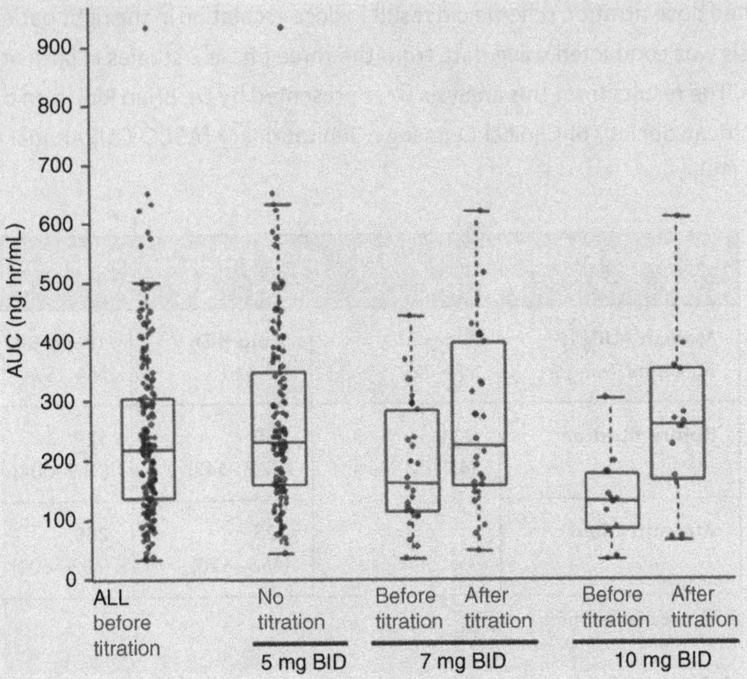

FIGURE 9.2 Axitinib plasma exposures before and after dose titration.

AUC, area under the curve; BID, twice a day.

Source: Rini BI, Escudier BJ, Michaelson MD, et al. Phase III AXIS trial for second-line metastatic renal cell carcinoma (mRCC): effect of prior first-line treatment duration and axitinib dose titration on axitinib efficacy. *J Clin Oncol*. 2012;30(5 suppl):354–354. doi:10.1200/jco.2012.30.5_suppl.354

Because the prior analysis justifying the basis for dose titration of axitinib was based on retrospective analysis of data from three phase 2 studies, there were concerns that the results might be prone to bias. Hence, a prospective study was designed to unequivocally evaluate the benefit of dose titration. The design for this study was developed jointly by Pfizer and key academic research investigators in renal cell carcinoma (17). In this phase 2, randomized, double-blind study that enrolled 213 patients, all patients were initially given the 5 mg BID starting dose. Based on individual patient tolerability, patients eligible for titration were randomly assigned to either active axitinib titration or placebo titration. For the primary end point of objective response there was a statistically significant higher response rate in the axitinib titration group compared to placebo titration; 54% versus 34% respectively ($p = .019$) (17). More mature data from the same study eventually demonstrated higher overall survival as well for the axitinib titration group compared to the placebo group; 42.7 months versus 30.4 months, respectively (18). This study provided prospective evidence in support of the benefit of the applied dose titration scheme for axitinib. This individualized dosing scheme is on the axitinib (Inlyta) label in all countries where the drug is

(*continued*)

CASE STUDY 2 (*continued*)

approved. Continued efforts are ongoing to further refine the dose titration scheme for axitinib to achieve even better patient tolerability.

Additional clinical studies are being conducted in collaboration with investigators in a variety of clinical settings. This includes single-agent use in neoadjuvant renal cell carcinoma, glioblastoma, hepatocellular carcinoma, neurofibromatosis type 2 and progressive vestibular schwannomas, soft tissue sarcomas, salivary gland cancers, adenoid cystic carcinoma, neuroendocrine carcinomas, melanoma, prostate cancer, and head and neck cancer. Axitinib is being tested in combination with a variety of agents including the PD-L1 inhibitor avelumab (Bavencio), the PD-1 inhibitor pembrolizumab (Keytruda), dalantercept, and temsirolimus, indicating the benefits of continued interaction between industry and academia, particularly in this unique case of the need to individualize dosing for axitinib.

EVOLVING COLLABORATIVE EFFORTS

Oftentimes, the overall goals of oncology drug development for academia and industry sectors are not aligned; this stems from the different lenses of the researchers in these sectors. For the academic researcher who is also the treating physician, the individual patient presenting in the clinic is the primary focus. For the industry researcher, demonstrating the efficacious and safe use of a candidate compound in a population of patients is desired. These intrinsic differences in vantage points and goals can lead to very different approaches in trial design and patient selection for clinical studies. For example, many industry sponsored trials have strict inclusion/exclusion criteria in an effort to generate cleaner and more interpretable data. Additionally, study protocols may be filled with assessments that may not be medically necessary for the patient, but may generate important scientific and clinical data for the industry researcher. For academic-treating physicians carrying out industry sponsored trials, the strict eligibility criteria may preclude their patients from receiving medications that may be beneficial to the patients. Similarly, the long list of additional assessments required in study protocols may prove to be too logistically cumbersome for physicians and patients to buy into enrolling in industry sponsored studies versus selecting a standard of care treatment. Therefore, there is a role for **investigator initiated trials (IITs)** to bring potentially effective therapeutics to their patients through differently designed studies that may allow for patients who would not otherwise be eligible or able to join traditional clinical studies, to potentially benefit from drugs in development. Research conducted through the use of IITs has changed much about the traditional collaborative roles held in the industry and academic sectors.

ROLE OF IITs: CASE STUDY WITH DART

IITs are studies proposed and conducted by academic researchers who are not affiliated with the biopharmaceutical company, but are studying the company's drug product or disease area of interest (19). All potential uses of the study medication cannot be explored through industry sponsored trials alone. Therefore, IITs can help to expand the knowledge of the drug product, including identifying new ways of using existing medications, optimizing dosing strategies, or better characterizing safety. Much of the work stemming from IITs has led to further development efforts by the industry partner and has contributed to expanding the labeling indications for existing therapies.

One area in which IITs are often most fruitful is investigating a rare tumor type (either by a histological or biomarker definition) for which the biology of the agent may be an ideal fit, but the overall market is likely smaller, limiting commercial opportunities. Both IITs and cooperative group studies play a key role in this space. One example of an ongoing study of rare tumors is Southwest Oncology Group (SWOG) 1609 (S1609), DART: **D**ual **A**nti-CTLA-4 and Anti-PD-1 Blockade in **R**are **T**umors (20). This clinical trial is studying the combination of two immunotherapy agents, ipilimumab and nivolumab, across more than 30 rare tumor histologic subtypes, and as of September 2017 had more than 700 sites and treated more than 120 patients in over 9 months.

DART was initially an investigator initiated study designed to more rationally investigate the utility of immune checkpoint blockade in rare tumors. Historically, these patients were seen often in phase 1 clinics and treated in dose escalation phase 1 clinical studies. However, while the rare tumor cancer patient may help inform dosing and toxicity of the novel agent, little clinical information related to the efficacy of that agent in that rare tumor type is gleaned from this approach. Thus, DART was devised as a study among a couple of phase 1 units to formally test the efficacy of ipilimumab and nivolumab across rare solid tumors in a basket design as part of a research collaboration with Bristol-Myers Squibb. However, increasing interest within SWOG and an opportunity to join National Cancer Institute-Molecular Analysis for Therapy Choice (NCI-MATCH) as a rare tumor "arm" led to the formal launch of the protocol within the NCI-National Clinical Trials Network (NCTN) network.

The study utilizes a Simon's two-stage design across each of the 30-plus rare histologic cohorts to investigate the overall response rate of ipilimumab with nivolumab across rare cancer subtypes, including cancers of unknown primary. Of note, a "not otherwise classified" (NOC) cohort was established to ensure that ultrarare cancers that were not classified among the 30-plus existing cohorts could also enroll. Finally, the translational medicine objectives of this study, which include whole-exome sequencing, RNAseq, cfDNA, proteomics, and immune-cell immunohistochemistry (IHC), will in many cases be the first of its kind for many of the tumor types in DART. With the potential for clinical efficacy in rare tumors and the further refinement of biomarker signatures across tumor types, the robust accrual of DART, despite being a rare tumor study, may open the door to other future rare tumor studies within the NCI-NCTN network. Another example of early phase clinical trials translating into a promising immunotherapeutic strategy involves pembrolizumab in microsatellite-unstable cancers.

EXPANDING THE USE OF THERAPIES WITH IITS: AN EXAMPLE WITH PEMBROLIZUMAB IN MICROSATELLITE INSTABILITY-HIGH (MSI-H) CANCERS

Pembrolizumab (Keytruda) is the first therapy that has been granted accelerated approval by the FDA for tissue- or site-agnostic indication. In May 2017, the FDA granted pembrolizumab accelerated approval for the treatment of adult and pediatric patients with unresectable or metastatic MSI-H or mismatch repair deficient (dMMR) solid tumors that have progressed on a prior treatment. This approval was based on data from five uncontrolled, single-arm clinical trials in 149 patients with 15 different cancer types who were prospectively determined to have MSI-H or dMMR cancers. The accelerated approval was based on an ORR of 39.6% (95% CI: 31.7–47.9) where responses lasted 6 months or more in the 78% of patients who responded to pembrolizumab. The ORR was similar whether the patients were diagnosed with colorectal cancer (which made up 90 of the 149 patients) or the other 14 cancer types at 36% versus 46% (21).

The main dMMR colorectal trial was initiated by researchers (Luis Diaz and Dung Le) from Johns Hopkins Sidney Kimmel Comprehensive Cancer Center (22). Although the use of anti-PD-1 antibodies has led to remarkable clinical responses in a number of cancers, including melanomas, non-small cell lung cancer, renal cell carcinoma, Hodgkin lymphoma, and more, its use in colorectal cancer has not turned out to be particularly promising. However, Diaz et al. hypothesized that patients with dMMR cancers with 10 to 100 times more somatic mutations would have prominent lymphocyte infiltrates, which would be susceptible to immune response. The inspiration for Diaz's study was a previously published study that enrolled patients with multiple cancer types reported by fellow Johns Hopkins researchers, Suzanne Topalian and Drew Pardoll, in 2012 where a single colorectal cancer patient responded well to treatment with nivolumab, another anti-PD-1 antibody (23,24). The difference with this colorectal patient who responded versus other colorectal cancer patients was that this patient also had Lynch syndrome, which is an inherited form of dMMR. From there, Diaz conducted the phase 2 study that evaluated the efficacy of pembrolizumab in 41 patients with dMMR colorectal cancer, mismatch repair proficient colorectal cancer, and dMMR cancers that were not colorectal. The results were striking: ORR was 40% in dMMR colorectal patients versus 0% in mismatch repair proficient colorectal patients. Patients with dMMR colorectal cancer had progression-free survival rates comparable to those of the dMMR noncolorectal cancer patients (78% vs. 67%).

This initial trial led by Hopkins researcher Diaz eventually led to the enrollment of other patients with different cancer types that shared this genetic trait, as reported earlier in 2017 in *Science* (22). The expansion led to the inclusion of 86 patients with 12 different tumor types with evidence of dMMR disease and progressive disease prior to enrollment. In this group of patients, 53% had objective radiographic responses with 21% achieving complete response. With even the positive results from the initial trial in dMMR colorectal patients by Diaz, Merck, the industry sponsor of Keytruda, conducted four clinical studies (NCT02460198, NCT01848834, NCT02054806, and NCT02628067) in multiple tumor types that are dMMR or MSI-H that led to the landmark tumor site and age agnostic approval of pembrolizumab. This example of an IIT that led to further industry sponsored studies and the eventual accelerated approval of the therapy based on the existence of a biomarker rather than the organ defining the disease has dramatically shifted the paradigm for collaboration between academia and industry partners, and more importantly the approach to oncology research and drug development that will, it is hoped, expand treatment options to previously difficult-to-treat cancers.

FUNDING STUDIES WITH INDUSTRY

Many companies fund extensive internal and external research and development (R&D) programs through partnerships with investigators in academia. This is a common method for funding IITs that are either directly **sponsored** by the company or sponsored by the investigator's institution with financial support from the company (see more in what follows). Often such research collaborations are facilitated through a **Medical Science Liaison** (**MSL**). These are individuals employed by the company to help shepherd new ideas and proposals through the funding process. It is a good idea to try to identify whether a company has a local MSL you can contact to initiate funding applications for research concepts.

Often companies will partner with academic investigators on research they wish to sponsor, either through subcontracts for laboratory work, or to engage in clinical trials. In many cases, companies will sponsor trials they are conducting in order to seek federal regulatory approval (e.g., through the FDA) to permit labeling and marketing of their product. Academic investigators also frequently function as study chairs or local PIs, or as medical monitors, or through scientific advisory boards and steering committees. It is important when establishing research relationships with industry—particularly those that involve remuneration—to be open in declaring them, as they may generate conflicts of interest that can affect scientific objectivity (25).

In addition, many government agencies, such as the National Institutes of Health (NIH), offer **Small Business Innovation Research** (**SBIR**) funding mechanisms for the express purpose of facilitating research collaborations between small or start-up companies and academic investigators. Other research collaborations between companies and government agencies may involve establishing a **Cooperative Research and Development Agreement** (**CRADA**), which is an agreement on the part of a federal government laboratory to provide resources, such as facilities, equipment, staffing, drugs, and so on, rather than funding, to support certain R&D efforts. The industry CRADA partner would contribute necessary funding and additional resources to support the project. A CRADA allows the nonfederal collaborating party the option to negotiate licensing for any invention or intellectual property developed through a collaborative research project.

Many oncology clinical trials are also funded through partnerships between industry, the NCI, and the NCTN. The NCTN consists of several major cooperative groups: Alliance, SWOG, NRG Oncology, Eastern Cooperative Oncology Group (ECOG)–American College of Radiology Imaging Network (ACRIN), and the Children's Oncology Group (COG). In addition, NCI of Canada (NCIC) is a frequent participant in supporting U.S. federally sponsored clinical trials, especially phase III trials. The NCI principally supports cooperative group trials through two agencies: the **Cancer Therapy Evaluation Program (CTEP)** and the **Division of Cancer Prevention (DCP)**, which respectively address trials either designed primarily to improve clinical outcomes or to reduce morbidity/improve patients' quality of life. Industry partners often support such trials by providing funding and/or drug supply to support the costs of running large clinical experiments. For example, the NRG HN004 trial (https://clinicaltrials.gov/ct2/show/NCT03258554) represents a partnership between CTEP, NRG Oncology, the FDA, and Astra-Zeneca to test the PD-L1 inhibitor durvalumab in head/neck cancer patients who are medically unfit for standard therapy with radiation and cisplatin.

Finally, several NCTN groups also have established research **foundations** to operate clinical trials that are not expressly sponsored through the NCI but rather through a partnership directly between a company and a cooperative group. Examples include the Alliance Foundation, Radiation Therapy Oncology Group (RTOG) Foundation, and Gynecologic Oncology Group (GOG) Foundation. The mechanism for procuring support for such trials typically involves trilateral partnership among the investigator(s) initiating the proposal, the potential industry sponsor, and the respective cooperative group committee leadership, in order to advance a trial concept.

INVESTIGATIONAL NEW DRUG (IND) APPLICATIONS

In order to evaluate a drug or biological product in human patients, an IND application is required of all sponsors (i.e., the individual or institution who is considered the **IND holder**) and sponsor-investigators (e.g., academic or industry) by the FDA (26). Generally, for the IITs that evaluate an existing drug that is approved and marketed, it is important to first understand whether the investigation can occur without an IND. If the investigation is not exempt from the IND process, an existing IND may be used to evaluate the marketed drug for a different indication; alternatively, a new IND may be submitted to support the study.

Any IIT where the intent of the findings would support a new indication or any labeling or advertising changes to an existing, commercially approved drug would require an IND (26). The FDA has issued a draft guidance document that provides guidance on when to submit an IND application and the components of the IND application for sponsor-investigators (27). An individual is considered a sponsor-investigator if he or she both initiates and conducts a study—in most cases with IITs investigating existing drugs as new regimens or for new indications, the academic researcher would be considered a sponsor-investigator and would need an IND prior to initiating the research.

There are six main components of a new IND application: information on the qualifications of the sponsor-investigator, the drug's Investigator's Brochure, a clinical trial protocol, chemistry manufacturing and control (CMC) information, pharmacology and toxicology information, and a summary of previous human experience. If the sponsor-investigator has the permission to initiate a study using an existing IND from the industry sponsor, then a letter of cross-reference authorization from the industry partner (e.g., commercial sponsor) can be submitted. In the event a new IND application is needed, some of the six required components may be pulled from other applications (e.g., CMC and pharmacology and toxicology information usually are available from the industry sponsor in the previous application). To determine whether an existing IND can be used for a new IIT, it is important for the academic researcher to work with the industry sponsor and its regulatory team to determine the best course of action.

FDA REGISTRATION

Positive results from IITs that can potentially expand the use of existing drugs or treatment regimens to other indications should be considered for regulatory **registration**. The decision and process for filing a Supplemental New Drug Application (sNDA) or Supplemental Biologics License Application (sBLA) to the FDA depend on the legal agreements between the academic researcher and his or her institution and with the industry partner. This often becomes a complicated process for navigating the cosharing of patent rights.

An example is the recent approval of Mylotarg (gemtuzumab ozogamicin) for the treatment of newly diagnosed CD33-positive acute myeloid leukemia (AML) (28). The basis for this approval was the IIT study ALFA-701 (NCT00927498), a multicenter, randomized, open-label phase 3 study conducted in 271 patients with newly diagnosed de novo AML (29). Patients received induction therapy consisting of daunorubicin and cytarabine with or without Mylotarg. Mylotarg had been previously withdrawn from the market, and the reintroduction of the drug occurred via the exploration of lower fractionated doses of Mylotarg in the IIT study. The New Drug Application submission was conducted by the sponsor (Pfizer Inc.) in collaboration with the investigators, and utilized data from the IIT study. Of note, two additional IIT trials enabled additional indications for Mylotarg. The AML-19 (NCT00091234) was an IIT study conducted in 237 patients with newly diagnosed AML unsuitable for intensive chemotherapy (30). MYLOFRANCE-1 was a phase 2, single-arm, open-label study IIT trial of Mylotarg in adults with CD33-positive AML in first relapse (31). This is an example of three separate indications gaining registrational approval based on data from IIT studies that were jointly submitted with the sponsor.

WORKING WITH TECHNOLOGY AND DEVICE COMPANIES

In addition to food and drugs, the FDA also regulates medical devices, which are approved through a similar but slightly different mechanism compared to drugs (510(k) clearance). Medical devices fall under several different classes (e.g., Class I, II, or III), depending on the degree of regulatory requirements, risk, and the potential for regulatory exemption. A description of this process is beyond the scope of our chapter; more details can be acquired via the FDA website (www.fda.gov/MedicalDevices/default.htm).

Similar to pharmaceutical companies, most technology and device companies sponsor R&D programs with opportunities to fund research in conjunction with academic investigators. Research support may be provided in the form of direct grants or often as **in-kind loans**, which usually entail provision of special or proprietary equipment to conduct research at an academic institution. For example, Varian Medical Systems supports both individual investigator applications through a recurring grant cycle, in addition to Master Research Agreements with several university departments to fund coordinated research programs to advance innovations in medical physics. Because of the differences in regulatory approval processes for devices, however, these companies do not sponsor large clinical trials to the same degree as pharmaceutical companies. Therefore, larger questions regarding the clinical impact of new technologies are often taken up either through cooperative groups, or by alternative study designs to classic phase III trials (e.g., comparative effectiveness or registry trials).

TRAINING RESEARCHERS

As the line between traditional academia and industry research continues to blur, training budding researchers who can better bridge the two sectors is immensely important. Clinical researchers generally have one or more of three advanced degrees—MD/DO, PhD, or PharmD—and postgraduate training opportunities for these graduates differ depending on the degree.

For the physician (MD/DO), the typical path of postgraduate training involves more hands-on clinical experiences through residency programs and fellowships. For specialty therapeutic areas such as medical or surgical oncology, completing a fellowship in clinical training is essential. Then, to enter the realm of clinical research, young physicians often may need formal training in research methodology, statistics, and patient-oriented outcomes research. Many academic institutions offer part-time courses or even master's programs in clinical research to provide more formal didactic training to enable physicians to gain these skills. Developing these skills can then help physicians become clinical researchers at academic institutions with an opportunity to be involved with clinical trials, including industry sponsored clinical trials. The experience of being an investigator physician in a clinical trial then allows the physician to gain access to industry opportunities as medical drug safety monitors or clinical development scientists. In essence, the exposure of physician researchers to academia and industry sectors is more sequential than in parallel.

Similarly, for the PhD graduate, postdoctoral research programs exist in academic institutions or private companies that are immediately available after conferral of the degree. Aside from the joint programs available with Rutgers University and various industry sponsors or University of North Carolina (UNC) with GlaxoSmithKline, there are very few postdoctoral programs that are jointly run by academic and industry partners. For PhD graduates, much of their experience has been in academia and most likely preclinical or basic science in nature. It is less common for PhD graduates to have direct clinical research experience through their graduate education, unless the PI was involved in clinical trials. Therefore, breaking into the clinical research space generally involves finding a postdoctoral program in industry in a clinical functional area to gain hands-on training in clinical research. It may be possible with some years of experience conducting clinical research in industry to then transition back into academia. In this case, introduction to clinical research in both sectors is also mostly sequential.

In contrast, more formal postdoctoral fellowship training programs for PharmD graduates exist that allow for immediate exposure to both academia and industry sectors. After graduation, there are often three routes available for PharmD graduates: retail or community pharmacy, pharmacy residency training, or postgraduate fellowship programs. A pharmacy residency helps to improve skills in patient care through experiences in both inpatient and outpatient settings, including general internal medicine, ambulatory care clinics, or specialty areas such as infectious disease and hematology/oncology. Conversely, a pharmacy fellowship is designed to prepare the PharmD graduate to become an independent researcher. In the United States, there are several major joint postdoctoral fellowships between well-known schools of pharmacies and industry sponsors, including: Rutgers, Massachusetts College of Pharmacy and Health Sciences (MCPHS), UNC, University of Southern California (USC), and University of California San Diego (UCSD). In these programs, the PharmD fellows focus on a functional area of practice and gain hands-on training with the industry sponsor while also having the opportunity to conduct academic research projects and participate in didactic courses in clinical research and professional/leadership development.

As an example, the UCSD oncology clinical pharmacology fellowship program is run jointly with Pfizer in La Jolla, California. The fellowship is 2 years in duration and aims to help the trainee develop skills in clinical pharmacology, including conducting clinical pharmacology studies and learning quantitative pharmacology to analyze and interpret PK and PD data. As the fellowship is oncology focused, it is necessary also to ensure that the fellow is clinically adept. Therefore, starting at the beginning of the fellowship, the PharmD trainee rotates through inpatient hematology/oncology service and outpatient oncology clinics at the UCSD Moores Cancer Center. After the full-time rotation experience, which lasts about 2 months, the fellow follows a medical oncologist outpatient in the phase 1 clinic longitudinally 1 day per week to continue to develop and practice clinical pharmacy skills, while also gaining exposure to phase 1 studies from an academic center point of view. In parallel, fellows also begin to take on projects at Pfizer, where they gain experience in clinical pharmacology study design, protocol writing, data analysis, and population PK and PKPD modeling. With the UCSD School of Pharmacy, the fellow has an opportunity to teach at the school, while also having opportunities to work on clinical pharmacology related IITs, usually also in collaboration with oncologists at Moores. For the duration of the fellowship program, the trainee is immersed in research projects both industry and academic, and thus gains invaluable insight into the cultures of both sectors, which may help to better position the fellow for improved and more fruitful collaborative efforts in the future.

CONCLUSION

From the case examples with trastuzumab and axitinib, it is clear that academia and industry collaboration has long existed and proven to be necessary in the approval of these agents. In light of the rapidity of delivering new therapeutics in treating hematologic and solid malignancies, the work of academic and industry researchers is becoming more integrated and collaboration between the two entities is crucial to more efficiently bring novel treatments to patients, as evidenced by the use of IITs including DART and the story of pembrolizumab. With the ever evolving roles of academic and industry researchers, adequate exposure and training programs for future researchers are needed to aid in fostering stronger relationships and better collaboration. Although some postgraduate training programs that offer experience in both sectors already exist, more are needed to better prepare physician, PhD, and PharmD graduates for oncology clinical research.

GLOSSARY

investigator initiated trials (IITs): studies done to bring potentially effective therapeutics to patients through differently designed studies that may allow patients, who would not otherwise be eligible or able to join traditional clinical studies, to potentially benefit from drugs in development.

sponsored: underwritten.

Medical Science Liaison (MSL): person employed by an industry (drug) company to establish and maintain relationships with physicians and practitioners often at academic institutions.

Small Business Innovation Research (SBIR): a mechanism for funding offered by many government agencies, such as the National Institutes of Health (NIH), for the express purpose of facilitating research collaborations between small or start-up companies and academic investigators.

Cooperative Research and Development Agreement (CRADA): a research collaboration agreement on the part of a federal government laboratory to provide resources, such as facilities, equipment, staffing, drugs, and so on, rather than funding, to support certain R&D efforts.

Cancer Therapy Evaluation Program (CTEP): an NCI entity that supports cooperative group trials designed primarily to improve clinical outcomes.

Division of Cancer Prevention (DCP): an NCI entity that supports cooperative group trials designed primarily to reduce morbidity/improve patients' quality of life.

foundation: a research entity established to operate clinical trials that are sponsored through a partnership directly between a company and a cooperative group.

IND holder: the individual or institution who makes an Investigational New Drug Application to the FDA.

registration: regulatory submission made when the use of an existing drug or treatment regimen can potentially be expanded to other indications.

in-kind loan: research support that usually entails provision of special or proprietary equipment

REFERENCES

1. Bazell R. *Her-2, The Making of Herceptin, a Revolutionary Treatment for Breast Cancer*. New York, NY: Random House; 2011.
2. Schechter AL, Stern DF, Vaidyanathan L, et al. The *neu* oncogene: an erb-B-related gene encoding a 185,000-Mr tumour antigen. *Nature*. 1984;312(5994):513–516. doi:10.1038/312513a0
3. Paul Carter BMF, Lewis GD, Sliwkowski MX. Development of herceptin, in HER2: basic research, prognosis and therapy. In: Y. Yarden, ed. *Breast Disease*. IOS Press, Amsterdam. 2000:103–111.
4. Downward J, Yarden Y, Mayes E, et al. Close similarity of epidermal growth factor receptor and v-erb-B oncogene protein sequences. *Nature*. 1984;307(5951):521–527. doi:10.1038/307521a0
5. Slamon DJ, Clark G, Wong S, et al. Human breast cancer: correlation of relapse and survival with amplification of the HER-2/neu oncogene. *Science*. 1987;235(4785):177–182. doi:10.1126/science.3798106
6. Baselga J, Tripathy D, Mendelsohn J, et al. Phase II study of weekly intravenous recombinant humanized anti-p185HER2 monoclonal antibody in patients with HER2/neu-overexpressing metastatic breast cancer. *J Clin Oncol*. 1996;14(3):737–744. doi:10.1200/jco.1996.14.3.737
7. Bang YJ, Cutsem EV, Feyereislova A, et al. Trastuzumab in combination with chemotherapy versus chemotherapy alone for treatment of HER2-positive advanced gastric or gastro-oesophageal junction cancer (ToGA): a phase 3, open-label, randomised controlled trial. *Lancet*. 2010;376(9742):687–697. doi:10.1016/s0140-6736(10)61121-x
8. Genentech. *My pathway: a study evaluating herceptin/perjeta, tarceva, zelboraf/cotellic, erivedge, alecensa, and tecentriq treatment targeted against certain molecular alterations in participants with advanced solid tumors*. 2017. https://clinicaltrials.gov/ct2/show/NCT02091141
9. Rugo HS, Herbst RS, Liu G, et al. Phase I trial of the oral antiangiogenesis agent AG-013736 in patients with advanced solid tumors: pharmacokinetic and clinical results. *J Clin Oncol*. 2005;23(24):5474–5483. doi:10.1200/jco.2005.04.192
10. Liu, G., Rugo HS, Wilding G, et al. Dynamic contrast-enhanced magnetic resonance imaging as a pharmacodynamic measure of response after acute dosing of AG-013736, an oral angiogenesis inhibitor, in patients with advanced solid tumors: results from a phase I study. *J Clin Oncol*. 2005;23(24):5464–5473. doi:10.1200/JCO.2005.04.143
11. Garrett M, Poland B, Brennan M, et al. Population pharmacokinetic analysis of axitinib in healthy volunteers. *Br J Clin Pharmacol*. 2014;77(3):480-492. doi:10.1111/bcp.12206
12. Rixe O, Bukowski RM, Michaelson MD, et al. Axitinib treatment in patients with cytokine-refractory metastatic renal-cell cancer: a phase II study. *Lancet Oncol*. 2007;8(11):975–984. doi:10.1016/S1470-2045(07)70285-1
13. Rini BI, Wilding G, Hudes G, et al. Phase II study of axitinib in sorafenib-refractory metastatic renal cell carcinoma. *J Clin Oncol*. 2009;27(27):4462-4468. doi:10.1200/JCO.2008.21.7034
14. Eto M, Uemura H, Tomita Y, et al. Overall survival and final efficacy and safety results from a Japanese phase II study of axitinib in cytokine-refractory metastatic renal cell carcinoma. *Cancer Sci*. 2014;105(12):1576–1583. doi:10.1111/cas.12546
15. Rini BI, Escudier BJ, Michaelson MD, et al. Phase III AXIS trial for second-line metastatic renal cell carcinoma (mRCC): effect of prior first-line treatment duration and axitinib dose titration on axitinib efficacy. *J Clin Oncol*. 2012;30(5_suppl):354–354. doi:10.1200/jco.2012.30.5_suppl.354
16. Rini BI, Escudier B, Tomczak P, et al. Comparative effectiveness of axitinib versus sorafenib in advanced renal cell carcinoma (AXIS): a randomised phase 3 trial. *Lancet*. 2011;378(9807):1931–1939. doi:10.1016/S0140-6736(11)61613-9
17. Rini BI, Melichar B, Ueda T, et al. Axitinib with or without dose titration for first-line metastatic renal-cell carcinoma: a randomised double-blind phase 2 trial. *Lancet Oncol*. 2013;14(12):1233–1242. doi:10.1016/S1470-2045(13)70464-9
18. Rini BI, Tomita Y, Melichar B, et al. Overall survival analysis from a randomized phase II study of axitinib with or without dose titration in first-line metastatic renal cell carcinoma. *Clin Genitourin Cancer*. 2016;14(6):499–503. doi:10.1016/j.clgc.2016.04.005
19. Suvarna V. Investigator initiated trials (IITs). *Perspect Clin Res*. 2012;3(4):119–121. doi: 10.4103/2229-3485.103591
20. National Cancer Institute. *Nivolumab and ipilimumab in treating patients with rare tumors*. 2016. https://clinicaltrials.gov/ct2/show/NCT02834013
21. Merck. *Keytruda: highlights of prescribing information*. 2014. https://www.merck.com/product/usa/pi_circulars/k/keytruda/keytruda_pi.pdf
22. Le DT, Durham JN, Smith KN, et al. Mismatch repair deficiency predicts response of solid tumors to PD-1 blockade. *Science*. 2017;357(6349):409–413. doi:10.1126/science.aan6733
23. Brahmer JR, Drake CG, Wollner I, et al. Phase I study of single-agent anti-programmed death-1 (MDX-1106) in refractory solid tumors: safety, clinical activity, pharmacodynamics, and immunologic correlates. *J Clin Oncol*. 2010;28(19):3167–3175. doi:10.1200/JCO.2009.26.7609
24. Topalian SL, Stephen Hodi F, Brahmer JR, et al. Safety, activity, and immune correlates of anti-PD-1 antibody in cancer. *N Engl J Med*. 2012;366(26):2443–2454. doi:10.1056/NEJMoa1200690
25. Tringale KR, Marshall D, Mackey TK, et al. Types and distribution of payments from industry to physicians in 2015. *JAMA*. 2017;317(17):1774–1784. doi:10.1001/jama.2017.3091
26. Food and Drug Administration. *Guidance for Clinical Investigators, Sponsors, and IRBs: Investigational New Drug Applications (INDs) — Determining Whether Human Research Studies Can Be Conducted Without an IND*. 2013. https://www.fda.gov/downloads/drugs/guidances/ucm229175.pdf
27. Food and Drug Administration. *Investigational New Drug Applications Prepared and Submitted by Sponsor-Investigators: Guidance for Industry*. 2015. https://www.fda.gov/downloads/Drugs/Guidances/UCM446695.pdf
28. Pfizer. *Mylotarg - Highlights of Prescribing Information*. 2017. https://www.accessdata.fda.gov/drugsatfda_docs/label/2017/761060lbl.pdf
29. Castaigne S, Pautas C, Terré C, et al. Effect of gemtuzumab ozogamicin on survival of adult patients with de-novo acute myeloid leukaemia (ALFA-0701): a randomised, open-label, phase 3 study. *Lancet*. 2012;379(9825):1508–1516. doi:10.1016/S0140-6736(12)60485-1

30. Amadori S, Suciu S, Selleslag D, et al. Gemtuzumab ozogamicin versus best supportive care in older patients with newly diagnosed acute myeloid leukemia unsuitable for intensive chemotherapy: results of the randomized phase III EORTC-GIMEMA AML-19 trial. *J Clin Oncol*. 2016;34(9):972–979. doi:10.1200/JCO.2015.64.0060
31. Pilorge S, Rigaudeau S, Rabian F, et al. Fractionated gemtuzumab ozogamicin and standard dose cytarabine produced prolonged second remissions in patients over the age of 55 years with acute myeloid leukemia in late first relapse. *Am J Hematol*. 2014;89(4):399–403. doi:10.1002/ajh.23653

III Population and Outcomes Research

10

Study Designs

MICHAEL MILLIGAN ■ AILEEN CHEN

Population and outcomes research is a multidisciplinary field of study that utilizes principles from epidemiology, economics, and policy research to determine how exposures in the form of health services affect outcomes of interest, such as survival, functional status, and patient satisfaction, among many others (1).

As outlined in Figure 10.1, this chapter reviews common study designs used in population and outcomes research. First, researchers define the distribution of disease or healthcare services in the populace through descriptive studies. By asking, "Why do certain individuals develop disease or undergo treatment, while others do not?" researchers generate testable hypotheses about the causes of such patterns. Next, observational studies are used to identify associations between healthcare interventions—also known as *exposures*—and the effects observed in patients—the *outcome of interest*. While these studies might strongly suggest a link between an exposure and outcome, real-world individuals are complex, and often introduce confounding factors that complicate any analysis. Therefore, in a final step, researchers perform meticulous experimental studies to isolate and test only the effects of a single healthcare intervention on a single outcome, thereby generating highly reliable conclusions.

DESCRIPTIVE STUDIES

PURPOSE

The primary goal of descriptive studies is to characterize the patterns of disease, treatment, and outcomes in a population. These insights can, in turn, be used to develop hypotheses to test in analytical studies.

DESIGN

Descriptive studies commonly characterize the so-called "three Ws"—*who, where,* and *when.* There are three main types of descriptive studies, all of which can address the three Ws. The first, and smallest, is a ***case report***. These studies provide detailed information about a single patient. Typically, case reports are notable for some reason. Perhaps a disease occurred in an individual

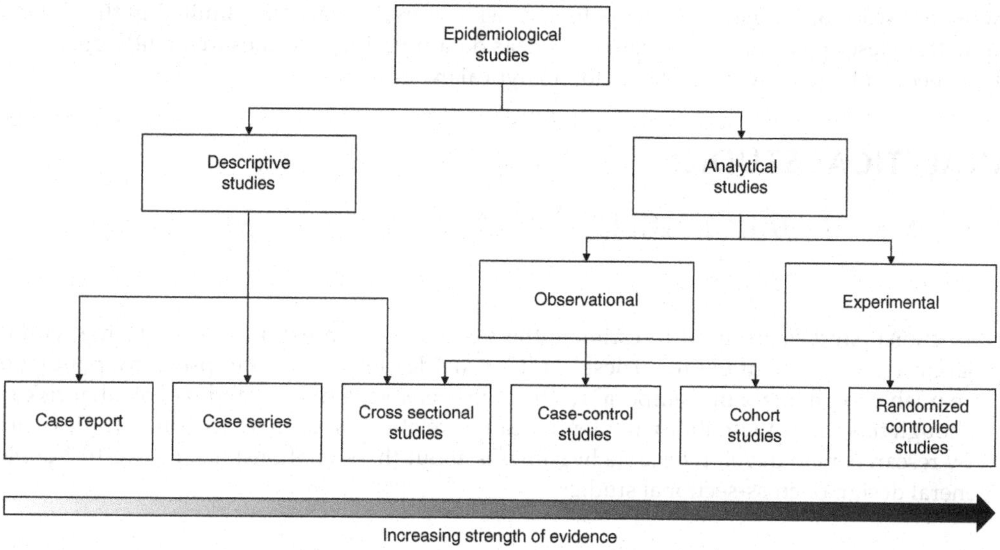

FIGURE 10.1 Organization of outcomes studies and their relative strength of evidence.

not commonly thought to be at risk, or an unexpected complication occurred following treatment with a new cancer agent. The second type, a ***case series,*** compiles detailed accounts of several cases. These studies often present data regarding the commonalities among affected individuals, information that might suggest—but cannot confirm—potential associations. The third type, known as a ***cross-sectional study,*** represents the most complex descriptive study design. Cross-sectional studies characterize a specific population at a given point in time. Cross-sectional studies are unique among descriptive studies, in that they can simultaneously characterize the occurrence of both an outcome and its potential explanatory factors. Using these data, we can begin to consider potential associations between an exposure and an outcome (see analytical studies section).

ANALYSIS

The analysis of descriptive studies tends to be straightforward. Case reports and case series provide an in-depth, written description of the facts surrounding a small number of individual cases. Cross-sectional studies go further and analyze the distribution of a disease, outcome, or risk factor within a ***population.*** Akin to taking a "snapshot in time," these studies are typically used to calculate the total number of individuals with a particular characteristic or condition in a population—a measure known as the ***prevalence.*** When a change in a particular characteristic or condition is captured over time, ***incidence*** (i.e., new cases in a population over a given time) can also be calculated. The National Health and Nutrition Examination Study (NHANES) and the U.S. Census are examples of cross-sectional studies that are often used to estimate prevalence of disease and risk factors in the United States (2).

When researchers first observe a change in the apparent prevalence or incidence of a disease, they rarely have enough information to point to a specific cause with any certainty. Thus, they must infer possible causes and put their hypotheses to the test. Therefore, the final analysis of any descriptive study should culminate in a well-reasoned, testable hypothesis.

ADVANTAGES AND DISADVANTAGES

Compared to analytical studies, descriptive studies tend to be less expensive and less time-consuming to perform. However, they are unable to statistically test any apparent associations between a disease or outcome and its potential risk factors, and are thus limited in their impact. Despite this, descriptive studies remain crucial, as data from these studies frequently provide the insights needed to generate hypotheses for analytical experiments.

ANALYTICAL STUDIES

CROSS-SECTIONAL STUDIES

Purpose

Cross-sectional studies are used to estimate the frequency of an exposure or outcome within a population at a given point in time. These studies provide only a static glimpse into a population, and are unable to untangle the temporal relationship between a disease and its potential risk factors. Though this limits their ability to identify causal relationships, cross-sectional studies can be used by researchers to develop testable hypotheses about these relationships. Figure 10.2 depicts the general design of cross-sectional studies.

Design

Though cross-sectional studies seek to define the distribution of exposures and outcomes in an entire population, it is rarely feasible to study every member of the population. As such, researchers typically study a well-defined ***sample*** of individuals and extrapolate the results to an entire target population. Because the validity of inferences about the population critically depends on the sampling methods, it is important to define these methods clearly and rigorously.

The first step in any cross-sectional study is to define the target population. Target populations can range from very broad—the entire adult population of the United States—to very narrow—women receiving breast cancer care at a single clinic. The next step is to select a sample of representative individuals. Ideally, samples would be drawn at random from the population, and many

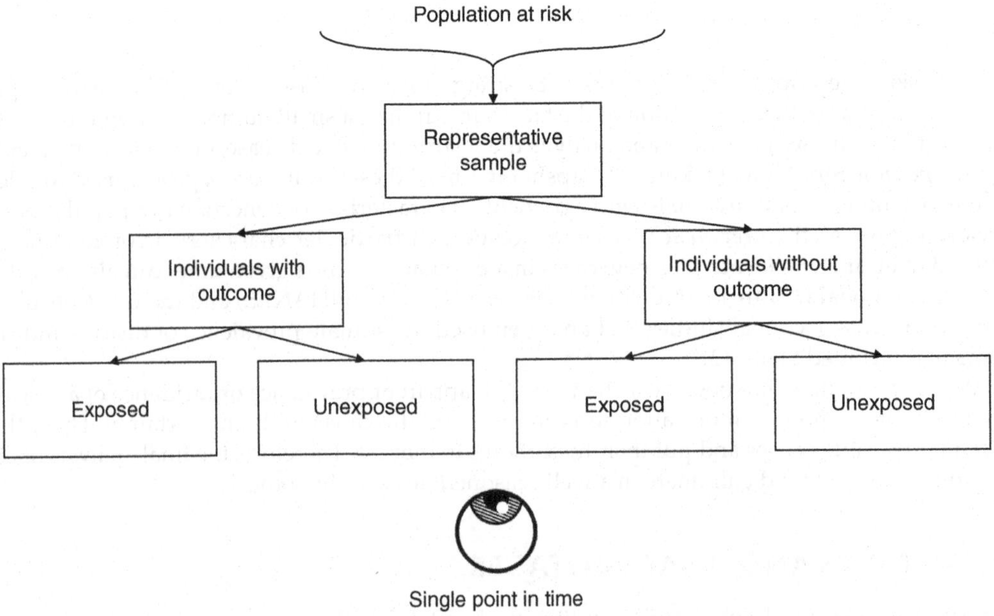

FIGURE 10.2 Outline of cross-sectional studies.

statistical methods explicitly or implicitly assume that samples are generated in this fashion. In practice, samples are commonly selected based on logistical simplicity—such as those people who choose to respond to a survey, or who naturally appear in a clinic (i.e., a convenience sample). In other cases, investigators may use their judgment to identify a mix of individuals felt to be representative of the larger population. While straightforward, these selection methods can potentially introduce bias into the study. Thus, to increase the likelihood that a sample is truly representative of the target population, researchers have developed a number of rigorous selection methodologies, such as simple random sampling, stratified random sampling, and others.

Once a representative sample is selected, information is collected about the attributes of interest. This can be performed using tools or instruments, such as questionnaires, along with clinical information, such as physical exam findings or laboratory data. No matter the type of data collected, it is crucial that researchers develop a specific definition of the attribute of interest and make a concerted effort to ascertain complete data for all cases within their sample.

Analysis

The primary goal of most cross-sectional studies is to estimate the prevalence of a factor (e.g., a disease, exposure, outcome, or some other characteristic) in a population. Prevalence is calculated by dividing the number of individuals with the factor of interest by the total number of individuals in the sample. Figure 10.3 presents this calculation using a 2-by-2 table. In Figure 10.3, the prevalence of the outcome in the entire sample would be calculated as $(a + c)/(a + b + c + d)$. Prevalence can also be calculated independently for those with different exposures. By dividing the prevalence in exposed individuals (e.g., the prevalence of lung cancer among smokers), by the prevalence in unexposed individuals (e.g., lung cancer in nonsmokers), one can calculate the ***prevalence ratio***. In Figure 10.3, the prevalence ratio is calculated as $(a/(a + b))/(c/(c + d))$. In contrast, the ***risk ratio*** (which is calculated identically) refers to the ratio of the probability of an incident condition or outcome in exposed and unexposed groups.

In addition, cross-sectional studies can simultaneously collect data about potential associated factors, and can be used to calculate an ***odds ratio***. In Figure 10.3, the odds ratio is calculated as (ad)/(bc). While the prevalence ratio is a useful measure of association in some situations—such as conditions in which exposure status does not affect prognosis—it is reported much less often in cross-sectional studies than the odds ratio (3). The odds ratio allows researchers to directly compare associations measured in different types of outcomes research studies.

As an example, consider the cross-sectional study of depression among cancer patients as reported by Walker and colleagues, described in the following (4). The total prevalence of clinical depression in this sample was 13.4% ((327 + 238)/(327 + 1717 + 238 + 1927)). Prevalence was 16.0% among females (327/(327 + 1727)) and 11.0% among males (238/(238 + 1927)). The estimated prevalence ratio of depression in women to men was 1.46 (16.0%/11.0%) and the odds ratio was 1.54 ((327/1727)/(238/1927)).

	Has outcome	Does not have outcome
Exposed	a	b
Unexposed	c	d

Prevalence in exposed (P_e)= a/(a + b)

Prevalence in unexposed (P_u)= c/(c + d)

Prevalence ratio (PR) = P_e/P_u

Odds ratio (OR) = ad/bc

FIGURE 10.3 Calculation of prevalence, prevalence ratio, and odds ratio in a cross-sectional study.

Advantages and Disadvantages

Cross-sectional studies are useful for describing the general outcomes and exposures in large populations, and they provide researchers an understanding of the health needs of society. Many studies utilize routinely collected data from established patient panels, so such studies are inexpensive and easy to perform. However, cross-sectional studies have a number of important limitations. First, samples are often selected from the target population without regard to an individual's exposure or outcome status, making it difficult to analyze rare attributes. Additionally, cross-sectional studies are typically conducted at a single time point and thus do not probe the time course between exposures and outcomes. Therefore, it can be challenging to establish a cause-and-effect relationship between the exposure and outcome.

Furthermore, cross-sectional studies may be affected by a number of measurable and unmeasurable forms of biases, such as ***selection bias, recall bias, response bias, observer bias,*** and ***misclassification bias***. For example, phone surveys may be less likely to reach individuals who work, and web-based surveys may be less likely to reach those without Internet access, leading to selection of samples that are not representative of the target population (i.e., selection bias) (5). Response bias is another problem, particularly with surveys, where the nature of questioning or conditions of the study (e.g., social pressures) elicits misleading data from subjects. Misclassification bias refers to errors in measurement (e.g., inability to accurately ascribe cause of death), especially when it is imbalanced between groups being compared. Other forms of bias are discussed later in this chapter and in Chapters 2 and 18.

Furthermore, prevalence may itself be a misleading indicator of disease. At any given point in time, diseases with a short natural history are less likely to be ascertained in a cross-sectional study. Patients with the most severe form of a disease with poor prognosis (e.g., stage IV cancer) may be less likely to be captured by a cross-sectional survey, compared to patients with milder forms of the disease. Therefore, prevalent cases identified in these studies may not accurately reflect the true spectrum of a disease.

Example

With improvements in disease detection and treatment, cancer patients are living longer (6), and there is increasing focus on comorbidities that disproportionately affect cancer patients. For example, Walker and colleagues conducted a study to better understand prevalence and covariates of depression in the cancer population (4). Defining their target population as patients with any of the most common cancers (breast, genitourinary, lung, colorectal, or gynecologic) living in the United Kingdom, the researchers identified a sample of 21,151 patients who received treatment at any of three outpatient cancer care centers in Scotland over a 3-year period. Among this cohort, 83% of all patients had undergone routine depression screening, and diagnoses of clinical depression were prevalent in 13.1% of patients with lung cancer, 10.9% with gynecologic cancer, 9.3% with breast cancer, 7.0% with colorectal cancer, and 5.6% with genitourinary cancer (4). Among those with lung cancer, depression was associated with female sex (odds ratio: 1.54, $p < .0001$) and younger age (odds ratio for patients < 50 years compared to those between 50 and 59 years: 1.41, $p < .0001$).

This study employed a large-scale, hospital-based, cross-sectional design to determine the prevalence of depression among patients with specific types of cancer. By shedding light on the population-level burden of depression among cancer patients, this study could be used to inform future experimental studies aimed at improving mental healthcare in cancer patients.

CASE–CONTROL STUDIES

PURPOSE

Case–control studies allow investigators to quickly assess a wide range of potential etiological factors of disease or results of healthcare interventions. Case–control studies enroll "cases"—individuals with a particular outcome of interest—and match them to "controls"—similar but unaffected individuals, and evaluate the association between the outcome and preceding exposures or treatments.

DESIGN

Case–control studies can be used to test a range of different hypotheses. For instance, in exploratory case–control studies, researchers with little insight as to potential etiological factors can investigate a vast number of different exposures. In more focused case–control studies, investigators can test the association between an outcome and exposure to a particular agent.

Once a hypothesis is developed, individuals known to have the outcome of interest (most commonly a disease or disease outcome) are selected as "cases." Cases can be drawn from different sources, including hospital registries and the general population.

Researchers must then find "controls"—individuals who meet the same eligibility criteria as cases, but who are unaffected by the outcome of interest. The selection of appropriate controls is crucially important. Ideally, population-based controls should be selected at random from the same population represented by the cases (e.g., students at a particular school or the general population of a region or nation).

Controls for case–control studies can either be matched or unmatched. In *unmatched* case–control studies, controls are enrolled without regarding the number or characteristics of the cases, and the number of cases does not necessarily equal the number of controls. Stratified analyses or logistic regression models can then be used to control for potential confounders. In matched case–control studies, controls are matched based on potential confounding factors (e.g., age, sex, race). It is important to avoid matching based on the exposure being investigated, as this would diminish the association between exposure and disease, a phenomenon known as *overmatching*. Finally, the exposure status of all cases and controls must be evaluated and compared. Figure 10.4 depicts the general design of case–control studies.

Nested case–control studies are a special type of case–control study in which all cases and controls are selected from a cohort study. Just like a standard case–control study, researchers compare

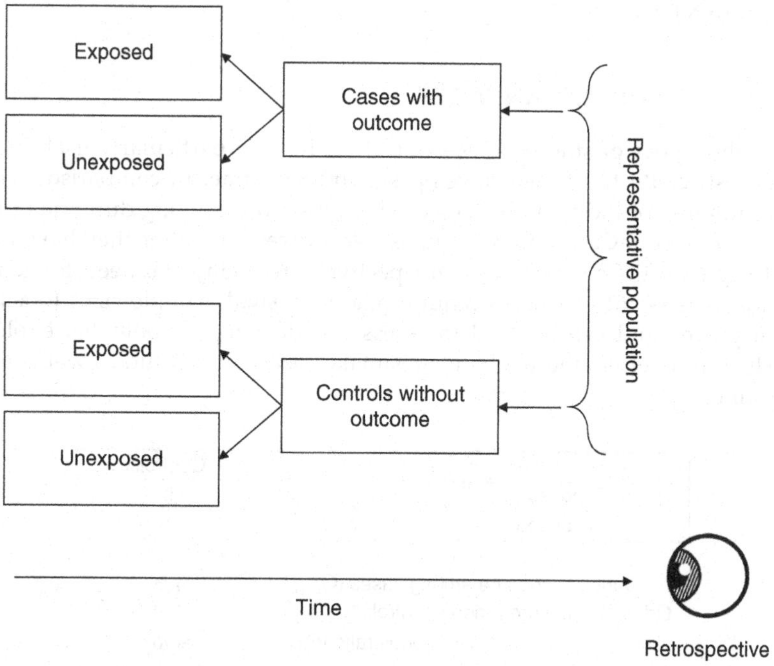

FIGURE 10.4 Outline of case–control studies.

the exposures between individuals who developed an outcome and individuals who did not. However, in these studies, the exposure status of all individuals was known prior to the development of the outcome, and researchers can infer causality between the exposure and outcome.

ANALYSIS

In case–control studies, cases are selected by their outcome status. Contrast this with cohort studies (next section), in which study participants are selected on the basis of their exposures or interventions. Cohorts are evaluated over time to determine the number of participants who develop an outcome, allowing researchers to calculate the incidence and ***relative risk*** of an outcome based on exposure status. Case–control studies reveal how much more (or less) likely an exposure or intervention is found among cases compared to controls, by measuring the odds ratio. Figure 10.5 presents a 2-by-2 table that can be helpful for organizing the results of a case–control study, along with the calculation of an odds ratio. Because cases are selected on their outcome rather than exposure status, the prevalence ratio (or risk ratio) cannot be known (i.e., $a/(a + b)$ is not a valid measure of the prevalence in case–control studies); therefore, the odds ratio is used. However, when controls are selected from a population at risk of developing the outcome, and the prevalence of the outcome is low (as is often the case with cancer diagnoses) the odds ratio approximates the relative risk (7). This so-called "rare disease assumption" increases the utility of case–control studies, by allowing them to estimate the relative risk, a measure of how much more likely a disease is to occur among exposed individuals.

As an example, a population-based case–control study in Denmark and Sweden enrolled 3,055 patients with non-Hodgkin lymphoma (NHL)—the cases—and 3,187 similar but disease-free individuals—the controls (8). Eight of the cases had been previously diagnosed with systemic lupus erythematosus (SLE—an exposure of interest), whereas only two control subjects had SLE. Among patients with NHL, the odds of being exposed to SLE were approximately 1 in 381, or 0.26% ($a = 8$, $c = 3047$, $a \div c = 0.0026$). Control subjects had the odds of being exposed to SLE of roughly 1 in 1,593, or 0.06% ($b = 2$, $d = 3185$, $b \div d = 0.0006$). Therefore, this study calculated an unadjusted odds ratio of SLE among patients with NHL to be 4.2 ($ad \div bc = 4.2$). Stated another way, patients with NHL were 4.2 times more likely to have been previously diagnosed with SLE than those without NHL (8).

ADVANTAGES AND DISADVANTAGES

Compared to other types of studies, case–control studies are particularly useful for evaluating rare outcomes, especially those that develop slowly over time. In comparison, cohort studies require a large number of individuals at risk to be followed for a long duration of time, a costly and complex proposition. Case–control studies select cases only after they have developed the outcome and evaluate their exposures retrospectively, reducing the need for lengthy follow-up. Furthermore, case–control studies require relatively small sample sizes to achieve reasonable statistical power, and can be used to assess a wide range of potential etiological factors simultaneously. Put together, these advantages make case–control studies well-suited for rapid hypothesis testing.

	Cases	Controls
Exposed	a	b
Unexposed	c	d

Odds of exposure among cases (O_{case}) = a/c

Odds of exposure among controls ($O_{control}$) = b/d

Odds ratio (OR) = ad/bc

FIGURE 10.5 Calculation of an odds ratio in a case–control study.

However, researchers must carefully interpret the results of case–control studies. Because cases and controls are arbitrarily selected from a larger population, the results are subject to multiple sources of bias, including selection bias, recall bias, and observer/interviewer bias. Furthermore, specific individuals included in a case–control study may not be representative of a wider population in terms of demographics, exposures, selective behaviors, propensity to participate, or a host of other factors. This can limit the generalizability of results to the overall or other populations. For example, hospital-based patients may have different exposures than the population at large, and these exposures may simultaneously influence multiple diseases, because tobacco smoking may be more common in hospitalized patients, and is associated with cardiac disease, stroke, and certain psychiatric disorders, in addition to lung cancer.

Additionally, when exposures are assessed through patient interviews or other qualitative measures, recall bias may reduce the validity of an apparent association. Furthermore, individuals with a disease may be more or less likely to remember certain exposures than their disease-free counterparts, and qualitative responses should be carefully analyzed and prospectively defined to minimize recall and interviewer bias.

EXAMPLE

Vaginal cancer is a rare disease occurring most commonly in older women. However, by 1970, physicians in Boston, Massachusetts, had diagnosed an unusual number of young women with vaginal clear cell adenocarcinoma in a 4-year period. A review of the cases failed to uncover any obvious etiological explanations, so Arthur L. Herbst and his colleagues initiated a case–control study to identify factors associated with the development of clear cell adenocarcinoma (9).

Each woman diagnosed with vaginal cancer was matched with four controls. Control patients were born at the same hospital within 5 days of their matched case. In total, the study identified 8 cases and 32 matched controls. Researchers examined medical records and inquired about a broad range of potential exposures. The study found that 7 of the cases and 0 of the controls were exposed to diethylstilbestrol (DES), and concluded that there was a "highly significant association between the treatment of mothers with estrogen diethylstilbestrol during pregnancy and the subsequent development of adenocarcinoma of the vagina in their daughters ($p < .00001$)" (10). After the results of this case–control study were published in the *New England Journal of Medicine*, the Food and Drug Administration (FDA) quickly moved to label pregnancy as a contraindication for DES therapy, later banning the drug outright in 1975. Though the strong association between DES exposure and vaginal cancers allowed conclusions to be made from only seven cases, in general, larger sample sizes are necessary.

In contrast, multiple forms of bias can plague and undermine inferences from case–control studies. For example, in 1981, Macdonald and colleagues reported a significant association between increased coffee consumption and the occurrence of pancreatic cancer in the *New England Journal of Medicine* (11). This putative link has not been confirmed subsequently in repeated investigations and meta-analyses of cohort studies (12,13). One problem is that patients may overestimate their exposure to a particular agent under study (regardless of whether the agent is truly carcinogenic) once they receive a cancer diagnosis (i.e., recall bias). Another is that investigators (and editors) are encouraged to report alarming but unexpected associations without subjecting them to higher standards of scientific rigor (i.e., observer bias) (14). Particular attention to such issues is recommended when designing and evaluating such studies.

COHORT STUDIES

PURPOSE

First coined by the epidemiologist W.H. Frost in 1935, a *cohort* is a group of people defined by a certain characteristic (15). The goal of a cohort study is to assess the relationship between a specific exposure or intervention and an outcome of interest. By following individuals over time, and observing the number who develop an outcome, cohort studies can be used to estimate the incidence of an outcome and to measure the strength of association between an exposure or intervention and an outcome.

DESIGN

Cohort studies begin with the selection of an appropriate sample of patients: the cohort. This sample should be representative of the population of interest and may come from a broad community (e.g., the general adult population in the United States) or from smaller groups of individuals felt to be at high risk of developing a particular outcome (e.g., heavy smokers). It is important to include only those participants who have not yet experienced the outcome of interest at the time of exposure. Otherwise, the temporal link between exposure and outcome would be broken.

Individuals in the cohort are evaluated for their exposure to a particular risk factor or intervention at baseline (e.g., chemotherapy), as well as whether they develop the outcome of interest (e.g., death from cancer) during follow-up. Cohort studies can be conducted in a prospective or retrospective manner. In prospective cohort studies, participants are enrolled before the outcome of interest has occurred. Participants are followed over time, and information about exposures and outcomes is periodically reassessed. The Framingham Heart Study and Nurses' Health Study are examples of prospective cohort studies (16,17).

Retrospective cohort studies utilize previously collected data in which the outcome of interest has typically already occurred. Investigators look backward in time at suspected risk factors or exposures that are related to the outcome. For example, many retrospective cohort studies in cancer patients are performed using data from the Surveillance, Epidemiology, and End Results (SEER) Program and National Cancer Database (NCDB). Figure 10.6 briefly reviews the design of cohort studies.

ANALYSIS

Incidence, defined as the frequency with which an outcome occurs, can be directly measured from cohort studies. An ***incidence rate*** divides the number of new cases by the number of people at risk

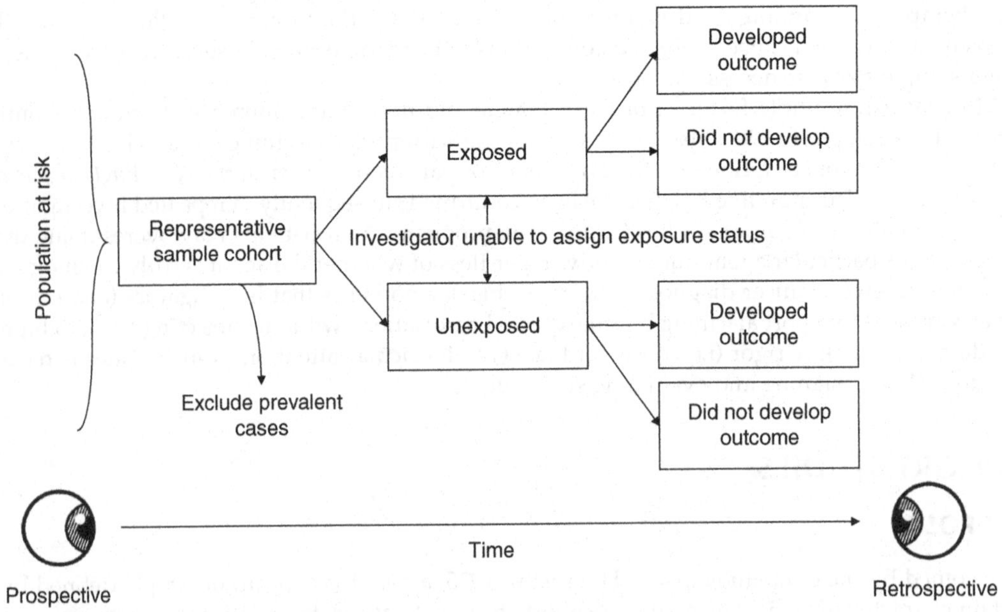

FIGURE 10.6 Outline of a cohort study.

	Developed outcome	Did not develop outcome
Exposed	a	b
Unexposed	c	d

Risk in exposed (R_e) = a/(a+b)

Risk in unexposed (R_u) = c/(c+d)

Relative risk (RR) = R_e/R_u

FIGURE 10.7 Analysis of risks among exposed and unexposed individuals in a cohort study.

in a given time frame. For instance, if 10 cases of prostate cancer were observed among a cohort in a single year, then the incidence of the disease is 10. If 1,000 men were included in the cohort, and all were followed throughout the entire year, then the incidence rate would be 1% per year (10 cases ÷ 1,000 people at risk).

The incidence rate of the outcome of interest can be determined for both exposed and unexposed individuals. Relative risk, a measure of how much more (or less) an outcome is likely to occur in exposed versus unexposed individuals, is calculated by dividing the incidence rates of the two groups. Figure 10.7 presents the now familiar 2-by-2 table for organizing the outcomes of a cohort and calculating the relative risk.

As an example of these calculations, consider the prospective cohort study described by Cheraghi and colleagues (18) that characterized the likelihood of developing sensorineural hearing loss within 6 months after the receipt of head and neck radiotherapy, with or without concomitant cisplatin-based chemotherapy. Among 20 patients exposed to radiation alone, 8 developed hearing loss, corresponding to an incidence of 40% (a = 8, a + b = 20, a ÷ (a + b) = 8 ÷ 20 = 40%). Meanwhile, among 9 patients exposed to radiation and chemotherapy, 7 developed hearing loss, indicating an incidence of 78% (7 ÷ 9 = 78%). For patients exposed to chemotherapy in addition to radiation, the relative risk of developing hearing loss was 1.9 (77% ÷ 40%). Of note, all 29 patients included in the cohort study were followed for the duration of the study.

In many cases, it is most useful to calculate incidence in terms of person-years at risk. If an individual remains in the study for a single year, then he or she would represent 1 person-year at risk, whereas another individual, remaining in the cohort for 10 years, would represent 10 person-years. Summing up the person-years contributed by all participants in a given group provides the denominator when calculating risk.

ADVANTAGES AND DISADVANTAGES

Cohorts are especially useful for analyzing rare exposures. Researchers select participants based on their exposure status and can thus create cohorts enriched for rare exposures. For instance, when assessing the association between asbestos exposure and lung cancer, one might consider analyzing a cohort of workers in asbestos manufacturing plants (19).

Another useful feature of cohort studies is their ability to simultaneously assess a number of different outcomes. By cataloging the various diseases that develop within a cohort, these studies can paint a more complete picture of the deleterious effects of an exposure. In addition to lung cancer, individuals in the asbestos manufacturing cohort were also found to have an increased risk of hypertensive cardiovascular disease and kidney cancer (20).

In contrast to cross-sectional studies, cohort studies can identify that an exposure preceded an outcome—information that can be used to help suggest causality. Though powerful, the quality of evidence provided by cohort studies is most often limited by confounding. Because researchers are unable to manually assign the exposure status to each participant (as they can in randomized controlled studies), those who are exposed to a risk factor may differ in important ways from their unexposed counterparts. Many factors—both measured and unmeasured—may correlate with the exposure, and these factors may in turn affect the outcome.

This problem—namely, selection bias—is perhaps the most critical limitation of cohort studies. Though many statistical methods have been developed to parse out the effects of confounders (see Chapters 12 and 13 for a more in-depth treatment of such techniques), cohort studies are unable to provide data as robust as randomized controlled studies (described in the next section and Chapter 21). However, cohort studies often require less up-front investment and can be performed more cheaply and easily. Furthermore, cohort studies may include more diverse populations and allow investigators to evaluate results of interventions under real-world conditions, compared to randomized studies. Additionally, cohort studies can be used to test exposures that may not be feasible or ethical to test in a randomized controlled study (e.g., effect of poverty on cancer outcomes).

EXAMPLE

One of the first prospective cohort studies published in the medical literature served to link tobacco smoking to lung cancer mortality. Published in 1954 by Richard Doll and A. Bradford Hill, two medical statisticians from the United Kingdom, the study surveyed British physicians about their smoking habits and followed them over time to assess their risk of lung cancer (21).

Among 10,017 male respondents older than 35 years of age, researchers found a heavy burden of smoking at baseline (only 12.7% of participants were nonsmokers). Over a 29-month follow-up period, 789 participants died, with 36 deaths attributed to lung cancer. Notably, all of the lung cancer deaths occurred among tobacco smokers. Doll and Hill then calculated an age-standardized rate of death for lung cancer, and found that it increased sharply with increasing tobacco use, from 0 per 1,000 person-years among nonsmokers to 1.14 per 1,000 person-years in men who smoked more than 25 grams of tobacco per day ($p < .001$).

Citing Doll and Hill's work, as well as several other large prospective cohorts, the 1964 *United States Surgeon General's Report on Smoking and Health* concluded, for the first time, that the harmful effects of tobacco smoking were incontrovertible. This report catalyzed sweeping changes in tobacco policy in the United States and is widely credited for its role in curbing smoking rates in the country (22).

RANDOMIZED CONTROLLED STUDIES

PURPOSE

Randomized controlled studies are considered the gold standard for generating evidence for confirming or rejecting a hypothesis. In these studies, participants are randomly assigned to a particular intervention. Through the randomization process, potential sources of bias are diminished and the connection between an intervention and outcome is isolated.

DESIGN

Researchers must first carefully outline the objectives of their randomized controlled study and define the target population, intervention, controls, and outcomes of interest. Interventions are the new behaviors, medications, or surgical procedures that investigators hypothesize may improve outcomes in their cohort. Controls represent the scenario to which the intervention is being compared. If a disease already has an established treatment, participants in the control group can receive this "standard of care." Outcomes can include either a sought-after end point—such as survival—or an intermediate response that is predicted to correlate with an end point—for instance, a reduction in tumor burden, or an improvement in functional status.

Once the objective of the study is laid out, researchers must identify a sample of individuals within which to conduct their study—the so-called study population. The study population should be ***generalizable*** to the target population in terms of demographics, behaviors, and clinical factors. It should also consist of individuals who are at risk for the outcome of interest and can be closely monitored. Researchers must establish eligibility criteria, specifying who from the study population to include in their experiment. The purpose of these criteria is to exclude individuals who are unable to provide informed consent, are likely to be harmed in the trial, or pose serious complications for data analysis (23). Once ineligible individuals are excluded, potential participants are approached to provide informed consent. Researchers must provide information about the purpose of the study, how it will be conducted, and the potential risks that each person might face.

Figure 10.8 depicts the general design of randomized controlled studies. In a classic dual-arm 1:1 randomized trial, the final study population—which includes all eligible and willing participants—are then randomized in equal numbers into intervention and control groups. Occasionally trials may consist of three or more arms (including 2 × 2 designs to test interactions between two interventions), or may involve unbalanced randomizations (such as 1:2 or other ratios). Randomization eliminates selection bias and typically (though not always) creates groups that are similar across both measured and, presumably, unmeasured risk factors. This last quality is of the utmost importance. As discussed further in Chapter 21, patients can be stratified by particularly important risk factors in the randomization process to further ensure that these characteristics are balanced between the intervention and control groups. After randomization, individuals are exposed to their assigned intervention or control, and followed prospectively to assess for the outcomes of interest.

To reduce the risk of measurement bias, participants and researchers should be unable to determine which individuals have been assigned to each group. A single-blind study is one in which participants do not know which group they belong to. In double-blind studies, neither the participants nor the researchers are aware of group assignments. Triple-blind studies further blind those performing ongoing monitoring and data analysis. Methods of blinding include the administration of placebos or sham procedures and the use of coded patient identifiers. In some instances, it may not be feasible to blind the study (e.g., when the intervention is highly effective or readily observable, like a mastectomy), and researchers should consider the potential role of bias in their interpretation. In settings where blinding is infeasible, it is particularly important to

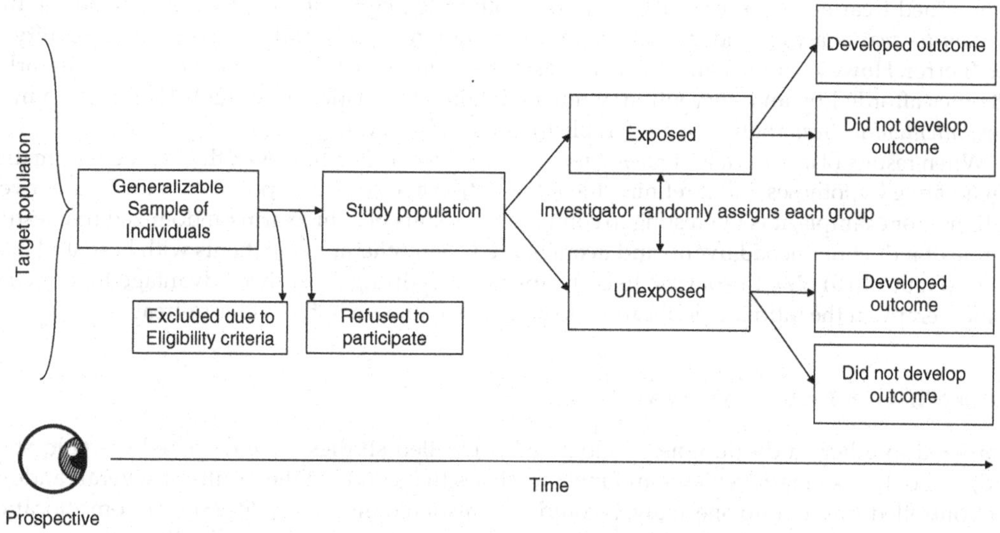

FIGURE 10.8 Outline of randomized controlled studies.

ensure that the relevant end point(s) are rigorously defined, and preferably both quantitative and unambiguous (such as mortality from any cause).

When investigating cancer therapies, the ultimate goal of many clinical trials is to increase the life span or quality of life of patients with cancer. However, due to constraints in the budget and time frame for clinical trials, it is not always feasible to analyze overall survival as a primary end point (24). Alternatively, many trials define clinically meaningful "intermediate" or "surrogate" outcomes, which are correlated with overall survival but occur earlier and more frequently, thus enabling conclusions to be reached sooner with lower costs (25). These issues are discussed further in Chapters 16 and 21. Common outcomes investigated in oncological randomized controlled trials include tumor response (typically assessed by radiology or symptom scales), progression-free survival (duration of time the patient survives after treatment without disease progression), treatment-related toxicity or other adverse events, and patient-reported outcomes (PROs), which are discussed in Chapter 22.

ANALYSIS

Randomized studies are analyzed similarly to cohort studies to assess a particular outcome. In general, the process of randomization balances potential confounders between the study groups, reducing the need to control for selection bias, compared to nonrandomized study designs. As described earlier, in a classic dual-arm randomized trial, researchers randomly allocate each individual in the study population to either an intervention or a control group. However, allocation alone does not ensure exposure. Individuals assigned to the intervention may not be fully compliant with the therapy, while those in the control group may seek the intervention outside the purview of the study. To account for these scenarios, there are two main ways in which randomized controlled trials can be analyzed: ***as treated*** and ***intention to treat***. These topics are addressed in greater detail in Chapter 26.

In *as-treated* analysis, individuals are analyzed according to their actual exposure status. Members of either group who did not comply with treatment or were lost to follow-up prior to initiating treatment are typically removed from the analysis. This method excludes many individuals who are almost certainly different from those who complied with the study. As such, while this method infers the effect of complete exposure to the intervention, it is susceptible to significant bias, and is typically utilized for sensitivity analysis to compare with *intention-to-treat* results.

Intention-to-treat analysis, in contrast, analyzes the outcomes of all people based on the group to which they were allocated. This method does not discern between those who remained on the assigned treatment, nor does it take into account the degree of compliance. Some argue that *intention-to-treat* analysis underestimates an intervention's effect and increases susceptibility to type II error. However, this method also represents a more realistic assessment of the "real-world" outcomes afforded by an intervention, while maintaining statistical rigor (26). Therefore, in most cases, *intention-to-treat* analysis is preferable to *as-treated* analysis.

When results of *as-treated* and *intention-to-treat* analyses differ, however, this can be informative in generating hypotheses about refining the intervention and/or study population for future investigations. For example, it is interesting to compare the results of a three-arm randomized trial testing the role of induction (neoadjuvant) and taxane-based chemotherapy in patients with head and neck cancer (Figure 10.9) (27). In contrast to early abstracts reporting a survival advantage to induction chemotherapy, in the ultimate publication no benefit was shown in the intent-to-treat analysis.

ADVANTAGES AND DISADVANTAGES

Compared to other study designs, randomized controlled studies are considered the gold standard, and only systematic reviews and meta-analyses that combine the results of several randomized controlled studies into one analysis could be considered more reliable (28). Random allocation of participants reduces selection bias and ensures that potential confounding factors are evenly

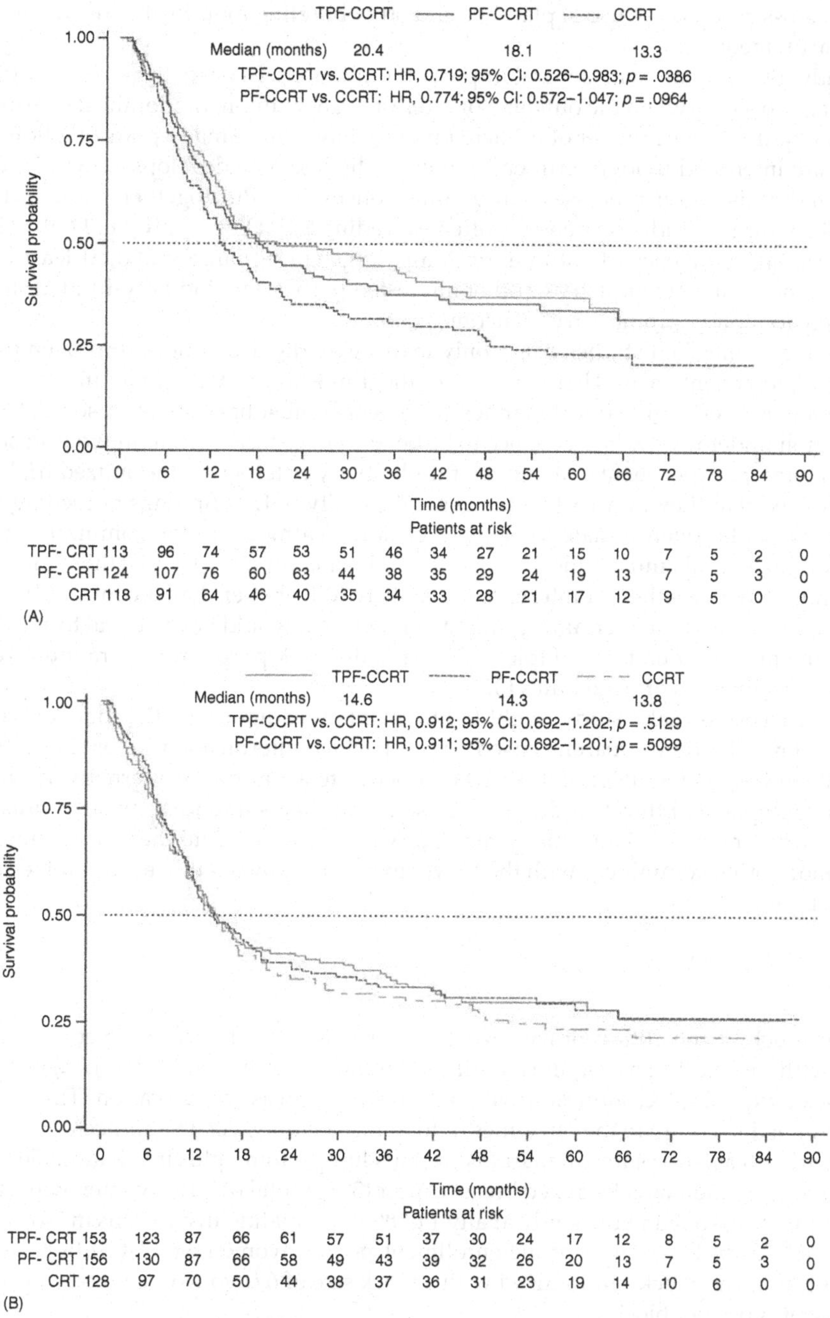

FIGURE 10.9 Comparison of as-treated (top) versus intention-to-treat (bottom) results from the randomized trial by Hitt et al. While patients treated with induction chemotherapy (TPF-CCRT and PF-CCRT) had better progression-free survival compared to patients treated with chemoradiotherapy only (CCRT), there was no significant difference in outcomes when data were analyzed based on the arm to which they were randomly assigned.

CI, confidence interval; HR, hazard ratio.

Source: Hitt R, Grau JJ, López-Pousa A, et al. A randomized phase III trial comparing induction chemotherapy followed by chemoradiotherapy versus chemoradiotherapy alone as treatment of unresectable head and neck cancer. *Ann Oncol*. 2013;25(1):216–225. doi:10.1093/annonc/mdt461

distributed across groups. The use of placebos and other blinding tools further decreases the likelihood of measurement bias.

These advantages come with several important limitations. In order to generate sufficient statistical power, especially when the outcome of interest is uncommon, randomized controlled studies typically require a large number of participants and may require many years of follow-up when researchers are interested in long-term end points or the outcome develops slowly. Additionally, regulatory and registration processes can be time-consuming. Put together, these factors make randomized controlled studies expensive, often exceeding $6,000 per individual (29). Along with this high price tag come conflicts of interest. Many large studies are funded, at least in part, by companies in the healthcare industry or other interested parties, and industry-funded studies may be more likely to report "proindustry" outcomes (30).

Randomized controlled studies commonly investigate the use of new, unproven treatments, which can lead to patient harm. Therefore, it is of the utmost importance that randomized studies be conducted in a careful and ethical manner. Researchers must have some reason to believe that the intervention under review has a chance to be beneficial, typically from previous observational studies or laboratory experiments. Moreover, the eligibility criteria for randomized trials are often so tightly defined that they may distort the generalizability of trial findings to the target population, and in particular overestimate the benefit of new treatments in the community writ large. Finally, randomized trials must adhere to the principle of equipoise. That is, there must be genuine uncertainty about whether an intervention is likely to be better than a control (31). If there is already wide consensus that a certain treatment is superior, it would be unethical to administer the inferior treatment. Consider, for example, the tongue-in-cheek proposal for a randomized trial to compare the effectiveness of parachutes (32).

Another concern is that a study might fail to maintain equipoise by the time it is completed. For instance, it may become apparent, based on prespecified interim analyses or results from other randomized studies, that an intervention is far superior to a control, or alternatively, that its side effects are unacceptable. Ethical studies require some mechanism to identify such situations and to intervene when required. Thus, many regulatory agencies mandate the establishment of data and safety monitoring committees with the power to periodically review results and terminate the study early, if needed.

EXAMPLE

Throughout much of the 20th century, breast cancer was treated with mastectomy, which was associated with morbidity and significant effects on quality of life and body image. Thus, there was interest in more limited surgeries that could result in breast conservation. The NSABP B-06 trial was designed to compare the outcomes of total mastectomy, versus lumpectomy (removal of the tumor with disease-free surgical margins), versus lumpectomy plus irradiation (50 Gy in 2 Gy fractions) among women with localized breast cancer (33). A total of 2,163 women with stage I or II breast cancer were enrolled in the study at any 1 of 89 participating institutions in North America, between 1976 and 1984. For most of the enrollment period, women were stratified by their presenting institution and block-randomized with a block size of 6 (two women receiving each of the three treatment types per block).

After 20 years of follow-up, in an *intention-to-treat* analysis (specified a priori by the study protocol), there were no differences in overall survival among the three groups ($p = .57$). Among women treated with total mastectomy, lumpectomy alone, and lumpectomy plus irradiation, 20-year survival was 47%, 46%, and 46%, respectively. In an *as-treated* analysis of women undergoing lumpectomy (excluding those who were converted to a total mastectomy alone), irradiation was found to significantly decrease the rate of local cancer recurrence (39.2% recurrence vs. 14.3%, $p < .001$). This effect was evident in women with cancer in their axillary lymph nodes (44.2% recurrence vs. 8.8%, $p < .001$), as well as those with cancer-free nodes (36.2% recurrence vs. 17.0%, $p < .001$) (34).

The results of NSABP B-06 suggested that breast-conserving therapy, with lumpectomy and irradiation, was a reasonable treatment option for women with localized breast cancer. Rather than putting all women through the morbidity of a mastectomy, surgeons and radiation oncologists could confidently individualize treatment for their patients, maximizing both survival and quality of life. More examples of clinical trials and their analyses are considered in Section IV.

CONCLUSION

Put together, the studies that comprise population and outcomes research provide a framework for rapid hypothesis generation and rigorous statistical testing. Descriptive studies can define the distribution of exposures and disease in a population, allowing researchers to construct specific cause-and-effect hypotheses. Case–control studies allow for an expeditious prioritization of these hypotheses, which can then be probed in more complex, yet more reliable cohort studies. Finally, randomized controlled studies allow researchers to intervene on an exposure and assess its isolated role in the outcome.

The outcomes of this approach can be readily appreciated in modern medicine. Consider the story of *Helicobacter pylori* and gastric adenocarcinoma. Descriptive studies in the 1970s showed that rates of gastric adenocarcinoma varied dramatically across different geographic regions. Then, in a cross-sectional study published in 1984, Marshall and Warren identified a heretofore unknown bacterium colonizing the stomachs of several patients with chronic gastritis—a known precursor of peptic ulcer disease and gastric adenocarcinoma (35). Subsequently, several case–control studies further revealed that patients with chronic gastritis and gastric adenocarcinoma were more likely to have *H. pylori* infection than healthy controls (36–38). Then, several nested case–control and cohort studies revealed that *H. pylori* exposure tended to precede the development of gastric cancer, strengthening the evidence of a causal relationship (39,40). Around the same time, researchers identified several antimicrobial regimens to effectively eradicate *H. pylori* infection (41). Most recently, several large-scale randomized controlled studies concluded that eliminating *H. pylori* led to a roughly 50% reduction in the risk of gastric cancer over a 15-year period (42). In this way, the use of carefully coordinated studies allowed researchers to uncover *H. pylori*'s causative role in stomach cancer and to develop a treatment, ultimately saving many lives.

GLOSSARY

case report: the smallest descriptive study, providing detailed information about a single patient.

case series: a type of descriptive study that compiles detailed accounts of several cases.

cross-sectional study: the most complex descriptive study design; characterizes a specific population at a given point in time.

population: a group of people.

prevalence: the total number of individuals with a particular characteristic or condition in a population.

incidence: new cases in a population over a given time.

sample: a defined segment of a population.

prevalence ratio: value arrived at by dividing the prevalence in exposed individuals by the prevalence in unexposed individuals.

risk ratio: a calculation that yields the ratio of the probability of an incident condition or outcome in exposed and unexposed groups.

odds ratio: calculation from cross-sectional study data that allows researchers to directly compare associations measured in different types of outcomes research studies.

selection bias: derives from selection of samples that are not representative of the target population.

recall bias: systematic error caused by differences in the accuracy of recall of past events by study participants.

response bias: skewing that arises when the nature of questioning or conditions of the study elicits misleading data from subjects.

observer bias: bias caused by tendency of researchers to see what they expect to see.

misclassification bias: skewing that arises from errors in measurement, especially when a measure is imbalanced between groups being compared.

relative risk: value calculated using data from cohort studies that reveal the number of participants who develop an outcome.

cohort: a group of people defined by a certain characteristic.

incidence rate: value regarding the frequency with which an outcome occurs; yielded by dividing the number of new cases by the number of people at risk in a given time frame.

generalizable: describes study data that are applicable to the target population in terms of demographics, behaviors, and clinical factors.

as treated: an analysis type applied to randomized controlled trials in which individuals are analyzed according to their actual exposure status.

intention to treat: an analysis type applied to randomized controlled trials that uses the outcomes of all people based on the group to which they were allocated.

REFERENCES

1. Clancy CM, Eisenber JM. Outcomes research: measuring the end results of healthcare. *Science*. 1998;282(5387):245–246. doi:10.1126/science.282.5387.245
2. National Center for Health Statistics. National Health and Nutrition Examination Survey: Overview. 2017. https://www.cdc.gov/nchs/nhanes/index.htm
3. Zocchetti C, Consonni D, Bertazzi PA. Relationship between prevalence rate ratios and odds ratios in cross-sectional studies. *Int J Epidemiology*. 1997;26(1):220–223. doi:10.1093/ije/26.1.220
4. Walker J, Hansen CH, Martin P, et al. Prevalence, associations, and adequacy of treatment of major depression in patients with cancer: a cross-sectional analysis of routinely collected clinical data. *Lancet Psych*. 2014;1(5):343–350. doi:10.1016/S2215-0366(14)70313-X
5. Szolnoki G, Hoffmann D. Online, face-to-face and telephone surveys—comparing different sampling methods in wine consumer research. *Wine Econ and Policy*. 2013;2(2):57–66. doi:10.1016/j.wep.2013.10.001
6. National Cancer Institute. 2016. SEER Cancer Statistics Review 1975-2015: Relative Survival Rates by Year of Diagnosis. https://seer.cancer.gov/csr/1975_2015/results_merged/topic_survival_by_year_dx.pdf
7. Cornfield J. A method of estimating comparative rates from clinical data. Applications to cancer of the lung, breast, and cervix. *JNCI*. 1951;6:1269–1275. doi:10.1093/jnci/11.6.1269
8. Smedby KE, Hjalgrim H, Askling J, et al. Autoimmune and chronic inflammatory disorders and risk of non-Hodgkin lymphoma by subtype. *JNCI*. 2006;98(1):51–60. doi:10.1093/jnci/djj004
9. Herbst AL, Scully RE. Adenocarcinoma of the vagina in adolescence: a report of 7 cases including 6 clear cell carcinomas (so called mesonephromas). *Cancer*. 1970;25:745–757. doi:10.1093/jnci/djj004
10. Herbst AL, Ulfelder H, Poskanzer DC. Adenocarcinoma of the vagina: association of maternal stilbestrol therapy with tumor appearance in young women. *N Engl J Med*. 1971;284(16):878–881. doi:10.1056/NEJM197104222841604
11. MacMahon B, Yen S, Trichopoulos D, et al. Coffee and cancer of the pancreas. *N Engl J Med*. 1981;304(11):630–633. doi:10.1056/nejm198103123041102
12. Hsieh CC, MacMahon B, Yen S, et al. Coffee and pancreatic cancer (Chapter 2). *N Engl J Med*. 1986;315(9):587–589. doi:10.1056/NEJM198608283150918

13. Turati F, Galeone C, Edefonti V, et al. A meta-analysis of coffee consumption and pancreatic cancer. *Ann Oncol.* 2012;23(2):311–318. doi:10.1093/annonc/mdr331
14. Feinstein AR, Horwitz RI, Spitzer WO, Battista RN. Coffee and pancreatic cancer. The problems of etiologic science and epidemiologic case-control research. *JAMA.* 198128;246(9):957–961. doi:10.1001/jama.1981.03320090019020
15. Comstock GW. Cohort analysis: W.H. Frost's contributions to the epidemiology of tuberculosis and chronic disease. *Soz Praventivmed.* 2001;46(1):7–12. doi:10.1007/bf01318793
16. Kannel WB. Fifty years of Framingham Study contributions to understanding hypertension. *J Hum Hypertens.* 2000;14(2):83–90. doi:10.1038/sj.jhh.1000949
17. Colditz GA, Hankinson SE. The nurses' health study: lifestyle and health among women. *Nat Rev Cancer.* 2005;5(5):388–396. doi:10.1038/nrc1608
18. Cheraghi S, Nikoofar P, Fandavi P, et al. Short-term cohort study on sensorineural hearing changes in head and neck radiotherapy. *Med Oncol.* 2015;32:200. doi:10.1007/s12032-015-0646-3
19. Enterline, PE, DeCoufle P, Henderson V. Mortality in relation to occupational exposure in the asbestos industry. *J Occup Med.* 1972;14:897–903.
20. Smith AH, Shearn VI, Wood R. Asbestos and kidney cancer: the evidence supports a causal association. *Am J Ind Med.* 1989;16(2):159–166. doi:10.1002/ajim.4700160207
21. Doll D, Hill AB. The mortality of doctors in relation to their smoking habits. *Br Med J.* 1954;1:1451–1455. doi:10.1136/bmj.1.4877.1451
22. Samet JM, Speizer FE. Sir Richard Doll, 1912–2005. *Am J Epidemiol.* 2006;164(1):95–100. doi:10.1093/aje/kwj210
23. Van Spall HGC, Toren A, Kiss A, et al. Eligibility criteria of randomized controlled trials published in high-impact general medical journals: a systematic sampling review. *JAMA.* 2007;297(11):1233–1240. doi:10.1001/jama.297.11.1233
24. Wilson MK, Karakasis K, Oza AM. Outcomes and endpoints in trials of cancer therapy: the past, present, and future. *Lancet Oncol.* 2014;16:e32–e42. doi:10.1016/S1470-2045(14)70375-4
25. Wilson MK, Collyar D, Chingos DT, et al. Outcomes and endpoints in cancer trials: bridging the divide. *Lancet Oncol.* 2015;16:e43–e52. doi:10.1016/S1470-2045(14)70380-8
26. Fergusson D, Aaron SD, Guyatt G, Hebert P. Post-randomisation exclusions: the intention to treat principle and excluding patients from analysis. *BMJ.* 2002;325:652–654. doi:10.1136/bmj.325.7365.652
27. Hitt R, Grau JJ, López-Pousa A, et al. A randomized phase III trial comparing induction chemotherapy followed by chemoradiotherapy versus chemoradiotherapy alone as treatment of unresectable head and neck cancer. *Ann Oncol.* 2013;25(1):216–225. doi:10.1093/annonc/mdt461
28. Murad MH, Asi N, Alsawas M, et al. New evidence pyramid. *Evid Based Med.* 2016;21:125–127. doi:10.1136/ebmed-2016-110401
29. Emanuel EJ, Schnipper LE, Kamin DY, et al. The costs of conducting clinical research. *JCO.* 2003;21(22):4145–4150. doi:10.1200/JCO.2003.08.156
30. Bhandari M, Busse JW, Jackowski D, et al. Association between industry funding and statistically significant pro-industry findings in medical and surgical randomized trials. *CMAJ.* 2004;170(4):477–480. https://www.ncbi.nlm.nih.gov/pmc/articles/PMC332713
31. Freedman B. Equipoise and the ethics of clinical research. *N Engl J Med.* 1987;317(3):141–145. doi:10.1056/NEJM198707163170304
32. Smith GC, Pell JP. Parachute use to prevent death and major trauma related to gravitational challenge: systematic review of randomised controlled trials. *BMJ.* 2003;327(7429):1459–1461. doi:10.1136/bmj.327.7429.1459
33. Fisher B, Bauer M, Margolese R, et al. Five-year results of a randomized clinical trial comparing total mastectomy and segmental mastectomy with or without radiation in the treatment of breast cancer. *N Engl J Med.* 1985;312(11):665–673. doi:10.1056/NEJM198503143121101
34. Fisher B, Anderson S, Bryant J, et al. Twenty-year follow-up of a randomized trial comparing total mastectomy, lumpectomy, and lumpectomy plus irradiation for the treatment of invasive breast cancer. *N Engl J Med.* 2002;347(16):1233–1241. doi: /10.1056/NEJMoa022152
35. Marshall BJ, Warren JR. Unidentified curved bacilli in the stomach of patient with gastritis and ulceration. *Lancet.* 1984;1(8390):1311–1315. https://doi.org/10.1016/S0140-6736(84)91816-6
36. Jaskiewicz K, Louwrens HD, Woodroof CW, et al. The association of *campylobacter pylori* with mucosal pathological changes in a population at risk for gastric cancer. *S Afr Med J.* 1989;75:417–419.
37. Correa P, Cuello C, Duque E, et al. Gastric precancerous process in a high-risk population: cohort follow-up. *Cancer Res.* 1990;50:4737–4740. http://cancerres.aacrjournals.org/content/50/15/4737.full-text.pdf
38. Talley NJ, Zinsmeister AR, DiMagno EP, et al. Gastric adenocarcinoma and *Helicobacter pylori* infection. *JNCI.* 1991;83(23):1734–1739. doi:10.1093/jnci/83.23.1734
39. Parsonnet J, Friedman GD, Vandersteen DP, et al. *Helicobacter pylori* infection and the risk of gastric carcinoma. *N Engl J Med.* 1991;365(16):1127–1131. doi:10.1056/nejm199110173251603
40. Wang RT, Wang T, Kun C, et al. *Helicobacter pylori* infection and gastric cancer: evidence from a retrospective cohort study and nested case-controls study in China. *World J Gastroenterol.* 2002;8(6):1103–1107. doi:10.3748/wjg.v8.i6.1103
41. McColl KEL. Clinical practice: *Helicobacter pylori* infection. *N Engl J Med.* 2010;362:1597–1604. doi:10.1056/nejmcp1001110
42. Lee YC, Chiang TH, Chou CK, et al. Association between *Helicobacter pylori* eradication and gastric cancer incidence: a systematic review and meta-analysis. *Gastroenterology.* 2016;150(5):1113–1124. doi:10.1053/j.gastro.2016.01.028

11

Basic Statistics for Clinical Cancer Research

LOREN K. MELL ■ HANJIE SHEN ■ BENJAMIN E. LEIBY

One of the most daunting challenges for cancer researchers at all levels is to master the statistical skills required to produce and evaluate high-quality science. Many trainees advance through degree programs without formal training in statistics or biostatistics, finding themselves at sea when it comes to navigating the technical aspects of data analysis. In particular, awareness of common analytical pitfalls is crucial to avoid disseminating erroneous or misleading information.

Consultation with a biostatistician early and often in the conduct of one's research is always advisable. However, this process is sometimes time-consuming and expensive, and many researchers are keen to draw their own conclusions about their data. Furthermore, many simple analyses are possible with an investment in learning some basic techniques. This knowledge also enables one to digest literature more rapidly and gives one a special appreciation for the strengths and limitations of different studies. Therefore, to the extent possible, we recommend becoming familiar with the fundamental concepts in statistics and data analysis, and collaborating with statisticians for more challenging and technical research endeavors.

This chapter gives a basic overview of fundamental concepts in biostatistics, methods for testing hypotheses and describing data, and considerations to be taken into account when applying specific statistical tests. In addition, as a reference guide, we provide a tabular summary of common statistical tests and the software commands that can be used to execute them. Last, we introduce and provide an overview of key modeling techniques that are described in more detail throughout the book. This foundation ideally will help in navigating the fundamentals of preclinical and human subjects research and clinical trials.

DESCRIBING DATA

RANDOM VARIABLES AND DISTRIBUTIONS

A **random variable** is a variable that can take on any numerical value generated by or representative of a random process. Random variables can be either **discrete** (i.e., taking on a value in a countable set) or **continuous** (i.e., taking on a value in an uncountable set). Examples of discrete random variables include the number of outpatient visits a patient makes, stage of cancer, and number of medical errors committed. Examples of continuous variables may include tumor size, prostate-specific antigen (PSA) and other blood tests, or length of time to tumor recurrence. Because many applications in clinical oncology treat random variables as continuous, our discussion primarily considers the continuous case, with emphasis on the discrete cases whenever appropriate.

A **population** refers to the set of individuals from which a random variable (or set of variables) could be drawn. A **sample** refers to the set of individuals from which the random variable(s) are actually drawn. In most situations, researchers are dealing with samples that are assumed to have been drawn at random from the population. Deviations from this assumption can affect the validity of one's inferences about the data, so it is important to be aware of the provenance of one's sample. In particular, a critical first step in describing data is to clearly define both the population and the methods used to collect the sample (i.e., sampling methods).

A **distribution** refers to the set of frequencies of each possible value of a random variable. Often this is displayed graphically using a **histogram**, to plot either a discrete (Figure 11.1A) or continuous (Figure 11.1B) variable. When the frequencies are cumulated with increasing values of the random variable, the result is a **cumulative distribution** (Figure 11.1C).

A probability distribution or **probability density function (pdf)** for a random variable x refers to a distribution in which the frequencies correspond to the relative likelihood of observing each possible value of x. A corresponding probability function for discrete distributions is termed the **probability mass function (pmf)**. For a pdf, the *probability* of a value lying on the interval [a,b] refers to the area under the pdf:

$$P(a \le x \le b) = \int_a^b f(x)\,dx$$

Examples of widely used pdfs in clinical cancer research are the **normal**, chi-square, and **Student's *t*-distribution**. These are described later in the chapter. A characteristic of pdfs is that the sum of the individual probabilities over the entire domain of x (i.e., integral) is 1.

Several basic measures are used to describe a distribution. These include measures of central tendency (e.g., **mean, median, mode**), measures of dispersion (e.g., **variance**, standard deviation, range), and **skew**. The mean, variance, and skew are considered the first, second, and third **moments** of a distribution. The fourth moment is called the kurtosis, which indicates the "fatness" or "thinness" of the distribution (Figure 11.2).

A mode for a continuous distribution $f(x)$ is defined as a value of x where $f(x)$ is (locally) maximized. A distribution may therefore have more than one mode. For a discrete distribution, the mode is the value of x with the largest frequency; this might not be unique. The median of a distribution is the value $x = M$ such that

$$\int_{-\infty}^{M} f(x)dx = \int_{M}^{\infty} f(x)dx = 0.5$$

For a continuous distribution, this value is unique. For a discrete distribution, the median could fall between two values of x that satisfy these criteria; in this case, the median is uniquely defined as the average of the two values.

The mean (μ)—also known as average or **expected value,** $E(x)$—of a discrete random variable x is the sum of its values divided by the sample size (n):

$$\mu = E(x) = \Sigma\,(x_i/n)$$

whereas for a continuous distribution f(x), the mean is defined as

$$\mu = E(x) = \int_{-\infty}^{\infty} x\,f(x)\,dx$$

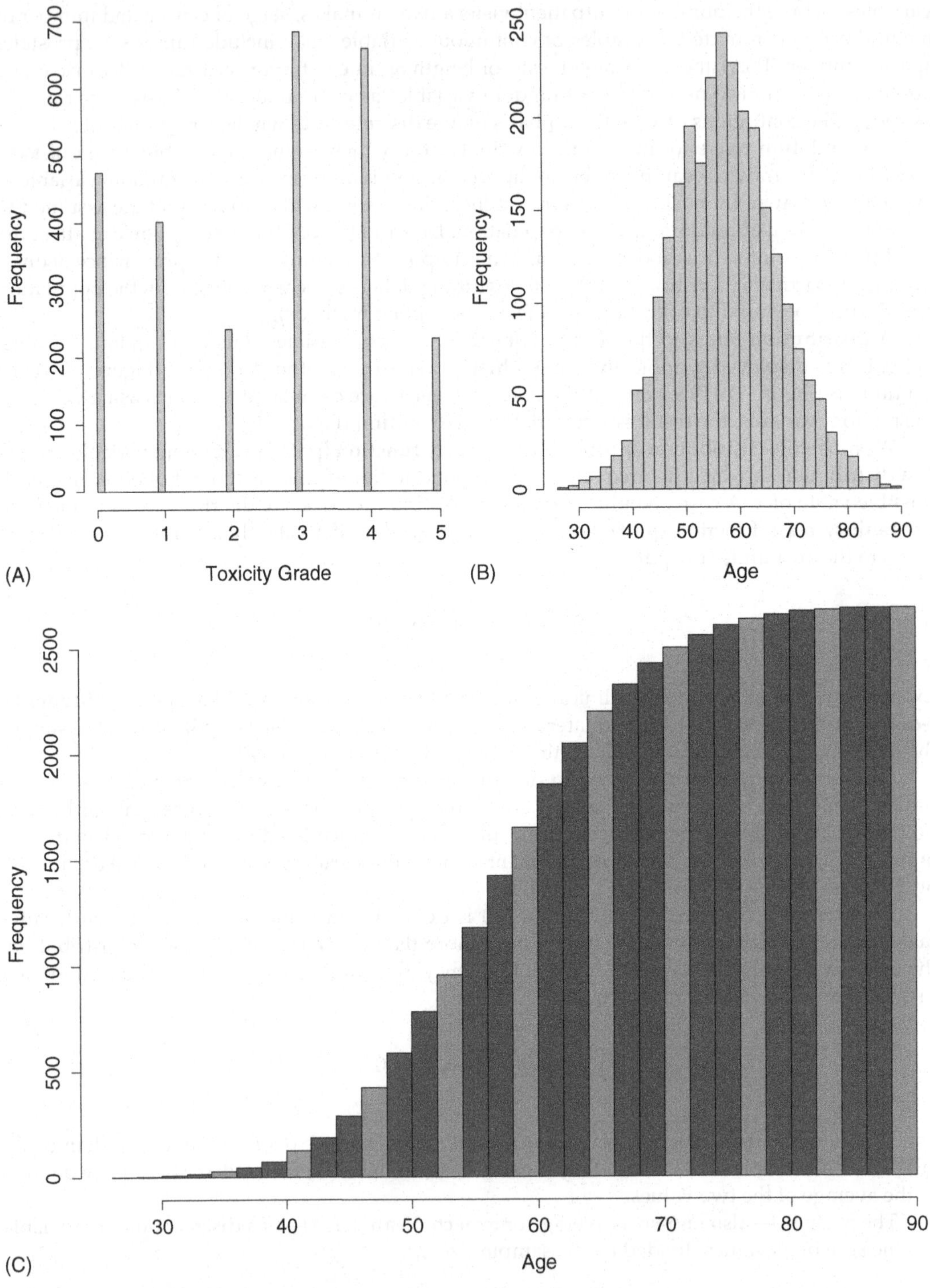

FIGURE 11.1 (A) Histogram from a sample distribution for a discrete variable (toxicity grade). (B) Histogram from a sample distribution for a continuous variable (age). (C) Cumulative histogram from a sample distribution (age).

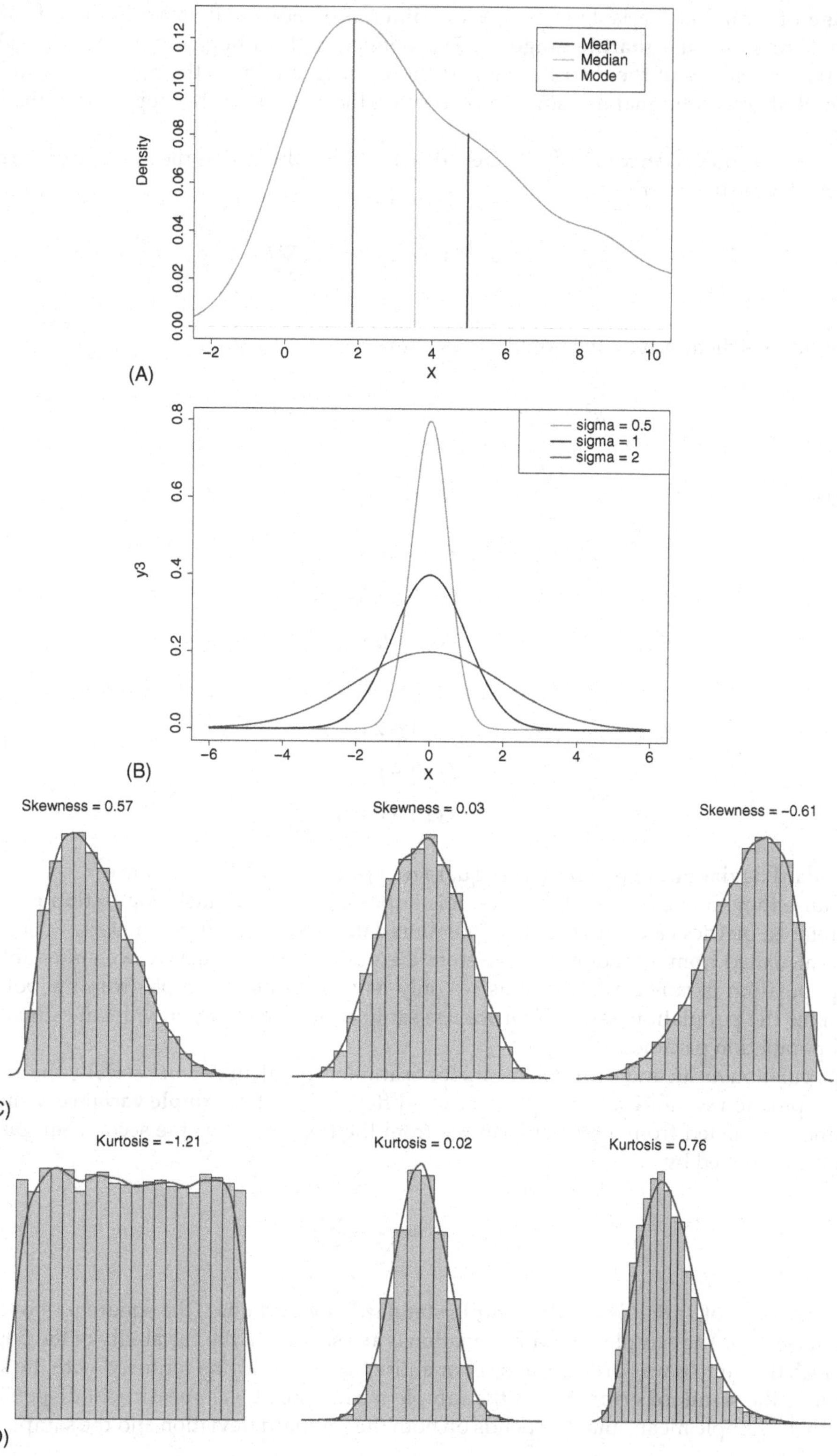

FIGURE 11.2 Moments of a distribution: (A) mean, median, and mode; (B) variance; (C) skew; (D) kurtosis.

The **range** of a random variable is simply the difference between its maximum and minimum values, whereas the **interquartile range (IQR)** is defined as the difference between the value that defines the upper 25% of the distribution and the value that defines the bottom 25% of the distribution. Both are additional measures of dispersion that are sometimes reported in the medical literature.

The **population variance** (σ^2) of a discrete distribution is defined as the average of the squared residuals after mean centering:

$$\sigma^2 = E((x-\mu)^2) = \frac{1}{N}\sum_{i=1}^{N}(x_i-\mu)^2$$

For a continuous distribution, the population variance is defined as

$$\sigma^2 = E((x-\mu)^2) = \int_{-\infty}^{\infty}(x-\mu)^2 f(x)\,dx$$

Note that:

$$\begin{aligned}\sigma^2 &= E((x-\mu)^2)\\ &= \int (x-\mu)^2 f(x)\,dx\\ &= \int (x^2-2\mu x+\mu^2) f(x)\,dx\\ &= \int x^2 f(x)\,dx - 2\mu \int x f(x)\,dx + \mu^2 \int f(x)\,dx\\ &= E(x^2) - 2\mu^2 + \mu^2\\ &= E(x^2) - \mu^2\\ &= E(x^2) - [E(x)]^2\end{aligned}$$

The **standard deviation** (σ) is simply the square root of the population variance.

Because they can be confused at times, it is important to distinguish **population parameters**, which refer to metrics calculated from population data, from sample parameters, which refer to metrics calculated from a random sample from the population. Frequently, we are unable to calculate population parameters directly, as we only have access to a sample from the population, not data for the population itself. Often we use sample parameters to provide an estimate of the desired population parameters.

A population mean and a sample mean, for example, are calculated in basically the same way, but the population variance and sample variance differ slightly. The **sample variance**, which refers to variance calculated from a random sample from the population, is the second sample central moment and defined by

$$s^2 = \frac{1}{N-1}\sum_{i=1}^{N}(x_i-\bar{x})^2$$

Another measure of variability is the **sample standard deviation** (i.e., the square root of the sample variance, or s). The sample standard deviation is an estimate of the variability of the population from which the sample was drawn. Another quantity that can easily be confused with the standard deviation is the **standard error (SE)** of the sample mean. The SE is a measure of dispersion with respect to the sample mean, and it depends on both the standard deviation and the sample size (n):

$$\text{SE} = s/\sqrt{n}$$

PLOTTING DATA

A key early stage in any data analysis is exploratory graphical analysis. Common plots are useful in identifying potential data errors, assessing normality of continuous variable distributions or transformations that would make the distribution normal, and getting a preliminary sense of whether group differences exist (Table 11.1). The most common plots for continuous outcomes are histograms (Figure 11.1) and box-and-whisker plots or boxplots (Figure 11.3). As discussed earlier, histograms are displays of the relative frequency of binned values of the outcome and produce an empirical estimate of the distribution of the variable. They provide a quick visual assessment of the shape of the distribution. Comparative histograms can be produced based on levels of some factor or predictor (e.g., treatment or genotype), and give an assessment of whether the distribution differs by level of the predictor either in terms of the center of the distribution or in some other way.

Boxplots are also useful in identifying characteristics of the distribution of an outcome and for comparative purposes. They are essentially graphical depictions of summary measures of the distribution (typically mean, median, quartiles), which give a sense of both the center and variability or spread of the data. In addition to their usefulness as exploratory plots, they are better for graphically summarizing continuous outcome data in publications than bar plots (Figure 11.3) with error bars for the standard deviation or standard error (often seen only in the positive direction).

When the goal is to identify the association between two continuous variables, **scatterplots** are a helpful first step (see Chapter 12). These represent simple relationships between two variables and can be useful for visually determining whether a linear association exists between two variables of interest, or whether some other relationship (e.g., logarithmic or quadratic) is a better fit to the data. In particular, scatterplots that show the relationship between **residuals**, or differences between observations and model predictions, are of great value for assessing model validity (see Chapter 12). When fitting regression models, plots of residuals versus variables of interest can be helpful in identifying violation of modeling assumptions and bias.

Bland–Altman plots (Figure 11.4) are frequently used to assess agreement between two different measurements of the same quantity. This might be the same measurement performed by different graders/readers or different machinery, or it can be the same instrument applied at different times in order to assess reliability and repeatability of the measurement. A Bland–Altman plot is essentially a scatterplot of the difference between the measurements on the y-axis versus the average of the measurements on the x-axis. The plot also includes horizontal lines for the mean difference and limits of agreement defined by the average difference +/− 1.96 standard deviations of the difference. This allows for examination of systematic bias, which would exist if the mean difference were substantially different from 0, and/or if there were a pattern such that there is not a random scatter of the differences within the limits of agreement.

Several other types of plots are commonly used in cancer research to describe data and interventions, or to depict effects of treatments and other factors on outcomes. **Receiver operating characteristic** (**ROC**) curves were discussed in Chapter 8 and are revisited again in Chapter 25. These are useful for graphically depicting key properties of a diagnostic test (namely, sensitivity and specificity). For graphically representing time-to-event outcomes (Chapter 16), **survival plots** and **cumulative incidence** plots are critical in describing event probabilities and effects of treatment on key end points. **Forest plots** (Chapters 16 and 28) are often used in reports of randomized trials, to graphically indicate treatment effect estimates and confidence intervals within key subgroups, and in meta-analyses to plot the study-specific treatment effect estimates along with a measure of variability of the estimate. They can also be used to summarize results of regression analysis, by graphically displaying both the effect estimates and confidence intervals.

Waterfall plots (Figure 11.5) are ordered bar charts that are typically used to describe the magnitude of change in an outcome that would be indicative of response. Each bar represents the magnitude of change for a continuous outcome for one patient. Typically, these are ordered from the worst to the best change. For example, if the outcome being displayed is change in a biomarker, the largest increase in the biomarker would be the first bar on the left with the bar above the 0 line

TABLE 11.1 LIST OF COMMON PLOTTING TECHNIQUES, WITH CORRESPONDING COMMANDS IN SELECT STATISTICAL SOFTWARE PACKAGES

Description of Problem	Data Type	Test	R Command/Package	SAS Procedure	Chapter
Display values between two variables for a set of data	Any	Scatterplot	plot()/graphics	sgplot procedure	12
A method for graphically depicting groups of the numerical variable through their quartiles	Any	Box-and-whisker plot	boxplot()/graphics	boxplot procedure	11
A graphical method to compare two measurement techniques	Any	Bland–Altman plot	bland.altman.plot()/ BlandAltmanLeh	gpplot procedure	11
A graphical display of estimated results from a number of scientific studies addressing the same question, along with the overall results	Any	Forest plot	forestplot()/rmeta	sgplot procedure	16, 27
A decision tree that strives to correctly classify members of the population	Any	Recursive partitioning analysis	rpart()/rpart	hpsplit procedure	11
A plot that illustrates the diagnostic ability of a binary classifier system	Binary	ROC curve	roc()/pROC	logistic procedure	8, 24
Response to treatment	Continuous, paired	Waterfall plot	waterfallplot()/ waterfall	sgplot procedure	11
Visualize the estimated probability of an event prior to a specified time	Censored	Cumulative incidence plot	plot.cuminc()/cmprsk	lifetest procedure	16
A series of declining horizontal steps that approach the true survival probability for the population	Censored	Kaplan–Meier survival plot	plot.survfit()/survival	lifetest procedure	16
Plot event probabilities for stratified data (e.g., meta-analysis)	Censored, stratified	Peto curve	–	lifetest procedure	11

ROC, receiver operating characteristic.

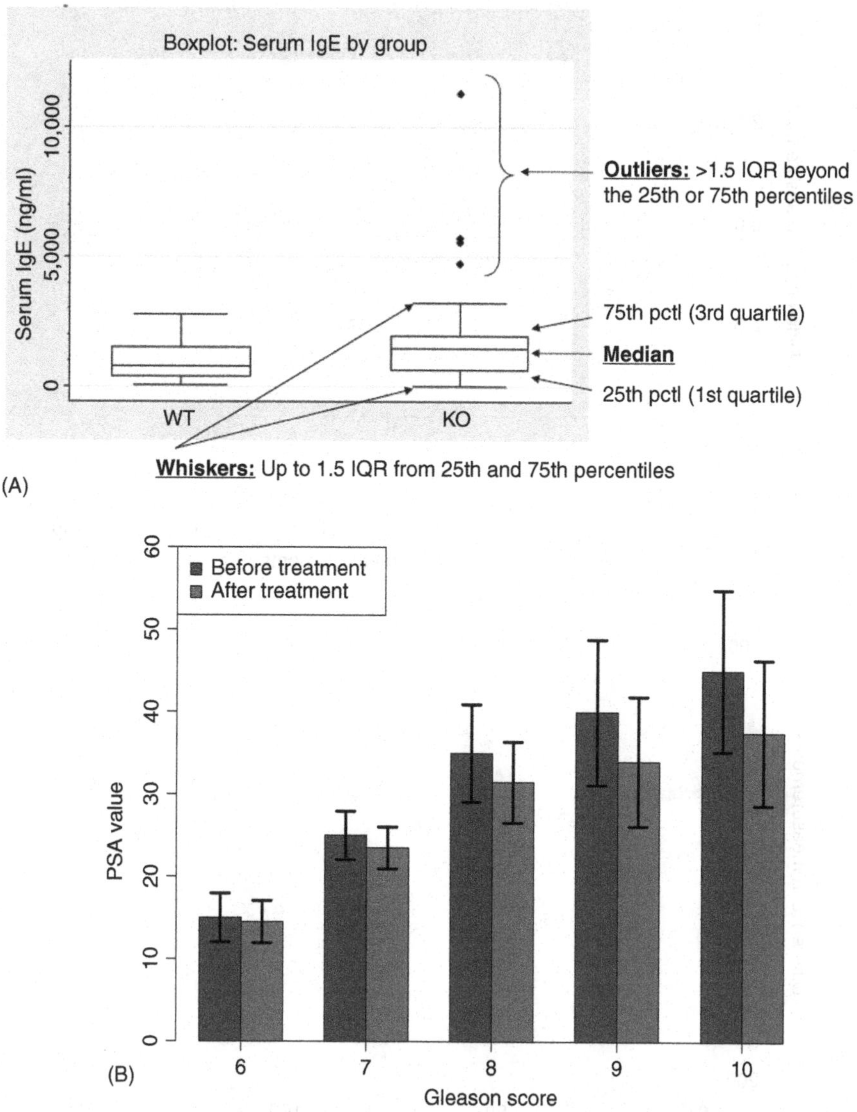

FIGURE 11.3 (A) Box-and-whisker plot; (B) bar plot.

IQR, interquartile range; PSA, prostate-specific antigen.

and the largest decrease in the biomarker would be the last bar on the right with the bar below the 0 line. Bars may also be colored to indicate a treatment group, or as in the example figure, the clinical response status.

TYPES OF DISTRIBUTIONS

All random variables have some distribution in the population. When considering continuous outcome variables, it is common to assume that the population distribution is a **normal distribution**. The normal distribution is defined by two parameters: the mean (μ) and the variance (σ^2). The defining characteristic of the normal distribution is its bell-shaped density function. The mean of the normal distribution is also its median and its most common value (mode). A **standard normal distribution** has mean 0 and variance 1. A normally distributed random variable can be converted

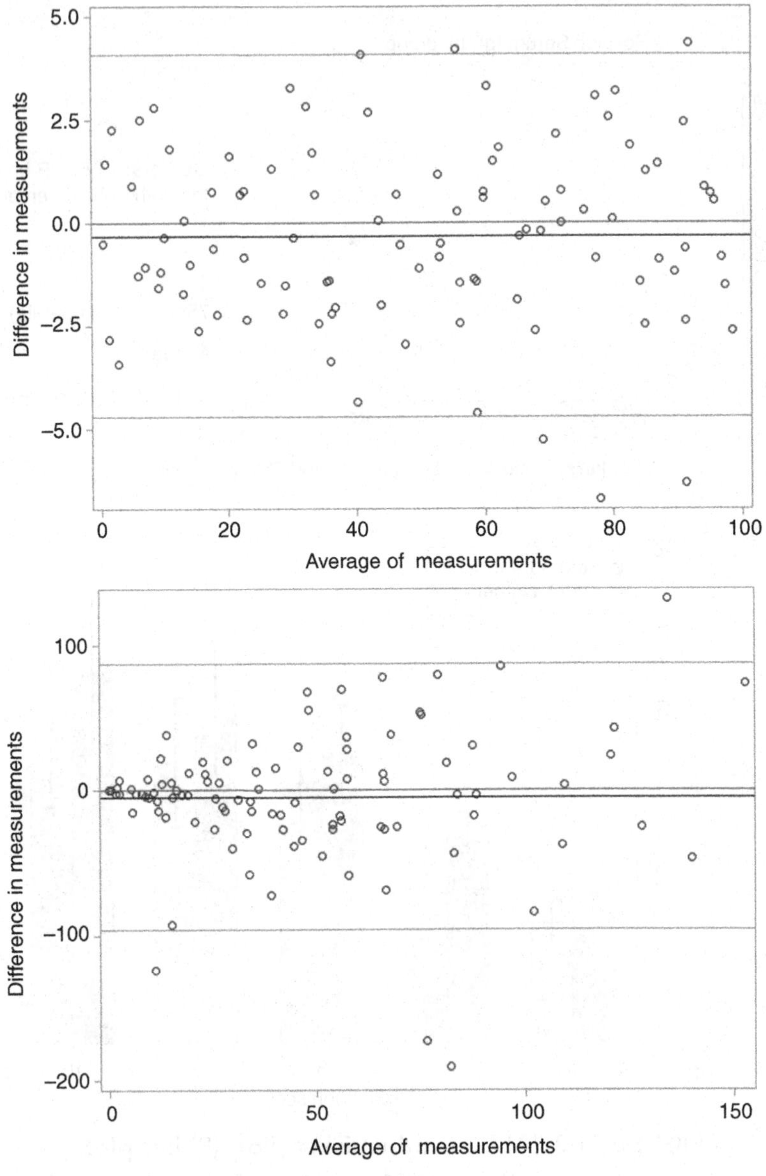

FIGURE 11.4 Bland-Altman plots showing (Above) little evidence of bias or pattern to the difference in measurement and (Below) evidence of disagreement in measures increasing with average measurement.

to a random variable with a standard normal distribution by subtracting its mean and dividing by its variance. The normal distribution has the following pdf:

$$f(x) = \frac{1}{\sqrt{2\pi\sigma^2}} e^{\frac{-(x-\mu)^2}{2\sigma^2}}$$

Student's t-distribution is similar to a normal distribution but has heavier tails—meaning a higher probability of being further from the mean than in a normal distribution with the same mean in variance. It is defined by a mean, variance, and degrees of freedom. As the degrees of

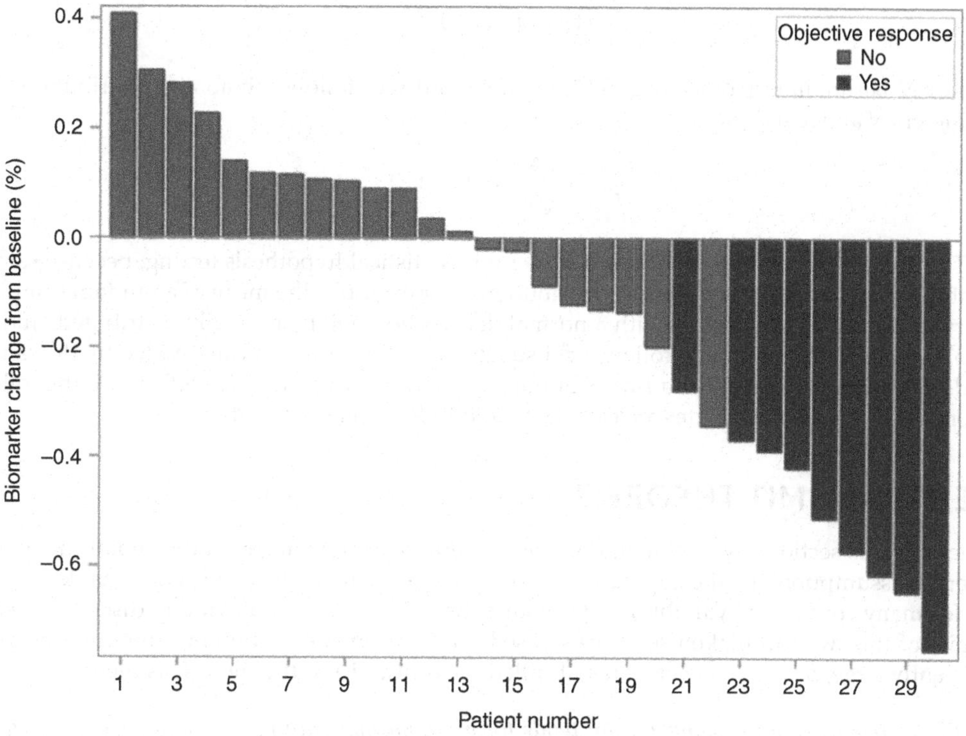

FIGURE 11.5 Waterfall plot.

freedom increase and approach infinity, the *t*-distribution converges to the normal distribution. If a variable that is normally distributed is divided by a variable that has a chi-square distribution (see the following), the resulting variable will follow a *t*-distribution.

Continuous random variables that exist only in the positive space ($x > 0$) are often assumed to follow a gamma distribution. The gamma pdf is

$$f(x) = \frac{\beta^a}{\Gamma(a)} x^{a-1} e^{-\beta x}$$

The distribution is defined by two parameters: a, the shape parameter, and β, the rate parameter. The gamma function is

$$\Gamma(a) = \int_0^\infty x^{a-1} e^{-x} dx$$

If a is an integer, then $\Gamma(a) = (a-1)!$.

A gamma distribution with $a = v/2$ and $\beta = 1/2$ is called a chi-square distribution with v degrees of freedom (χ_v^2). When a normally distributed variable with mean 0 is squared, it follows a standard chi-square distribution. If $X_1 \sim \chi_{v_1}^2$ and $X_2 \sim \chi_{v_2}^2$, then $\frac{X_1/v_1}{X_2/v_2} \sim F(v_1, v_2)$, that is, the ratio of two random variables with a chi-square distribution follows an F-distribution with numerator degrees of freedom v_1 and denominator degrees of freedom v_2.

Dichotomous outcomes follow a Bernoulli distribution, which is a discrete distribution defined by a single parameter: the probability of the event (π). The pmf for a Bernoulli outcome is

$$p(x) = \pi^x (1-\pi)^{1-x}$$

A set of N Bernoulli outcomes (e.g., N flips of a coin) will follow a binomial distribution with parameters N and π and pmf:

$$p(x) = \binom{N}{x} \pi^x (1-\pi)^{N-x}$$

The aforementioned distributions are useful in statistical hypothesis testing, because sample quantities tend to follow one of these distributions. For example, the mean of a random sample of observations from a population with a normal distribution will be normally distributed, and the sample standard deviation will follow a chi-square distribution. The mean divided by the sample standard deviation will follow a t-distribution. In analysis of variance (ANOVA; see the following), ratios of variance estimates are calculated and follow an F-distribution.

CENTRAL LIMIT THEOREM

In the previous sections, we discussed the distribution of sample means and standard deviations under the assumption that the population is normally distributed. This is not a reasonable assumption for many continuous variables and not an appropriate assumption for any discrete variable. In spite of this, we can make use of tests based on the normal distribution if the sample size is sufficiently large, due to a powerful result called the **central limit theorem**. This theorem states:

> *The distribution of the sample mean tends toward a normal with mean μ and variance σ^2/n ($N(\mu, \sigma^2/n)$) as n becomes arbitrarily large, regardless of the type of distribution from which the random variable is drawn.*

Although modern computing has made reliance on the central limit theorem unnecessary for many settings, tests appropriate for normal data applied to non-normally distributed variables will still yield valid inference when the sample size is sufficiently large.

DRAWING COMPARISONS AND TESTING HYPOTHESES

HYPOTHESIS TESTING

Classical statistical inference (e.g., frequentist inference) relies on the concepts of population and sample presented earlier. A true value of the parameter of interest (e.g., a mean, or a difference in means representing the average effect of a treatment) exists in the population. We learn about the population by taking random samples and making an estimate of the population parameter. For example, if we take a random sample of 100 from a particular population and calculate the sample mean, we can use this as an estimate of the population mean. This sampling could be done repeatedly, and each time we would end up with a different sample estimate of the population parameter. In any particular study, however, we have only one sample. To perform a statistical test, we compare our sample estimate to the distribution of possible estimates assuming that some null hypothesis is true.

In most statistical testing, the null hypothesis is one that assumes there is no effect or no difference present. For example, suppose we want to get preliminary evidence of the efficacy of a new prostate cancer therapy. We start by hypothesizing that the mean change in PSA in a study for a new treatment is 0. Our null hypothesis is thus framed as

$$H_0 : \mu = 0$$

We then test the treatment on n patients and calculate the average change in PSA. To perform a statistical test, we ask the question, "If the null hypothesis were true, how likely are we to observe the mean change in PSA that we did observe, or something even less consistent with the null hypothesis (i.e., a larger difference)?" We can calculate this probability based on the theoretical distribution of a test statistic, which is simply a function of sample estimates. In the example, we could use a *t*-statistic:

$$t = \frac{\overline{x}}{s/\sqrt{n}}$$

where $\overline{x}$ is the sample mean, s is the sample standard deviation, and n is the sample size. Assuming the null hypothesis is true, this statistic has a *t*-distribution with mean 0, variance 1, and $n - 1$ degrees of freedom. We perform a statistical test by comparing our observed statistic to a *t*-distribution with $n - 1$ degrees of freedom. We calculate a ***p* value** by estimating the area under the curve for values that exceed our observed statistic.

If we are interested only in changes that are greater than 0 (i.e., alternative hypothesis $H_1 : \mu > 0$), we perform a one-sided test to obtain a *p* value (Figure 11.6A). If we would like to reject the null hypothesis if the difference is large in either the positive or negative direction (i.e., alternative hypothesis $H_1 : \mu \neq 0$), we perform a two-sided test (Figure 11.6B), and multiply the area to the right of the test statistic by 2. The *p* value is interpreted as the probability that we would observe the value at least as large as the test statistic under the null hypothesis, *under the assumption that the null hypothesis is true.* We compare our *p* value to a predetermined significance level, called α, which is typically set at 0.05 or less. If the *p* value is less than α, we reject the null hypothesis in favor of the alternative hypothesis. Otherwise, we "fail to reject" the null hypothesis—meaning we cannot say for sure the null hypothesis is true, but the observed data are consistent with it being true. The statistical test can also be performed by determining the critical value of the *t*-distribution corresponding to the alpha level. The critical value is the value of the test statistic with area under the curve α to the right for a one-sided test and $\alpha/2$ to the right for a two-sided test. If the absolute value of the test statistic is greater than the critical value, the null hypothesis is rejected.

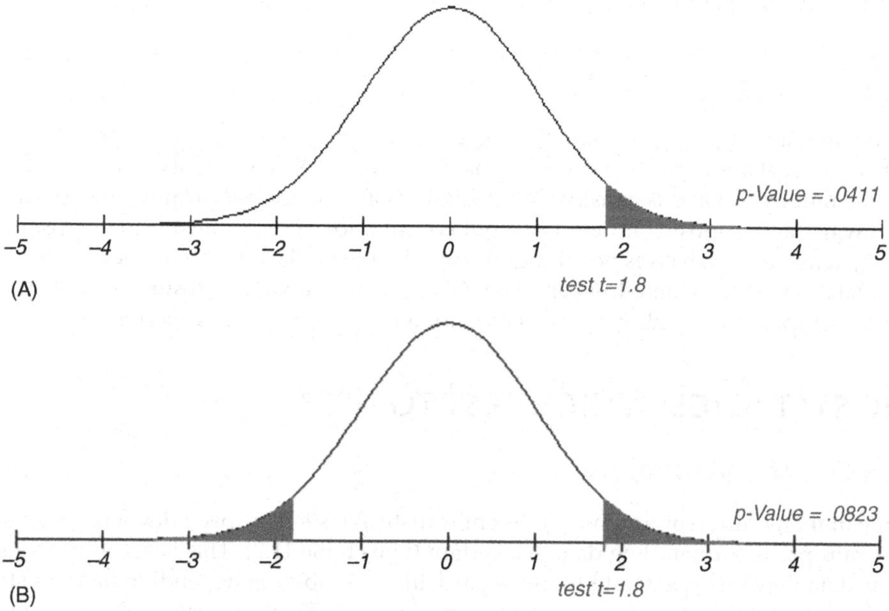

FIGURE 11.6 (A) One-sided t-test; (B) two-sided t-test.

Critical values with corresponding areas under the pdf in most cases can be easily found in lookup tables published online. Practically, most researchers use software programs that automatically report p values corresponding to the particular value of a test statistic, making manual lookup steps unnecessary. However, it may be a worthwhile exercise to undertake a manual calculation of a test statistic and manually look up the corresponding p value for the proper distribution, to understand the basic statistical process at work behind the scenes.

CONFIDENCE INTERVALS

Hypothesis testing is performed under the assumption that a specific null hypothesis is true and determining how consistent our data are with that specific null hypothesis. We can invert this question and ask: What null hypotheses are consistent with our data? That is, for what set of null values would we fail to reject the null hypothesis, for a given α level? This set of values constitutes a $(1 - \alpha)$ confidence interval. Thus, a 95% confidence interval contains all values not rejected at a 5% significance level.

TYPE I/II ERROR AND POWER

Because we do not know the truth about the parameter in the population, we can make one of two errors in testing. If the null hypothesis is in fact true, we can incorrectly reject the null hypothesis when by chance we observe test statistics in the tails of the distribution. This is called type I error. The probability of a type I error is α. Classical statistical tests are set up to minimize type I error and control it at the level α.

The second type of error occurs when we fail to reject the null hypothesis, even though the alternative hypothesis is true. This is called type II error. The probability of a type II error is β, and $1 - \beta$ is called the power. Power is determined by (a) the significance level of the test; (b) the size of the sample; and (c) the specific value of true parameter value in the alternative space. As α increases, the probability of rejecting the null hypothesis for a given sample size and true parameter value increases. As the sample size increases, the power for a given α level and true parameter value increases. Finally, as the true parameter moves further away from the null value, the power for a given α level and sample size increases.

SAMPLE SIZE CALCULATIONS

When planning studies, sample sizes may be estimated to provide a certain power to detect a specific true effect at a prespecified α level. Typically, having 80% probability or higher of correctly rejecting the null hypothesis is considered adequate. Software for performing power calculations is readily available for most common tests, but consultation with a statistician is recommended, particularly when the analysis is not straightforward and standard tests may not apply (e.g., longitudinal data, Chapter 15; time-to-event data, Chapter 16; equivalence testing, Chapter 27). For a real-world example of a sample size calculation for a phase III trial, see Chapter 22.

BASIC STATISTICS: WHICH TEST TO USE?

SCALES OF MEASUREMENT

Data come in many different formats. Different statistical tests have been developed that are particularly appropriate for handling data of a certain type (Table 11.2). This is because, as discussed earlier, the data may be expected to follow a particular distribution depending on their structure. Often, it is convenient to transform data from one scale to another, such as from a non-normal distribution to a normal distribution; several methods are discussed in Chapter 12. In general,

TABLE 11.2 LIST OF COMMON STATISTICAL TESTS AND PROCEDURES, WITH CORRESPONDING COMMANDS IN SELECT STATISTICAL SOFTWARE PACKAGES

Description of Problem	Data Type	Test	R Command/Package	SAS Procedure	Chapter
Simple description of the data, measures of central tendency, and dispersion	Any	Summary statistics	summary()/stats	univariate procedure	11
A type of table in a matrix format that displays the frequency distribution of the multiple variables	Binary	Contingency table	ftable()/stats	freq procedure	11
Test for independence between two or more variables	Binary, independent	Chi-square test	chisq.test()/stats	freq procedure (chisq)	11
Test for nonrandom associations between two variables	Binary or categorical	Fisher's exact test Barnard's exact test	fisher.test()/stats barnard.test()/Barnard	freq procedure (fisher) freq procedure (barnard)	11
Test for differences among three or more matched sets of frequencies or proportions	Binary, dependent	Cochran's Q	cochran.qtest()/ RVAideMemoire	freq procedure	27
Test for statistically significant change in proportions that have occurred on a dichotomous trait at two time points on the same population	Binary, paired	McNemar's test	mcnemar.test()/stats	freq procedure (mcnem)	11
Test for difference in mean of two independent samples	Continuous, independent	Unpaired *t*-test	t.test()/stats	ttest procedure	11
Test for quality of means among three or more groups	Continuous	ANOVA (*f*-test)	anova()/stats	anova procedure	11, 12

(continued)

TABLE 11.2 LIST OF COMMON STATISTICAL TESTS AND PROCEDURES, WITH CORRESPONDING COMMANDS IN SELECT STATISTICAL SOFTWARE PACKAGES (*continued*)

Description of Problem	Data Type	Test	R Command/Package	SAS Procedure	Chapter
Measure inter-rater reliability	Continuous	Kappa test	cohen.kappa()/psych wkappa()/psych	freq procedure (kappa)	11
Test for association between two variables measured on at least one interval scale	Continuous	Pearson product-moment correlation test	cor.test()/stats (method="pearson")	freq procedure (measures)	11
Test for difference in mean of two dependent samples	Continuous, dependent	Paired *t*-test	t.test()/stats	ttest procedure	11
Test for quality of means among three or more groups	Continuous, dependent	Repeated measures ANOVA	anova()/stats	anova procedure	11, 15
Test for significant differences on a continuous dependent variable by a categorical independent variable	Ordinal, independent	Kruskal–Wallis test	Kruskal–Wallis test/stats	npar1way procedure	11
Test for comparing average of two samples that come from the same population and whether two sample means are equal or not	Ordinal, independent	Mann–Whitney *U* test	wilcox.test()/stats	npar1way procedure	11
Measure the ordinal association between two measured quantities	Ordinal, independent	Kendall's tau	cor.test()/stats (method="kendall")	freq procedure (kentb)	11
Test for differences among multiple groups	Ordinal	Friedman test	friedman.test()/stats	freq procedure (cmh2 noprint)	11

(*continued*)

TABLE 11.2 LIST OF COMMON STATISTICAL TESTS AND PROCEDURES, WITH CORRESPONDING COMMANDS IN SELECT STATISTICAL SOFTWARE PACKAGES (*continued*)

Description of Problem	Data Type	Test	R Command/Package	SAS Procedure	Chapter
Test for comparing two dependent samples or two samples from the same population	Ordinal, dependent	Wilcoxon signed rank test	wilcox.test()/stats	npar1way procedure	11
Test for association between two ranked samples	Ordinal	Spearman rank test	cor.test()/stats (method="spearman")	freq procedure (measures)	11
Test for overall degree of association in a series of 2 × 2 tables	Stratified cumulative incidence, categorical data	Mantel–Haenszel test	mantelhaen.test()/stats	freq procedure (mhchi)	11, 13
Test for difference in survival curves	Censored	Log-rank test	survdiff()/survival	lifetest procedure	16
Test for difference in survival curves	Censored	Peto's test	logrank_test()/coin	lifetest procedure	11
Test for comparing survival distribution from two samples	Censored	Gehan's test	gehan.test() / npsm	lifetest procedure	11
Test for difference in cumulative incidence curves	Censored	Gray's test	summary.crr()/cmprsk	lifetest procedure	16

ANOVA, analysis of variance.

statistical tests are more powerful when more assumptions can be made about the nature of the data distribution. The trade-off, however, is that if one or more assumptions are invalid, then the resulting inferences may be invalid and misleading. Before embarking on a statistical experiment, it is crucial to specify the scale of both the dependent variable(s) (i.e., the primary outcome(s)) and independent variable(s) (i.e., explanatory factor(s)) with which you will be working. In particular, the scale of the chosen outcome variable will determine the appropriate statistical test(s) and/or modeling technique(s) to employ.

The **binary** or dichotomous scale is the simplest data structure, in which each data point can be represented (isomorphically) as either 0 or 1. Some investigators will mean-center their binary data, so that data take on values of either −0.5 or 0.5. A simple example of a binary outcome might be the presence or absence of a disease, whereas a binary explanatory variable would be male/female sex. Often, it is convenient to convert data from other scales, such as a **continuous** or categorical scale, to the dichotomous scale for ease of analysis. For example, a continuous outcome like a quantitative biomarker could be reclassified as binary, by being above or below a certain threshold. Dummy variables, frequently used as explanatory variables in regression models, are also represented in this fashion and may be converted from a categorical representation (see Chapter 12).

Data measured on the **continuous scale** could theoretically take on any value over a certain domain; for example, body mass index (BMI)—defined as the ratio of one's mass (kg) to squared height (m^2)—could, in theory, be any positive number. A feature of continuous data is that a unit change in the variable has the same meaning regardless of the location; that is, a unit change in BMI from 20 to 21 is the same unit change as going from 30 to 31. In contrast, **ordinal data** typically take on discrete values without a clear meaning to a unit change. For example, survey data, such as a pain scale from 0 to 10, typically have an ordinal structure: a value of 10 is worse than 5, which is worse than 1, but a unit change in the variable has no clear meaning.

The term **nominal (categorical) data** refers to values that cannot be adequately represented by an ordinal number, such as ethnicity, or anatomic tumor site. Like ordinal data, there is no meaning to a unit change, but unlike ordinal data, there is no clear orientation or hierarchy to the data. Often it is best to discretize categorical variables into a binary scale for analysis. Finally, the term censored data refers to data, usually represented on a continuous scale, that are incomplete, such as because an observation period was cut off, or the meaning of the variable ceases to matter beyond a certain threshold. Time-to-event data (discussed in Chapter 16) are typically right-censored, because a study often must end before the true event time can be observed for all subjects; for subjects who do not have an event, it is only known that the event time is at least as long as the observed value. Analogously, left-censored data are data with values only known to be at least as low as the observed value; for example, some blood tests may become unreliable at extremely low values and could be better modeled by left-censoring the data.

A key assumption underlying the validity of many statistical tests is that the values obtained from each individual measurement are **statistically independent**, meaning there is no systematic correlation between the values; the value of one measurement does not affect the value of another. Solitary random samples from unique individuals, for example, usually are assumed to be independent. When the observations are dependent, or cannot be assumed to be independent, different statistical methods are used for hypothesis testing that can account for the correlation or clustering between measurements. Situations where data may be dependent include repeated measures or longitudinal observations within the same individual (Chapter 15), or observations within relatives, coworkers, or other cohorts belonging to a defined cluster.

BINARY (DICHOTOMOUS) DATA

CONTINGENCY TABLES AND CHI-SQUARE TEST

A **contingency table** is a type of table in matrix format that displays the frequency distribution of multiple variables. These tables are commonly used in medical research and survey research. They

TABLE 11.3 EXAMPLE OF A CONTINGENCY TABLE FOR A BINARY VARIABLE

	Level 1	Level 2	Level 3	Total
OBSERVED DATA				
Group 1	O_{11}	O_{12}	O_{13}	$O_{1.}$
Group 2	O_{21}	O_{22}	O_{23}	$O_{2.}$
Total	$O_{.1}$	$O_{.2}$	$O_{.3}$	O_{all}
EXPECTED DATA				
Group 1	E_{11}	E_{12}	E_{13}	$E_{1.}$
Group 2	E_{21}	E_{22}	E_{23}	$E_{2.}$
Total	$E_{.1}$	$E_{.2}$	$E_{.3}$	E_{all}

Note: $E_{ij} = \frac{T_i \times T_j}{N}$, where T_i is the total in the *i*th row of A, T_j is the total in the *j*th column of A, and *N* is the table grand total of A.

can be used to test for correlation between two or more independent binary variables; for example, see Table 11.3.

The chi-square test of independence is used to determine whether there is a significant relationship between two categorical variables. The frequency of each category for one nominal variable can be compared across the categories of the second nominal variable. The data can be displayed in an $r \times c$ contingency table where each row represents a category for one variable and each column represents a category for the other variable. The chi-square test statistic can be calculated by $\chi^2 = \sum \frac{(O-E)^2}{E}$, where *O* represents the observed frequency and *E* is the expected frequency under the null hypothesis, which is computed by $E = \frac{r \times c}{N}$, where *N* is the sample size. The statistic is $\sim\chi^2$ (*df*), where *df* (degrees of freedom) = $(r - 1)*(c - 1)$. The value of the statistic can be compared against critical values of the chi-square distribution to test the null hypothesis.

CONTINUITY CORRECTIONS (YATES CORRECTION)

The **Yates correction** is a correction made to account for the fact that chi-square tests can be biased upward for a 2 × 2 contingency table. The corrected chi-square statistic can be calculated as

$$\chi^2_{Yates} = \sum_{i=1}^{N} \frac{(|O_i - E_i| - 0.5)^2}{E_i}$$

where O_i is an observed frequency, E_i is an expected (theoretical) frequency according to the null hypothesis, and *N* is the number of distinct events. The effect of Yates correction is to

TABLE 11.4 TABLE USED FOR YATES CORRECTION

	Group 1	Group 2	Total
Level 1	a	b	n_1
Level 2	c	d	n_2
Total	n_3	n_4	n

prevent overestimation of statistical significance for small data. For a specific 2 × 2 table shown in Table 11.4, we can find that

$$\chi^2_{Yates} = \frac{n\left(|ad - bc| - n/2\right)^2}{n_1 n_2 n_3 n_4}$$

MANTEL–HAENSZEL TEST

The Mantel–Haenszel test is a test of the association between two binary variables, while controlling for a third confounding nominal variable. Essentially, the Mantel–Haenszel test examines the weighted association of a set of 2 × 2 tables. This test is commonly used in case–control studies for assessing relationships between a dichotomous outcome and explanatory variables across different strata (such as age and demographic groups).

FISHER'S AND BARNARD'S EXACT TESTS

The usual approach to contingency tables is to apply the chi-square statistic to each cell of the table. However, when samples are small, the distribution of statistic is not well approximated by the chi-square distribution. Hence, the p values for the hypothesis tests cannot be trusted (and are often biased against the null hypothesis). In this case, one should consider using an **exact test** to assess the null hypothesis of no difference between binary outcomes across two or more groups. A typical rule of thumb is that one should apply an exact test if there are five or fewer events/counts per cell in a contingency table. Table 11.2 shows a list of commands that can be used to perform exact tests in R and SAS.

Fisher's exact test is commonly used in such situations. This approach looks at a contingency table that displays how different treatments or factors have produced different outcomes. The null hypothesis is that treatments do not affect outcomes. Barnard's exact test is a computationally intensive but more powerful exact test for 2 × 2 contingency tables. The precise formulas for exact tests are rather complicated. We recommend using Fisher's exact test if the row totals and the column totals are both fixed by the design of the study, the sample size is small, or more than 20% of cells have an expected cell count less than 5.

A famous experiment proposed by Sir R.A. Fisher himself was designed to test the validity of a particular English lady's claim that she could discern, by taste alone, whether a cup of tea with milk had the tea poured first or the milk poured first. Eight cups of tea were prepared and presented to her in random order. Four had the milk poured first, and four had the tea poured first. The lady tasted each one and rendered her opinion. Example results are summarized in Table 11.5. Under the null hypothesis that the lady has no discerning ability (i.e., the four cups she calls tea first are a random sample from the eight), if she selects four at random, the probability that three of these four are actually tea first comes from the hypergeometric distribution, $P(n_{11} = 3)$:

TABLE 11.5 TABLE USED FOR FISHER'S EXACT TEST

	Lady's statement	
Poured first	Tea first	Milk first
Tea	$n_{11} = 3$	$n_{12} = 1$
Milk	$n_{21} = 1$	$n_{21} = 3$

$$\frac{\binom{4}{3}\binom{4}{1}}{\binom{8}{4}} = 0.229$$

A p value from this test is the probability of getting a result at least as extreme as the outcome we actually did observe, if the null hypothesis were true. In this example, the p value = $P(n_{11} = t_0)$, where t_0 is the observed value of n_{11}, in this case 3.

The only result that could be more extreme would be if the woman had selected all four of the cups that are truly tea first, which has the probability

$$\frac{\binom{4}{4}\binom{4}{0}}{\binom{8}{4}} = 0.014$$

The p value can be calculated as 0.229 + 0.014 = 0.243, which is only weak evidence against the null hypothesis. In other words, if the lady were purely guessing, she would have approximately 24% chance of obtaining a result at least as extreme as what was observed, so there is not enough evidence to reject our null hypothesis that the lady is purely guessing.

NORMALLY DISTRIBUTED AND CONTINUOUS DATA

A basic and common problem in medical statistics is to test whether the mean value of a particular measure significantly differs across two or more groups. For this class of problems, often it is convenient to assume (under the null hypothesis) that the two measures are independently distributed and drawn from either a normal or t-distribution. This assumption is usually valid for data that are measured on a continuous scale, especially when applied to large samples, as the resulting distributions tend be normal (bell-shaped).

UNPAIRED *t*-TEST

An **unpaired *t*-test** is commonly used to assess whether the population means of two independent groups are statistically different from each other. The test statistic follows a Student's t-distribution and is calculated as

$$t = \frac{\bar{x}_1 - \bar{x}_2}{\sqrt{s^2\left(\frac{1}{n_1} + \frac{1}{n_2}\right)}}$$

and

$$s^2 = \frac{\sum_{i=1}^{n_1}(x_i - \overline{x}_1)^2 + \sum_{j=1}^{n_2}(x_j - \overline{x}_2)^2}{n_1 + n_2 - 2}$$

where $\overline{x}_1$ and $\overline{x}_2$ are the means of two samples, s^2 is the pooled sample variance, n_1 and n_2 are the sample size, and t is a quantile from Student's t-distribution with $n_1 + n_2 - 2$ degrees of freedom.

Consider, for example, the observed weight gain for 19 female rats between 28 and 84 days after birth, where $n_1 = 12$ were fed a high protein diet and $n_2 = 7$ were fed a low protein diet. The mean weight gain on the high protein diet is $\overline{x}_1 = 120$ and the mean weight gain on the low protein diet is $\overline{x}_2 = 101$. Suppose the t-statistic calculated in this case is $t = 1.89$. The critical value from the t-distribution with 17 degrees of freedom at the 0.05 significance level is 2.11. Because our observed value of the t-statistic is less than 2.11, we would fail to reject the null hypothesis that the diet had no effect on the weight of the rats in the two groups being compared.

ANOVA AND *F*-TEST

ANOVA is a method for comparing outcomes measured on the continuous scale across three or more groups. For comparing multiple observations within individuals across three or more groups, a technique called repeated measures ANOVA is used. The null hypothesis in an ANOVA test is that there is no difference in means across all groups being compared, which is compared against the alternative hypothesis that not all means are equal. The method uses the F-statistic, named after Sir Ronald Fisher, which represents the ratio of two variances.

For example, suppose that we wish to compare the systolic blood pressure (SBP) among three groups of patients, and we want to know whether there is evidence that the mean SBP is significantly different in one or more of the groups. The ANOVA hypotheses are

$$H_0 : \mu_1 = \mu_2 = \mu_3 \text{ vs. } H_1 : \text{not all means are equal.}$$

For sample data organized as in Table 11.6, the F-test statistic can be calculated by the formula

$$F = \frac{\sum_i n_i(\overline{x}_i - \overline{x})^2/(k-1)}{\sum_j \sum_i (x_j - \overline{x}_i)^2/(N-k)}$$

where $i = 1, 2, \ldots, k$, k is the number of groups, and N is the total sample size. The value of the F-statistic can then be compared against the critical value of the F-distribution with $k - 1$ numerator and $N - k$ denominator degrees of freedom. Importantly, for significant values of the test statistic, the F-test just described does not determine which group (or groups) has the means that differ; only that one can reject the null hypothesis that they are all equal. One may wish to conduct tests

TABLE 11.6 TABLE USED FOR ANOVA

	Group 1	Group 2	Group 3
Sample Size	n_1	n_2	n_3
Sample Mean	$\overline{x}_1$	$\overline{x}_2$	$\overline{x}_3$
Sample Standard Deviation	s_1	s_2	s_3

ANOVA, analysis of variance.

between two groups to interrogate hypotheses regarding a particular group; however, one should take care to correct for multiple hypothesis testing (see the following).

Note that ANOVA can also be used as a method to compare two or more statistical models (see Chapter 12). Essentially, ANOVA and linear regression are equivalent methods to compare differences in outcomes across a categorical independent variable. ANOVA can be used to determine whether a regression model is significantly different from a random model (null model), or whether additional variables add value to an existing regression, by comparing the degree of additional variation explained by their inclusion in the model. This comes from a partitioning of (i.e., *analysis* of) the different components of the variation around the overall mean value that occurs in the data (i.e., total sum of squared residuals, SS_T): one part is the variation explained by a statistical model (or model sum of squares, SS_M) and the other part is variation resulting from random errors (or error sum of squares, SS_E). The value SS_M/SS_T is called the **R-squared (R^2)** value, which is the proportion of the total variation explained by a model; hence, a good model generally has a high R^2, though an adjusted R^2 value,

$$Adjusted\,R^2 = 1 - \frac{(1-R^2)\,(n-1)}{n-k-1}$$

is often used to correct for models that include too many predictors.

The total sample variance, mean square for the model (MSM), and mean square error (MSE) are defined as $s_T^2 = SS_T/(n\text{-}1)$, $s_T^2 = SS_T/(k\text{-}1)$, and $s_E^2 = SS_E/(n\text{-}k)$, respectively. The null hypothesis of no difference in the outcome across categories can be tested using the *F*-statistic

$$F = \text{MSM}/\text{MSE}$$

or, in other words, by analyzing the ratio of the variation explained by the model to the variation explained by random error. When this ratio exceeds the critical value for the appropriate *F*-distribution, the null hypothesis is rejected.

PAIRED OR CORRELATED DATA

Many standard statistical tests (e.g., paired *t*-test, chi-square, ANOVA) assume that the observations being obtained are statistically independent from one another. When this is not the case, applying standard tests may give invalid or misleading results. Importantly, standard tests may underestimate the true variation that exists in the population, because the variation between correlated observations is usually less than between independent observations. Second, true effects could be missed if the natural variation between subjects in the sample is much larger than the natural variation within subjects. Thus, both type I and type II errors can be inflated if the proper statistical approach is not used.

PAIRED *t*-TEST

A **paired sample *t*-test** is used to test for differences in the population means from two samples, when observations in one sample can be paired with the other (e.g., values are taken within the same individuals before and after some intervention). Other common applications of the paired sample *t*-test include case–control studies and repeated measures designs. The test statistic follows the Student's *t*-distribution and is calculated by

$$t = \frac{\sum d}{\sqrt{\dfrac{n\left(\sum d^2\right) - \left(\sum d\right)^2}{n-1}}}$$

where $\sum d$ is the sum of the differences between two samples and n is the sample size.

REPEATED MEASURES ANALYSIS OF VARIANCE

Repeated measures ANOVA is the equivalent of the one-way ANOVA, but for related or independent groups, which is an extension of the dependent *t*-test. A repeated measures ANOVA is also referred to as a within-subjects ANOVA or ANOVA for correlated samples. Detailed discussion of this approach is beyond the scope of this chapter; further information is provided in Glantz (1).

ORDINAL AND CATEGORICAL (NOMINAL) DATA

Parametric statistical methods are those that rely on assumptions about parameters (e.g., means and variances) with a defined distribution (e.g., normal or chi-square) in a defined population. In contrast, **nonparametric** statistical methods do not depend on assumptions about the population distribution of the data being compared. Because ordinal structures preserve ranking in the data but do not convey any intrinsic meaning about unit changes, parametric models may not be valid in this context, in which case it is desirable instead to use nonparametric methods, such as **rank tests**. As mentioned previously, nonparametric models often sacrifice power in exchange for greater validity (a sort of **bias–variance trade-off**; see the following).

MCNEMAR'S TEST

McNemar's test is a nonparametric test to assess for changes in a dichotomous variable according to a factor within the same population. Unlike the chi-square test, McNemar's test evaluates consistency in responses across two variables, rather than for independence between proportions. McNemar's test can only be applied to a 2 × 2 contingency table, but the **Stuart–Maxwell test** is an extension for larger contingency tables. For example, suppose we wanted to determine whether a specific drug reduces anxiety associated with cancer therapy. Consider Table 11.7. McNemar's chi-square test statistic with one degree of freedom is calculated as

$$\chi^2 = \frac{(B-C)^2}{B+C}$$

MANN–WHITNEY U TEST

The **Mann–Whitney *U* test** is a nonparametric statistical test to evaluate the equality of two sample means when the data are ordinal or when the assumptions of an unpaired *t*-test do not hold. The Mann–Whitney *U* statistic can be calculated by

$$U = n_1 n_2 + \frac{n_2(n_2+1)}{2} - \sum_{i=n_1+1}^{n_2} R_i$$

TABLE 11.7 TABLE USED FOR MCNEMAR'S TEST

	Before Drug	After Drug	Total
Anxiety Present	A	B	A + B
Anxiety Absent	C	D	C + D
Total	A + C	B + D	A + B + C + D

where n_1 and n_2 are the sizes of the two samples, and R_i is the rank of the sample size, which is the sum of all observations' ranks (index of ordinal position) in group i.

KRUSKAL–WALLIS TEST

The **Kruskal–Wallis test** is a nonparametric test to assess differences in a continuous dependent variable across values of a categorical independent variable. It is used when it cannot be assumed that the dependent variable is normally distributed with equal variance across groups of a one-way ANOVA (i.e., ANOVA based on one independent variable). The test determines whether the medians of two or more groups are different. The test statistic (H) used is

$$H = \left[\frac{12}{n(n+1)} \sum_{i=1}^{c} \frac{T_i^2}{n_i} \right] - 3(n+1)$$

where n is the sum of sample sizes for all samples, c is the number of samples, T_i is the sum of ranks in the ith sample, and n_i is the size of the ith sample.

WILCOXON RANK SUM AND SIGNED RANK TESTS

Wilcoxon's rank test is a nonparametric test to compare outcomes for two independent (for the rank sum test) or dependent (for the signed rank test) samples, when the assumption of normality does not hold and/or the use of a t-test is inappropriate. Suppose, for example, we were interested in testing for a difference between the median values of a pain score (scaled from 0 to 10) for two different treatments applied sequentially to the same set of 30 patients, with the null hypothesis that the type of treatment does not affect the median pain score. Suppose the distribution of the pain score is heavily skewed toward the higher values of the scale. To compute the Wilcoxon statistic (W), first the pain score under treatment 2 is subtracted from the score under treatment 1 for each individual to get the set of differences. Then the differences are placed in rank order from 1 to 30 by absolute value (ignoring the positive or negative sign) and given a new value corresponding to the rank multiplied by the sign of the difference (positive or negative). Finally, the W-statistic is calculated by summing all of the signed ranks and the resulting test statistic is compared to critical values of the Wilcoxon distribution.

COCHRAN'S Q TEST

Cochran's Q test is an extension of McNemar's test for testing differences among three or more matched sets of frequencies or proportions (i.e., where an outcome can be classified as a "success" or "failure"). The null hypothesis for Cochran's Q is that the proportion of "successes" is equal for all groups, with the alternative hypothesis that the proportion is different for at least one group. The test statistic is

$$Q = k(k-1)\frac{\sum_{j=1}^{k}\left(x_{.j} - \frac{N}{k}\right)^2}{\sum_{i=1}^{b} x_{i.}(k - x_{i.})}$$

where b is the number of blocks, k is the number of treatments, $x_{.j}$ is the column total for the jth treatment, $x_{i.}$ is the row total for the jth block, and N is the grand total. The null hypothesis is rejected when the Q statistic exceeds the critical value for a chi-square distribution with $k - 1$ degrees of freedom.

FRIEDMAN'S TEST

Friedman's test is a nonparametric test for detecting differences in an outcome across multiple groups or treatments. Essentially, it is used in place of the ANOVA test when the distribution of outcome in the population is unknown. Friedman's test can be regarded as an extension of the sign test when there are multiple treatments. The null hypothesis is that the treatments all have identical effects. Friedman's test statistic can be calculated as

$$FM = \left[\frac{12}{(N * k * (k+1))}\right] \sum R^2 - [3 * N * (k+1)]$$

where N is the number of subjects, k is the number of treatments, and R is the total rank for each of the three treatments.

MEASURES OF CORRELATION

PEARSON PRODUCT-MOMENT CORRELATION

The **Pearson product-moment correlation coefficient** is a measure of the strength of a linear association between two variables X and Y, denoted by r:

$$r = \frac{cov(X,Y)}{\sigma_X \sigma_Y}$$

where *cov* is the covariance, σ_x is the standard deviation of X and σ_y is the standard deviation of Y, and r ranges in value from +1 to −1. A value of 0 indicates that there is no association between the two variables, a positive value indicates a positive association between X and Y, and a negative value indicates a negative association. Basically, this approach identifies a best-fit line through a scatterplot of the two variables, with r indicating how far away the data points lie with respect to the line.

SPEARMAN RANK COEFFICIENT AND KENDALL'S TAU

Spearman's correlation coefficient is a nonparametric measure of rank correlation (statistical dependence between the rankings of two variables). It assesses how well the relationship between two variables can be described using a monotonic function. For a sample size n, the n original scores X_i, Y_i are converted to ranks $X_{(i)}$, $Y_{(i)}$, and the Spearman correlation can be calculated by

$$r_s = \frac{cov(X_{(i)}, Y_{(i)})}{\sigma_{X_{(i)}} \sigma_{Y_{(i)}}}$$

where $cov(X_{(i)}, Y_{(i)})$ is the covariance and $\sigma_{X_{(i)}}$ and $\sigma_{Y_{(i)}}$ are the standard deviations of the rank variables. Similarly, **Kendall's tau** (τ) is a nonparametric measure of relationships between columns of ranked data. The tau correlation coefficient returns a value of 0 (no relationship) to 1 (perfect relationship). Considering paired data $(x_1, y_2), \ldots, (x_n, y_n)$, we define τ as

$$\tau = \frac{C - D}{n(n-1)/2}$$

where C is the number of concordant pairs, D is the number of discordant pairs, and n is the number of pairs.

KAPPA TESTS

Cohen's kappa (κ) is a statistic that measures inter-rater reliability (interobserver agreement). Inter-rater reliability happens when independent data raters give the same score to the same data item. This statistic is calculated as

$$\kappa = \frac{p_0 - p_e}{1 - p_e}$$

where p_0 is the relative observed agreement among raters and p_e is the hypothetical probability of chance agreement. For categories *k*, there are *N* items with n_{ki} the number of times rater *i* predicted category *k*:

$$p_0 = \frac{\#in\ Agreement}{N}$$

$$p_e = \frac{1}{N_2}\sum_k n_{k1} n_{k2}$$

Fleiss's kappa is an extension of Cohen's kappa to assess inter-rater agreement when the number of raters is greater than two. Weighted kappa statistics are sometimes used to give differing amounts of weight to large versus small disagreements; they can be calculated using a table of weights that apply to the extent of disagreement between raters.

CENSORED DATA

The **log-rank test** is a nonparametric statistical test to compare two or more samples involving censored data. It is often used in survival analysis to compare event times across groups of individuals (see Chapter 16). The **Gehan–Breslow–Wilcoxon test** is an alternative and less frequently used nonparametric statistical test to compare survival distribution from two samples. It does not require the assumption of a consistent hazard ratio, but does require that one group consistently have a higher risk than the other. Peto's log-rank test is generally the most appropriate method, but the modified Wilcoxon test (Prentice) is more sensitive when the ratio of hazards is higher at early survival times than at late ones (2).

Gray's test (see Chapter 16) is a common method for testing for differences in the cumulative incidences (subdistribution hazards) between two or more groups with competing risks. **Breslow's method** is an approach to handling ties in time-to-event data, which is commonly used in the Fine–Gray model and other competing risks approaches. The Mantel–Haenszel test is also sometimes applied to the analysis of stratified cumulative incidence data.

MULTIPLE HYPOTHESIS TESTING

A classic pitfall in data analysis can occur when multiple statistical tests are performed, either explicitly or implicitly, undermining the validity of the primary hypothesis test (3). Various resulting biases, such as confirmation bias and the Texas sharpshooter effect, were discussed in Chapters 2 and 10. A hypothesis test should be specified a priori, including a declaration of what one intends to conclude will constitute evidence to support or reject the null hypothesis. Once a study is complete, however, it is tempting to subject the data to additional post hoc hypothesis tests in an attempt to find new or additional evidence to support one's hypothesis. Each additional test, however, raises the probability that at least one test will reject its null hypothesis—simply because of cumulative type I error. In such cases, the overall type I error should be adjusted, and more stringent criteria for statistical significance of p values applied, using methods discussed in the following (Table 11.8).

TABLE 11.8 LIST OF SPECIALIZED STATISTICAL TESTS AND PROCEDURES, WITH CORRESPONDING COMMANDS IN SELECT STATISTICAL SOFTWARE PACKAGES

Description of Problem	Test/Procedure	R Command/Package	SAS Procedure	Chapter
Test for normality in frequentist statistic	Anderson–Darling test	ad.test()/ADGofTest	univariate procedure	12
Multiple hypothesis adjustment	Bonferroni test	p.adjust() / stats (method="bonferroni")	anova procedure	11
Structural stability	Chow test	chow.test()/gap	model procedure	
A measure of internal consistency	Cronbach's α	alpha()/psych	corr procedure	11
Test for autocorrelated residuals	Durbin–Watson test	dwtest()/lmtest	autoreg procedure	12
Missing data	Expectation–maximization algorithm	amelia()/Amelia	mi procedure	11
Compare area under an ROC curve (used for model validation and calibration)	Harrell's C	compare()/compareC	-	11
Multiple hypothesis adjustment	Holm test	p.adjust()/stats (method="holm")	multtest procedure	11
Goodness of fit	Hosmer–Lemeshow test	hoslem.test()/ ResourceSelection	logistic procedure	11
Test for heterogeneity in treatment effects across trials (used in meta-analysis)	I^2 statistic	rma()/meta	-	27
Cross-validation	LOOCV	loocv()/DMwR	glmselect procedure	11
Simulation	Markov chain Monte Carlo	mcmc (R package)	mcmc procedure	23

(continued)

TABLE 11.8 LIST OF SPECIALIZED STATISTICAL TESTS AND PROCEDURES, WITH CORRESPONDING COMMANDS IN SELECT STATISTICAL SOFTWARE PACKAGES (*continued*)

Description of Problem	Test/Procedure	R Command/Package	SAS Procedure	Chapter
Missing data	Multiple imputation	amelia()/Amelia	mi procedure	11, 23
Test for independence between residuals and time	Schoenfeld residuals test	cox.zph()/survival	lifetest procedure	16
Test for normality in frequentist statistic	Shapiro–Wilk test	shapiro.test()/stats	univariate procedure	12
Test for whether specific groups' means are different	Tukey post hoc test	TukeyHSD()/stats	anova procedure	11
Test for independence in a contingency table	Yates correction (Yates chi-square test)	chisq.test()/stats	freq procedure (chisq)	11

HSD, honestly significant difference; LOOCV, leave-one-out cross-validation; ROC, receiver operating characteristic.

BONFERRONI CORRECTION

The **Bonferroni correction** is a method for adjusting results from multiple independent statistical tests. The method adjusts the significance level a used to assess statistical significance, such that $a_{new} = \frac{a}{k}$ for a set of k independent statistical tests with a as the original significance level. This approach shifts the original a to a new value, a_{new}, used to determine statistical significance over a set of multiple tests. The rationale is that the probability of rejecting at least one null hypothesis is increased with each independent test, if we consider each test as a simple draw from a binomially distributed random variable with $p = a$ and $n = k$. For example, if we plan to run three independent tests of a null hypothesis, each with $a = 0.05$, if there is actually no difference (i.e., the null hypothesis is correct) in every case, then although there is a 5% chance of finding a significant result in each test individually, across the set of three tests the long-run type I error rate will be higher than 5%. In order to correct for this problem, we would run each individual test with a significance level set at $a_{new} = \frac{a}{3} = .0167$.

HOLM TEST

The **Holm–Bonferroni "step-down" method** is a modification of the Bonferroni correction that deals with familywise error rates (FWERs) for the multiple testing problem. Although the Bonferroni correction reduces the type I error when performing multiple tests and is simple to calculate, it is conservative and suffers from a lack of statistical power. In contrast, the Holm–Bonferroni method is also fairly simple and is more powerful than the Bonferroni correction. The first step is to rank the multiple (i.e., k) p values in order from smallest to largest. Then, the significance level of the highest ranked (i.e., smallest) p value is adjusted using the Bonferroni method described earlier (i.e., $a_1 = \frac{a}{k}$). If the smallest p value is less than the new significance level, we can reject the first null hypothesis. In the second step, the second smallest p value is adjusted by "stepping down" the adjustment by 1, that is, $a_2 = \frac{a}{k-1}$. The third smallest p value is adjusted as $a_3 = \frac{a}{k-2}$, and so on such that the largest p value is essentially unadjusted $\left(a_k = \frac{a}{k-(k-1)} = a\right)$. At the end, through repeating the Holm–Bonferroni step-down procedure for all of the tests, the adjusted p values can be used to obtain results of multiple null hypothesis tests.

TUKEY'S POST HOC TEST

An ANOVA test can indicate if a difference exists in means across three or more groups, but does not prove where the differences lie. Tukey's post hoc test can be used to find out which specific groups have different mean values, by comparing all possible pairs of means and adjusting the type I error. The test statistic (honestly significant difference [HSD]) is

$$HSD = \frac{M_i - M_j}{\sqrt{\frac{MS_w}{n}}}$$

where $M_i - M_j$ is the difference between the pairs of means, MS_w is the mean square within, and n is the number per group or treatment. Following ANOVA, two groups' means are selected for comparison. Tukey's statistic is calculated for each comparison and checked against a table of critical values with the appropriate degrees of freedom.

OTHER SPECIALIZED STATISTICS

CRONBACH'S a

Cronbach's a is a measure of the reliability of a composite score. It is often used in survey and quality of life (QOL) research to assess the reliability of an assay or instrument, that is, how well the instrument measures what it should. Cronbach's a is applicable under the assumption that one has multiple items measuring the same underlying construct, and is calculated as

$$a = \frac{N \cdot \bar{C}}{\bar{V} + (N-1) \cdot \bar{C}}$$

where N is the number of items, $\bar{C}$ is the average covariance between item pairs, and $\bar{V}$ is the average variance between item pairs. A value of $a > 0.9$ implies excellent reliability, whereas a value of $a < 0.5$ indicates poor reliability.

STATISTICAL MODELING

The goal of statistical modeling is to isolate and quantify the effect of one or more variables on one or more outcomes of interest. Generally this is achieved using **regression models** (Chapters 12, 13, and 16; Table 11.9); however, various applied machine learning methods (Table 11.10) use a slightly different framework to approach this problem, as discussed in Chapter 17. A gross generalization

TABLE 11.9 LIST OF REGRESSION TECHNIQUES, WITH CORRESPONDING COMMANDS IN SELECT STATISTICAL SOFTWARE PACKAGES

Description of Problem	Data Type (Outcome)	Test	R Command/ Package	SAS Procedure	Chapter
Binary outcomes	Binary	Logistic regression	glm()/stats	logistic procedure	13
Dependent variable can take only two values	Binary	Probit model	glm()/stats (family = binomial(link = "probit")	probit procedure	13
Dependent variable is categorical	Binary	Logit model	(family = binomial(link = "logit")	logistic procedure	13
A technique where the response is the result of a series of Bernoulli trials	Binary/ Categorical	Binomial regression	glm()/stats (family = "binomial")	genmod procedure/ countreg procedure	13
Continuous outcomes	Continuous	(Multiple) Linear regression	lm()/stats	reg procedure	12
Modeling multiple outcomes simultaneously	Continuous	MANOVA, MANCOVA	manova()/ stats	glm: manova procedure	11
Response variable has a Poisson distribution (log-linear model)	Count variable	Poisson regression	glm()/stats (family = binomial(link = "poisson")	genmod procedure/ countreg procedure	13
Model/feature selection	Categorical	LASSO regression	glmnet()/ glmnet	glmselect procedure	11
Survival model	Survival (hazard function)	Cox proportional hazards model	coxph()/ survival	phreg procedure	16
Competing risk	Cumulative incidence (sub-distribution hazards)	Fine–Gray model	crr()/cmprsk	phreg procedure	16
Competing risk model	Time to event (competing risks)	Generalized competing event regression	gcecox()/ gcerisk gcefg()/ gcerisk	-	16
Clustered survival data	Survival/ Time to event	Frailty model	frailtyPenal()/ frailtypack	phreg procedure	11

LASSO, least absolute shrinkage and selection operator; MANCOVA, multivariate analysis of covariance; MANOVA, multivariate analysis of variance.

TABLE 11.10 LIST OF MACHINE LEARNING TECHNIQUES, WITH CORRESPONDING COMMANDS IN SELECT STATISTICAL SOFTWARE PACKAGES

Description of Problem	Test	R Command/ Package	SAS Procedure	Chapter
An interconnected group of nodes, akin to the vast network of neurons in a brain	Artificial neural network	neuralnet()/ neuralnet	neural procedure	17
A method used to find a linear combination of features that characterizes two or more classes of objects or events	Linear discriminant analysis	lda()/MASS	discrim procedure	17
A technique for feature extraction and dimension reduction	Principal component analysis	prcomp()/stats	factor procedure	17
An ensemble learning method for classification	Random forest	randomForest()/ randomForest	hpforest procedure	17
A probabilistic model for representing normally distributed subpopulations within an overall population	Gaussian mixture model	Mclust()/mclust	-	17
A supervised learning method for classification	Support vector machine	svm()/e1071	fmm procedure	17
An unsupervised learning method for clustering	*k*-means clustering	kmeans()/stats	fastclus procedure	17
Estimate the parameters of a generalized linear model with a possible unknown correlation between outcomes	GEE	gee()/gee	genmod procedure	15
A generalization of ordinary linear regression that allows for response variables whose error distribution models are other than a normal distribution	Generalized linear models	glm()/stats	genmod procedure/glm procedure	12, 13

GEE, generalized estimating equation.

is that regression models seek to identify[1] a parametric, functional form that represents the "true" relationship between a dependent variable or end point and a set of explanatory variables, with discrepancies between observations and model predictions represented as independent random

[1] *A parametric model is said to be* ***identifiable*** *if the values of the parameters in the model can be estimated from the data; that is to say, the mapping from parameters to probability distributions is one-to-one, so it is possible to identify the underlying population parameter uniquely.*

errors (see more on mixed effects in the following). Key assumptions are typically that the errors are uncorrelated with each other and also with the other explanatory variables in the model.

The goal of a regression analysis is to identify or estimate the value of model parameters from the given set of observations. Due to their greater mathematical flexibility, regression models frequently hypothesize a functional relationship that is linear (at least, after a simple transformation) in the model parameters. **Maximum likelihood estimation** (MLE) is a general technique to identify the values of model parameters with the greatest likelihood to give rise to the observed set of data, along with estimates of the uncertainty surrounding each parameter estimate.

Many of the most common statistical modeling techniques used in clinical cancer research, including generalized linear modeling (e.g., multiple linear regression, logistic regression, probit regression) and proportional hazards regression, are discussed in depth later in this book. Other more advanced topics, especially those with less frequent application to oncology research (e.g., multivariate ANOVA [MANOVA] and analysis of covariance [ANCOVA and MANCOVA], hierarchical models, isotonic regression, Bayesian model averaging, frailty models, and time series regression including autoregressive integrated moving average [ARIMA] models) are better expanded upon in advanced textbooks. However, many general principles apply to the conduct of regression and other modeling approaches; in particular, model specification and model evaluation are critical aspects of any statistical analysis. These concepts will be useful to review before embarking on deeper applications.

MODEL SPECIFICATION AND BUILDING

A first step in statistical modeling is to specify its form. This means delineating the precise statistical model to be used, the dependent variable, the set of explanatory variables to be included in the model, and the hypothesized error structure. The latter is a particularly crucial and often not well-described aspect of statistical modeling in clinical cancer research. Poor model specification, however, will lead to poor inferences. It is thus important to consider that any inferences attendant to a given statistical analysis implicitly assume that the model is correctly specified. Data transformations such as **mean centering** and **normalization** can facilitate interpretation of model output, to take out the effects of scaling variables to different units of measurement. Sometimes, the optimal model form is not clear a priori, so either a **top-down approach** (which starts with available explanatory variables and systematically excludes insignificant contributors to the model) or **bottom-up approach** (i.e., a parsimonious model) is initially specified based on a scientific rationale, then sequentially augmented with additional variables that are observed to enhance the model. Stepwise regression (discussed in Chapter 12) is among the most widely used methods for variable selection in statistical modeling. **Least absolute shrinkage and selection operator** (LASSO) and **least angle regression** are advanced techniques to assist in variable selection in modeling.

A key purpose of a multivariable model is to control for effects of confounding variables, or **confounders**, which are measurable variables that are correlated with both the primary outcome and the explanatory variable of interest. When a critical confounder is not measurable, investigators may seek to identify one or more **instrumental variables**, which are variables that are correlated with unmeasured confounders, but are assumed to be independent of the error term in the model. An example might be the distance to a specialized treatment center, which could influence the treatment a patient receives but is unlikely to be correlated with unmeasured health characteristics that would otherwise affect the outcome. **Propensity scores** are another modeling technique to adjust for confounding; these methods aim to predict the probability of a patient being assigned to the treatment of interest, which can help remove effects of selection and thus reduce bias in the effect estimates. When effects of one predictor could vary in the presence of another, **interaction terms** may be included in the model. Increasingly, linear predictors have been extracted from regression models and used to generate risk scores in statistical modeling. These are especially useful in predictive modeling approaches designed to detect treatment effect interactions, such as generalized competing event (GCE) regression (Chapter 16).

TESTING MODEL FIT AND FUNCTION

Ideally, a functional model should not only fit the data well, but should also explain future observations with a high degree of accuracy. There are two key concepts related to the performance of a model: bias and variance. For any given level of total error, as a model becomes less biased, the variance will increase, and vice versa—a relationship called the bias–variance trade-off. This follows from the decomposition of the total error from a statistical model (i.e., the difference between predicted and observed values) into three components: model bias, model variance, and irreducible error. A biased model with low variance will give similar answers under repeated sampling, but overall will be inaccurate in its predictions; an unbiased model with high variance will give widely different predictions but on average will yield accurate results.

Overfitting a model with too many explanatory variables can lead to poor model performance and inefficiency; this issue is discussed further in Chapter 17. A general rule of thumb to avoid this problem is to ensure that the sample has at least 10 events per parameter being estimated in the model; the higher the number of events per degree of freedom, the more stable the model will be. Several assays should also be performed, such as error or residual plots, to ensure that the error distributions conform to the model specification. Ridge regression is a technique to address the problem of multicollinearity (Chapter 12), which can result from overfitting. This is an intentionally biased form of regression designed to reduce the model error that results from having too many correlated explanatory variables.

Several basic indices are used to assess model fit. The **Akaike information criterion** (**AIC**) and **Bayesian information criterion** (**BIC**) are two methods to compare models. The AIC is calculated by obtaining the overall likelihood value (L) from the model, and is computed as

$$\text{AIC} = 2k - 2\ln(\text{L})$$

where k is the number of fitted parameters in the model; a lower AIC value indicates the preferred model. Similarly,

$$\text{BIC} = k\ln(n) - 2\ln(\text{L})$$

where k is the number of parameters and n is the sample size; a lower BIC value is comparatively better. Both AIC and BIC penalize the inclusion of additional parameters in the model to address overfitting, but BIC does so to a greater degree. The R^2 and adjusted R^2 are measures used to evaluate the proportion of variation in the data explained in a linear regression model. **Harrell's C-index** is a measure of **goodness of fit** often used in evaluating the performance of binary predictive models, such as logistic regression. The C-index reports the probability that a randomly selected patient who experienced an event had a higher score than a patient who had not experienced the event. It is equal to the area under the ROC curve, and ranges from 0.5 to 1. A C-index with a confidence interval that includes 0.5 indicates poor model fit; however, the C-index only gives a general idea about the fit of a statistical model. Another test of goodness of fit is the **Hosmer–Lemeshow test**, which tests model agreement/calibration, but does not take overfitting into account and can be inefficient (low power) for the purpose of assessing model fit.

A fitted model should have both internal and external validity. **Internal validation** refers to the process of ensuring that a model performs well within the sample from which it was derived, whereas **external validation** refers to testing the performance of the proposed model on an independent dataset that was not used to generate the parameter estimates. Often a single sample will be used for both model training and validation. Some investigators use split-sample validation methods, wherein the sample is randomly partitioned into a subset (usually 50%–67% of the original sample) for model training, with the remaining set reserved strictly for testing model fit and function. Other investigators used repeated "**bootstrap**" sampling with replacement to generate separate datasets for training and testing. Finally, **leave-one-out cross-validation** (**LOOCV**), **leave-multiple-out cross-validation** (**LMOCV**), **jackknife**, or **K-fold cross-validation** routines are commonly used for model training and testing—such methods are especially useful in small, potentially skewed datasets that are limited by outliers or fewer number of events.

MIXED EFFECTS MODELING

When assessing the effect of a factor or treatment on an outcome, there are two types of errors to consider: errors that are constant with respect to different values of the factor of interest, and errors that vary with different values of the factor. When the errors are constant across values of a factor, such that the group means are fixed (nonrandom) values across the sample, then one is able to consider that all possible values or levels of a factor are represented, and this is considered a **fixed effects model**. In contrast, when the errors vary according to different values of a factor, the group means are considered to be random, and the observed values of the factor represent only a sample of its possible values; this is a **random effects model**. When both effects are present, a **mixed effects model** (or **mixed model**) is applicable, which can be represented as

$$Y = X\beta + \zeta u + e$$

where the terms β and u correspond to fixed and random effects, respectively; X and ζ are the matrices of regressors (which are observed); and e is the error term. In this case, while we seek to estimate the fixed effect β, the random effect u is assumed to come from a distribution, and we seek to estimate the distribution of the random effects.

Mixed models have many applications, especially in the analysis of clustered data (Chapter 15) and meta-analysis (Chapter 28); in the latter case, each study is considered as a data cluster. Under a fixed effects model, the true effect is assumed to be identical for all values of the factor, and the effect size only varies due to sampling error. This has the effect of discounting information provided from smaller data clusters, since the same information is contained in the larger clusters. Under a random effects model, each cluster provides different information about the true overall effect, regardless of its size; one might think of each cluster as something closer to a single data point. A fixed effects model might be more applicable if (a) one can assume that each data cluster is, for all intents and purposes, identical to one another, and (b) one is not particularly concerned with generalizing the effect to other populations. In contrast, a random effects model might be more applicable if (a) the data clusters are likely to differ substantively from one another in the way the data were collected, and (b) we seek to generalize the analysis to the broader population.

MISSING DATA

Missing data is a problem affecting many analyses. Various methods are available to handle this problem. Briefly, we introduce several here. Further discussion of these issues appears in Chapters 15 and 23. **Mean imputation** is the simplest method: missing values are imputed by the mean of the observed values. The method is quite easy to apply, but it tends to underestimate standard deviations and variance. Also, this method may reduce the variability in data. **Regression imputation** involves imputing missing values using predictions from a regression equation. In this method, complete observations can be used to predict the missing observations. The assumption is that the imputed values fall on a regression line, which implies that the correlation is 1 to 1 between the missing outcome and predictors. Comparing with mean imputation, regression imputation will overestimate the correlation and underestimate variance and covariance. **Multiple imputation** is a useful statistical technique for dealing with incomplete datasets that include missing values. Imputation, analysis, and pooling are three main phases in multiple imputation. At first, the missing data are imputed m times to generate m complete datasets. And then, the m complete datasets are analyzed. The final step is to combine m analysis results and obtain the final inference.

The expectation–maximization (EM) algorithm is an iterative method of MLE for incomplete data. The idea for the EM algorithm is to calculate the maximum likelihood estimates for the incomplete data problem by applying the complete data likelihood instead of the observed likelihood. Computationally more tractable complete likelihood can be created by augmenting the observed data with manufactured data. We then replace the incomplete data at each iteration by their conditional expectation given the observed data and the current estimation of parameter (E-step). The new estimation of parameter is obtained from these replaced sufficient statistics as though they had come from the complete sample (M-step). Alternating E- and M-steps, the sequence of estimates often converges under a very general condition.

CONCLUSION: A NOTE ON TERMINOLOGY

Often the terminology in statistics can be confusing because the lay public will use terms interchangeably that mean different things to a statistician. For example, the public might casually refer to the "odds" or "likelihood" of an event as the same thing, but these are different statistical concepts. Probability was discussed earlier in this chapter when discussing density functions, and is defined as an area under the pdf. Odds, in contrast, represents the ratio of a probability, p, to its complement, $1 - p$, that is, odds $= p/(1 - p)$.

Likelihood is a **conditional probability** (see Chapter 24) that is a function of a parameter and a random variable: $L(\beta \mid x) = P(x \mid \beta)$, that is, the probability a parameter β given the observed value of a random variable. Sometimes investigators will refer to a probability as a "**rate**," when the latter term should really be used in reference to a timescale (such as per year). Similarly, **risk** is the probability of an event occurrence, with specific related definitions particularly relevant to cancer epidemiology (Chapter 13). Hazard, however, is a very different quantity specific to survival analysis (Chapter 16). Finally, incidence and prevalence are distinct terms that correspond to new and existing cases, respectively, with formal definitions (see Chapter 13).

One will often find that people confuse their *sample* with the *population* it is supposed to represent, even though these concepts are distinct. Occasionally one will see the word "parameter" used in reference to what is actually an explanatory variable; the terminology can be confusing, because often the parameter estimate of interest is actually the value of the multiplier, or coefficient, of the explanatory variable in the model, and the *parameter* is actually the unknown population quantity one is seeking to estimate. In general, a statistic is an observable and estimable quantity, whereas a parameter is not. Other confusing terms can be multivariable versus multivariate (Chapter 12); often people will use the latter when they mean the former. Another turn of phrase one often encounters is when investigators refer to a nonsignificant p value that is close to the significance threshold as one that is "borderline" or "almost reaches statistical significance." This is a misleading statement that means the same as "not statistically significant" and should be avoided, as practically it has the potential to increase type I error. One may encounter this terminology when investigators wish for a certain outcome, or have something ulterior to gain as a result of the statistical test. For further information on advanced statistics in oncology, please consult several excellent texts (4–10).

GLOSSARY

random variable: a variable that can take on any numerical value generated by or representative of a random process.

discrete: describes a random variable that takes on a value in a countable set.

continuous: describes a random variable that takes on a value in a uncountable set.

population: the set of individuals from which a random variable (or set of variables) could be drawn.

sample: the set of individuals from which a random variable is actually drawn.

distribution: the set of frequencies of each possible value of a random variable.

histogram: a graph that displays the relative frequency of binned values of an outcome and produces an empirical estimate of the distribution of a variable.

cumulative distribution: results when the frequencies are cumulated with increasing values of the random variable.

probability density function (pdf): for a random variable x, refers to a distribution in which the frequencies correspond to the relative likelihood of observing each possible value of x.

probability mass function (pmf): A probability function for discrete distributions in which the frequencies correspond to the relative likelihood of observing each possible value of x.

Student's *t*-distribution: a widely used probability density function similar to a normal distribution but with heavier tails (a higher probability of being further from the mean than in a normal distribution with the same mean in variance); defined by a mean, variance, and degrees of freedom.

mean (average value, expected value): a measure of central tendency used to describe a distribution; the first moment of a distribution.

median: a measure of central tendency used to describe a distribution.

mode: a measure of central tendency used to describe a distribution; a value of x where f(x) is (locally) maximized.

variance: a measure of dispersion; the second moment of a distribution.

skew: a measure of dispersion; the third moment of a distribution.

moment: element of a distribution.

expected value: see *mean*.

average value: see *mean*.

range: the difference between the maximum and minimum values of a random variable.

interquartile range (IQR): the difference between the value that defines the upper 25% of a distribution and the value that defines the bottom 25% of the distribution.

population variance (s^2): the average of the squared residuals of a discrete distribution after mean centering.

standard deviation: the square root of the population variance.

population parameters: metrics calculated from population data.

sample variance: variance calculated from a random sample from the population.

sample standard deviation: an estimate of the variability of the population from which the sample was drawn.

standard error (SE): a measure of dispersion with respect to the sample mean that depends on both the standard deviation and the sample size.

scatterplot: graphic that represents simple relationships between two variables; useful for visually determining whether a linear association exists between two variables of interest.

residuals: differences between observations and model predictions.

receiver operating characteristic (ROC) curve: plot useful for graphically depicting key properties of a diagnostic test.

survival plot: graphic critical in describing event probabilities and effects of treatment on key end points.

cumulative incidence plot: graphic critical in describing event probabilities and effects of treatment on key end points.

forest plot: graphic often used in reports of randomized trials to indicate treatment effect estimates and confidence intervals within key subgroups; used in meta-analyses to plot the study-specific treatment effect estimates along with a measure of variability of the estimate.

waterfall plot: an ordered bar chart typically used to describe the magnitude of change in an outcome that would be indicative of response.

normal distribution: a distribution defined by two parameters: the mean (μ) and the variance (s^2); displays a bell-shaped density function.

standard normal distribution: a normal distribution that has mean 0 and variance 1.

dichotomous: describes an outcome with only two possibilities.

central limit theorem: theorem which states that the distribution of the sample mean tends toward a normal with mean μ and variance s^2/n ($N(\mu, s^2/n)$) as n becomes arbitrarily large, regardless of the type of distribution from which the random variable is drawn.

***p* value:** value calculated by estimating the area under the curve for values that exceed an observed statistic.

binary (dichotomous) scale: the simplest data structure, in which each data point can be represented (isomorphically) as either 0 or 1.

continuous scale: scale on which data can theoretically take on any value over a certain domain.

ordinal data: data that typically take on discrete values without a clear meaning to a unit change.

nominal (categorical) data: values that cannot be adequately represented by an ordinal number.

statistically independent: the condition of having no systematic correlation between values.

contingency table: a type of table in matrix format that displays the frequency distribution of multiple variables.

Yates correction: a continuity correction made to account for the fact that chi-square tests can be biased upward for a 2 × 2 contingency table.

exact test: used to assess the null hypothesis of no difference between binary outcomes across two or more groups when the distribution of statistic is not well approximated by the chi-square distribution.

unpaired *t*-test: commonly used to assess whether the population means of two independent groups are statistically different from each other.

ANOVA: a method for comparing outcomes measured on the continuous scale across three or more groups.

R-squared (R^2) value: the proportion of the total variation explained by a model.

paired sample *t*-test: used to test for differences in the population means from two samples, when observations in one sample can be paired with the other.

parametric: describes statistical methods that rely on assumptions about parameters with a defined distribution in a defined population.

nonparametric: describes statistical methods that do not depend on assumptions about the population distribution of the data being compared.

rank test: a nonparametric statistical method.

McNemar's test: a nonparametric test to assess for changes in a dichotomous variable according to a factor within the same population.

Stuart–Maxwell test: an extension of McNemar's test for larger contingency tables.

Mann–Whitney *U* test: a nonparametric statistical test to evaluate the equality of two sample means when the data are ordinal or when the assumptions of an unpaired *t*-test do not hold.

Kruskal–Wallis test: a nonparametric test to assess differences in a continuous dependent variable across values of a categorical independent variable.

Wilcoxon's rank test: a nonparametric test to compare outcomes for two independent or dependent samples when the assumption of normality does not hold and/or the use of a *t*-test is inappropriate.

Cochran's Q test: an extension of McNemar's test for testing differences among three or more matched sets of frequencies or proportions.

Friedman's test: a nonparametric test for detecting differences in an outcome across multiple groups or treatments.

Pearson product-moment correlation coefficient: a measure of the strength of a linear association between two variables X and Y.

Spearman's correlation coefficient: a nonparametric measure of rank correlation (statistical dependence between the rankings of two variables).

Kendall's tau (τ): a nonparametric measure of relationships between columns of ranked data.

Cohen's kappa (κ): a statistic that measures inter-rater reliability.

Fleiss's kappa: an extension of Cohen's kappa to assess inter-rater agreement when the number of raters is greater than two.

log-rank test: a nonparametric statistical test to compare two or more samples involving censored data.

Gehan–Breslow–Wilcoxon test: a nonparametric statistical test to compare survival distribution from two samples.

Gray's test: a common method for testing for differences in the cumulative incidences (subdistribution hazards) between two or more groups with competing risks.

Breslow's method: an approach to handling ties in time-to-event data.

Bonferroni correction: a method for adjusting results from multiple independent statistical tests.

Holm–Bonferroni "step-down" method: a modification of the Bonferroni correction that deals with familywise error rates (FWERs) for the multiple testing problem.

Cronbach's α: a measure of the reliability of a composite score.

regression model: statistical model intended to identify a parametric, functional form that represents the true relationship between a dependent variable or end point and a set of explanatory variables.

maximum likelihood estimation (MLE): a general technique to identify the values of model parameters with the greatest likelihood to give rise to the observed set of data, along with estimates of the uncertainty surrounding each parameter estimate.

model specification: delineation of the precise statistical model to be used, the dependent variable, the set of explanatory variables to be included in the model, and the hypothesized error structure.

mean centering: a data transformation done to facilitate interpretation of model output, to take out the effects of scaling variables to different units of measurement.

normalization: a data transformation done to facilitate interpretation of model output, to take out the effects of scaling variables to different units of measurement.

top-down approach: statistical modeling technique which starts with available explanatory variables and systematically excludes insignificant contributors to the model.

bottom-up approach: statistical modeling technique initially specified based on a scientific rationale, then sequentially augmented with additional variables that are observed to enhance the model.

least absolute shrinkage and selection operator (LASSO): an advanced technique to assist in variable selection in modeling.

least angle regression: an advanced technique to assist in variable selection in modeling.

confounding variables (confounders): measurable variables that are correlated with both the primary outcome and the explanatory variable of interest.

instrumental variables: variables that are correlated with unmeasured confounders, but are assumed to be independent of the error term in the model.

propensity scores: a modeling technique to adjust for confounding.

interaction terms: terms included in a model when effects of one predictor could vary in the presence of another.

bias–variance trade-off: relationship stating that for any given level of total error, as a model becomes less biased, the variance will increase, and vice versa.

overfitting: supplying a statistical model with too many explanatory variables.

Akaike information criterion (AIC): an index used to assess model fit and compare models.

Bayesian information criterion (BIC): an index used to assess model fit and compare models.

Harrell's C-index: a measure of goodness of fit often in evaluating the performance of binary predictive models.

goodness of fit: describes how well a statistical model handles the variables and data used.

Hosmer–Lemeshow test: a test of goodness of fit which tests model agreement/calibration.

internal validation: the process of ensuring that a model performs well within the sample from which it was derived.

external validation: the process of testing the performance of a proposed model on an independent dataset that was not used to generate the parameter estimates.

"bootstrap" sampling: validation method that uses replacement to generate separate datasets for training and testing.

leave-one-out cross-validation (LOOCV): a routine commonly used for model training and testing; especially useful in small, potentially skewed datasets that are limited by outliers or fewer number of events.

leave-multiple-out cross-validation (LMOCV): a routine commonly used for model training and testing; especially useful in small, potentially skewed datasets that are limited by outliers or fewer number of events.

jackknife: a routine commonly used for model training and testing; especially useful in small, potentially skewed datasets that are limited by outliers or fewer number of events.

K-fold cross-validation: a routine commonly used for model training and testing; especially useful in small, potentially skewed datasets that are limited by outliers or fewer number of events.

fixed effects model: model in which the errors are constant across values of a factor, such that the group means are fixed (nonrandom) values across the sample and all possible values or levels of a factor are represented.

random effects model: model in which the errors vary according to different values of a factor, the group means are considered to be random, and the observed values of the factor represent only a sample of its possible values.

mixed effects model (mixed model): model that combines both fixed and random effects.

mean imputation: the simplest method by which to impute missing values by the mean of the observed values.

regression imputation: method of handling missing observations that involves imputing missing values using complete observations to predict the missing observations via a regression equation.

multiple imputation: a statistical technique for dealing with incomplete datasets that include missing values.

likelihood: a conditional probability that is a function of a parameter and a random variable.

rate: a reference to a timescale.

risk: the probability of an event occurrence.

REFERENCES

1. Glantz SA. *Primer of Biostatistics*. New York, NY: McGraw Hill Professional; 2012.
2. Peto R. Rank tests of maximal power against Lehmann-type alternatives. *Biometrika*. 1972;59(2):472–475. doi:10.1093/biomet/59.2.472
3. Lagakos SW. The challenge of subgroup analyses–reporting without distorting. *N Engl J Med*. 2006;354(16):1667–1669. doi:10.1056/NEJMp068070
4. Green S, Benedetti J, Smith A, Crowley J. *Clinical Trials in Oncology*. Boca Raton, FL: Chapman and Hall/CRC; 2010.
5. Pintilie M. *Competing Risks: A Practical Perspective*. Chichester, UK: John Wiley & Sons; 2006.
6. Casella G, Berger RL. *Statistical Inference*, 2nd ed. Pacific Grove, CA: Duxbury; 2002.
7. Rao C. *Linear Statistical Inference and Its Applications*, 2nd ed. New York, NY: Wiley; 1973.
8. Gibbons JD, Subhabrata C. Nonparametric statistical inference. In: Lovric M, ed. *International Encyclopedia of Statistical Science*. Heidelberg, Berlin: Springer; 2011:977–979.
9. Lehmann EL, Casella G. *Theory of Point Estimation*. New York, NY: Springer Science & Business Media; 2006.
10. Lehmann EL, Joseph PR. *Testing Statistical Hypotheses*. New York, NY: Springer Science & Business Media; 2006.

12

Statistical Modeling for Clinical Cancer Research

SANJAY ANEJA ■ JAMES B. YU

The previous chapter described how to detect significant differences that may exist between single variables within different groups of data. An important limitation of these analyses in general is the inability to account for potential confounding variables (confounders). **Confounders** are variables outside the study variable, which are associated with the study variable and also predict the outcome of interest (see also Chapter 13). Statistical models are useful if one is interested in investigating the relationship between variables for assessment of association and for prediction.

An example of a common confounding variable on clinical outcomes within oncology is age. Understandably, older patients have higher mortality rates. Employing statistical models, however, can allow one to adjust for the confounding effect of increased age on survival to estimate the efficacy of clinical interventions on mortality more accurately. In this way, statistical models also provide the added benefit of assessing the relationship among a set of multiple variables on investigational outcomes.

This chapter first briefly outlines a common research question that could be effectively solved using a statistical model. We then discuss mathematical modeling and give context to the importance of mathematical models in oncology research. We demonstrate how posing research questions in different ways may alter the ideal modeling technique, and how to choose the most appropriate technique to best fit your research question.

Although there are innumerable modeling techniques that can feasibly be applied to oncologic data, this chapter focuses on techniques most commonly used to model structured, low-dimensional, time-independent, uncensored data. Time series methods are not addressed in depth in this book, but techniques for conducting time-to-event analysis on censored data (Chapter 16) and for modeling high-dimensional unstructured data (Chapter 17) are discussed later. The main focus of this chapter is the most common family of modeling techniques employed in oncology research, namely regression algorithms. We describe **linear regression**, which is the fundamental regression technique in statistics. We describe how to employ simple linear regression, transformations, and multivariable regression. Although this is an introduction to only one common mathematical modeling technique within oncology research, the techniques described are applicable to several other more advanced regression techniques.

STATISTICAL MODELING

Statistical models are important tools across multiple scientific disciplines. The broadest definition of a statistical model is a set of mathematical expressions that attempt to simplify real-world phenomena with hopes of exposing important aspects of reality. The important aspects which statistical models attempt to describe are often the underlying mechanism behind a process, or surrogate variables which can be used to help us predict or forecast a process.

Arguably, statistical models are a form of empiric mathematical models (vs. mechanistic models). Empiric models are those that attempt to use available information to predict a process and guide behavior. An example of an empiric model within oncology is a nomogram that utilizes clinical variables to predict risk of metastasis. In contrast to mechanistic models, which focus on the true drivers of the outcome of interest, empiric models are more concerned about the ability of the model to predict reality regardless of inputs. This is an important distinction, because mechanistic models can reveal causal relationships between variables and outcomes, whereas empiric models more conservatively find associative ones.

Statistical models have an important place in clinical cancer research. They can both reduce bias and increase the flexibility of clinical data to answer unique clinical questions. Statistical models are one of the primary methods for bias reduction when comparing groups of patients. Specifically, such models are necessary for observational studies, where treatment groups cannot be randomized or equally balanced with respect to potential confounders. Similarly, statistical models often identify the extent to which covariates affect study outcomes, and provide context to interpret the effect of variables of interest. For example, if the stage of cancer affects outcomes, one could argue that increased research into screening may be warranted. Additionally, statistical models allow for variance reduction caused by known confounding variables, to better appreciate the relationship between experimental variables and the outcome of interest. Models also can be used to induce equivalence in comparison groups within randomized clinical studies. Although randomization theoretically induces equivalence, in practice minor imbalances may require statistical adjustment. Last, statistical models allow us to ascertain the applicability of results to specific subpopulations. For example, testing for statistically significant interactions between a treatment effect and gender would shed light on whether a treatment could be applicable to both men and women.

We center our discussion of statistical models on linear regression, an extremely powerful method for statistical modeling. We illustrate the utility of different regression algorithms with an example pertaining to breast mammography and cancer outcomes. We discuss the different regression techniques that can be used to model different types of outcome variables.

SAMPLE RESEARCH QUESTION

Suppose we are interested in understanding the relationship between mammographic tumor size and pathologic tumor size for patients diagnosed with early-stage invasive breast cancer. We were given a data set of 300 diagnostic mammograms with tumor size estimates made by diagnostic radiologists and subsequent pathologic tumor sizes for the same lesions after surgical resection. For the sake of simplicity, let us assume that surgical resection occurred immediately after diagnostic mammography, all surgeries resulted in complete resection, and that tumor size is simply measured as the largest diameter of the tumor.

This research question highlights the pragmatic benefit of regression techniques compared to the hypothesis testing techniques discussed in previous chapters. Although hypothesis testing could tell a researcher whether or not an association existed between radiographic and pathologic breast tumor size, there was limited information on the nature of that relationship that could be employed in practice. In this type of problem, researchers may be interested not only in the association between radiographic tumor size and pathologic tumor size, but also in predicting pathologic tumor size from radiographic measurements.

When specifying regression models, one variable is usually taken to be the dependent variable and the remaining variables are considered the independent (explanatory) variables. The independent variables are used to predict or explain the dependent variables. In our example, radiographic tumor size is the independent variable and pathologic tumor size is the dependent variable. A representation of the data is in Table 12.1.

Choosing the best regression technique depends primarily on the nature of the dependent variable and how it is distributed. In our current example, the dependent variable (pathologic tumor diameter) is continuous, meaning the variable theoretically has an uncountable and infinite number of values. To characterize the distribution of the variable, we can create a histogram of the dependent variable values, to identify whether or not the outcome variable appears normally distributed. A histogram of the data is seen in Figure 12.1. The data appear to be normally distributed. If we were unsure whether the dependent variable was normally distributed, we could employ statistical tests to assess for normality, such as the **Shapiro–Wilk test** or **Anderson–Darling test** (see Chapter 11).

ORDINARY LEAST SQUARES (LINEAR) REGRESSION

For a normally distributed continuous dependent variable, linear regression is often the most effective modeling technique. In **ordinary least squares (OLS)** regression, the model describes the

TABLE 12.1 MAMMOGRAPHIC TUMOR DIAMETER AND PATHOLOGIC TUMOR DIAMETER

Patient ID	Mammographic Tumor Diameter (cm)	Pathologic Tumor Diameter (cm)
1	1.00	1.05
2	2.50	2.45
3	3.00	3.12
4	1.31	1.41
5	1.21	1.11
6	1.67	1.78
7	6.30	6.22
8	4.50	4.51
9	2.00	2.02
10	1.10	1.19
299	2.10	1.95
300	2.00	2.15

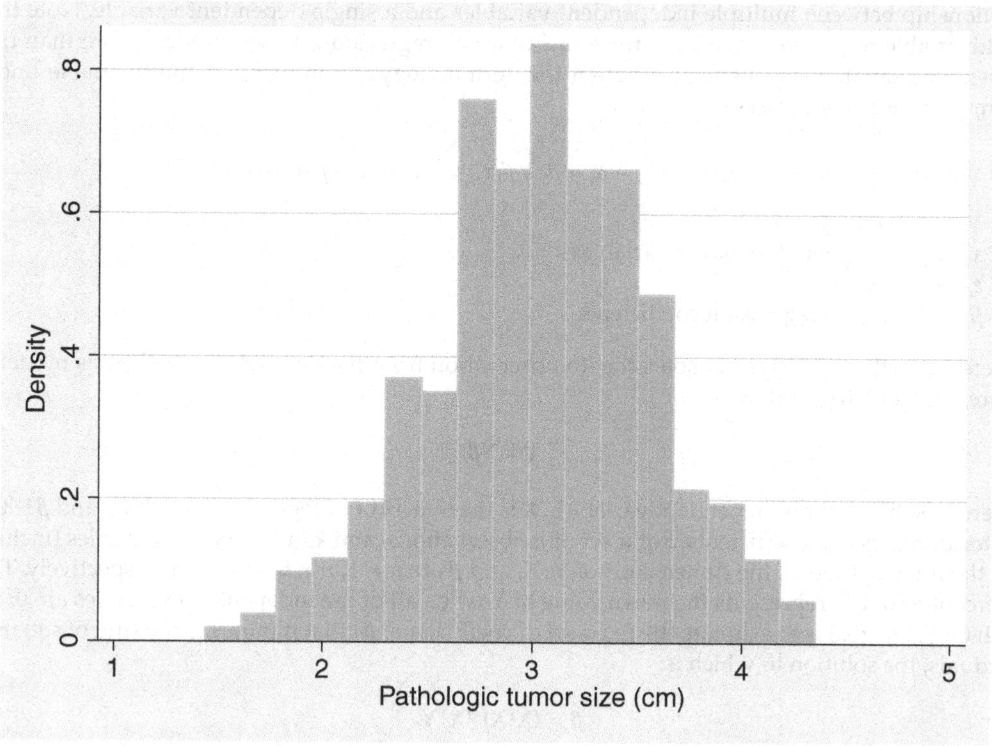

FIGURE 12.1 Distribution of pathologic tumor size.

mean of the normally distributed dependent variable as a function of the explanatory or independent variable(s). Formally this equation is noted as:

$$Y_i = \beta_0 + \beta_1 x_i + \varepsilon_i$$

Y_i = dependent variable
x_i = independent variable
ε_i = error term
β_0 and β_1= regression coefficients.

The subscript i denotes the ith observation from the data set. Note that the term *linear* refers to this functional relationship being linear in the regression coefficients (i.e., the parameters β_0 and β_1). The objective of OLS regression is to identify fixed estimates of β_0 and β_1 ($\widehat{\beta_0}$ and $\widehat{\beta_1}$, respectively) that minimize the function:

$$\Sigma\varepsilon_i^2 = \Sigma(Y_i - \beta_0 - \beta_1 x_i)^2$$

with respect to β_0 and β_1. That is, for a given set of observed explanatory (x_i) and dependent (Y_i) variables, we want to find the set of regression coefficients defining a line that minimizes the overall sum of squared errors, or residuals (i.e., deviations from the line). The solution (given in matrix form in the following) provides the best linear unbiased estimator of the effect of x on Y.

MULTIPLE (MULTIVARIABLE) LINEAR REGRESSION

OLS regression models the simple relationship between a singular independent variable and dependent variable, limiting its application in clinical practice. **Multiple linear** or **multilinear** regression (often called multivariable linear regression) extends the OLS model to explain the relationship between multiple independent variables and a single dependent variable. Note that multivariable regression is distinct from **multivariate regression**, which models more than one dependent variable simultaneously; often this terminology is confusing. A multivariable linear regression model is expressed as:

$$Y_i = \beta_0 + \beta_1 x_{1i} + \beta_2 x_{2i} + \ldots + \beta_n x_{ki} + \varepsilon_i$$

Y_i = dependent variable
$x_{1i}, x_{2i}, \ldots, x_{ki}$ = independent variables
ε_i = error term
$\beta_0, \beta_1, \ldots, \beta_n$ = regression coefficients,

where again the subscript i denotes the ith observation from the data set. Typically, this model is expressed in matrix notation:

$$\mathbf{Y} = \mathbf{X}\boldsymbol{\beta},$$

where **Y** is the vector of dependent variables, **X** is the matrix of independent variables, and $\boldsymbol{\beta}$ is the vector of regression coefficients. For a set of n observations, and k independent variables (including the intercept term), the dimensions of **Y**, **X**, and $\boldsymbol{\beta}$ are $n \times 1$, $n \times k$, and $k \times 1$, respectively. The intercept term (β_0) represents the mean value of **Y** when all of the independent variables are 0. As with OLS, the goal is to estimate the fixed set of coefficients ($\hat{\boldsymbol{\beta}}$) that minimizes the sum of squared residuals, the solution to which is:

$$\hat{\boldsymbol{\beta}} = (\mathbf{X}^T\mathbf{X})^{-1}\mathbf{X}^T\mathbf{Y}.$$

This set of coefficients defines a hyperplane (n-dimensional plane) describing the relationship between the dependent and independent variables. A common goal in clinical cancer research, as discussed in Chapter 13, is to measure the effect of a particular variable of interest on a particular outcome of interest, while controlling for other independent variables that might also be affecting the outcome. The value of the corresponding regression coefficient (and its standard error) provides an estimate (and degree of certainty around this estimate) of the amount the dependent variable will change in response to a unit change in the independent variable of interest.

ASSUMPTIONS OF LINEAR REGRESSION

Before we proceed to solving our research problem, it is important to understand the specific assumptions and limitations of linear regression.

LINEARITY

The first assumption is that a linear relationship exists between the independent and dependent variables, meaning the change in the dependent variable is constant with respect to increasing values of the independent variable. This can be assessed graphically using scatterplots or a plot of residuals versus predicted values. Later, we discuss techniques to model nonlinear relationships among data.

NORMALITY

An assumption of linear regression is that the residual values are normally distributed. This assumption can be assessed qualitatively by visually examining histograms (as seen earlier), or quantitatively using the Shapiro–Wilk or Anderson–Darling test. The null hypothesis in these latter tests is that the random variable of interest is drawn from a normal distribution. A rejection of the null hypothesis is evidence that the variable is not normally distributed.

COLLINEARITY

Multiple linear regression assumes that the independent variables are not too highly correlated. This can be tested using a variety of different methods, including a correlation matrix, variance inflation factors, or tolerance testing. This becomes more important when performing multivariable regression using a large number of covariates. We discuss this in more detail in the last section of the chapter.

AUTOCORRELATION

Linear regression assumes that there is no autocorrelation among dependent and independent variables. Autocorrelation can be assessed graphically using a **correlogram** or **autocorrelation plot**, or quantitatively using the **Durbin–Watson test**. Autocorrelation is often seen in time-dependent data, where the value of the dependent variable is related to its (lagged) value from previous time points. An example of this would be a research question looking at the relationship between tumor size and time, where the current tumor size is not independent of the previous tumor size. Techniques for handling autocorrelated data, such as time series analysis (e.g., autoregressive and moving average models) are discussed briefly in Chapter 11.

HOMOSCEDASTICITY

Homoscedasticity assumes that the random variations in the relationship between the independent and dependent variables are relatively stable for all values. This intuitively is thought of as a lack of variation in scatter of the data across a set of predictor variables. An example of potentially heteroscedastic data would be a set of primary care visits stratified by age. During childhood, individuals typically visit primary care physicians in a standard frequency because of required vaccinations and school-related physicals; however, in adulthood there likely is a larger variation in the number of primary care visits based on patient preference and overall health status. Homoscedasticity can be assessed using scatterplots or more formally by the **Breusch–Pagan test**.

EXAMPLE: OLS REGRESSION

First, we generate a scatterplot of the data (Figure 12.2). A scatterplot can help ensure that the data are distributed in a relatively linear fashion and satisfy the assumption of homoscedasticity. If the scattered data appeared to follow an exponential rather than a linear pattern, we would want to investigate alternative regression models or data transformation techniques; these are discussed later in this chapter and elsewhere in the book.

The regression coefficients quantify the relationship between our dependent variable and independent variables. As discussed previously, β_0 represents the (potentially hypothetical) mean value of the dependent variable when the independent variables are 0. In our example, β_0 represents the mean pathologic tumor size when the mammographic tumor size is 0 cm. In some cases, one may want this value to remain fixed (i.e., to fit a no-intercept model), rather than estimated. For example, in theory, if there is no tumor, then both the mammographic and pathologic tumor sizes should be 0, implying that $\beta_0 = 0$. In this case, we might only want to study the true correspondence between these two values starting from this objective point.

However, in reality, the limits of mammographic detection imply that some tumors will achieve a certain pathologic size before reaching the point of mammographic detection; we may want to estimate what this point is. So, when taking a sample of patients known to have the disease, we can define a model in which the true pathologic value may be greater than 0, even when the mammographic size is 0. This raises another point, which is that the linear model can still be valid, even if its assumptions only hold over a finite domain defined by the independent variable(s). For example, negative values of mammographic size are nonsensical, yet are

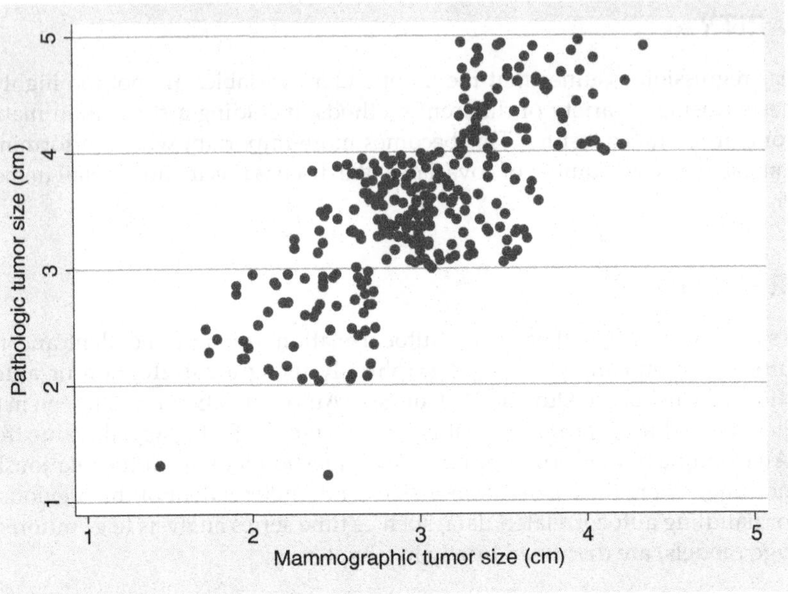

FIGURE 12.2 Scatterplot of pathologic tumor size (dependent variable) vs. mammographic tumor size (independent variable).

theoretically accommodated within an OLS model. It is a good idea, therefore, to make sure the resulting range of the dependent variable also makes sense. If the estimate of β_0 happened to be negative, for example, this would not make sense and would call into question the model's validity. In this case, one should consider either a no-intercept model, or transforming to the logarithm scale (log transformations are often helpful when dealing with variables that are strictly positive).

In regression modeling, the value of β_1 is often of greatest interest, representing the relative change in the mean of the dependent variable associated with a unit change in our primary independent variable. In our example, β_1 represents the change in the mean pathologic tumor size associated with a 1 cm increase in mammographic tumor size. A positive regression coefficient would suggest a relative increase compared to mammographic tumor size and a negative regression coefficient would suggest a relative decrease in mammographic tumor size.

Clinical cancer researchers typically use statistical software packages, such as SAS (JMP), STATA, or R to generate regression output. In our example, we can see the output of our linear regression analysis, with estimated regression coefficients β_0 = 0.455 and β_1 = 1.02 (Table 12.2; Figure 12.3). Additionally, we see that a graphical representation of our linear regression equation overlaid on the scatterplot confirms that the parameters make sense. The output suggests, as we might expect, that once reaching a threshold pathologic size of about 0.45 cm, there is roughly a one-to-one correspondence between change in mammographic and pathologic tumor size. Practically, we can use the equation generated from our linear regression to predict the expected pathologic size for a given mammographic size:

$$\text{Mean pathologic tumor size} = 1.02 * (\text{mammographic tumor size}) + 0.455.$$

Another important step in our analysis is to examine the uncertainty surrounding our estimated slope ($\widehat{\beta_1}$) and intercept ($\widehat{\beta_0}$), which is represented by their standard errors: 0.529 and 0.163, respectively (Table 12.2). Specifically, we can test for the independence between pathologic and mammographic tumor size and for the presence of a nonzero y-intercept. Intuitively, we understand that if the mammographic and pathologic tumor size were independent of one another, changes in mammographic tumor size would have no effect on pathologic tumor size, so the

TABLE 12.2 LINEAR REGRESSION OUTPUT FOR EXAMPLE CASE

Source	SS	df	MS		
Model	82.6597107	1	82.6597107		
Residual	66.3175607	298	.22254215		
	Coefficient Estimate	**Standard Error**	**t-Statistic**	***p* Value**	**95% Confidence Interval**
β_1 (mammographic)	1.018947	.0528702	19.27	0.000	1.0149009, 1.122993
β_0 (intercept)	.454708	.1625459	2.80	0.005	.1348249, .7745912

regression coefficient β_1 would be 0. Moreover, if mammography were a perfect instrument with no lower bound for tumor detection, the regression coefficient β_0 would also be 0. Similar to one-sample problems described in earlier chapters, we can perform pairwise *t*-tests of the null hypotheses H_0: $\beta_1 = 0$ and H_0: $\beta_0 = 0$. The *t*-statistics are calculated by dividing the respective coefficient estimate by its standard error and then comparing it to critical values of the *t*-distribution with $n - k = 300 - 2 = 298$ degrees of freedom. A statistically significant result was found for both tests (Table 12.2), indicating the presence of a positive association between mammographic tumor size and pathologic tumor size, and a significant nonzero threshold for mammographic detection.

DATA TRANSFORMATION

Often the residuals do not satisfy the assumption of normality, or the relationship between independent and dependent variables does not satisfy the assumption of linearity. When dealing

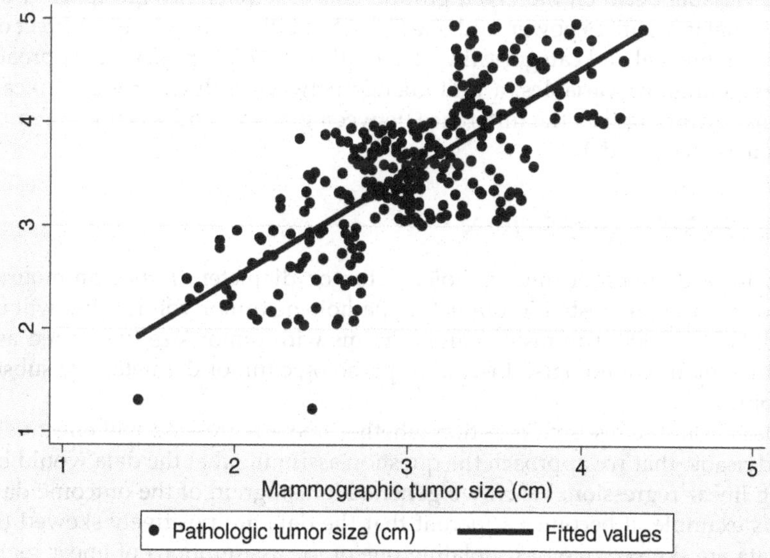

FIGURE 12.3 Linear regression analysis: scatterplot with regression line overlain.

with complex biological and clinical data, it becomes important to increase the flexibility of our regression methods. One common method to satisfy the assumption of linearity and normality is through transformation of the data. There is a variety of different data transforms that statisticians can employ to help normalize data.

The most widely employed technique is the log transformation (i.e., base e logarithm). Log-transforming one or more variables is often justified theoretically—for example, if the dependent variable is known to change exponentially with a given variable of interest. Scientific knowledge of the relationships one expects to observe can thus help one anticipate necessary data transformations and specify a better regression model. Log-linear (log-lin), **lin-log**, and **log-log** models refer to generalized linear modeling approaches that involve a log transformation of the dependent variable, independent variable of interest, or both, respectively.

Other transformations that are less often used are square root transformations, square transformation, and reciprocal transformations. One particularly useful method is the Box–Cox transformation:

$$\tau(x;\lambda) = \begin{cases} \dfrac{x^{\lambda}-1}{y}, \lambda \neq 0 \\ \ln(x), \lambda = 0 \end{cases}$$

where λ is a fitted parameter. This transformation has been used, for example, to model radiation effects on bone marrow for patients undergoing chemotherapy and radiation (1). This transformation is particularly useful for handling data that have zeros and negative values, as the logarithm function is defined only for positive values. Note that the log transformation is a special case where the Box–Cox parameter is 0.

Another method to consider when handling non-normally distributed data is to create **dummy variables.** Dummy variables are binary (0 or 1) indicators of the presence or absence of a certain condition. Often it is advisable to group ordinal variables, like stage and grade, or categorical variables, like race and disease site, into dummy categories. For example, one could create dummy variables indicating stage I–II versus stage III–IV, or define several levels of grouping, such as grade 3 (yes/no) versus grade 2 (yes/no) versus grade 1 (yes/no). In a regression model, for a variable with g potential groups, one would define $g - 1$ dummy variables, with the omitted category serving as the reference group. An advantage of using dummy variables is their ease of interpretation in regression output, as the effect corresponds to the difference in mean values of the dependent variable between the given group versus the reference group. A disadvantage of this approach is that it sacrifices power, and one loses the ability to measure the effect of gradations in the variable. For ordinal and categorical variables, this is often a preferable approach, however, because unlike continuous variables, a unit change between ordinal groups typically does not have any intrinsic meaning (i.e., the difference between grades 1 and 2 is not the same as the difference between grades 2 and 3).

SAMPLE RESEARCH QUESTION

Suppose that, instead of predicting pathologic tumor diameter from mammographic tumor diameter, we were more interested in predicting pathologic tumor volume. We will use the same hypothetical data set of 300 diagnostic mammograms with tumor size (measured as by greatest diameter) defined by the radiologist. Instead of pathologic tumor diameter, we substitute pathologic tumor volume.

It is not clear from the research question whether linear regression will effectively model the data, so it is advisable that we approach the question assuming that the data would be effectively modeled using linear regression. When we generate a histogram of the outcome data as we did in the previous example, it becomes apparent that the data are positively skewed (Figure 12.4). Because the data are skewed, we risk violating one of the assumptions of linear regression mentioned previously. This highlights the importance of developing a methodical approach to regression problems, which does not assume a de facto ideal regression technique.

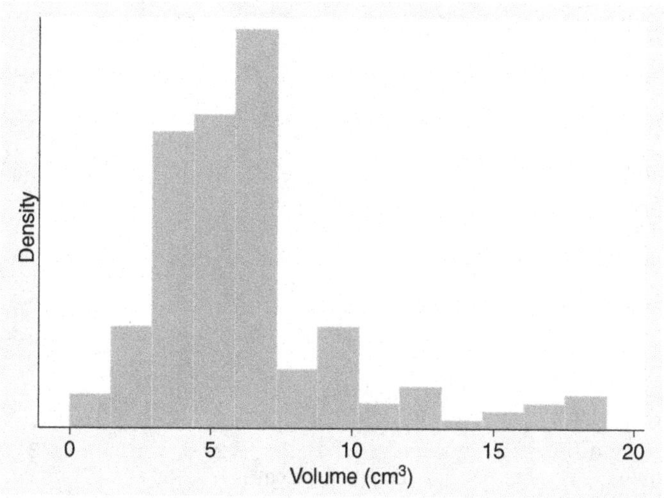

FIGURE 12.4 Histogram of pathologic tumor volume.

Ideally, we would like the distribution of our outcome variable to mimic our previous example. The solution is to transform the outcome data by applying a similar function across all values. Nevertheless, it is recommended that one evaluate different types in order to find the best approximation of the outcome data to normality. More importantly, it is necessary to identify situations in which one would employ data transformation. Transformation often allows us to achieve linearity (for subsequent linear regression), homogeneity of variance, and normality (of skewed data). Note also that one can transform both the dependent and independent variable(s), if necessary; these are still linear models, because they are a linear function of the parameters.

In our example, when we do a log transformation of the pathologic tumor volume for our 300 patients and generate a histogram, we see that the distribution of the log(pathologic tumor volume) appears to be more normal (Figure 12.5). Although linear regression with untransformed data may reveal statistically significant results and possibly identify similar relationships between the two variables, log transformation of the data will generate a more accurate model for estimation, given our assumptions.

After the data undergo log transformation, the process of developing a regression model mirrors our previous example of linear regression. The major difference is in the interpretation of the coefficients from the regression model. In our previous example, the coefficients of the regression provided easily interpretable relationships between our dependent and independent variables. In a transformed regression, however, it is important to remain cognizant that the coefficients generated describe the relationship between the (transformed) independent variables and the (transformed) dependent variables.

Depending on the complexity of the transformation, the interpretation of the coefficients may become increasingly difficult. For example, the coefficients generated from our log-transformed regression represent the relationship between mammographic tumor size and the log(pathologic tumor volume):

$$\log(Y_i) = \beta_0 + \beta_1 x_i + \varepsilon_i$$

$$Y_i = \exp(\beta_0 + \beta_1 x_i + \varepsilon_i)$$

$$Y_i = e^{\beta_0}\ e^{\beta_1 x_i} e^{\varepsilon_i}$$

$$Y_i = e^{\beta_0}\ e^{\varepsilon_i}\ (e^{x_i})^{\beta_1}.$$

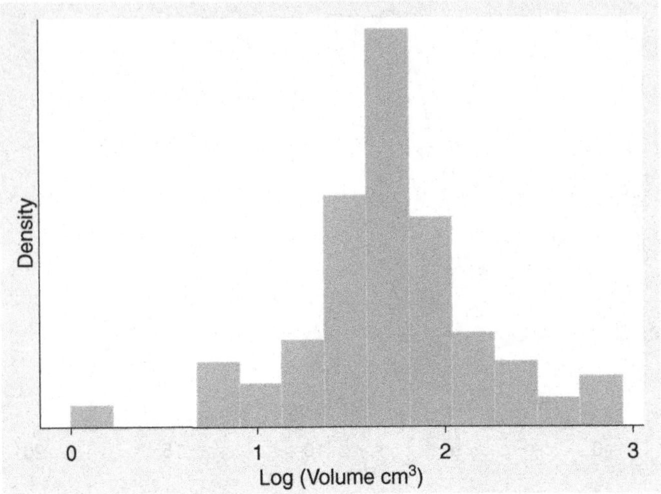

FIGURE 12.5 Histogram of log-transformed pathologic tumor volume.

So, for the log-linear model, the error and intercept terms are multiplicative rather than additive, and the primary effect (i.e., the coefficient β_1) is a power of the exponentiated independent variable. In the log-log model, β_1 is a power of the independent variable:

$$\log(Y_i) = \beta_0 + \beta_1 \log(x_i) + \varepsilon_i$$

$$Y_i = \exp(\beta_0 + \beta_1 \log(x_i) + \varepsilon_i)$$

$$Y_i = e^{\beta_0}\ e^{\beta_1 \log(x_i)} e^{\varepsilon_i}$$

$$Y_i = e^{\beta_0}\ e^{\varepsilon_i}\ (e^{\log(x_i)})^{\beta_1}$$

$$Y_i = e^{\beta_0}\ e^{\varepsilon_i}\ (x_i)^{\beta_1}.$$

In this context, β_1 is called the elasticity of the regression function.

It is important to keep in mind the nature of your research question and the ultimate goal of your model in order to balance interpretability and accuracy. If one is interested in identifying relationships between variables and is less concerned with accuracy, interpretability might be of greater importance than accuracy. In our example, if we were more interested in understanding whether there was a relationship between mammographic tumor size and pathologic tumor volume, we might decide that a more interpretable transformation is preferred. However, if we were more interested in getting the most accurate tumor volume predictions, then the ideal transformation should be chosen without considering interpretability.

EXAMPLE: MULTIVARIABLE REGRESSION

In our initial linear regression example, we modeled the relationship between mammographic tumor size (diameter) and pathologic tumor size (diameter). Multivariable regression would be useful if in addition to mammographic tumor size we had information which we felt would improve our ability to model pathologic tumor size. For the next example, we will assume that in addition to mammographic tumor size, we also have demographic data including patient age and race.

Given the increasingly large amount of data available within oncology, multivariable regression is a cornerstone of clinical oncology research. Similar to our previous examples, one must first identify the ideal regression model to employ. Given that linear regression was effective at modeling the relationship between mammographic tumor size and pathologic tumor size in a "univariable" regression, we will employ a similar approach to multivariable linear regression.

There are a number of different variations of multivariable regression. A majority of the differences can be attributed to the criteria used to select covariates to include in the model. One of the more widely used multivariable regression techniques is **stepwise regression**. This approach is often useful when faced with a large number of possible independent variables and we wish to identify the subset of variables that relate significantly to the dependent variable of interest (outcome). Compared to our previous example of linear regression, where we were interested in identifying the correct mathematical equation to model the relationship between a dependent and an independent variable, the multivariable case introduces the additional complexity due to the plurality of independent variables. In addition to identifying the correct mathematical equation to model the relationship between independent and dependent variables, we first must identify which subset of dependent variables should be included in the model.

In stepwise regression, one adds and removes significant factors individually into the regression model in an order of relative importance. Significance of factors is determined using two univariate probability cutoffs. The first is an exclusion probability (P_e), which specifies the baseline significance required for inclusion in the stepwise regression process. The second is a removal probability (P_r), which specifies the significance required to prevent removal from the stepwise model once a variable is included. Although P_e and P_r can often be the same number (e.g., $p = .05$), often P_e is made larger to prevent the accidental exclusion of significant factors (e.g., $P_e = .15$ or .20). Occasionally, more liberal cutoffs for P_r are also recommended.

Forward selected stepwise regression and backward selected stepwise regression are two variations of stepwise regression often seen in oncology research. Forward selected stepwise regression involves starting with an empty regression model. Variables with univariable probabilities $>P_e$ are removed from the analysis. The remaining independent variables are ranked according to their univariable probability cutoffs with respect to the dependent variable. The independent variable that is most significant (lowest P value) is entered into the regression model first. During each iteration, the most significant of the remaining independent variables is included in the regression model and statistical significance is recalculated. At the completion of each iteration, variables in the model with probabilities $>P_r$ are removed prior to the next iteration.

Backward selected stepwise regression begins in a similar fashion to forward selected stepwise regression. First, variables with univariate probabilities $>P_e$ are removed from the analysis. Unlike forward selection, backward selected stepwise regression begins with a full regression model with all candidate factors for which univariable probabilities $<P_e$. Rather than adding additional variables with each iteration, backward selected stepwise regression involves removing variables in the model with probabilities $>P_r$ until all variables within the model have a probability $<P_r$. One theoretical advantage of backward selected stepwise regression is the potential for fewer iterations during model development. Given that most statistical analyses are done using high-speed computer processors, this has little practical importance. The differences in methods between forward and backward stepwise regression can be seen in Table 12.3.

Although our discussion has focused on linear regression, the multivariable selection techniques described previously can be applied across many more advanced regression types. There are a few practical considerations one must consider, however, when fitting a multivariable regression model. At first glance it may appear that including numerous variables in a regression model would be beneficial. However, including unnecessary variables in a model can reduce statistical efficiency and produce regression terms with large standard errors. It also has a greater chance of identifying spurious associations with variables that are not truly important to the model. For this reason, we often recommend construction of the most **parsimonious model**, which includes only the most important and statistically significant covariates, preferably with a strong scientific rationale for inclusion in the model.

Missing data can also affect regression calculations. In more complex multivariable regressions with numerous covariates, there is an increased likelihood of having missing data for some

TABLE 12.3 FORWARD AND BACKWARD SELECTED STEPWISE REGRESSION PROCEDURES

Forward Selected	Backward Selected
1. Determine P_r and P_e 2. Remove variables from analysis where $p > P_e$ on univariate analysis 3. Begin with empty model 4. Add most significant variable among covariates and estimate probabilities 5. Add second most significant variable among covariates and estimate probabilities 6. Among included variables if estimated probabilities $>P_r$, then remove from analysis 7. Repeat steps 4–6 until all included variables have estimated probabilities $<P_r$	1. Determine P_r and P_e 2. Remove variables from analysis where $p > P_e$ on univariate analysis 3. Begin with full model with all remaining variables and estimate probabilities 4. Among included variables if estimated probabilities $>P_r$, then remove from analysis and reestimate probabilities 5. Repeat step 4 until all included variables have estimated probabilities $<P_r$

or all of the covariates. Most statistical packages will automatically drop any individuals who have a missing value for any of the data points included in the model, sometimes without warning. Because regression estimates cannot be calculated unless data are present for all covariates, using data sets with large amounts of missing data could result in significant selection bias. Thus, particular care in handling missing data needs to be taken when conducting large multivariable regressions. In these situations, we recommend limiting the regression to covariates for which there is not a significant amount of missing data (though this can risk biasing the model), or employing more advanced imputation techniques to account for missing data.

Multicollinearity is another common issue when completing multivariate regression. When two covariates are highly collinear, there is a risk of overfitting the multivariable regression, leading to inefficiency in the model. An example of two collinear variables are waist size and percentage body fat. If one were to control for both effects in a multivariable regression model, it would be difficult to know which of the two variables was contributing to the outcome.

One final consideration for any statistical modeling is that of an **interaction**. When two variables "interact," it means that they together have more-than-additive effects, that is, the primary effect of interest differs in the presence or absence of a certain condition. Colloquial terms could be *synergy* or *antagonism*. For example, let us consider the impact of both the size of a tumor and its grade on the likelihood that the tumor will recur after treatment. Let us assume that the greater the size of a tumor, the more likely it is that a cancer will recur. What if we also learn that for each increased grade of tumor (for example, going from grade 1 to grade 2), there is also a likelihood of recurrence? An example of a positive interaction would be that the impact of tumor size was *greater* for each increase in grade. In other words, a tumor increasing from 1 to 2 cm was much more risky if a tumor was a higher grade compared to a lower grade. An example of a negative interaction would be if the impact of tumor size was less or opposite for each increase in grade; for example, if for grade 1 tumors larger tumors were more likely to be cured, compared to smaller tumors for grade 4.

Interactions are important to test, as they can reveal important insights as to the interconnectedness of variables. Practically, interactions can be tested empirically (i.e., between variables that are of clinical interest or are suspected to interact based on clinical knowledge), or interactions can be hinted at if regression coefficients change sign or magnitude to a large degree during the course of stepwise regression. These interactions can be tested formally using statistical software. Interaction terms can be added to a statistical model by creating a new variable that is the product of the two variables being interacted (this is often easier to implement using dummy variables). Care must be taken in interpreting the model coefficients, however, as the effects of both the variable of interest and its interaction term must be added together to interpret the overall effect. This issue receives further attention later in the book when we discuss clinical trials.

CONCLUSION

In this chapter we introduced linear regression modeling, a fundamental technique in oncology research. Although our discussion focused primarily on OLS and multivariable linear regression, the techniques described are applicable for other regression models, including logistic, Poisson, and binomial regression (see Chapter 13). A list of cancer research studies using various regression models is included in Table 12.4. The span of research questions included highlights the wide applicability of regression across oncology research. For more advanced discussions regarding regression, we recommend several texts (2–5).

TABLE 12.4 ONCOLOGY STUDIES EMPLOYING VARIOUS FORMS OF REGRESSION MODELING

Authors	Cancer Type	Regression Type	Dependent Variable	PMID
Aizer et al.	Glioblastoma	Logistic regression	Omission of radiation	24122361 (6)
Miller et al.	Nonmelanoma skin cancer	Linear regression	Cancer incidence	8176018 (7)
Aneja et al.	Multiple	Negative binomial	Radiation oncologist workforce	21493013 (8)
Rajagopalan et al.	Vaginal cancer	Logistic regression	Receipt of chemoradiation	25281493 (9)
Shi et al.	Breast cancer	Linear regression	Cancer costs	23796402 (10)
Hopman et al.	Multiple	Linear regression	Patient perception survey	24891136 (11)
Lee et al.	Multiple	Linear regression	Job satisfaction	25919702 (12)
Klein et al.	Breast cancer	Linear regression	Oncotype DX Recurrence score	23503643 (13)
Manninen et al.	Leukemia	Logistic regression	AML diagnosis	24023658 (14)
Liang et al.	Multiple	Logistic regression	Genetic biomarkers	23777239 (15)
Lamm et al.	Lung cancer	Logarithmic transform linear regression	Lung cancer risk	26690190 (16)
Fang et al.	Melanoma	Logarithmic transform logistic regression	Disease progression	25779565 (17)
Suppli et al.	Breast cancer	Poisson regression	Antidepressant use	25349294 (18)
Byrne et al.	Multiple	Poisson regression	Clinical trial participation	23897588 (19)

AML, acute myeloid leukemia.

GLOSSARY

confounders: variables outside the study variable, which are associated with the study variable and also predict the outcome of interest

linear regression: a fundamental regression technique in statistics.

Shapiro–Wilk test: a statistical test used to assess for normality.

Anderson–Darling test: a statistical test used to assess for normality.

ordinary least squares (OLS) regression: modeling technique that describes the mean of the normally distributed dependent variable as a function of the explanatory or independent variable(s).

multiple linear (multilinear) regression: statistical procedure that extends the OLS model to explain the relationship between multiple independent variables and a single dependent variable.

multivariate regression: statistical procedure that models more than one dependent variable simultaneously.

correlogram: means of graphically assessing autocorrelation.

autocorrelation plot: means of graphically assessing autocorrelation.

Durbin–Watson test: means of quantitatively assessing autocorrelation..

homoscedasticity: an assumption that the random variations in the relationship between the independent and dependent variables are relatively stable for all values.

Breusch–Pagan test: a means of assessing homoscedasticity.

lin-log: a generalized linear modeling approach that involves a log transformation of the independent variable of interest.

log-log: a generalized linear modeling approach that involves a log transformation of both the dependent variable and the independent variable of interest.

dummy variables: binary (0 or 1) indicators of the presence or absence of a certain condition.

stepwise regression: a multivariable regression technique used when there is a large number of possible independent variables, to identify the subset of variables that relate significantly to the dependent variable of interest (outcome).

parsimonious model: statistical model that includes only the most important and statistically significant covariates.

interaction: results when two variables together have more-than-additive effects.

REFERENCES

1. Mell LK, Schomas DA, Salama JK, et al. Association between bone marrow dosimetric parameters and acute hematologic toxicity in anal cancer patients treated with concurrent chemotherapy and intensity-modulated radiotherapy. *Int J Radiat Oncol Biol Phys*. 2008;70:1431–1437. doi:10.1016/j.ijrobp.2007.08.074
2. Olive D. *Linear Regression*. New York, NY: Springer Science+Business Media; 2017.
3. Tai BC, Machin D. *Regression Methods for Medical Research*. Oxford, UK: John Wiley & Sons; 2013.
4. Rabe-Hesketh S, Everitt, B. *Handbook of Statistical Analyses Using Stata*. 3rd ed. New York, NY: Chapman and Hall/CRC; 2003.
5. Steyerberg EW, Eijkemans MJ, Harrell FE, Jr, Habbema JD. Prognostic modelling with logistic regression analysis: a comparison of selection and estimation methods in small data sets. *Stat Med*. 2000;19(8):1059–1079. doi:10.1002/(SICI)1097-0258(20000430)19:8<1059::AID-SIM412>3.0.CO;2-0

6. Aizer AA, Ancukiewicz M, Nguyen PL, et al. Underutilization of radiation therapy in patients with glioblastoma: predictive factors and outcomes. *Cancer*. 2014;120(2):238–243. doi:10.1002/cncr.28398
7. Miller DL, Weinstock MA. Nonmelanoma skin cancer in the United States: incidence. *J Am Acad Dermatol*. 1994;30(5 Pt 1):774–778. doi:10.1016/S0190-9622(08)81509-5
8. Aneja S, Smith BD, Gross CP, et al. Geographic analysis of the radiation oncology workforce. *Int J Radiat Oncol Biol Phys*. 2012;82(5):1723–1729. doi:10.1016/j.ijrobp.2011.01.070
9. Rajagopalan MS, Xu KM, Lin JF, et al. Adoption and impact of concurrent chemoradiation therapy for vaginal cancer: a National Cancer Data Base (NCDB) study. *Gynecol Oncol*. 2014;135(3):495–502. doi:10.1016/j.ygyno.2014.09.018
10. Shi HY, Chang HT, Culbertson R, et al. Breast cancer surgery volume-cost associations: hierarchical linear regression and propensity score matching analysis in a nationwide Taiwan population. *Surg Oncol*. 2013;22(3):178–183. doi:10.1016/j.suronc.2013.05.004
11. Hopman P, Rijken M. Illness perceptions of cancer patients: relationships with illness characteristics and coping. *Psychooncology*. 2015;24(1):11–18. doi:10.1002/pon.3591
12. Lee SY, Kim SJ, Shin J, et al. The impact of job status on quality of life: general population versus long-term cancer survivors. *Psychooncology*. 2015;24(11):1552–1559. doi:10.1002/pon.3828
13. Klein ME, Dabbs DJ, Shuai Y, et al. Prediction of the oncotype DX recurrence score: use of pathology-generated equations derived by linear regression analysis. *Mod Pathol*. 2013;26(5):658–664. doi:10.1038/modpathol.2013.36
14. Manninen T, Huttunen H, Ruusuvuori P, Nykter M. Leukemia prediction using sparse logistic regression. *PLoS One*. 2013;8(8):e72932. doi:10.1371/journal.pone.0072932
15. Liang Y, Liu C, Luan XZ, et al. Sparse logistic regression with a L1/2 penalty for gene selection in cancer classification. *BMC Bioinformatics*. 2013;14:198. doi:10.1186/1471-2105-14-198
16. Lamm SH, Ferdosi H, Dissen EK, et al. A systematic review and meta-regression analysis of lung cancer risk and inorganic arsenic in drinking water. *Int J Environ Res Public Health*. 2015;12(12):15498–15515. doi:10.3390/ijerph121214990
17. Fang S, Wang Y, Sui D, et al. C-reactive protein as a marker of melanoma progression. *J Clin Oncol*. 2015;33(12):1389–1396. doi:10.1200/JCO.2014.58.0209
18. Suppli NP, Johansen C, Christensen J, et al. Increased risk for depression after breast cancer: a nationwide population-based cohort study of associated factors in Denmark, 1998–2011. *J Clin Oncol*. 2014;32(34):3831–3839. doi:10.1200/JCO.2013.54.0419
19. Byrne MM, Tannenbaum SL, Gluck S, et al. Participation in cancer clinical trials: why are patients not participating? *Med Decis Making*. 2014;34(1):116–126. doi:10.1177/0272989X13497264

13

Cancer Epidemiology: Measuring Exposures, Outcomes, and Risk

RISHI DEKA ■ LOREN K. MELL

The field of epidemiology broadly deals with characterizing the impact of diseases on populations (1). This may involve identifying causes of disease due to behaviors or environmental exposures, describing trends in and factors influencing disease **incidence** and **prevalence**, or studying the impact of interventions on treatments on the course of disease in society (2). Cancer epidemiology addresses applications specific to oncology and in some sense bears a connection to *all* studies under the umbrella of clinical cancer research. This is because the principal concern of an epidemiologist is to employ methods to study **effects of exposures** on **outcomes**, a common goal of nearly all who conduct research (2).

A key distinction between cancer epidemiology, and population sciences more broadly, and the types of studies described in the sections of this book on translational research and clinical trials, is that population sciences frequently deal with exposures that can be observed but not directly controlled. It is not difficult to make correct inferences from perfect data, but it takes care and sophistication to generate such data. Imperfect data, in contrast, require more care and sophistication to interpret properly. In a way, epidemiology is the science of making proper inferences from imperfect data.

Our understanding of the causes of cancer, its prevention, and its treatment owes a great deal to cancer epidemiologists. In 1713, Italian Bernardino Ramazzini reported the absence of cervical cancer in nuns (3). This observation was an important step forward toward identifying and understanding the importance of hormones and sexually transmitted infections and cancer risk. In 1775, Englishman Percivall Pott described an occupational cancer in chimney sweeps (3). He noted that scrotal cancer was caused by soot collecting in the skin folds of the scrotum. His research led to more studies that identified occupational health exposures and to public health measures aimed to reduce a person's cancer risk at work.

Englishman Richard Doll's studies on the consequences of tobacco in the 1950s paved the way for the modern-day field of cancer epidemiology (4). Doll was one of the first epidemiologists to document a link between smoking and lung cancer. Overall, Doll's research highlighted that many diseases—both major and minor—are related to smoking. Doll also studied the risks of radiation epidemiology. This included the consequences of fallout, risks to veterans who had participated in nuclear testing exercises, and indoor radon. Finally, Doll identified asbestos as a cause of lung cancer through his work on textile factory workers.

A number of recent epidemiologic studies have revealed new risk factors for a variety of cancers. For example, obesity has been identified as an independent risk factor for endometrial cancer (5). It is well known that alcohol consumption and cigarette smoking are independently associated with risk of head and neck cancer, as exemplified by a 2014 study from the Netherlands (6). Moderate alcohol consumption is also consistently associated with increased risk of breast cancer, particularly hormone receptor positive subtypes (7).

MEASURES USED IN CANCER EPIDEMIOLOGY

In order to identify associations between exposures and outcomes, we must first quantify what we mean by an event occurrence, by computing measures of disease frequency (2). A **count** is the simplest and most frequently used measure in epidemiology (2). This is simply the number of cases of a disease or another health outcome under consideration. Ratios, proportions, and **rates** are used to describe the relationship between the number of cases of a disease (or health outcome) and the size of the population or subpopulations in which they occurred (2). For example, if among 1,000 lung cancer fatalities, 700 are men and 300 are women, then the male to female sex ratio for lung cancer fatalities is

$$\frac{\text{Number of male cases}}{\text{Number of female cases}} = \frac{700}{300} = 2.33.$$

Ratios include proportions and rates (2). Proportions show how a part is related to the whole. For example, the number of men with prostate cancer out of the total number of males in the United States is as follows:

$$\frac{\text{Number of men with prostate cancer}}{\text{Total U.S. male population}}.$$

A rate is a measure of how quickly an event of interest happens (2). Unlike a proportion, a rate contains a dimension of time. For example, the incidence rate is the number of new cases of prostate cancer, which develops per 1,000 person-years of follow-up time:

$$\frac{\text{Number of new cases of prostate cancer}}{\text{Total time disease-free subjects observed}} \times 1000.$$

Prevalence measures existing cases of a disease at a particular time (2). There are two types of prevalence: point and period. **Point prevalence** measures the frequency of a disease at a given point in time:

$$\frac{\text{Number of observed prostate cancer cases at time T}}{\text{Population size at time T}}.$$

Period prevalence denotes the number of cases of a disease during a specified time (2). It includes prevalent cases at the beginning of the time period and incidence cases that develop during the same period:

$$\frac{\text{Number of prevalent cases} + \text{number of incident cases}}{\text{Population size during time period}}.$$

Mathematically, the relationship between incidence and prevalence is

$$P = IR \times D,$$

where P is prevalence, IR is the incidence rate, and D is the average length of time that an individual has the disease of interest.

Risk is the probability or chance that an individual will develop a disease or health event over a specified time, and is conditional on baseline characteristics; it also assumes that an individual does not have disease at the start of follow-up (2,8). Risk can be estimated from either **cumulative incidence** or the incidence rate. Cumulative incidence is the most common way to measure risk and is always a proportion between 0 and 1. Cumulative incidence is the proportion of a fixed population that becomes diseased over a specific period:

$$\frac{\text{Number of new cases of prostate cancer}}{\text{Number of disease-free subjects at start of follow-up}}.$$

For example, assuming a follow-up of 10 years and no deaths, if 100 men develop prostate cancer out of a cohort of 1,000 who initially did not have the disease, then the 10-year risk of prostate cancer is

$$\textit{Cumulative incidence} = \frac{10}{1{,}000} = 10\% \text{ over } 10 \text{ years.}$$

The incidence rate is useful for risk prediction with dynamic populations; it is non-negative and assumes no upper bound. The numerators for both the cumulative incidence and incidence rate are the same. The difference between the two is that the incidence rate's denominator incorporates time, person-years of follow-up. The relationship between cumulative incidence and the incidence rate is

$$CI = \Sigma IR_i x_{Ti}$$

where CI is the cumulative incidence, IR_i is the incidence rate, and T_i is the specified time.

The **standardized incidence rate (SIR)** is used to determine if the occurrence of cancer is high or low in a population of interest (2). The SIR is obtained by dividing the observed number of cancer cases by the "expected" number of cases in the study population of interest (2). The observed number of cases refers to the number of cases in the study population of interest. The expected number of cases is computed using age-specific rates from a reference population, weighted according to the age structure of the study population. An SIR greater than 1 indicates that the incidence for a certain type of cancer is higher than expected for that type of cancer based on state/countrywide age-specific incidence rates. A **risk ratio** is based on the ratio of two measures of disease frequency (2). A relative comparison provides information on the strength of the association between exposure and outcome. Mathematically, the risk ratio is the following:

$$RR = R_e/R_u$$

where R_e is the cumulative incidence, incidence rate, or prevalence in the exposed group and R_u is the cumulative incidence, incidence rate, or prevalence in the unexposed group. If there is no relationship between exposure and outcome, the value of the risk ratio is 1.0; a value greater than 1.0 means that the exposed group is at a higher risk of developing the disease, whereas a value less than 1.0 means that the exposed group is at a lower risk of developing the disease. Although the risk ratio is most commonly used to assess associations, the **risk difference** can also be used. The risk difference is simply the risk of the unexposed group subtracted from the risk of the exposed group.

Measures of disease frequency are used to evaluate associations between exposure and outcome. Common measures include counts, ratios, proportions, and rates. Risk is the **probability** or chance that an individual will develop a disease or health outcome over a specific time. The risk ratio is the ratio of the cumulative incidence, incidence rate, or prevalence between two groups. It is used to assess the risk of disease between exposed and unexposed subjects.

ASSOCIATION AND CAUSATION

The goal of epidemiology is to learn about the distribution and causes of diseases. A **cause** produces an effect, result, or consequence; causation indicates that one event is the result of another event (2). Specifically, a cause is a characteristic, condition, or event that precedes disease and without which the disease would not have occurred. A two-step process is used to determine causal relationships. First, it must be ascertained that the observed result is valid or true. Thus, the observed estimate must be free of **bias** (systematic error in the way the study was conducted), **confounding** (distorted results from comparing dissimilar groups), and **random errors** (probability that the results are simply due to chance). If the results are valid, then it must be determined whether the exposure actually caused the outcome.

There are three characteristics of a cause (2). The first is association. If there is no association between exposure and outcome, then causality can be rejected. The second is time order. The cause must precede the disease. The time between exposure and disease can be short or long. The third is direction. There must be an asymmetrical relationship between exposure and outcome; a symmetrical relationship is noncausal. Smoking causes lung cancer but lung cancer does not cause an individual to smoke. In general, the term **risk factor** is preferred to *cause* due to the inherent difficulty in making causal claims. For example, risk factors for prostate cancer include age, race, lifestyle, marital status, and family history. Due to a greater understanding in the etiology of disease, these risk factors are not direct causes but rather serve to identify more proximate causes of prostate cancer.

Historical causation theories stem from Robert Koch's germ theory in the late 1800s (2). Koch's postulates demonstrated that a disease is caused by a certain organism:

1. The organism will occur in every case of the disease and can explain the pathological and clinical changes associated with the disease.
2. The organism must be shown to be distinct from any others that might be found with the disease.
3. If the organism is isolated and repeatedly grown in culture, it will induce a new case of disease in a susceptible animal.

In the 1960s, the **web of causation** (Figure 13.1) described that disease occurrence can be explained by a complex web of interconnected factors, including both host and environmental factors (2). The current guidelines for causal inference are attributed to two sources. The first is from the 1964 Report of the U.S. Advisory Committee to the Surgeon General of Public Health (2). This work concluded that smoking causes lung cancer and was the first application of causal criteria to a major health issue. Criteria for determining causation from the U.S. Advisory Committee included consistency, strength, specificity, temporality, and coherence.

The best-known criteria for determining causation were set forth in 1965 by Bradford Hill. Hill's nine guidelines build on the earlier work of U.S. scientists and include the following (2):

1. Strength of an association
2. Consistency
3. Specificity
4. Temporality
5. Biological gradient
6. Biological plausibility

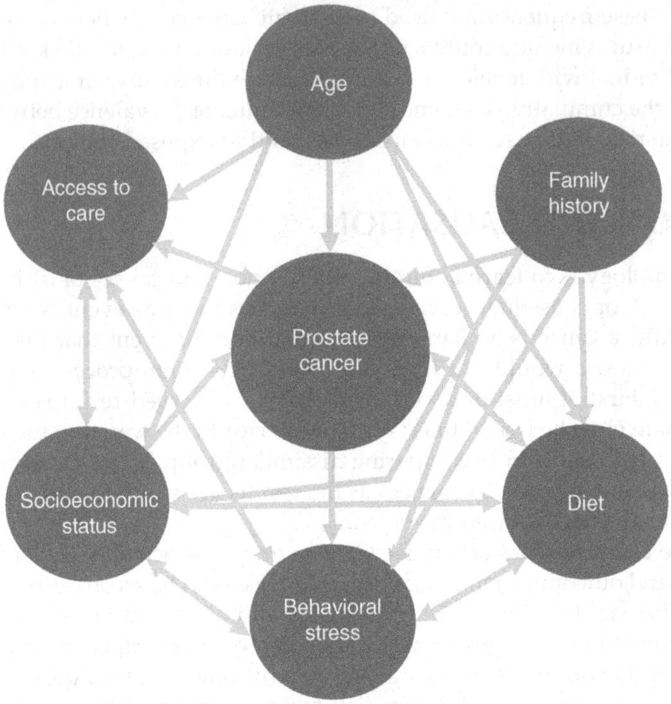

FIGURE 13.1 Prostate cancer web of causation.

7. Coherence
8. Experimental evidence
9. Analogy

The first guideline for determining causation is the strength of an association. True causes must exhibit association. According to Hill, large associations (risk ratios or **odds ratios** [ORs]) are more likely to be causal than small ones. Large associations are more likely to be causal because they are unlikely to be completely due to bias/confounding. The second criterion is consistency. Associations are more likely to be causal if they are repeatedly observed by different persons in different places, circumstances, and times. Meta-analysis can be used to check for consistency.

For example, the relationship between smoking and lung cancer was found in many studies with different locations, populations, and time periods. The third guideline, specificity, is that one cause should lead to one effect. The temporality criterion states that cause must precede disease. The biological gradient guideline indicates that a relationship is more likely to be causal if its strength increases as the exposure level increases. This means that there is a dose–response effect. The sixth criterion notes that there should be an existing biological model to explain an association. However, understanding of biological mechanisms often lags behind identification of causal inference. The seventh guideline, coherence, is similar to biological plausibility. The causal interpretation of results should not conflict with generally known facts of the natural history and biology of disease. The eighth criterion, experimental evidence, indicates that well-designed experimental studies should provide strong evidence for/against causation. However, randomized controlled trials are not feasible or ethical for many exposure–disease relationships; thus, lack of experimental evidence should not necessarily be considered evidence against causation. Finally, analogy concerns the use of analogies or similarities between the observed association and other associations. For example, Hill noted that the effect of rubella during pregnancy is known; thus similar evidence about the relationships between other viral diseases and pregnancy outcomes can

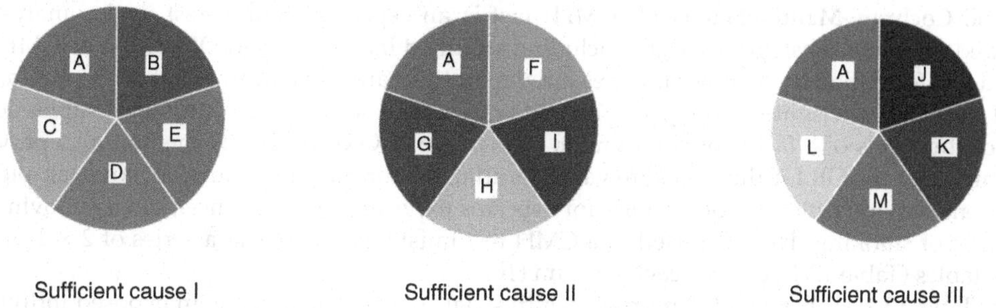

FIGURE 13.2 Causal pies. There are three sufficient causes of a cancer (I, II, and III). Each sufficient cause consists of five component causes. Component cause A is in all three sufficient causes. Thus, component cause A is a necessary cause. An example of a necessary cause is smoking, which causes lung cancer.

be accepted. Overall, the most commonly used guidelines for causal inference are strength of an association, biological gradient, biological plausibility, and consistency.

Although the Hill criteria for causal inference are most commonly used, Kenneth Rothman presented a **causal pie** model in 1976 to bridge the gap between theories about causation and the practice of epidemiology (Figure 13.2). Each pie represents a theoretical causal mechanism, called a **sufficient cause** (1). A sufficient cause is a set of factors that inevitably produce disease. Each factor in a sufficient cause is called a **component cause**. A single component cause does not cause disease itself. A component cause that belongs to *every* sufficient cause is a **necessary cause**.

Consider the causal pies in Figure 13.2, which represent a disease with three sufficient causes, that is, three pathways to disease. Each sufficient cause consists of five component causes (A–J). Component cause A is a necessary cause because it is included in each sufficient cause model. None of the other component causes is necessary because each is not part of every sufficient cause. A **strong cause** is a component cause in a large proportion of cases. For example, smoking is a strong cause of lung cancer because smoking plays a causal role in a large proportion of cases.

Of importance to epidemiologists is the fact that *association does not imply causation*. A cause produces an effect, result, or consequence. Causal inference is complex and requires careful judgment and interpretation of evidence. Although causation theories have changed over time, the criteria of association, biological gradient, biological plausibility, and consistency are most commonly used to determine causation.

SELECTED STATISTICAL TESTS IN CANCER EPIDEMIOLOGY

Many common statistical tests in cancer epidemiology are common to other fields; for example, **chi-square tests**, **Wilcoxon rank tests**, and **analysis of variance (ANOVA)** are frequently used analytic methods that were discussed in Chapter 11. In cancer epidemiology, **trend data** are also often used to report cancer rates over time (9). Chi-square tests are often used to evaluate trends in proportions over time, although this approach may be suboptimal if **autocorrelation** (Chapter 12) is present. **Vector autoregression** is a time series projection method that is used to model contemporary trend data (9). This type of modeling can be performed with Joinpoint Trend Analysis Software (9). First, the analyst inputs the minimum and maximum number of joinpoints. A *joinpoint* is where several different lines are connected together. The program starts with the minimum number of joinpoints and tests whether an additional joinpoint is statistically significant and must be added to the model. This allows to test whether an apparent change in trend is statistically significant. The actual tests of significance use a Monte Carlo permutation method. Ultimately, this software fits the simplest joinpoint model that the trend data allow and tests whether these trends change significantly over time.

The **Cochran–Mantel–Haenszel (CMH) test** is an especially useful test in the analysis of stratified or matched categorical data, including stratified incidences and ORs (10). The CMH test provides information on whether the measured quantities are equal or unequal across strata. The CMH test takes a weighted average of the odds ratios for a set of 2 × 2 contingency tables across each of the levels of a factor or confounder. In the case of ORs, the CMH method also provides an estimate of the OR for the exposure variable, adjusted for the strata variable. For example, the CMH can provide estimates of the ORs for asbestos exposure to lung cancer, after removing the influence of smoking. The data used in a CMH test must be stratified in a series of 2 × 2 contingency tables (Table 13.1), one for each stratum (10).

In Table 13.1, A, B, C, and D represent individual counts. The odds of an exposed individual contracting disease is

$$OR_e = \frac{A}{B}.$$

The odds of an unexposed individual contracting disease is

$$OR_u = \frac{C}{D}.$$

Their ratio (i.e., OR) is

$$\frac{OR_e}{OR_u} = \frac{AD}{BC}.$$

The common OR of the *i*th contingency tables is then calculated as (10)

$$OR_{cmh} = \frac{\sum\left(\frac{A_i D_i}{T_i}\right)}{\sum\left(\frac{B_i C_i}{T_i}\right)}.$$

The ratio thus obtained provides a weighted average of the OR across the different strata of the confounding variable, producing a single, summary measure of association (10). The CMH test statistic has an (asymptotic) chi-square distribution, which can be used to assess the statistical significance of the common OR versus the null hypothesis of no association. A p value of less than .05 indicates that the association between two variables is significant even after stratifying for a confounding variable, whereas a p value of greater than .05 indicates that the relationship between

TABLE 13.1 2 × 2 CONTINGENCY TABLE FOR CMH TEST FOR THE ITH CONTINGENCY TABLE.

Exposure	Disease Present Yes (Cases)	Disease Absent No (Controls)	Total
Yes	A_i	B_i	$(A + B)_i$
No	C_i	D_i	$(C + D)_i$
Total	$(A + C)_i$	$(B + D)_i$	T_i

CMH, Cochran–Mantel–Haenszel.

two variables is no longer significant after stratifying for a confounding variable. In the latter case, an association between the two variables is actually due to the influence of the confounder (see more in what follows).

MODELING EXPOSURES AND OUTCOMES

With observational data, because the treatments and other exposures of interest are not directly controlled, inferences about their effects on outcomes are subject to bias due to influences of other factors (11). In general, the approach to controlling these factors involves the use of a statistical model, as discussed in Chapters 11 and 12, in order to isolate the exposure of interest and acquire an unbiased measure of its effect (12). Many types of factors can influence the effects of exposures on outcomes (Figure 13.3). These include **moderators, mediators, confounders**, and **covariates**. The goal of statistical models in epidemiology is to mitigate the biasing effects of confounders and covariates, and elucidate the role of effect modifiers and mediators of disease, which may be actionable or targetable as a method to control disease.

A *moderator*, or effect modifier, is a variable that influences the way and degree to which an exposure affects an outcome; for example, the effect of asbestos on mesothelioma risk is augmented in the presence of smoking, a moderator. A *mediator* is a variable that is proximal and causal to the outcome of interest and directly impacted by the exposure; for example, obesity can lead to a rise in unopposed estrogen, which mediates as a risk factor for endometrial cancer. A *covariate* is a variable that affects the outcome without necessarily being associated with the exposure. When a covariate is completely uncorrelated with the exposure, estimates of the effect of an exposure will be unbiased, but may be imprecise due to the variation the other factor introduces. For example, peripheral neuropathy can be related to both chemotherapy and diabetes, without the exposure (chemotherapy)—or its effect—being related to the covariate (diabetes). However, one's ability to discriminate the effect of chemotherapy on neuropathy may be more difficult in a population with a high prevalence of diabetes. When a covariate is correlated with both the outcome *and* the exposure, it is called a *confounder*.

Confounders are a particularly important problem because excluding them from a model or otherwise failing to account for their impact can bias estimates of the effect of an exposure. Confounders can be measurable or unmeasurable. It is always desirable, to the extent possible, to control for *measurable* confounders in one's analysis; *unmeasurable* confounders typically refer to subjective factors like selection bias, which are controlled by randomization. A classic example of

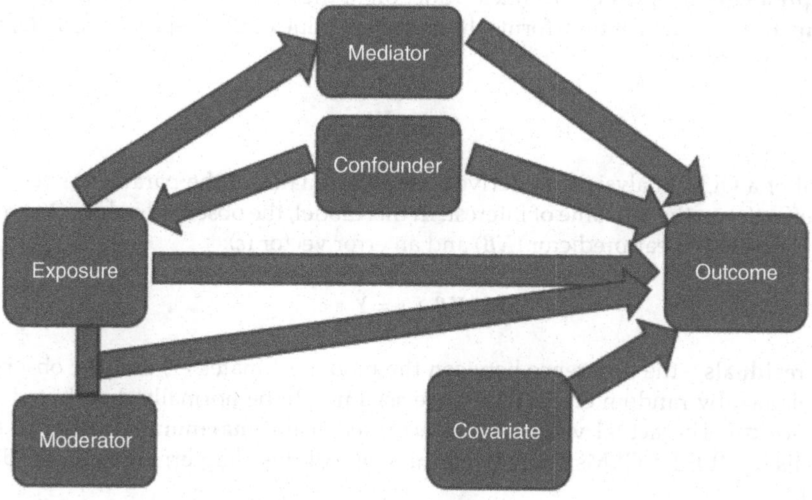

FIGURE 13.3 Factors influencing the effect of exposures on outcomes.

a confounder is the influence of tumor size on the relationship between blood transfusions (exposure) and tumor progression (outcome). On the surface, it might appear that blood transfusions make tumors grow. However, this relationship only appears because larger tumors tend to bleed more (necessitating transfusions) and also tend to grow faster (leading to disease progression). Specifically, this is an example of **confounding by indication**, wherein the reason for the exposure is linked to the severity of the outcome itself, a sort of tautology or circular logic. This kind of confounding can also undermine purported associations between more intensive treatment and poorer disease control or complications, and more subtle relationships, such as effects on cancer control with drugs used for nonmalignant conditions (13). Other types of confounding can bias analyses simply through strong collateral associations; for example, high-profile "destination" treatment centers sometimes advertise their ability to achieve superior results under their care, yet only those patients with the greatest resources and least debilitating illness are able to travel long distances to receive treatment.

Several methods to control for confounding include **restriction**, **stratified analysis** (aka **fully interacted models**), **matched analysis**, and **multivariable analysis** (11). Under restriction, study participation is restricted to individuals who lie within a specified category or categories of the confounder. Stratification analysis is the evaluation of the potential association within homogeneous categories or strata of the confounding variable(s) of interest. In matched analysis, subjects are selected in such a way that potential confounders are distributed equally among the study groups. Multivariable analysis involves the construction of multivariable models, which directly adjust for confounders as independent covariates.

GENERALIZED LINEAR MODELING

In statistical modeling, regression analysis is used to estimate the relationship between a dependent variable and one or more independent variables. **Generalized linear modeling** involves a systematic approach to linear regression in which the dependent variable is allowed to assume a non-normal distribution. In general, generalized linear models (GLMs) consist of the following aspects (14):

1. A random component specifying the conditional distribution of the $n \times 1$ response vector, **Y**, given the $n \times k$ matrix of explanatory variables, **X**. n is the number of observations and k is the number of explanatory variables (including an intercept term)
2. A distribution of **Y** belonging to an exponential family (e.g., binomial, Gaussian [normal], inverse Gaussian, Poisson, gamma)
3. A **linear predictor** ($X\beta$), which is a linear function of the $k \times 1$ regressor vector ($\boldsymbol{\beta}$)
4. A **link function** g(.), which transforms the expected value of the response variable, $\boldsymbol{u} = E(Y)$, to the linear predictor:

$$g(\boldsymbol{u}) = \boldsymbol{X\beta}$$

The goal of a GLM analysis is to derive a set of estimates of the parameters (i.e., $\boldsymbol{\beta}$) that are driving the effect(s) on the outcome of interest. In this model, the observed values (Y) are explained by both the estimated linear predictor ($\boldsymbol{X\hat{\beta}}$) and an error vector ($\varepsilon$):

$$Y = \boldsymbol{X\hat{\beta}} + \varepsilon = \hat{Y} + \varepsilon.$$

That is, the **residuals**—the difference between the model estimates ($\hat{Y}$) and the observed values (Y)—are explained by random error (which are assumed to be normally distributed with mean 0 and variance σ^2). The actual value of $\boldsymbol{\hat{\beta}}$ is acquired using **maximum likelihood estimation** (MLE). Details of MLE for GLMs are beyond the scope of this chapter; for technical details, consult Fox (14).

ASSUMPTIONS WHEN USING GLMS

When using GLMs, several assumptions underlying their validity must be assessed (14):

1. The dependent variable assumes a distribution from an exponential family. This can be evaluated using a **modified Park test** to identify the potential distribution.
2. There is a linear relationship between the transformed response in terms of the link function and the explanatory variables. A **scatterplot** can be used to check if nonlinearity is present.
3. There is homogeneity of variance of the residuals (i.e., **homoscedasticity**; Chapter 12); that is, the variance of residuals should be constant. This can be checked graphically using a plot of residuals versus estimated values. Ideally, this should be random (show no clear discernible pattern). Statistically, the White test for homogeneity can be used to test this assumption.
4. Residuals are normally distributed. Graphically, a plot of residuals against normal quantiles should lie along a 45-degree line. This assumption can be tested statistically with a **Shapiro–Wilk test** (Chapter 12) for normality.

LOGISTIC, CONDITIONAL LOGISTIC, AND PROBIT REGRESSION

Logistic regression is a type of linear regression that evaluates the relationship between a categorical dependent variable and a set of independent variables using a logit link function (14). The dependent variable is binomial, meaning that it can take on values of "0" or "1" (e.g., alive/dead or diseased/nondiseased). Logistic regression is often used to predict the risk of developing a disease based on observed patient characteristics.

Consider the following example, in which the dependent variable, **Y**, takes on a value of 1 if a patient has prostate cancer or 0 if a patient does not have prostate cancer. A set of independent variables, **X**, includes prostate-specific antigen (PSA) level, age, race, and family history. The logistic regression model that explains the relationship between these variables and the risk of prostate cancer is

$$logit\{\Pr(Y=1 \mid \mathbf{X})\} = \log\left\{\frac{(\Pr(Y=1) \mid \mathbf{X})}{(1-\Pr(Y=1 \mid \mathbf{X})}\right\} = \mathbf{X\beta} = \beta_0 + \beta_1X_1 + \beta_2X_2 + \beta_3X_3 + \beta_4X_4,$$

where $\boldsymbol{\beta} = <\beta_0, \beta_1, \beta_2, \beta_3, \beta_4>$ is a vector of regression coefficients representing the log odds associated with the intercept and each of the four independent variables. The exponentiated $\boldsymbol{\beta}$ vector ($\exp(\boldsymbol{\beta})$) gives a vector of ORs for each covariate.

Conditional logistic regression is used for matched case–control studies where a case is matched to a number of controls based on one or more matching factors (14). While similar to the logistic regression, the conditional logistic regression contains effects for different strata (one for each case–control pair or matched set), and excludes the intercept term (i.e., β_0). An additional assumption is that the OR for each explanatory variable is the same in all strata. The conditional logistic regression model is specified as

$$logit\{\Pr(Y=1 \mid \mathbf{X})\} = \mathbf{X\beta} + a_i,$$

where $\boldsymbol{\beta}$ is the vector of regression coefficients that represent log odds and α_i are the stratum constants.

For example, multiple logistic regression can be used to calculate an adjusted OR for lung cancer by smoking status, age, and sex. In the example logistic regression model, the referent categories are male, age 40–49, and never smoked for the sex, age, and smoking status categorical variables. In STATA, the *logit* command is used to estimate a logistic regression. The command is the following:

logit cancer female i.smokingstatus i.age

The "i." before the smoking status and age variables indicates that each subcategory within that variable should be included in the model as a series of indicator variables (i.e., past smoker or not, 1–19 cigarettes or not, 20+ cigarettes or not, age 50–59 or another age, age 60–69 or another age, age 70–79 or another age).

The STATA command returns the output for the model seen in Table 13.2. The model indicates that past smoking, and in particular smoking more than 20 cigarettes or more per day, increase the odds of being diagnosed with lung cancer. Furthermore, increasing age and male sex also increase the odds of a lung cancer diagnosis. Overall, the risk of lung cancer increases with age after adjusting for smoking status and gender (when compared to those aged 40–49). Females are at a decreased risk of lung cancer compared to males after adjusting for smoking status and age. Third, the risk of lung cancer increases with the number of cigarettes consumed after adjusting for age and gender.

Regression diagnostics are often used to assess the validity of a model (15). A logistic regression assumes a linear relationship between the logit of the outcome and explanatory variables as well as normality of the residuals (15,16). For example, the model described in the following uses data for prostate cancer patients from the Veterans Health Administration. Patients with prostate cancer are often administered androgen deprivation therapy (ADT) as a constituent therapy. In this instance, multiple logistic regression was used to model ADT administration as a function of substance abuse, smoking status, Charlson Comorbidity Index (CCI) score, race, income, and age. To assess the linearity assumption, the *margins* command in STATA is first used to estimate the predicted probabilities of ADT use based on the CCI score (15). The *marginsplot* is then used to plot the probability of ADT use against CCI score (15). As shown in Figure 13.4A, there is a linear

TABLE 13.2 STATA OUTPUT FOR A LOGISTIC REGRESSION MODEL OF RISK FACTORS FOR LUNG CANCER (SMOKING HISTORY, NUMBER OF CIGARETTES SMOKED, AGE, AND SEX)

Cancer	Odds Ratio	Standard Error	z	P > lzl	[95% CI]	
Past Smoker	4.455837	.5669614	11.74	0.000	3.47234	5.717896
1–19 cigarettes	12.23355	1.633652	18.75	0.000	9.416386	15.89355
20+ cigarettes	35.17525	3.874248	32.33	0.000	28.34554	43.65054
Age 50–59	1.335118	.2428156	1.59	0.112	.9347884	1.906893
Age 60–69	1.726414	.2961679	3.18	0.001	1.233447	2.416403
Age 70–79	2.353807	.4079567	4.94	0.000	1.675878	3.305972
Females	.719927	.0595784	−3.97	0.000	.6121337	.8467021

CI, confidence interval.

relationship between the logit of ADT use and CCI score. The second assumption is normality of the residuals. The *predict* command is used to generate the residuals (15). This is followed by the *qnorm* command to plot quantiles of the residuals against quantiles of a normal distribution (15):

logit adt i.substanceabuse i.smokingstatus i.cciscore i.race i.income i.age

margins, at (cciscore = (0 1 2 3 4 5 6 7 8 9 10 11 12 13))

marginsplot

predict r, resid

qnorm r

As can be seen in Figure 13.4B, the plot of the residuals against the normal quantiles lies along the 45-degree line, which indicates normality of the residuals (15). Finally, model fit for the logistic regression can be assessed through the **Hosmer–Lemeshow goodness-of-fit test** (16). The statistic compares expected to observed event rates in subgroups of the model population (16). The null hypothesis is a good model fit. In the ADT example, a p value of 0.13 indicates that a logistic regression does indeed fit the data. For more on model validation tests for multivariable logistic regression, see Ottenbacher et al. (17). Finally, as revealed in Figure 13.4C, there is no pattern in the plot of the residuals against income.

Probit regression is similar to logistic regression, in that it models the relationship between a binomial dependent variable and a set of independent variables. The difference is that the dependent variable in probit regression assumes an inverse Gaussian distribution (compared to a logit assumption in logistic regression) (14). The probit and logistic models usually produce similar results. However, unlike a logistic regression with ORs, coefficients from the output of a probit regression are not as easy to interpret. Instead, the marginal effects of the regressors—the change in the probability of the outcome variable given a change in the value of a regressor—are directly interpreted from the probit model. Thus, in cancer epidemiology, logistic analysis based on log odds is commonly preferred to probit regression.

One particular application of logistic and probit regression is in **propensity score** modeling. Propensity scores are often used in observational clinical cancer research to obtain an unbiased estimate of a treatment effect, when treatment selection can be assumed to be largely attributable to measurable factors. The idea is that the propensity to receive a given treatment depends on a number of observable covariates, and thus a logistic or probit model can be built to predict the probability of receiving a given treatment, such that this factor is controlled when modeling a treatment effect (or any effect of interest) on an outcome. It is often implemented as an alternative approach to multivariable modeling. Essentially, the two approaches constitute a similar model specification but for a slightly different error structure (nested, in the case of propensity scores). The results one obtains using a propensity score specification versus a standard multivariable model specification are similar, making the advantages of using propensity scores uncertain (18). Propensity score models may also be biased in the setting of heavy confounding (18). However, propensity scores can be desirable and may have advantages when the number of events per covariate is low, such as for rare outcomes, as is sometimes the case in cancer epidemiology studies. When specifying a propensity score, it is best to ensure that the covariates used to model propensity are not included again in the multivariable specification (as the interpretation of the coefficient estimate is unclear in this context). In general, we recommend considering propensity scores instead of standard multivariable models when:

- The study design is observational
- A treatment effect is the primary effect of interest (it is best to examine both model specifications in that case, as inferences could differ)
- The number of events per model parameter is low, or multicollinearity is a significant problem (as for the primary model fitting, propensity scoring reduces the number of parameters estimated)

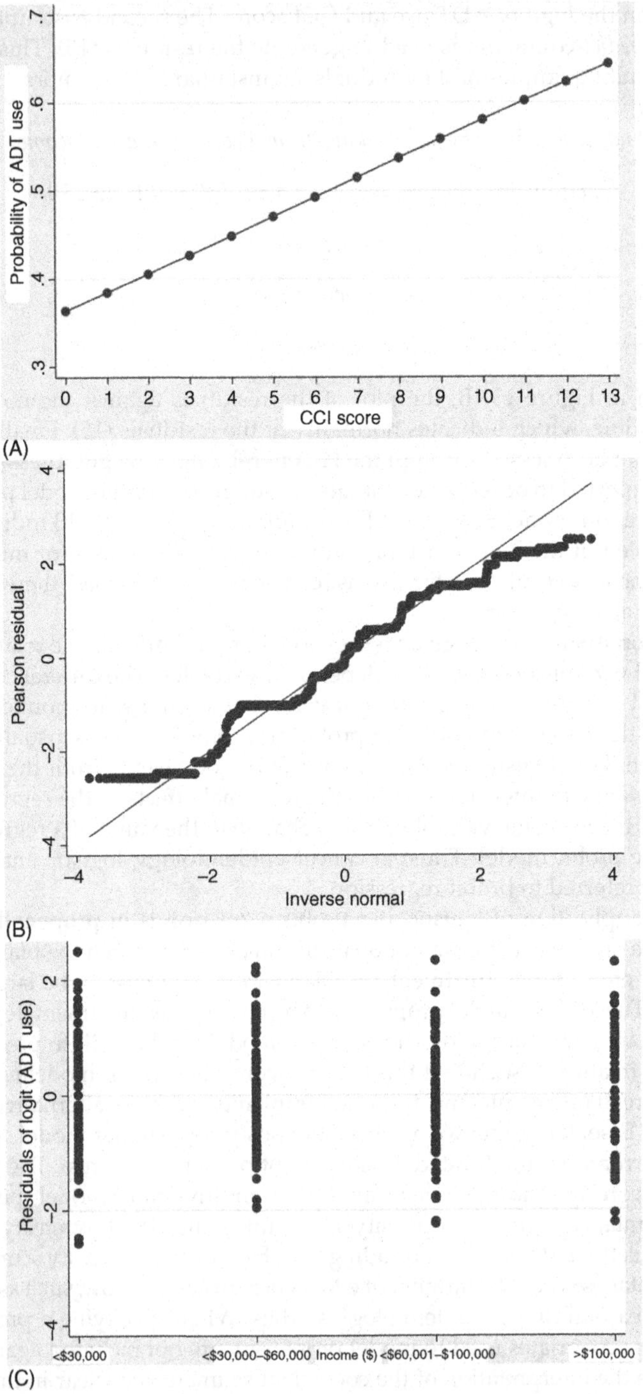

FIGURE 13.4 (A) Test of the linearity assumption. The logit of the outcome is plotted against values of the explanatory variable, CCI, which graphically verifies the conformity of the relationship to a linear gradient. (B) Q–Q plot to test the normality assumption. Quantiles of the residuals from the model follow a linear path vs. the quantiles of the normal distribution (except at the tails). (C) Plot of residuals as a function of the explanatory variable income; note the lack of a pattern under varying levels of income.

ADT, androgen deprivation therapy; CCI, Charlson Comorbidity Index.

- Treatment selection is largely explained by measurable factors (if not, then the model is biased regardless of the model specification)

POISSON, LOG-BINOMIAL, AND NEGATIVE BINOMIAL REGRESSION

If there are only two possible outcomes, then a logistic, conditional logistic, or probit regression can be used (14). However, if there are more than two events, then **Poisson regression** can be used (14). Poisson regression is commonly used when the outcomes of interest are counts, rates, or ratios. This approach is also used to model effects on incidence rates and prevalence. The unit of analysis in a Poisson regression is a **log rate** (14), with expected value:

$$E(\log(\text{rate})) = \boldsymbol{X\beta}.$$

The regression coefficients ($\boldsymbol{\beta}$) represent the increase in the log rate of the outcome per unit increase in the covariate, adjusted for all other covariates.

Log-binomial and **modified Poisson regression** can be used to directly estimate risk ratios and risk differences (19). The difference between the log-binomial model and the logistic regression model is the link between the independent variables and the probability of outcome. In a log-binomial model, the log link function is used (20). Although the log-binomial model generally computes unbiased estimates of the adjusted risk ratio, there are a couple of limitations associated with its use (20). First, the log-binomial model can sometimes estimate narrower confidence intervals for the adjusted risk ratios. Second, model convergence can be an issue, which results in an inability of the log-binomial to provide actual estimates. In that case, modified Poisson regression, which is Poisson regression with robust error variance, can be used. Modified Poisson regression has a major assumption that the variance equals the mean, where $E(y) = \mu$ is the mean of the response variable and ϕ is the dispersion parameter:

$$\text{Var}(y) = \phi^* E(y) = \phi^* \mu, \text{ assuming } \phi = 1.$$

This assumption can be assessed statistically through the scale factor: the scaled deviance or the scaled Pearson dispersion parameters. If either scale factor is greater than one, then a **negative binomial model** is used to account for overdispersion where the variance is not equal to the mean.

NONLINEAR REGRESSION: TUMOR CONTROL AND NORMAL TISSUE COMPLICATION PROBABILITY MODELS

Frequently, investigators are interested in developing clinical risk assessment tools to predict the effects of treatment decisions on outcomes. In particular, one may be interested in modeling the effects of increased dose on the probability of an outcome, such as tumor control probability (TCP) or normal tissue complication probability (NTCP). Typically, such dose–response models assume that the event probability follows the path of a sigmoidal function (Figure 13.5). Specific applications of NTCP modeling for predicting long-term morbidity of therapy are considered in Chapter 14.

Effects of covariates on probability of an outcome can be modeled using GLMs with logit or probit link functions, as described previously. For outcomes represented on an interval (continuous) scale, such as blood biomarkers, multiple linear regression is sometimes applicable as well (Chapter 12). With TCP and NTCP models, however, investigators are frequently interested in identifying the values of parameters associated with a sigmoidal curve represented as a function of a single predictor, such as dose to a given organ of interest. In this setting, the model is not specified in terms of a linear combination of parameters, and nonlinear estimation (i.e., MLE) techniques are thus required. Examples of nonlinear estimation techniques include the Gauss–Newton method, Levenberg–Marquardt–Fletcher algorithm, and gradient (e.g., steepest descent) methods.

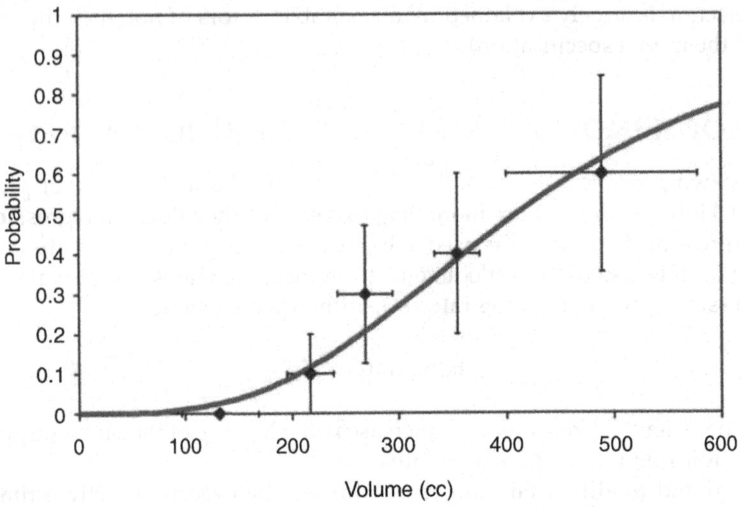

FIGURE 13.5 Example of a sigmoidal function used in outcome probability modeling. The probability of a toxicity event is plotted against increasing volume of an organ receiving radiation dose.

Source: Roeske JC, Bonta D, Mell LK, et al. A dosimetric analysis of acute gastrointestinal toxicity in women receiving intensity-modulated whole-pelvic radiation therapy. *Radiother Oncol.* 2003;69(2):201–207. doi:10.1016/j.radonc.2003.05.001

For example, the **Lyman–Kutcher–Burman (LKB) model**, which is often used in NTCP modeling, uses a probit-like function to specify key parameters associated with a sigmoidal dose–response curve. The key parameters in the LKB model are D_{50}, which is the dose at which the probability of an outcome is 50%, *m*, which represents the "slope" of the sigmoidal curve, and *a*, which represents a "volume parameter":

$$\text{TCP or NTCP} = \frac{1}{\sqrt{2\pi}}\int_{-\infty}^{t} e^{-\frac{x^2}{2}}\,dx,$$

where

$$t = \frac{D - D_{50}}{m * D_{50}}$$

and

$$D = (\sum v_i d_i^{a})^{1/a}.$$

Dose (D) to a volume of interest, such as an organ or tumor volume, is expressed as an equivalent uniform dose (EUD), which is taken as a summation over its subregions. The dose to and volume of the *i*th voxel are represented as d_i and v_i, respectively. Large values of *a* indicate weak volume dependence, where only the high doses to a small region of interest are critical to probability. Values of *a* between 0 and 1 indicate strong volume dependence, and extreme negative values of *a* indicate that only low doses to a small region of interest critically affect the outcome probability. For NTCP models, *a* is typically assumed (or estimated) to be positive, whereas for TCP models, it is assumed (or estimated) to be negative. The observed outcomes and dose values can be fitted to the LKB model, and the values of the model parameters are estimated using one of the nonlinear MLE techniques described previously.

Similar TCP and NTCP specifications can be represented as logit-type functions. Such methods are useful for constructing **volume–response** models, which quantify the trade-off between the probability of an outcome and the volume of a structure that is affected (such as by a resection, or radiation dose). For example, Roeske et al. (21) used the following function to model the relationship between bowel dose and gastrointestinal toxicity in patients undergoing radiation with or without chemotherapy for pelvic malignancies:

$$\text{TCP or NTCP} = \frac{1}{1+\left(\frac{V_{50}}{V}\right)^{k}},$$

where V_{50} and k values are fitted parameters. Analogous to the D_{50}, the V_{50} is the volume of a structure receiving a specified dose (such as the prescription dose) at which the probability of an outcome is 50%. Note that higher values of V_{50} in this model flatten and shift the curve rightward, indicating increasing insensitivity of the structure to volume effects (as it takes a higher dose to result in 50% probability of the outcome). A higher value of the parameter k results in increasing steepness or sharpness to the curve, with small fluctuations in volume receiving dose resulting in rapid rise/fall in probability over the critical part of the domain (Figure 13.5).

One limitation of classical TCP/NTCP models is that the spatial relationship between dose deposition and organ or tumor function is lost. This is an important obstacle to describing dose–response effects in heterogeneous-function organs such as the brain, liver, bone marrow, and lung, among others. Modern approaches to TCP and NTCP modeling increasingly involve more sophisticated, space-preserving models, such as facial recognition and other machine learning approaches; these applications are discussed further in Chapter 17.

GLOSSARY

incidence: measure of new cases of a disease.

prevalence: measure of existing cases of a disease at a point in time.

effect: measure of impact of a variable or treatment on an event or outcome of interest.

outcome: result of an experiment, trial, or study.

count: the number of cases of a disease or another health outcome under consideration.

rate: a measure of how quickly an event of interest happens.

incidence rate: measure of new instances of an event of interest per unit time.

point prevalence: measures the frequency of a disease at a given point in time.

period prevalence: measure of the number of cases of a disease during a specified time.

risk: the probability or chance that an individual will develop a disease or health event over a specified time.

cumulative incidence: the proportion of a fixed population that becomes diseased over a specific period.

standardized incidence rate (SIR): incidence measure adjusted for background event rate in a population of interest.

risk ratio: the ratio of two measures of disease frequency between two groups.

risk difference: the difference in risk between an exposed and unexposed group.

probability: risk or chance that an individual will develop a disease or health outcome over a specific time.

cause: something that produces an effect, result, or consequence; characterized by association, time order, and direction.

bias: systematic error in the way a study was conducted.

confounding: distortion in results that stems from comparing dissimilar groups.

random error: probability that the results are simply due to chance.

risk factor: term for a circumstance that predisposes an individual to a disease or contributes to the development of that disease.

web of causation: notion that disease occurrence can be explained by a complex web of interconnected factors, including both host and environmental factors.

odds ratio: measure of association strength.

Chi-square test: statistical test used to compare frequencies or proportions in two or more groups.

Wilcoxon rank test: statistical test used to compare two independent groups with ordinal data or with nonnormally distributed observations.

analysis of variance (ANOVA): statistical test used to determine whether any differences exist among two or more groups on one or more factors.

linear predictor: a linear function representing the inner product of a vector of variables (covariates) and their associated parameters (coefficients).

link function: a function that transforms the expected value of the response variable to the linear predictor.

residuals: the difference between the model estimates and the observed values.

maximum likelihood estimation: a type of parameter estimation that attempts to find the parameter values that maximize the likelihood function given the observations.

modified Park Test: a statistical test used to identify the distribution of a dependent variable in a generalized linear model.

scatterplot: a graph in which the values of two variables are plotted along two axes which can reveal if correlation is present.

homoscedasticity: homogeneity of variance of the residuals.

causal pie: model that bridges gaps between theories about causation and the practice of epidemiology.

sufficient cause: a set of factors that inevitably produce disease.

component cause: a factor in a sufficient cause; a single component cause does not itself cause disease.

necessary cause: a component cause that belongs to every sufficient cause.

strong cause: a component cause in a large proportion of cases.

trend data: data reported over time.

vector autoregression: a time series projection method used to model contemporary trend data.

Cochran–Mantel–Haenszel (CMH) test: a statistical test that provides information on whether incidence data are equal or unequal across strata.

moderator (effect modifier): a variable that influences the way and degree to which an exposure affects an outcome.

mediator: a variable that is proximal and causal to the outcome of interest and directly impacted by the exposure.

confounder: a covariate that is correlated with both the outcome and the exposure.

covariate: a variable that affects the outcome without necessarily being associated with the exposure.

confounding by indication: type of confounding wherein the reason for the exposure is linked to the severity of the outcome itself.

restriction: method to control confounding in which study participation is restricted to individuals who lie within a specified category or categories of the confounder.

stratification analysis (fully interacted model): method to control confounding in which potential associations are evaluated within categories or strata of the confounding variable.

matched analysis: method to control confounding in which subjects are selected in such a way that potential confounders are distributed equally among the study groups.

multivariable analysis: technique to control for confounding which involves the construction of multivariable models that directly adjust for confounders as independent covariates.

generalized linear modeling: a systematic approach to linear regression in which the dependent variable is allowed to assume a non-normal distribution.

logistic regression: a type of linear regression that evaluates the relationship between a categorical dependent variable and a set of independent variables using a logit link function.

conditional logistic regression: regression method used for matched case–control studies where a case is matched to a number of controls based on one or more matching factors.

regression diagnostics: means of assessing the validity of a model.

Hosmer–Lemeshow goodness-of-fit test: method of assessing model fit for a logistic regression.

probit regression: method similar to logistic regression in that it models the relationship between a binomial dependent variable and a set of independent variables, but uses a dependent variable that assumes an inverse Gaussian distribution.

propensity scores: often used in observational clinical research to obtain an unbiased estimate of a treatment effect, when treatment selection can be assumed to be largely attributable to measurable factors.

Poisson regression: statistical method is commonly used when the outcomes of interest are counts, rates, or ratios; also used to model effects on incidence rates and prevalence.

log rate: the unit of analysis in a Poisson regression.

log-binomial regression: statistical method that can be used to directly estimate risk ratios and risk differences.

modified Poisson regression: statistical method with robust error variance that can be used to directly estimate risk ratios and risk differences.

negative binomial model: means of accounting for overdispersion where the variance is not equal to the mean.

Lyman–Kutcher–Burman (LKB) model: method that uses a probit-like function to specify key parameters associated with a sigmoidal dose–response curve; often used in NTCP modeling.

volume–response models: models that quantify the trade-off between the probability of an outcome and the volume of a structure that is affected.

REFERENCES

1. Rothman KJ. *Epidemiology: An Introduction*. 2nd ed. Oxford, UK: Oxford University Press; 2012.
2. Aschengrau A, Seage GR. *Essentials of Epidemiology*. Burlington, MA: Jones & Bartlett; 2007.
3. American Cancer Society. History of cancer epidemiology. https://www.cancer.org/cancer/cancer-basics/history-of-cancer/cancer-epidemiology.html. 2018.
4. Samet JM, Speizer FE. Sir Richard Doll, 1912–2005. *Am J Epidemiol*. 2006;164(1):95–100. doi:10.1093/aje/kwj210
5. Onstad MA, Schmandt RE, Lu KH. Addressing the role of obesity in endometrial cancer risk, prevention, and treatment. *J Clin Oncol*. 2016;34(35):4225–4230. doi:10.1200/JCO.2016.69.4638
6. Maasland DH, Van den Brandt PA, Kremer B, et al. Alcohol consumption, cigarette smoking, and the risk of subtypes of head-neck cancer: results from the Netherlands cohort study. *BMC Cancer*. 2014;14:187. doi:10.1186/1471-2407-14-187
7. Liu Y, Nguyen N, Colditz GA. Links between alcohol consumption and breast cancer: a look at the evidence. *Womens Health*. 2015;11(1):65–77. doi:10.2217/whe.14.62
8. Gordis L. *Epidemiology*. 5th ed. Philadelphia, PA: Saunders; 2013.
9. Siegel RL, Miller KD, Jemal A. Cancer statistics. *CA Cancer J Clin*. 2018;68(1):7–30. doi:10.3322/caac.21442
10. Wassertheil-Smoller S, Smoller J. *Biostatistics and Epidemiology: A Primer for Health and Biomedical Professionals*. 4th ed. New York, NY: Springer; 2015.
11. Garrido MM, Kelley AS, Paris J, et al. Methods for constructing and assessing propensity scores. *Health Serv Res*. 2014;49(5):1701–1720. doi:10.1111/1475-6773.12182
12. Faries D, Leon AC, Haro JM, Obenchain RL. *Analysis of Observational Health Care Data Using SAS*. Cary, NC: SAS Institute; 2012.
13. Zanders MM, Vissers PA, van de Poll-Franse LV. Association between metformin use and mortality in patients with prostate cancer: explained by confounding by indication? *J Clin Oncol*. 2014;32(7):701. doi:10.1200/JCO.2013.53.5161
14. Fox J. *Applied Regression Analysis and Generalized Linear Models*. Thousand Oaks, CA: Sage; 2015.
15. Mitchell MN. *Interpreting and Visualizing Regression Models Using Stata*. College Station, TX: Stata Press; 2012.
16. Kleinbaum DG, Klein M. *Logistic Regression: A Self-Learning Text* (Statistics for Biology and Health). 3rd ed. New York, NY: Springer; 2010.
17. Ottenbacher KJ, Ottenbacher HR, Tooth L, Ostir GV. A review of two journals found that articles using multivariable logistic regression frequently did not report commonly recommended assumptions. *J Clin Epidemiol*. 2004;57(11):1147–1152. doi:10.1016/j.jclinepi.2003.05.003
18. Stürmer T, Joshi M, Glynn RJ, et al. A review of the application of propensity score methods yielded increasing use, advantages in specific settings, but not substantially different estimates compared with conventional multivariable methods. *J Clin Epidemiol*. 2006;59(5):437–447. doi:10.1016/j.jclinepi.2005.07.004
19. Richardson DB, Kinlaw AC, MacLehose RF, Cole SR. Standardized binomial models for risk or prevalence ratios and differences. *Int J Epidemiol*. 2015;44(5):1660–1672. doi:10.1093/ije/dyv137
20. McNutt LA, Wu C, Xue X, Hafner JP. Estimating the relative risk in cohort studies and clinical trials of common outcomes. *Am J Epidemiol*. 2003;157(10):940–943. doi:10.1093/aje/kwg074ww
21. Roeske JC, Bonta D, Mell LK, et al. A dosimetric analysis of acute gastrointestinal toxicity in women receiving intensity-modulated whole-pelvic radiation therapy. *Radiother Oncol*. 2003;69(2):201–207. doi:10.1016/j.radonc.2003.05.001

14

Survivorship: Effects of Cancer Treatment on Long-Term Morbidity

ZORIMAR RIVERA-NÚÑEZ ■ KAVEH ZAKERI ■ SHARAD GOYAL

In Chapter 13, we discussed general concepts in the field of cancer epidemiology, and in particular, methods to estimate effects of exposures on outcomes. Various types of models were introduced and discussed, especially logistic and logit-type models of tumor control and normal tissue complication probability. These concepts have broad applications across the field of oncology, particularly for assessing dose–response effects of exposures on organs and tumors. Such models are critical for designing optimal therapeutic approaches and estimating the impact of new interventions.

In this chapter, we consider the problem of adverse effects on long-term morbidity and toxicity. This is particularly apropos in the setting caused by unwanted radiation dose delivery to the heart. This is of particular concern in breast cancer, because many patients survive their cancer but are subject to potentially serious late effects of therapy. This scenario is common in what is known as the **survivorship** setting, which affects more than 10 million people annually in the United States living with the aftereffects of cancer treatment (1). Investigation of radiation heart dose also sheds light on the importance of recognizing that exposures are often not "all or nothing," the importance of accurate and precise measurement of the exposure, the importance of considering comorbid illness and competing events, and the pitfalls of investigating a treatment that is evolving faster than long-term evidence can be generated.

RADIATION, BREAST CANCER, AND HEART DISEASE

Radiation therapy (RT) plays a critical role in the management of breast cancer. It is estimated that there are more than 3.5 million women living in the United States with a history of invasive breast cancer, and approximately 250,000 women were diagnosed in 2016 (2). In addition, an estimated 82.6 million adults in the United States have one or more types of cardiovascular disease, which accounted for 800,937 deaths or 30.8% of all deaths in the United States in 2016 (3). RT has been shown to reduce the risk of cancer recurrence and decrease mortality among breast cancer patients (4,5). Given the high prevalence of cancer in the general population, cancer survivors face many challenges, including the risk of cancer recurrence and cardiovascular events during survivorship.

The most recent meta-analysis on RT and breast-conserving surgery from the Early Breast Cancer Trialists' Collaborative Group analyzed data from 17 randomized trials, involving 10,801 women, and showed that RT reduced the 10-year risk of first recurrence from 35% to 19% and reduced the 15-year risk of breast cancer mortality from 25% to 21%. However, these reductions have been diminished by an increased heart disease incidence and mortality. The most common reported outcomes have been ischemic heart disease (IHD) and myocardial infarction (6–8).

Efforts to determine the risk of radiation-induced heart disease (RIHD) have been a main area of research for the past 10 years in the relatively new field of cardio-oncology. The field of cardio-oncology offers an interdisciplinary and integrative management approach to cancer patients with cardiovascular risks, specifically designed to mitigate risks of oncologic therapies and provide early detection and treatment of those at the greatest risk of cardiotoxicity (9). New developments in the field of cardio-oncology pertaining to RT and breast cancer will assist in (a) better informing patients about their risks, (b) management decisions for individual patients, (c) RT planning support, and (d) for cancer survivors, better follow-up and interventions.

According to Taylor and Kirby, there are three main factors in estimating the absolute RIHD risk for each woman: (a) risk per unit dose, (b) cardiac radiation dose, and (c) risk per unit in unexposed patients (10). First, evidence from population-based and randomized data suggests that the risk of heart disease increases linearly with increasing cardiac radiation dose. The importance of the population-based dose–response relationship is the inclusion of individual patient information including heart disease risk factors. Second, worldwide data suggest that the mean radiation dose may be around 5Gy in left-sided RT and 3Gy in right-sided RT (11). The delivered dose varies by country, patient anatomy, and technique. The precision of this estimate is critically important because it is used to estimate the risk per unit dose. Third, women with preexisting heart disease risk factors will have higher absolute risk than women with no risk factors for heart disease will. Accurate measurement of each of these parameters is essential in the interpretation of the RIHD in breast cancer patients. This chapter discusses sources of measurement error in the estimation of RIHD risk in current data and alternatives to current methods.

MEASUREMENT ERROR

The overall goal of an epidemiologic study is accuracy in estimation: to estimate the value of the parameter of interest with little error. Sources of error can be classified as either *random* or *systematic*. Random error refers to what cannot be predicted, because of either random variation or lack of knowledge about determinants. A major source of random error (noise) in epidemiological studies comes from *sampling variation* (12). The primary way to mitigate the effects of sampling error is to increase the sample size. However, sampling is not the only source of random error. Inaccuracies in key variable data collection also increase random error in epidemiological studies.

Errors in measurement can introduce bias and diminish the power of epidemiological studies. There are two key aspects of study validation in epidemiology: internal validity and external validity. **Internal validity** refers to the inferences drawn from the study that apply to the study population, while **external validity** refers to applications to individuals outside of the study population (generalizability). Naturally, the external validity of a study depends on its internal validity. We discuss validity issues that have an effect on the estimation of risk of RIHD and some ways to minimize measurement error (Figure 14.1).

MEASURING HEART DOSE

One of the major sources of measurement error in studies assessing RIHD is in the heart dosimetry calculations. RT doses have changed over the years as a consequence of new technology developments and cognizance of radiation-induced cardiotoxicity. For patients with long follow-up, the treatment techniques used may be relatively outdated; therefore, the reported cardiac doses may not represent typical doses delivered today. Although rates of cardiotoxicity are falling and

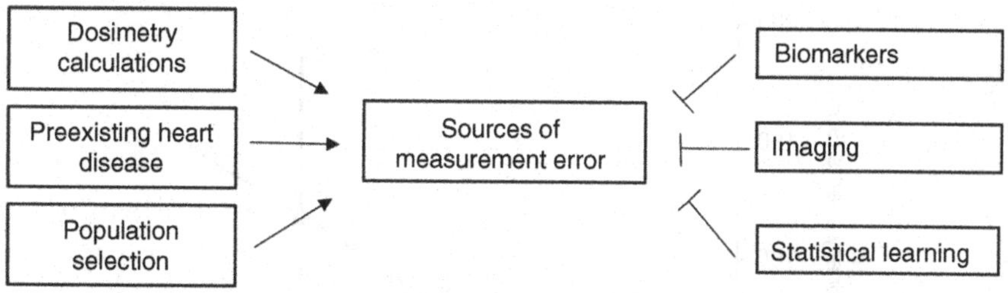

FIGURE 14.1 Main sources of measurement error and potential ways to minimize them in the study of radiation-induced heart disease.

methods of delivering and quantifying dose of radiation to the heart have become more sophisticated, reducing cardiotoxicity remains one of the primary aims of improving radiation techniques for patients with left-sided breast cancer.

A landmark case-control study by Darby et al. published in the *New England Journal of Medicine* in 2013 studied the relation of the risk of IHD after breast cancer RT (7). This study has been a significant contribution to the field because it was the first time a dose–response curve for RIHD was described. Comparing cases to controls, they reported that the risk of IHD linearly increased by 7.4% with each incremental Gy of mean radiation dose to the heart. However, their estimation of radiation dosimetry has some limitations. First, the authors used the CT scan of one woman with "typical anatomy" combined with individual radiation regimes to estimate the cardiac radiation for the entire population of 2,168 patients. In addition, the authors manually transformed hand calculations and fields estimated by photographs when performing modern CT-based estimations of cardiac dosimetry, leading to additional uncertainty in estimating cardiac dose. This same group found that this method of dose estimation has major uncertainties (13).

DOSE–RESPONSE MODEL OF RIHD

Darby et al. (7) described a linear increase of a major coronary event at a rate of 7.4% per Gy (Figure 14.2). There was no threshold minimum level of radiation below which there was no damage, and the increased risk started 5 years after RT and persisted for at least two decades. In a separate analysis, they categorized RT exposures as < 2 Gy, 2–4 Gy, 5–9 Gy, and > 10 Gy, and found that the percentage increased in major coronary events compared to zero cardiac dose was 10%, 30%, 40%, and 116%, respectively. Note that this study included women with both right- and left-sided breast cancers. The risk of coronary events was related to radiation dose, regardless of whether the tumor was in the left or right breast. Women with left-sided breast cancer had more coronary events than women with right-sided cancers did, but they also had higher mean heart doses on average (6.6 vs. 2.9 Gy). If the proportion of patients misclassified in their exposure (radiation dose) does not depend on disease status, this is called *nondifferential* misclassification. The direction on bias produced by nondifferential misclassification tends to be in the direction of the null value.

ROLE OF PREEXISTING HEART DISEASE AND OTHER COMORBIDITIES

The risk of developing heart disease is largely (75%–90%) explained by the presence or absence of traditional heart disease risk factors (14). Patients who have a diagnosis of heart disease might be at higher risk of subsequent RIHD than other women are. The appropriate selection of the control population in studies of RIHD becomes critical to examine preexisting heart disease and to avoid possible selection bias. Selection of controls from the same population as cases were drawn would be ideal but often not possible. For example, often cancer cases are sampled from cancer registries, whereas controls are sampled from physician/hospital data. Hence, key patient characteristics

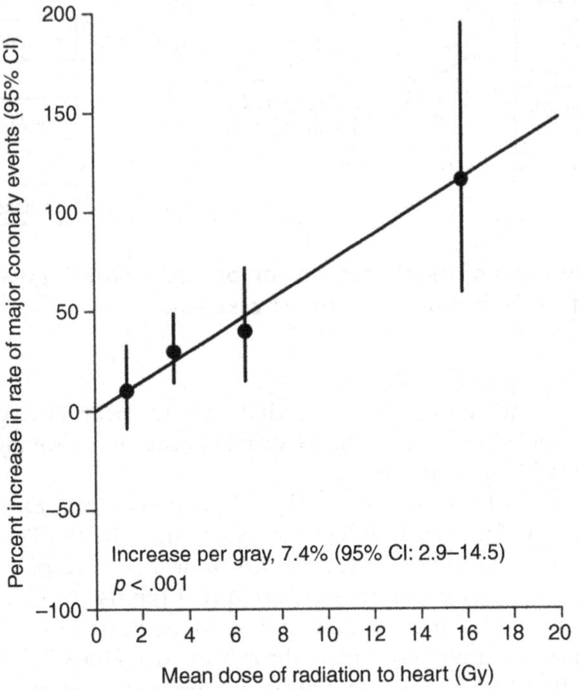

FIGURE 14.2 Rate of major coronary events according to mean radiation dose to the heart, as compared with the estimated rate with no radiation exposure to the heart.

Source: Reprinted from Darby SC, Ewertz M, McGale P, et al. Risk of ischemic heart disease in women after radiotherapy for breast cancer. *N Engl J Med.* 2013;368:987–998. doi:10.1056/NEJMoa1209825

acting as confounders may differ for cases and controls. After the study design stage, stratifying analyses to explore the effect of preexisting heart disease is an important step. After stratifying their analysis by the presence or absence of preexisting cardiac disease risk factors, Darby et al. (7) reported that the absolute radiation-induced cardiac disease risks are greater for women with preexisting cardiac risk factors than for other women.

Other comorbidities, such as chronic obstructive pulmonary disease (COPD), are common confounders and effect modifiers (see Chapter 13). Accounting for comorbidities is an essential and often overlooked step in establishing the validity of studies. For example, **confounding by nonspecificity** (see Chapter 16) is a crucial problem that can undermine a study's conclusions. Comprehensive comorbidity measures, such as the **Charlson Comorbidity Index (CCI)**, Elixhauser score, and **Adult Comorbidity Evaluation (ACE-27) index**, are helpful to adjust for effects of background illness on both events of interest and competing events and can enhance a study's efficiency (15). In general, the greater the efficiency, the fewer observations required to achieve performance of a particular model. However, the selection of an appropriate comorbidity index from those available will depend on the type of data available, study population, and specific outcome of interest (16). In addition to summary comorbidity measures, competing risk methods can be applied when a competing event precludes the occurrence of the event under study (17).

ROLE OF THERAPY

Another source of error can arise due to the use of systemic therapies for breast cancer, such as anthracyclines, that also cause cardiotoxicity. Such adjunctive therapies can alter patients' baseline risk for cardiotoxicity. For example, anthracycline-induced cardiac dysfunction occurs in 10% to 65% of patients depending on dose during breast cancer treatment (18). There is limited evidence regarding how treatments interact with regard to the risk of cardiovascular disease. Sensitivity analyses and stratification by treatment can be used to minimize bias due to background variation in RIHD studies.

ROLE OF SOCIOECONOMIC AND DEMOGRAPHIC RISK FACTORS

Sociodemographic factors, including age and race, are important confounders in the study of RIHD. Age is a risk factor for both heart disease and breast cancer (19,20). Disproportionate rates of heart disease in racial and ethnic minority populations are seen in the United States. Certain minority groups also have higher risk of hypertension, diabetes, and obesity, which can contribute to the differences in heart disease risk.

One method used to minimize bias in epidemiological studies is **matching**. Matching refers to the selection of a reference group—unexposed subjects in a cohort study and control subjects in a case–control study—that is identical or closely so to the study group with respect to the distribution of one or more potentially confounding factors. The matching process reduces heterogeneity due to matching factors and unmeasured risk factors. In the case of age, race, and ethnicity, these include both genetic and nongenetic factors. In order to properly account for the matching process, data analysis should include stratified analysis by the matching variables. Each matching category should be treated as a unique stratum, at least during exploratory analysis. **Residual confounding** may still exist, depending on the selected reference group or data collection strategies, since, for example, race and ethnicity are often self-reported.

MODERN ANALYTIC TECHNIQUES

Newer analytic techniques, including statistical learning, biomarkers, and novel imaging technologies, are contributing to new understanding of the role of radiation exposure in cardiac disease. These methods can be used to augment existing strategies, reduce error in risk estimation, and improve the management of breast cancer patients and their risk of heart disease.

STATISTICAL LEARNING

Statistical learning is a branch of data science that makes predictions using complex data through statistical models (21). Statistical learning methods consist of computational algorithms to relate a set of predictor variables to an outcome. Traditionally, regression models have been used to study associations between specific variables and clinical outcomes. For example, logistic regression can be used to estimate the probability of developing heart disease, given varying levels of physical activity (22). These models focus on the predictor variables that are used to test associations. However, rather than testing associations, statistical learning methods can be used to predict heart doses from current data, without traditional assumptions of regression analysis. Statistical learning offers great flexibility in modeling approaches by not requiring specific model structures but instead searching for the best fit, given certain constraints. The use of such methods (see Chapters 11, 12, and 17) may provide clinicians with more accurate patient-specific risk estimates for RIHD (23).

BIOMARKERS

Many biomarkers are used to predict clinical outcomes across a diverse span of treatments and cancer populations. Hence, there is a growing interest in their use for detecting cardiac injury (24). Identifying biomarkers of early damage and heart disease development is a current challenge in cardio-oncology. Biomarkers are useful in general to increase the specific evaluation of a particular outcome or, better, to adjust for baseline risk using quantitative and mechanistic evidence.

For example, classic biomarkers of heart disease, such as troponin (TnI), can be used to predict the risk of future adverse cardiac events in cancer patients after chemotherapy (23). However, toxicity mechanisms between chemotherapy drugs and irradiation may be different, and careful validation of these biomarkers in RT patients is required. NT-pro-brain natriuretic peptide (BNP), cardiac troponin, and C-reactive protein are widely used for the detection of cardiac injury in cancer patients.

BNP is an endogenous peptide produced initially by ventricular cardiomyocytes as a 134-aa pre-pro-peptide, which is cleaved into a 108-aa precursor molecule stored in secretory granules (proBNP) (25). Upon release, proBNP is cleaved by a specific protease into an inactive N-terminal fraction (NT-proBNP) (76-aa) and BNP (32-aa) active hormone. BNP concentration has already become a widely accepted index of cardiac failure or cardiac remodeling.

Troponin has been extensively studied as a marker of cardiotoxicity (26). Release of cardiac troponins reflects early damage of myocytes and is indicative of myocardial necrosis. However, hemodynamic changes occurring in a later stage can also lead to subclinical ischemia. Troponins could also play a role in late cardiac dysfunction. C-reactive protein is another established marker of acute phase reactions. Another potential biomarker is miRNA expressed by heart cells. Multiple studies have reported the use of miRNA as circulating biomarkers for diagnosis and prognosis of cardiovascular disease (27).

IMAGING

Like biomarkers, quantitative imaging can greatly enhance the specificity of the data collected, reducing measurement error and lending insight into biological impact of exposures. For example, the effect of radiation in individual breast cancer patients has been studied using various cardiovascular imaging techniques. Marks et al. prospectively studied 114 patients between 1998 and 2001 to assess changes in regional and global cardiac function using single-photon emission computerized tomography (SPECT) scans after RT for left-sided breast cancer (28). They found that the incidence of new perfusion defects 6, 12, 18, and 24 months after RT was 27%, 29%, 38%, and 42%, respectively, and that new defects occurred in approximately 10% to 20% and 50% to 60% of patients with less than 5% and greater than 5% of their left ventricle included within the RT fields, respectively ($p = .33$ to .00008).

Multi-parametric MRI (MP-MRI) allows the assessment of several possible pathologies in a single examination, including ventricular dysfunction, impaired myocardial perfusion, and abnormalities in the coronary artery anatomy (29). Other advantages of cardiac MRI include the lack of ionizing radiation, lack of attenuation artifacts, and its high spatial resolution. Furthermore, although SPECT provides information about ischemia, infarction, and ventricular function, it provides no detail of coronary artery anatomy. *MRI stress functional imaging* (stress echocardiography) allows the evaluation of regional contractility in all segments of the left ventricle. Stress function MRI has high spatial and temporal resolution in addition to better inter- and intra-observer agreement. The high spatial resolution viability imaging allows for the in vivo assessment of the myocardium.

PROBLEMS IN STUDY DESIGN: INNOVATION TO EXTINCTION

Over the past century, advances in RT technique and delivery have incrementally reduced cardiac dose. In the early part of the 20th century, kilovoltage treatment machines used to treat left-sided breast cancers with tangential beams delivering mean heart doses >10 Gy (30). By the 1980s, 3-D CT-based radiation planning paved the way for the use of deep inspiration breath hold, prone positioning, and intensity-modulated radiation therapy (IMRT) as additional techniques to reduce cardiac dose (31–33). These stepwise technological advancements over the past century represent a remarkable achievement in the reduction of a major toxicity of RT.

Modern studies report mean cardiac doses <1 Gy for standard breast tangential fields (31,34,35). Contemporary cooperative group clinical trials specify per-protocol mean heart doses <4 Gy for breast and regional nodal radiation (36). Compared to treatment with x-rays, proton beam radiation can further reduce mean heart doses to <1 Gy even when the internal mammary chain (IMC) is covered (37). As discussed earlier, the study by Darby et al. found a linear 7.4% increase in the rate of major coronary events per mean Gy of radiation dose to the heart, without a lower threshold at which RT would not increase the risk of toxicity (7). Yet, sustained innovation and progress result in an ever-decreasing event rate, which represents both a signal of success and a barrier to further advances. Against the backdrop of a fixed boundary (e.g., lower limit for toxicity rates of 0%), each incremental reduction in toxicity becomes exponentially more costly and difficult to achieve (Figure 14.3), a phenomenon that has been termed **innovation to extinction** (38).

This phenomenon creates two primary challenges: (a) Similar effect sizes in successive trials result in diminishing returns, and (b) small absolute gains require exponentially larger sample sizes. A common pitfall occurs when propagating the same effect size from a previous trial to the next successive trial with the expectation of obtaining a similar absolute improvement in outcome. As we approach the lower boundary of zero mean heart dose, sample sizes needed to demonstrate clinical benefits increase exponentially (Figure 14.4).

In resource-constrained environments, the cost-effectiveness and feasibility of research efforts should be carefully considered. The pursuit of small clinical benefits may be justifiable for common diseases affecting large numbers of patients, as may be the case with treatment of the IMC in breast cancer. However, a point of clinical futility does exist; determining this threshold can be challenging. A potential solution to the problem of diminishing returns is to conduct cost-effectiveness analyses of clinical trials. What is the cost of the clinical trial, what is the magnitude of the benefit from the intervention, and how many patients would stand to benefit? Detailed cost-effectiveness analyses (see Chapter 19) addressing these questions can help prioritize the funding of clinical trials.

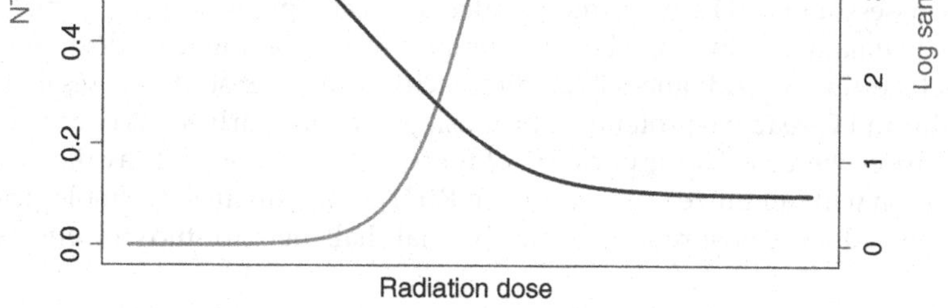

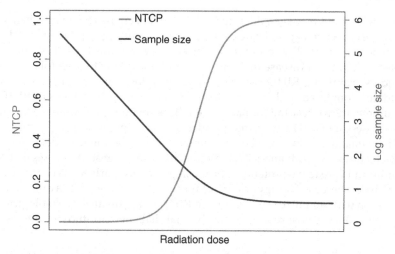

FIGURE 14.3 At the low end of the NTCP model, decreasing radiation dose leads to marginal reductions in toxicity and exponential increases in sample size, illustrating the concept of diminishing returns. The sample size represents the number needed to detect a difference in toxicity comparing the plotted NTCP probability to a control group receiving no radiation.

NTCP, normal tissue complication probability.

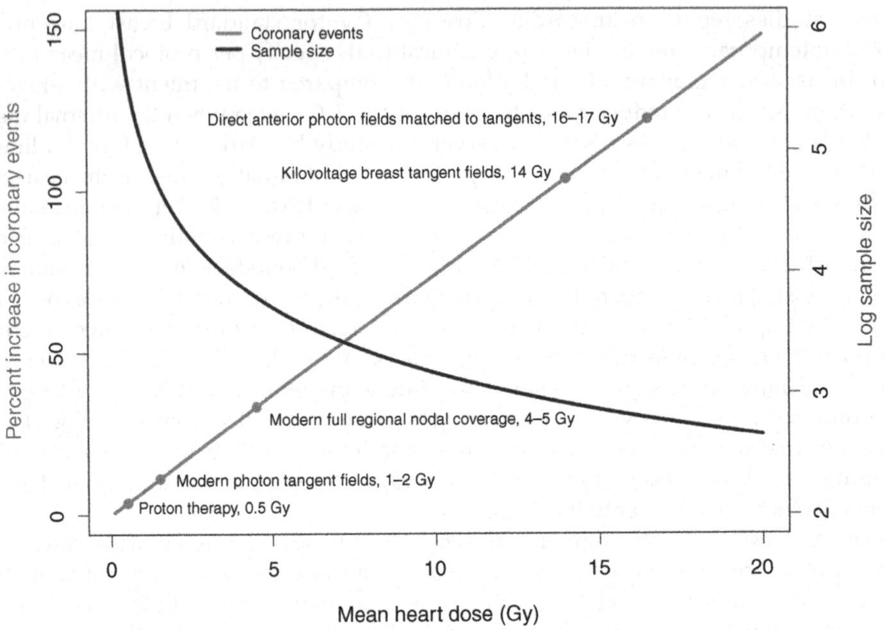

FIGURE 14.4 Radiation dose to the heart is associated with cardiac toxicity. Stepwise advances in radiotherapy have reduced heart doses to clinically insignificant doses for many women with left-sided breast cancer, illustrating the concept of "innovation to extinction."

CONCLUSION

As technology and patient management improve, cancer survivors face many challenges, including the risk of cancer recurrence and cardiovascular events during survivorship. RT significantly reduces recurrence and mortality from breast cancer. However, this benefit has been diminished by an increased risk in heart disease incidence and mortality. Due to long follow-up of patients, published studies examining RIHD risk include cardiac doses and other relevant data that are relatively outdated compared to those used today. Hence, current estimates of RIHD potentially include measurement error leading to inaccurate risk estimation. Major sources of measurement error in studies assessing RIHD are dosimetry calculation and preexisting heart disease. Statistical learning and new imaging technology help to minimize error coming from dosimetry calculations included in RIHD estimates. Advances in cardiotoxicity biomarker studies assessing NT-pro-BNP, cardiac troponin, and C-reactive protein are promising to assess early signs of cardiovascular dysfunction after cancer therapy. The application of these methods alongside available radiation and patient information will minimize error in current RIHD risk estimates. Technological innovations that progressively reduce exposure can pose additional challenges to studying effects of exposures on outcomes.

GLOSSARY

survivorship: status of persons living with the aftereffects of treatment.

internal validity: refers to the inferences drawn from a study that apply to the study population.

external validity: refers to applications to individuals outside of a study population (generalizability).

confounding by nonspecificity: occurs when inferences may be undermined by the fact that an observed effect could be due in whole or part to confounders driving risk for the competing event.

Charlson Comorbidity Index (CCI): a comprehensive comorbidity measure where each comorbidity category (from the International Classification of Disease [ICD]) has a weight based on the adjusted risk of mortality, and the sum of all weights results in a single comorbidity score for a patient.

Adult Comorbidity Evaluation (ACE-27) index: a comprehensive comorbidity measure for patients with cancer where comorbidities are graded based on severity (severe, moderate, mild), and defined by the highest ranked single ailment.

matching: describes the selection of a reference group (unexposed subjects in a cohort study and control subjects in a case control study) that is identical or closely so to the study group with respect to the distribution of one or more potentially confounding factors.

residual confounding: confounding that may exist despite proper reference group selection and data collection strategies.

innovation to extinction: name for the fact that against the backdrop of a fixed boundary, each incremental reduction in toxicity becomes exponentially more costly and difficult to achieve.

REFERENCES

1. Hewitt M, Greenfield S, Stovall E, eds. *From Cancer Patient to Cancer Survivor: Lost in Transition*. Washington, DC: National Academies Press; 2006.
2. Miller KD, Siegel RL, Lin CC, et al. Cancer treatment and survivorship statistics, 2016. *CA Cancer J Clin*. 2016;66(4): 271–289. doi:10.3322/caac.21349
3. Writing Group Members, Mozaffarian D, Benjamin EJ, et al. Executive summary: heart disease and stroke statistics--2016 update: a report from the American Heart Association. *Circulation*. 2016;133(4):447–454. doi:10.1161/CIR.0000000000000366
4. Darby S, McGale P, Correa C, et al. Effect of radiotherapy after breast-conserving surgery on 10-year recurrence and 15-year breast cancer death: meta-analysis of individual patient data for 10,801 women in 17 randomised trials. *Lancet*. 2011;378:1707–1716. doi:10.1016/s0140-6736(11)61629-2
5. McGale P, Taylor C, Correa C, et al. Effect of radiotherapy after mastectomy and axillary surgery on 10-year recurrence and 20-year breast cancer mortality: meta-analysis of individual patient data for 8135 women in 22 randomised trials. *Lancet*. 2014;383:2127–2135.doi:10.1016/S0140-6736(14)60488-8
6. McGale P, Darby SC, Hall P, et al. Incidence of heart disease in 35,000 women treated with radiotherapy for breast cancer in Denmark and Sweden. *Radiother Oncol*. 2011;100(2):167–175. doi:10.1016/j.radonc.2011.06.016
7. Darby SC, Ewertz M, McGale P, et al. Risk of ischemic heart disease in women after radiotherapy for breast cancer. *N Engl J Med*. 2013;368:987–998. doi:10.1056/NEJMoa1209825
8. Zagar TM, Cardinale DM, Marks LB. Breast cancer therapy-associated cardiovascular disease. *Nat Rev Clin Oncol*. 2016;13:172–184. doi:10.1038/nrclinonc.2015.171
9. Goyal S, Haffty BG. Cardiovascular toxicities of breast cancer treatment: emerging issues in cardio-oncology. *Front Oncol*. 2015;5:66. doi:10.3389/fonc.2015.00066
10. Taylor CW, Kirby AM. Cardiac side-effects from breast cancer radiotherapy. *Clin Oncol*. 2015;27:621–629. doi:10.1016/j.clon.2015.06.007
11. Taylor CW, Wang Z, Macaulay E, et al. Exposure of the heart in breast cancer radiation therapy: a systematic review of heart doses published during 2003 to 2013. *Int J Radiat Oncol Biol Phys*. 2015;93:845–853. doi:10.1016/j.ijrobp.2015.07.2292
12. Rothman KJ, Greenland S, Lash TL. *Modern Epidemiology*. 3rd ed. Philadelphia, PA: Wolters Kluwer Health/Lippincott Williams & Wilkins; 2012.
13. Lorenzen EL, Brink C, Taylor CW, et al. Uncertainties in estimating heart doses from 2D-tangential breast cancer radiotherapy. *Radiother Oncol*. 2016;119:71–76. doi:10.1016/j.radonc.2016.02.017
14. Vasan RS, Sullivan LM, Wilson PW, et al. Relative importance of borderline and elevated levels of coronary heart disease risk factors. *Ann Intern Med*. 2005;142:393–402. doi:10.7326/0003-4819-142-6-200503150-00005
15. Austin SR, Wong YN, Uzzo RG, et al. Why summary comorbidity measures such as the Charlson Comorbidity Index and Elixhauser Score work. *Med Care*. 2015;53:e65–e72. doi:10.1097/MLR.0b013e318297429c
16. Yurkovich M, Avina-Zubieta JA, Thomas J, et al. A systematic review identifies valid comorbidity indices derived from administrative health data. *J Clin Epidemiol*. 2015;68:3–14. doi:10.1016/j.jclinepi.2014.09.010
17. Wolbers M, Koller MT, Stel VS, et al. Competing risks analyses: objectives and approaches. *Eur Heart J*. 2014;35:2936–2941. doi:10.1016/j.jclinepi.2014.09.010

18. Swain SM. Doxorubicin-induced cardiomyopathy. *N Engl J Med*. 1999;340:654–655. doi:10.1056/nejm199902253400813
19. Dhingra R, Vasan RS. Age as a risk factor. *Med Clin North Am*. 2012;96:87–91. doi:10.1016/j.mcna.2011.11.003
20. Ward EM, DeSantis CE, Lin CC, et al. Cancer statistics: breast cancer in situ. *CA Cancer J Clin*. 2015;65:481–495. doi:10.3322/caac.21321
21. Kang J, Schwartz R, Flickinger J, et al. Machine learning approaches for predicting radiation therapy outcomes: a clinician's perspective. *Int J Radiat Oncol Biol Phys*. 2015;93:1127–1135. doi:10.1016/j.ijrobp.2015.07.2286
22. Shortreed SM, Peeters A, Forbes AB. Estimating the effect of long-term physical activity on cardiovascular disease and mortality: evidence from the Framingham Heart Study. *Heart*. 2013;99:649–654. doi:10.1136/heartjnl-2012-303461
23. Tian S, Hirshfield KM, Jabbour SK, et al. Serum biomarkers for the detection of cardiac toxicity after chemotherapy and radiation therapy in breast cancer patients. *Front Oncol*. 2014;4:277. doi:10.3389/fonc.2014.00277
24. Kehl DW, Iqbal N, Fard A, et al. Biomarkers in acute myocardial injury. *Transl Res*. 2012;159:252–264. doi:10.1016/j.trsl.2011.11.002
25. Mavinkurve-Groothuis AM, Kapusta L, Nir A, et al. The role of biomarkers in the early detection of anthracycline-induced cardiotoxicity in children: a review of the literature. *J Pediatr Hematol Oncol*. 2008;25:655–664. doi:10.1080/08880010802244001
26. Henri C, Heinonen T, Tardif JC. The role of biomarkers in decreasing risk of cardiac toxicity after cancer therapy. *Biomark Cancer*. 2016;8:39–45. doi:10.4137/BIC.S31798
27. Mirzaei H, Ferns GA, Avan A, et al. Cytokines and microRNA in coronary artery disease. *Adv Clin Chem*. 2017;82:47–70. doi:10.4137/BIC.S31798
28. Marks LB, Yu X, Prosnitz RG, et al. The incidence and functional consequences of RT-associated cardiac perfusion defects. *Int J Radiat Oncol Biol Phys*. 2005;63:214–223. doi:10.1016/j.ijrobp.2005.01.029
29. Florian A, Jurcut R, Ginghina C, et al. Cardiac magnetic resonance imaging in ischemic heart disease: a clinical review. *J Med Life*. 2011;4:330–345. doi:10.1016/j.ijrobp.2005.01.029
30. Taylor CW, Nisbet A, McGale P, Darby SC. Cardiac exposures in breast cancer radiotherapy: 1950s-1990s. *Int J Radiat Oncol Biol Phys*. 2007;69:1484–1495. doi:10.1016/j.ijrobp.2007.05.034
31. Kirby AM, Evans PM, Donovan EM, et al. Prone versus supine positioning for whole and partial-breast radiotherapy: a comparison of non-target tissue dosimetry. *Radiother Oncol*. 2010;96:178–184. doi:10.1016/j.radonc.2010.05.014
32. Osman SO, Hol S, Poortmans PM, Essers M. Volumetric modulated arc therapy and breath-hold in image-guided locoregional left-sided breast irradiation. *Radiother Oncol*. 2014;112:17–22. doi:10.1016/j.radonc.2014.04.004
33. Jagsi R, Moran J, Marsh R, et al. Evaluation of four techniques using intensity-modulated radiation therapy for comprehensive locoregional irradiation of breast cancer. *Int J Radiat Oncol Biol Phys*. 2010;78:1594–1603. doi:10.1016/j.ijrobp.2010.04.072
34. Bartlett FR, Colgan RM, Carr K, et al. The UK HeartSpare Study: randomised evaluation of voluntary deep-inspiratory breath-hold in women undergoing breast radiotherapy. *Radiother Oncol*. 2013;108(2):242–247. doi:10.1016/j.radonc.2013.04.021
35. Thorsen LB, Thomsen MS, Berg M, et al. CT-planned internal mammary node radiotherapy in the DBCG-IMN study: benefit versus potentially harmful effects. *Acta Oncol*. 2014;53:1027–1034. doi:10.3109/0284186X.2014.925579
36. National Surgical Adjuvant Breast and Bowel Project Foundation Inc. A randomized phase III clinical trial evaluating post-mastectomy chestwall and regional nodal XRT and post-lumpectomy regional nodal XRT in patients with positive axillary nodes before neoadjuvant chemotherapy who convert to pathologically negative axillary nodes after neoadjuvant chemotherapy. ClinicalTrials.gov Identifier: NCT01872975. https://clinicaltrials.gov/ct2/show/NCT01872975. Last updated May 17, 2017.
37. MacDonald SM, Patel SA, Hickey S, et al. Proton therapy for breast cancer after mastectomy: early outcomes of a prospective clinical trial. *Int J Radiat Oncol Biol Phys*. 2013;86:484–490. doi:10.1016/j.ijrobp.2013.01.038
38. Kent DM, Trikalinos TA. Therapeutic innovations, diminishing returns, and control rate preservation. *JAMA*. 2009;302:2254–2256. doi:10.1001/jama.2009.1679

15

Longitudinal and Observational Data

JEFF BURKEEN ■ SCOTT KEITH ■ JONA HATTANGADI-GLUTH

Longitudinal studies are studies in which the outcome variable is repeatedly measured in the same individuals on several different occasions, often for years or decades. These studies can be experimental or observational in design, with data being collected on any combination of outcomes, either in a qualitative or quantitative fashion. With longitudinal studies, the observations of a single individual over time are not independent as observations between independent individuals might be. Therefore, it is necessary to apply special statistical techniques that apply to the fact that the repeated observations of each individual are correlated. This chapter covers longitudinal study design with a focus on observational data, advantages and disadvantages of these study designs, examples, implementation, statistical methods, as well as analytic issues.

LONGITUDINAL STUDY DESIGNS

Longitudinal studies in oncology should be designed with chief research questions and goals in mind. Important contributions of patient function, comorbid health conditions, disease status, treatment type, and behavioral and environmental factors may be important considerations as well, depending on the study goals. It may be burdensome to quantify the various determinants of health to the same degree, as it might be important to report the primary questions of the study. Overall cost and usefulness may control the amount of accuracy for estimation and thus the feasibility of the study, directing questions to the priorities dictated by the primary research hypotheses. By setting goals concentrating on primary research questions and hypotheses, investigators can set priorities and determine what information is essential to reaching the goals, and other concerns regarding methodology can be put into perspective.

Design concerns in longitudinal observational studies can be categorized into target population, exposure(s) of interest, outcomes, and potential confounders. To ensure the best design in light of practical considerations, the primary investigators require a workforce with the tools to contribute to successful design of the longitudinal study. This includes leaders in the field with access to patients in the target population (or to important subgroups within the population);

experts in relevant diseases and outcomes or other exposures of interest (i.e., behavioral, environmental, or biological factors) and other important processes; as well as staff who are trained in collecting data, analyzing data, and performing statistics that are critical for avoiding errors and bias in estimation and inference used to address the research questions and hypotheses. The research group must have extensive knowledge of financial and human resource topics. Overall, the research workforce generally will not need prior training in medical disciplines, but must pay attention to detail and be intent on learning and adhering to the study protocols.

The target population may vary as it relates to the goals and interests of the study. The patient sample that can be feasibly studied will dictate inclusion and exclusion criteria. Limiting the population by location, disease characteristics, or patient characteristics and exposures may improve the ability to conduct an efficient study, but this limits how well the sample from the study population reflects the target population. The enrollment of individuals across the entire range of characteristics present in the target population, such as patient health, including the frailest, will increase generalizability of the results of the study. Oncologic longitudinal studies need to determine the assortment of the study population and decide whether to over-recruit particular subpopulations to have adequate power for conducting important subgroup analyses within the exposure groups. In most situations, additional means are needed for minority recruitment (1).

Characterizing changes in outcomes and exposures over time generally requires frequent contacts with the enrollees in the study. Certain cancer outcomes may be assessed using chart records, and others may require prospective in-person examinations. The need for a diverse sample representative of the target population must be weighed against the ability to obtain consent and maintain follow-up contact with the sampled patients. These are competing goals because random sampling (i.e., each individual having the same likelihood of being sampled) from the target population in this context is often impossible; convenience sampling may be the only practical option. Intensive assessments and the requirement for years of follow-up can decrease participation and increase dropout, further limiting generalizability and posing a threat to the validity of the findings.

Power calculations are needed to estimate the sample size required to have sufficient probability of detecting associations between the exposures of interest and the primary outcomes. Power depends on a number of things, including the acceptable type I error rate (α), the multiplicity of testing if there is more than one primary hypothesis (i.e., multiple primary exposures or primary outcomes), the size of the effects the primary exposures of interest have on the primary outcomes, the strength and perhaps the structure of the correlations among outcome observations from the same individual over time, and the variability in the primary outcome variables—which, if discrete or count variables, will depend on the outcome event proportion or rate. A multitude of distinct health outcomes may happen at rates at varying times per year, which can severely limit power. Therefore, sample sizes of hundreds to thousands may be needed to have enough expected events to overcome that limitation and allow investigators to conduct their study within a reasonable study period.

Longitudinal studies are typically structured to examine multiple outcomes. The choices of primary research questions and hypotheses are important when assessing multiple outcomes. Importantly, the research should be powered for the most influential and ideal questions of the study. By doing this, the sample size to be recruited will be greatly influenced, which is typically the primary factor in the viability and cost of the study. Nonetheless, there is a large methodological benefit to analyzing multiple endpoints, in that hazard ratios can be determined. Examining the association among multiple health outcomes can help determine the utility for and influences on individual- and community-level endpoints, such as patient outcomes and healthcare utilization.

To highlight, the Women's Health Initiative (2) included a longitudinal observational study component and was able to determine the incidence of fractures, breast cancer, cardiovascular outcomes, and cognition changes because of the care taken to design the study for answering these questions and the investments made by study sponsors, investigators, participants, and other stakeholders to accrue years of follow-up data on a large and diverse sample (3). Overall, the results have provided a stronger idea of the importance that these major comorbidities play in the overall health of elderly women (3–6).

ADVANTAGES AND DISADVANTAGES OF LONGITUDINAL STUDIES

Advantages. Longitudinal observational studies, when conducted prospectively, offer numerous benefits and advantages over cross-sectional studies. These include (a) determining and relating results to certain exposures and better describing these as it relates to occurrence and timing, (b) following changes over time in subjects within the group, (c) preventing bias in recall in study member by gathering prospective data and before information of a possible later event or outcome happening, and (d) the utility to modify the study via the cohort effect—allowing for testing of the individual time factors of the cohort (ranges of birth dates), period (current time span), and age of the subject—and accounting for the influence of each individually (7).

Disadvantages. Various difficulties are inherent in longitudinal studies, specifically because these studies happen over prolonged time periods. Some disadvantages inherent to longitudinal studies may include (a) inadequate and unconventional follow-up examinations of individuals and follow-up loss as time passes, (b) imprecision in conclusions if using statistical methods that do not explain the association of observations from the same individual, and (c) increased time and monetary requirements associated with this approach (7).

EXAMPLES OF LONGITUDINAL STUDIES

There are many examples of longitudinal studies in multiple disciplines and fields of medicine, but this section focuses on those centered on oncology. Changes in cognition attributed with central nervous system (CNS) and pediatric cancer treatments have long been established in the research literature (8,9). However, additional evidence has suggested that treatments for non-CNS tumors can have both acute and long-term effects on cognition, after exposure to chemotherapy in cross-sectional studies (10–12). Longitudinal neuropsychological studies have played a critical role in further characterizing these cognitive changes, specifically for patients with breast cancer after chemotherapy (Table 15.1) (13–17). Similar to prior cross-sectional studies, longitudinal studies imply that a small group of patients develop difficulties with cognition following treatment, to varying degrees among the studies.

A 2016 longitudinal study examined quality of life (QOL) and neurocognitive assessments as secondary endpoints in patients treated with whole brain radiotherapy (WBRT) in addition to stereotactic radiosurgery (SRS) versus SRS alone (18). The timing of the neurocognitive and QOL assessments was approximately every 3 months after treatment (Table 15.2). The Functional Assessment of Cancer Therapy-Brain (FACT-BR) questionnaire was used for patient self-reported QOL (19), and neutral analyses of changes in cognition (e.g., speech impairment) and physician-assessed toxicities (e.g., nausea) were collected. Two hundred and thirteen participants with a mean age of 61 years were analyzed. Though there was no difference in overall survival, QOL was higher at 3 months with SRS alone, including overall QOL ($p = .001$). For long-term survivors, decline in cognition was less after SRS alone at 3 ($p = .007$) and 12 months ($p = .04$) (18). These findings suggested that for patients eligible to receive SRS, SRS alone may be a preferred therapy regimen versus SRS combined with WBRT.

IMPLEMENTATION OF A LONGITUDINAL STUDY

Conducting longitudinal studies is difficult because such a study requires an appropriate structure that endures the test of time for the study duration. Importantly, there is a need to have a detailed and clearly written study protocol so that the gathering of information and documentation are similar among the multitude of study sites, keeping in mind that they are standardized and consistent over time. Data are noted, and accurateness increased, by utilizing recognized organization systems for individual data points (20). Data on various variables should be collected when

TABLE 15.1 LONGITUDINAL RESEARCH ARTICLES FOCUSED ON COGNITION OUTCOMES FOR PATIENTS WITH BREAST CANCER AFTER TREATMENT

Article	Patients	Schedule for Assessments	Results
Stewart et al. (13)	CTX (*N* = 61; MA, 57.5 years); hormonal therapy (*N* = 51; MA, 57.9 years)	Baseline (before treatment) and follow-up (after treatment)	Patients receiving CTX with increased risk of cognition deficits (increased threefold)
Collins et al. (14)	CTX (*N* = 53; MA, 57.5 years); hormonal therapy alone (*N* = 40; MA, 57.6 years)	Following surgery but prior to CTX; circa 1 month of finishing CTX or 5–6 months after initial assessments	CTX with the addition of hormones associated with decreases in verbal memory and processing speed
Hammerlink et al. (15)	Premenopausal (*N* = 11); induced menopause (*N* = 31); postmenopausal (*N* = 49, MA, 48.4 years); each patient received one of two neoadjuvant CTX courses; received TX or AI (*N* = 62)	Before treatment, near conclusion of neoadjuvant CTX and 1 year following baseline	Addition of hormones did not lead to changes regarding patient cognition
Mehlsen et al. (16)	Breast cancer patients (*N* = 34; MA, 48.6 years); patients with MI (*N* = 12; MA, 50.4 years); patients without MI (*N* = 12; MA, 39.3 years)	Assessed at baseline; patients with breast cancer, 1 week prior to CTX; MI patients, 4 days following hospitalization; follow-up 6 months for cancer patients, 3 months for MI patients, and 3–4 months for patients without MI	Between the three groups, no differences associated with cognition were found
Hedayati et al. (17)	CTX (*N* = 18; MA, 52 years); hormone therapy (*N* = 45; MA, 61 years); no adjuvant therapy (*N* = 14; MA 61 years); control patients (*N* = 69; MA, 51 years)	Prior to diagnosis, following surgery, before adjuvant therapy; 6 months after start of adjuvant therapy	Patients receiving adjuvant treatment displayed decreased memory; CTX patients displayed decreased memory and response speed

CTX, chemotherapy.

embarking on such a study in order to address all the research questions, characterize the population, and avoid sources of bias in analyses, such as confounding, which can be a serious threat to the validity of observational studies, since treatments and other exposures of interest are not randomly assigned. These variables include aspects related to the patients on study and their living situation (21). Moreover, the commitment and agreement of groups and investors supporting the study are important and have to be enabled and upheld via methods of consistent preparation and contact.

The frequency and extent of sampling should depend on the specific primary research question, properties of the primary outcomes and exposures in the population affecting power, and a variety of other concerns. Consent and ethical guidelines are important to longitudinal observational studies. The utmost action should be taken to keep patients on study, with the performance of exit interviews supplying additional understanding as to the reason for study departures (20). Increasing quality assessment is available with the Consolidated Standards of Reporting Trials

TABLE 15.2 LONGITUDINAL TESTING SCHEDULE FOR ALLIANCE BRAIN SRS VERSUS SRS + WBRT TRIAL

ASSESSMENTS		OBSERVATION									
		Week (W) 6	W 12	Month (M) 6	M 9	M 12	M 16	M 24	M 36	M 48	M 60
Quality of Life: FACT-BR	TREATMENT	X	X	X	X	X	X	X	X	X	X
Functional independence tests		X	X	X	X	X	X	X	X	X	X
Neurocognitive tests		X	X	X	X	X	X	X	X	X	X

(CONSORT) guidelines, which include a defined and organized 33-point checklist created and instituted by Tooth et al. in 2004 (22).

After appropriate study planning, bringing longitudinal research projects online may require a large amount of time, effort, and resources, particularly if the study is being launched and implemented at multiple institutions. Understanding the importance of study onboarding improves the type of data eventually collected, which will help the accuracy of the results. Consistent overview of data quality and keeping an eye out for areas of worry is very important (21). Longitudinal research is ever changing and may require training or retraining of contributors, as necessary.

STATISTICAL CONSIDERATIONS

Collecting longitudinal data can be challenging. First, it requires measuring subjects at least twice, which costs more per subject than single cross-sectional measurements, and subjects who are lost to follow-up (dropout) or are dead or unable to further participate (attrition) cannot be replaced. So, cooperation of those who participated at baseline must be strongly encouraged at each time point to improve the power and validity of any study.

Multiple statistical approaches are used in longitudinal studies via software packages such as R (available for free at https://cran.r-project.org), Statistical Analysis Software (SAS), Stata, and Statistical Package for the Social Sciences (SPSS). These packages offer procedures and functions for conducting both univariate and multivariate analyses, including those designed for longitudinal analysis.

Figure 15.1 presents a hypothetical scenario regarding the collection of longitudinal data. For the two subjects, data are collected for 1 year monthly, but one subject drops out prior to the 8 months visit and therefore the data that would have been collected for that patient for months 8 through 12 are not a part of the analysis. The observations appear approximately linear for both individuals over time. Allowing both individuals to have their own linear model fit, the vertical distance from the observations of the study subject to the subject's line is signified as the "within-subject" residual deviations that quantify the differences in the results. If there were only data for one individual, this would equal the residual error terms in a regression equation. Commonly, single patients are assumed to signify a random unique sample from an appropriate population that is targeted and the interest that is important is the *typical* linear trajectory (or its slope) and perhaps the *typical* magnitudes of the within-subject and between-subject deviations in the longitudinal observational studies.

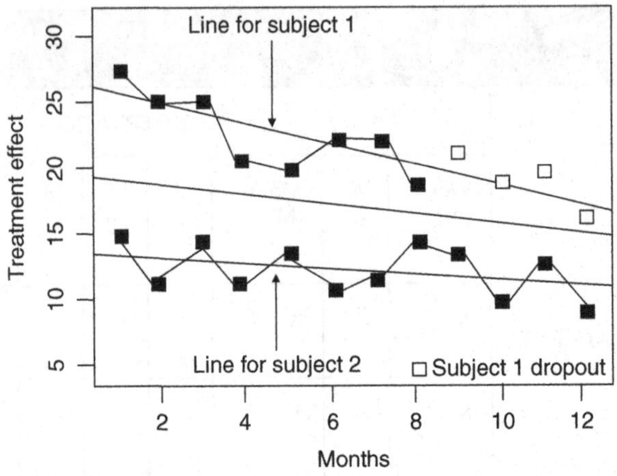

FIGURE 15.1 A hypothetical representation of longitudinal data for two subjects. Both subjects have their own individual trajectory. Subject 1 dropped out of the study at 8 months; open squares represent potential responses of Subject 1 that might have been observed if this subject had not dropped out.

In the center of Figure 15.1, the dashed line highlights the overall average of the linear time paths of the subjects included in the analysis. This line estimates the population average for the observations of all subjects in the targeted study group as it relates to time. To highlight, 3 months on the dashed line are estimated by the cross-sectional average of the linear trajectory values at 3 months for both individuals and is assumed to represent the average in the population at 3 months. As such, Figure 15.1 shows the "average line," which indicates the path and the average of the population as a function of time.

Longitudinal studies require advanced statistical modeling techniques, especially when the data are observational and adjustment for confounding variables is necessary. **Conditional models**, commonly fitted using **linear mixed-effects (LME) regression**, condition population parameter estimates explicitly on each subject changes over time while taking account of differences in frequency and timing of repeated measures and for events where data may be missing (23). In Figure 15.1, the within-subject differences are the deviation between individual observations, *Yij*, and the individual linear trajectory. In this figure,

$$b_{i,0} + b_{i,1} \cdot X_{ij}$$

is a linear expression that can characterize the linear trajectory of the Y_{ij}'s over time, where X_{ij} indicates the measurement of time j on subject i. The patients each have an individual-specific intercept ($b_{i,0}$) and slope ($b_{i,1}$). Again, within-subject differences are calculated by the importance of the residual differences between the observations and the individual trajectory, $Y_{ij} - (b_{i,0} + b_{i,1} \cdot X_{ij})$.

Statistical software is used to optimize the intercepts and slopes to minimize the within-subject variation (or some function of it) across time for each individual. The between-subject variation is highlighted by the differences among the estimated intercepts from an average intercept and variation among the estimated slopes from an average slope (23). Therefore, in LME there may be regression factors that differ among presumably randomly selected patients (i.e., random effect parameters), while some regression parameters are fixed and common to all individuals (i.e., fixed effect parameters). In Figure 15.1 it is clear that the subjects require a unique intercept for a reasonable model fit, but they may not require their own slope. This would be the case if we fit a random intercept linear mixed model, which would constrain the model to have parallel trajectories for all subjects:

$$Y_{ij} = \beta_0 + \beta_1 \cdot X_{ij} + b_{i,0} + \varepsilon_{ij},$$

where the intercept for subject i is given by $\beta_0 + b_{i0}$, while their slope is simply β_1, since there is no additional random individual slope parameter, $b_{i,1}$ in the random intercept model.

A **marginal model**, commonly fitted using **generalized estimating equations (GEEs)**, is a popular approach to both linear and **generalized linear modeling** of longitudinal data. It is different from conditional modeling in that there are no individual-level parameters to be estimated, which translates to easier interpretation of population mean parameter estimates when applied to discrete outcomes (24,25). Both approaches can accommodate many possible within-subject covariance structures beyond independent, including **exchangeable** (i.e., assumes the same non-zero correlation among observations from the same individual), **autoregressive** (i.e., the degree of correlation between observations from the same individual depends on the length of time or another measure of distance between the observations), and **unstructured** correlation, because longitudinal data within subjects generally cannot be assumed to be independent and may be correlated in complicated ways. The variances of a marginal model estimated by GEE can be obtained using the (Huber-White) sandwich estimator, which converges to the same values regardless of the form of the covariance matrix, suggesting that, unlike for conditional modeling, the analyst need only specify the correct mean response model to estimate valid standard errors of marginal model parameters.

The marginal model specification is similar to the familiar linear and generalized linear regression models of the mean response (μ_{ij}) for subject i at time j as a linear combination of the explanatory variables ($\mathbf{X}_{ij}$) and a set of corresponding regression parameters (β):

$$g(\mu_{ij}) = \mathbf{X}_{ij}'\beta$$

where the function g(·) is called a **link function**. Examples of common nonlinear link functions include natural log (for continuous or count responses) and logit or probit (for binary responses; see also Chapter 13). An identity link function (i.e., a function that makes no transformation) returns the ordinary linear model.

As you can see from the equation, applying the inverse link function to this equation provides a way of relating the population mean response to the explanatory variables through β, which does not depend on any individual-level parameter estimates. This is a key advantage of marginal models over conditional models when the outcomes are discrete. Conditional models can estimate both fixed effect parameters across individuals (like β) and individual random effect parameters (like $\boldsymbol{b}_i$) by generalized linear mixed modeling (GLMM) in this random intercept conditional model equation:

$$g(\mu_{ij}) = \mathbf{X}_{ij}'\beta + b_i$$

However, because we have to invert the link function to estimate the mean response, any link function that is not an identity function will cause a distortion to the random effect parameter distribution such that the population mean response cannot be represented by the fixed effect parameters alone (25). Thus, the choice of whether to use a conditional or marginal model (i.e., to use GLMM or GEE) depends on whether the research question refers to changes in mean response *within* an individual over time or to changes in mean response *between* individuals in the target population over time.

For example, Manzano et al. studied over 30,000 gastrointestinal cancer patients undergoing nearly 70,000 hospitalizations using a combination of cancer registry and Medicare claims data (26). They used GEE with a logistic link function to construct a marginal model of readmission patterns after hospitalization, since the probability of hospitalization within subjects is likely to be highly correlated. They found that the odds of unplanned readmissions were up to 50% greater in patients with multiple comorbidities (odds ratio 1.53 for Charlson comorbidity index ≥ 3 vs. 0). The flexibility of this approach and its utility in making direct population estimates and valid inferences, regardless of the link function applied, makes marginal modeling by GEE a popular choice for analyzing how exposures of interest and covariates relate to correlated outcomes in longitudinal observational data.

ANALYTIC CONSIDERATIONS

There are various analytic issues with the implementation of longitudinal observational studies. This section outlines these issues.

NONRANDOM ASSIGNMENT

In oncology, we are often interested in comparing the effects or associations of different interventions or treatments. Randomized controlled studies are the gold standard for determining whether one treatment's effect is superior (or non-inferior) to another. However, for practical, developmental, or ethical reasons, randomized studies are not always possible. In these situations, well-conducted observational studies can provide useful information on treatments or other exposures associated with outcomes to influence decision making and develop hypotheses for controlled trials. One common challenge in analyzing observational data is that treatments are not assigned randomly. Therefore, it is possible that characteristics of patients, providers, or healthcare systems, both observed and unobserved, can influence not only treatment assignment but also outcomes. For example, sicker patients might be less likely to receive aggressive treatment and they may also be more likely to have a poor outcome, regardless of treatment received. Analyses not accounting for such favorable selection into the more aggressive treatment will thus be biased by confounding and overestimate the benefit of the treatment.

ATTRITION AND HANDLING MISSING DATA

Attrition is a typical issue in longitudinal observation studies with cancer patients. For example, palliative oncology reports have recognized attrition rates up to 60% in this population (27–29). Various reasons in trials studying cancer outcomes have included patient comorbidities, death, severe symptoms, impaired cognition, poor performance status, increased age, low socioeconomic status, belonging to a particular minority group, long study time, and physician input, in addition to others (30–32). A recent longitudinal publication in palliative patients with locally advanced and metastatic cancer demonstrated that decline in cognition, poor physical symptoms, worse performance status, and short duration from cancer diagnosis were factors contributing to the likelihood of patient attrition as well (33). In addition, patients may drop out due to the burdens of multiple study procedures or even dissatisfaction stemming from interactions with study personnel.

The main concern with attrition is that missing data could bias study results. This concern is heightened in studies of comparative effectiveness when the level of missing data is different between study groups. Therefore, all studies must address how missing data were handled in analyses and may have affected the results. It is important to be aware that many statistical programs and packages will automatically or by default eliminate from the analysis all observations that have any missing values on the variables considered. In many cases, it may not be readily apparent from the output that this was done. Thus, caution must be used to ascertain the extent of missing values in the data and address the bias caused by the missing data before moving forward with analysis. Further details about missing data are discussed in Chapters 11 and 22.

Many approaches exist to handle missing data to avoid bias. One approach involves omitting all observations without complete data (i.e., **complete case analysis** after list-wise deletion). This approach is simple and likely valid if the number of missing observations is small relative to the overall sample size, the variables missing a considerable amount of data are not critical outcomes or exposures of primary interest, the mechanism driving the omissions is essentially random conditional on other variables used in modeling the data, and the conditional or marginal model fitted to the longitudinal observation data to address the research question is adequate (i.e., an appropriate LME, GLMM, GEE model). However, if there are many missing values causing omission of many observations over time, this approach can lead to substantial loss of statistical power and biased results, especially if the discarded observations differ systematically from those retained, in a way that cannot be explained by the observed study variables, in which case arriving at valid model results might not be possible (25).

An alternative (and often preferred) approach to handling missing data is **imputation**. Single imputation refers to assigning a fixed value that is assumed to be representative of the true value missing—perhaps a predicted value from a regression model based on the observed data. Similar to complete case analysis, this approach may be acceptable if the number of missing observations is small and the variables are not critical. For example, in some studies, body mass index (BMI, defined as [weight in kg] / [height in m]^2) is an important explanatory variable. If weight is missing at some observation time, however, the BMI would then be missing as well. In this case, an investigator may choose to impute the predicted value of the missing weight from an LME regression model of weight across the sample, perhaps conditioned on the sex and other time-varying or time-fixed factors important for predicting weight and available for the subject missing the data, to approximate that person's BMI at that time.

As a general approach, single imputation is fairly simple and avoids having to completely discard from a model all of a subject's observations at a time when there are missing data on variables used in the model (including their non-missing data at those observation points in the study). However, a principal disadvantage of single imputation is that it generally underestimates the true variation in the variables being imputed, attributing a degree of certainty to the imputed values that is not truly there. Multiple imputation (MI) addresses this problem by *repeatedly* simulating distributions of likely values for the missing data points modeled using non-missing data across study variables and time, imputing those simulated observations to "complete" the dataset, fitting the marginal or condition model addressing the research hypothesis to each "complete" dataset to generate a set of model results for each parameter and its variance estimate, and aggregating the replicated estimates using established formulas (34). Even results from 5 or 10 iterations of imputed "complete" datasets can be sufficient for addressing the variability in the imputed observations.

A common computation approach to MI uses Markov chain Monte Carlo (MCMC). This method assumes that the multiple missing variables follow a joint distribution (e.g., a multivariate normal distribution), then uses Bayesian prediction methods to obtain imputed values that are likely to represent well the true, but unobserved, values (35). However, depending on the number of iterations and size of the dataset under study, this approach can be computationally expensive. Other common MI approaches can use regression models and Monte Carlo simulation to assign imputed values, based on the data structure, as an extension to the approach for single imputation described earlier. For example, a binary variable missing some data could be modeled using logistic regression, in this way taking advantage of the information embedded in the non-missing values, and imputing binary random variables for the missing values using a Bernoulli random number generator conditioned on the predicted values (i.e., the propensity scores) from this model and then repeating this process and aggregating model parameter estimate results on the imputed "complete" datasets as already explained.

MI is generally accepted as the most reliably valid method for handling missing data, assuming that the data are missing at random conditional on the variables used in the model (see Chapter 16 for more details). It can be thought of as a method for representing the uncertainty of missing data in regression models and it can function like a **sensitivity analysis** for various assumptions about the true values of the missing data. Although its complexity and computation time are nontrivial disadvantages of MI, it can be facilitated readily for longitudinal data in most commonly available statistical packages by adding a few more steps to the analysis and modeling plans. Further details on these methods using SAS software (Cary, NC) are provided elsewhere (35).

As with any statistical approach, the validity of the results of each imputation method requires careful and appropriate modeling. Whichever approach is used, it is important to clearly specify the magnitude of the missing data problem, rationale for the approach chosen to address it, and the sensitivity of inferences to the problem. Any report should describe the number of patients excluded for missing data and the number and proportion of missing values for each variable of interest. Second, reports should examine differences between patients with complete or incomplete data across exposure and outcome variables over time. Finally, reports should discuss whether and how missing data might have biased study results, even when valid approaches were used to handle missing data.

CONCLUSION

In summary, carefully designed and well-executed studies using longitudinal observational data are needed to advance our understanding of many unanswered questions in oncology. Several common features characterize a well-developed longitudinal observational study. These include clearly defined hypotheses and research questions, careful selection of patients, collaboration with investigators with relevant statistical and methodological expertise, caution not to overinterpret small but statistically significant differences as clinically meaningful differences, and recognition of limitations when trying to evaluate causality. Understanding these issues is of critical importance to appropriate evaluation of evidence and to guide future practice and policy. For more in-depth guidance on the statistical analysis topics covered in this chapter, as well as other topics that were not addressed in detail (such as selecting correlation structures, distributional assumptions, and model diagnostics), we suggest the textbook by Fitzmaurice, Laird, and Ware (25).

GLOSSARY

longitudinal studies: studies in which the outcome variable is repeatedly measured in the same individuals on several different occasions, often for years or decades.

conditional models: condition population parameter estimates explicitly on each subject changes over time while taking account of differences in frequency and timing of repeated measures and for events where data may be missing.

linear mixed-effects (LME) regression: common fitting technique for conditional models.

marginal model: a popular approach to both linear and generalized linear modeling of longitudinal data in which there are no individual-level parameters to be estimated.

generalized estimating equations (GEEs): common fitting technique for marginal models.

exchangeable: within-subject covariance structure that assumes the same non-zero correlation among observations from the same individual.

autoregressive: within-subject covariance structure in which the degree of correlation between observations from the same individual depends on the length of time or another measure of distance between the observations.

unstructured: within-subject covariance structure in which longitudinal data within subjects generally cannot be assumed to be independent and may be correlated in complicated ways.

link function: function in a marginal model specification.

complete case analysis: an approach to handling missing data to avoid bias that involves omitting all observations without complete data.

imputation: an approach to handling missing data in which replacement values are assigned to missing data randomly or by means of an algorithm.

sensitivity analysis: analysis that is undertaken allowing for various assumptions about the values of parameters or missing data.

REFERENCES

1. Ahles TA, Correa DD. Neuropsychological impact of cancer and cancer treatments. In: Holland JC, ed. *Psycho-Oncology*. 2nd ed. New York, NY: Oxford University Press; 2010;251–257.
2. Anderson FS, Kunin-Batson AS. Neurocognitive late effects of chemotherapy in children: the past 10 years of research on brain structure and function. *Pediatr Blood Cancer*. 2009;52:159–164. doi:10.1002/pbc.21700
3. Cauley JA, Wampler NS, Barnhart JM, et al. Incidence of fractures compared to cardiovascular disease and breast cancer: the Women's Health Initiative Observational Study. *Osteoporos Int*. 2008;19:1717–1723. doi:10.1007/s00198-008-0634-y
4. Rapp SR, Espeland MA, Shumaker SA, et al. Effect of estrogen plus progestin on global cognitive function in postmenopausal women: the Women's Health Initiative Memory Study: a randomized controlled trial. *JAMA*. 2003;289:2663–2672. doi:10.1001/jama.289.20.2663
5. Robbins J, Aragaki AK, Kooperberg C, et al. Factors associated with 5-year risk of hip fracture in postmenopausal women. *JAMA*. 2007;298:2389–2398. doi:10.1001/jama.298.20.2389
6. Rossouw JE, Anderson GL, Prentice RL, et al. Risks and benefits of estrogen plus progestin in healthy postmenopausal women: principal results from the Women's Health Initiative randomized controlled trial. *JAMA*. 2002;288:321–333. doi:10.1001/jama.288.3.321
7. Caruana EJ, Roman M, Hernandez-Sanchez, et al. Longitudinal studies. *J Thor Dis*. 2015;7:E537–E540. doi:10.3978/j.issn.2072-1439
8. Mar Fan HG, Houédé-Tchen N, Yi QL, et al. Fatigue, menopausal symptoms, and cognitive function in women after adjuvant chemotherapy for breast cancer: 1- and 2- year follow-up of a prospective study. *J Clin Oncol*. 2005;23:8025–8032. doi:10.1200/JCO.2005.01.6550
9. Schilling V, Jenkins V, Morris R, et al. The effects of adjuvant chemotherapy on cognition in women with breast cancer—preliminary results of an observational study. *Breast*. 2005;14:142–150. doi:10.1016/j.breast.2004.10.004
10. Tannock IF, Ahles TA, Ganz PA, et al. Cognitive impairment associated with chemotherapy for cancer: report of a workshop. *J Clin Oncol*. 2004;22:2233–2239. doi:10.1200/JCO.2004.08.094
11. Vardy J, Wefel JS, Ahles TA, et al. Cancer and cancer-therapy related cognitive dysfunction: an international perspective from the Venice Cognitive Workshop. *Ann Oncol*. 2008;19:623–629. doi:10.1093/annonc/mdm500
12. Wefel JS, Vardy J, Ahles TA, et al. International Cognition and Cancer Task Force recommendations to harmonise studies of cognitive function in cancer patients. *Lancet Oncol*. 2011;12:703–708. doi:10.1016/S1470-2045(10)70294-1
13. Stewart A, Collins B, Mackenzie J, et al. The cognitive effects of adjuvant chemotherapy in early stage breast cancer: a prospective study. *Psychooncology*. 2008;17:122–130. doi:10.1002/pon.1210
14. Collins B, Mackenzie J, Stewart A, et al. Cognitive effects of chemotherapy in post-menopausal breast cancer patients 1 year after treatment. *Psychooncology* 2009;18:134–143. doi:10.1002/pon.1379
15. Hermelink K, Henschel V, Untch M, et al. Short-term effects of treatment-induced hormonal changes on cognitive function in breast cancer patients: results of a multicenter, prospective, longitudinal study. *Cancer*. 2008;113:2431–2439. doi:10.1002/cncr.23853
16. Mehlsen M, Pedersen AD, Jensen AB, et al. No indications of cognitive side-effects in a prospective study of breast cancer patients receiving adjuvant chemotherapy. *Psychooncology*. 2009;18:248–257. doi:10.1002/pon.1398
17. Hedayati E, Alinaghizadeh H, Schedin A, et al. Effects of adjuvant treatment on cognitive function in women with early breast cancer. *Eur J Oncol Nurs*. 2012;16:315–322. doi:10.1016/j.ejon.2011.07.006
18. Brown P, Jaeckle K, Ballman KV, et al. Effect of radiosurgery alone vs radiosurgery with whole brain radiation therapy on cognitive function in patients with 1 to 3 brain metastases: a randomized clinical trial. *JAMA*. 2016;316(4):401–409. doi:10.1001/jama.2016.9839
19. Weitzner MA, Meyers CA, Gelke CK, et al. The Functional Assessment of Cancer Therapy (FACT) scale. Development of a brain subscale and revalidation of the general version (FACT-G) in patients with primary brain tumors. *Cancer*. 1995;75:1151–1161. doi:10.1002/1097-0142(19950301)75:5<1151::AID-CNCR2820750515>3.0.CO;2-Q
20. van Weel C. Longitudinal research and data collection in primary care. *Ann Fam Med*. 2005;3(Suppl 1):S46–S51. doi:10.1370/afm.300
21. Newman AB. An overview of the design, implementation, and analyses of longitudinal studies on aging. *J Am Geriatr Soc*. 2010;58(Suppl 2):S287–S291. doi:10.1111/j.1532-5415.2010.02916.x
22. Tooth L, Ware R, Bain C, et al. Quality of reporting of observational longitudinal research. *Am J Epidemiol*. 2005;161:280–288. doi:10.1093/aje/kwi042
23. Brown H,Prescott R. *Applied Mixed Models in Medicine*. New York, NY: Wiley; 1999.
24. Edwards LJ. Modern statistical techniques for the analysis of longitudinal data in biomedical research. *Pediatr Pulmonol*. 2000;30:330–344. doi:10.1002/1099-0496(200010)30:4<330::AID-PPUL10>3.0.CO;2-D

25. Fitzmaurice GM, Laird NM, Ware JH. *Applied Longitudinal Analysis*. 2nd ed. New York, NY: Wiley; 2011.
26. Manzano JM, Yang M, Zhao H, et al. Readmission patterns after GI cancer hospitalizations: the medical versus surgical patient. *J Oncol Pract*. 2018;14(3):e137–e148. doi:10.1200/jop.2017.026310
27. Preston NJ, Fayers P, Walters SJ, et al. Recommendations for managing missing data, attrition and response shift in palliative and end-of-life care research: part of the MORE-Care research method guidance on statistical issues. *Palliat Med*. 2103;27:899–907. doi:10.1177/0269216313486952
28. Stromgren AS, Sjogren P, Goldschmidt D, et al. A longitudinal study of palliative care-patient-evaluated outcome and impact of attrition. *Cancer*. 2005;103:1747–1755. doi:10.1002/cncr.20958
29. Ahlner-Elmqvist M, Bjordal K, Jordhoy MS, et al. Characteristics and implications of attrition in health-related quality of life studies in palliative care. *Palliat Med*. 2009;23:432–440. doi:10.1177/0269216309104057
30. Applebaum AJ, Lichtenthal WG, Pessin HA, et al. Factors associated with attrition from a randomized controlled trial of meaning-centered group psychotherapy for patients with advanced cancer. *Psychooncology*. 2012;21:1195–1204. doi:10.1002/pon.2013
31. Hui D, Glitza I, Chisholm G, et al. Attrition rates, reasons, and predictive factors in supportive care and palliative oncology trials. *Cancer*. 2013;119:1098–1105. doi:10.1002/cncr.27854
32. Jordhoy MS, Kaasa S, Fayers P, et al. Challenges in palliative care research; recruitment, attrition and compliance: experience from a randomized controlled trial. *Palliat Med*. 1999;013:299–310. doi:10.1191/026921699668963873
33. Perez-Cruz PE, Shamieh O, Paiva CE, et al. Factors associated with attrition in a multicenter longitudinal observational study of patients with advanced cancer. *J Pain Symp Manag*. 2018;55:938–945. doi:10.1016/j.jpainsymman.2017.11.009
34. Rubin DB. Multiple *Imputation for Nonresponse in Surveys*. New York, NY: Wiley; 1987.
35. Yuan YC. Multiple imputation for missing data: concepts and new development (Version 9.0). https://support.sas.com/rnd/app/stat/papers/multipleimputation.pdf 2018.

16

Time-to-Event Analysis

LOREN K. MELL ■ KAVEH ZAKERI ■ HANJIE SHEN

Among the most common tasks undertaken by clinical cancer researchers is to determine the effect of a given factor or intervention on a particular outcome of interest, where the outcome is observed over a period of time. Examples include testing for disparities in overall survival among different demographic groups, developing predictive models and nomograms to predict the risk of cancer recurrence, or testing the effect of a novel therapy on progression-free survival (PFS). These situations typically involve monitoring for events that may or may not occur before the conclusion of the study, or before patients drop out of participation. In this case, event times for at least some individuals are not known exactly, and are censored, meaning that event times are only known to be greater than (**right-censored**) or less than (**left-censored**) a particular value.

The most common example is survival time, where a subject may still be alive at the conclusion of the study, in which case all that is known is that the subject survived at least to time *t*, where *t* represents the time from enrollment to last follow-up. In this case the observed survival times are right-censored. Situations calling for analysis of left-censored data are less common, so this chapter focuses on analysis of right- censored data; for further information on analysis of left-censored data, see Glantz (1).

An assumption underlying the validity of time-to-event data analysis is that the processes determining whether data are censored are uncorrelated with the survival times. That is to say, censoring should be random, or **noninformative censoring** (2). For example, if subjects with higher income were more likely to comply with follow-up visits and had a lower likelihood of cancer progression, one would obtain a biased estimate of the effect of income on progression (in this case, one would underestimate the negative effect of low income). This is an important consideration in the initial stages of prospective study design and in retrospective data analysis.

Time-to-event studies may be either uncontrolled (e.g., case series, phase I, and nonrandomized phase II clinical trials) or controlled (e.g., cohort studies, randomized trials). A **controlled study** is designed to compare two groups who differ only in a key factor or intervention of interest. **Uncontrolled studies** are generally appropriate for estimating outcomes (the probability of an event), whereas controlled studies are required to both estimate effects on a given outcome and draw meaningful conclusions regarding the treatment effects. Ideally, estimates of both outcomes and effects should be unbiased and as accurate and precise as possible. However, all studies (including randomized trials) are subject to forms of bias and are constrained in their accuracy and precision, at least to some extent, because sample sizes are also finite. The responsibility of the principal investigator and his/her team is to draw proper inferences from the data, taking into account the magnitude and direction of any biases and confounding that might affect their conclusions. This chapter provides a framework for investigators to produce quality time-to-event analyses and for readers to critically interpret such studies. Initially, we present the statistical models underlying the theory. Later we provide practical examples to facilitate understanding of the concepts.

STATISTICAL MODEL OF TIME-TO-EVENT DATA

The event function, or cumulative distribution function, describes the probability of an event of interest occurring prior to time t. For a random variable T representing the observed event times in a given set of subjects, we define this function as $F(t) = Pr(T \le t)$. $F(t)$ is the complement of the survival function, $S(t)$, which describes the probability of a subject not experiencing the event (i.e., surviving) at least to time t. An example of plots of estimated $S(t)$ and $F(t)$ is shown in Figure 16.1 (3,4).

Several important identities follow initially:

$$S(t) = 1 - F(t) \qquad \textbf{[1]}$$

and

$$F'(t) = f(t) = -S'(t) \qquad \textbf{[2]}$$

$S(t)$ and $F(t)$ are complements, and because both are non-negative, they are bounded between 0 and 1, with a slope of the same magnitude but in the opposite direction (which accounts for their inverted shapes). The probability density function, $f(t)$, represents the first derivative of $F(t)$, their relationship being represented as

$$F(t) = \int_0^t f(u)du \qquad \textbf{[3]}$$

An important related function in time-to-event analysis is the hazard function, $\lambda(t)$, which represents the instantaneous change in the probability of occurrence of an event of interest. The definition is provided in Equation 4 (see Appendix).

The cumulative hazard function, $\Lambda(t)$, is defined as follows:

$$\Lambda(t) = \int_0^t \lambda(u)du = -\ln(S(t)) \qquad \textbf{[5]}$$

Conversely, the survival function can be rewritten using Equation **[5]** as

$$S(t) = \exp\int_0^t -\lambda(u)du = \exp(-\Lambda(t)) \qquad \textbf{[6]}$$

This is a useful equation for converting hazard estimates to survival estimates (and vice versa).

ESTIMATING TIME-TO-EVENT FUNCTIONS

Note that, typically, when we model *outcomes*, we are using a set of observed data to estimate $S(t)$ (or $F(t)$), and when we model *effects*, we are estimating parameters that influence the hazard function (or subdistribution hazard function, defined later). When we consider an *estimator*, we mean a statistic representing a certain theoretical quantity of interest, which we are seeking to estimate the value of, given a certain set of data.

The most common method for estimating event functions used in the oncology literature is the Kaplan–Meier (KM) method (2). The central assumptions underlying the validity of the KM estimator are: (a) censoring is noninformative, (b) event probabilities are the same for subjects

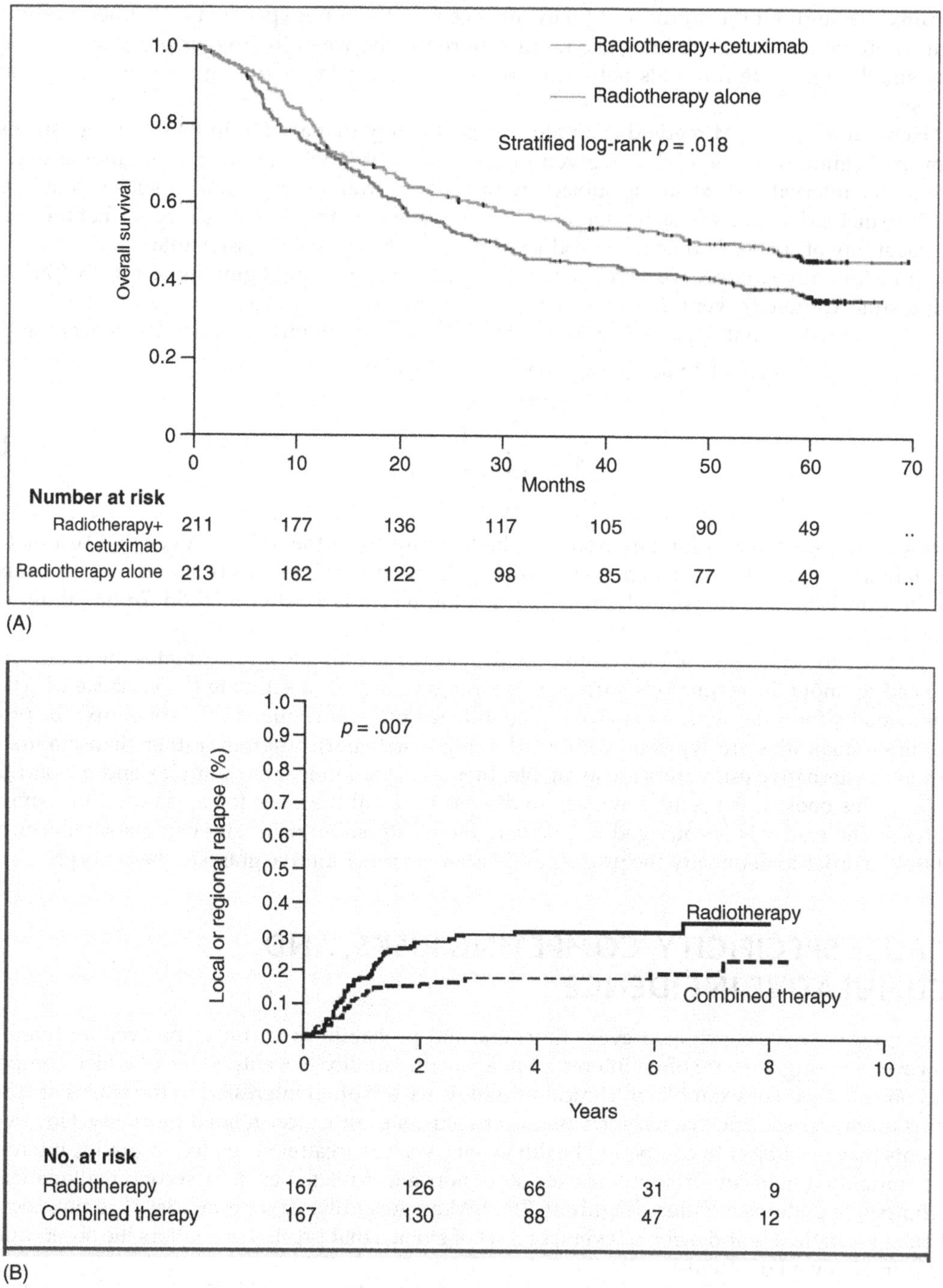

FIGURE 16.1 Example plots of (A) the survival function, $S(t)$, and (B) the cumulative incidence function, $F_k(t)$, for experimental and control groups. Note the inclusion of hashmarks in (A), indicating censoring, and that the numbers at risk are plotted on the *x*-axis.

Source: Reprinted from Bonner JA, Harari PM, Giralt J, et al. Radiotherapy plus cetuximab for locoregionally advanced head and neck cancer: 5-year survival data from a phase 3 randomised trial, and relation between cetuximab-induced rash and survival. *Lancet Oncol.* 2010;11(1):21–28. doi:10.1016/S1470-2045(09)70311-0; Bernier J, Domenge C, Ozsahin M, et al. Postoperative irradiation with or without concomitant chemotherapy for locally advanced head and neck cancer. *N Engl J Med.* 2004;350(19):1945–1952. doi:10.1056/NEJMoa032641

recruited throughout the study, and (c) events occur at the times specified (5). Other methods, such as life tables, are sometimes used, but differences between the two approaches are typically small, unless the intervals between assessments are relatively long, or sample sizes are very small.

Heuristically, the KM method evaluates the probability that a set of individuals will survive from the beginning to the end of a given interval without having an event, by tallying events within each interval and excluding subjects with an event from the risk pool for subsequent intervals. The method then treats each interval as independent given the event history, so that the overall probability of survival equals the product of probabilities over successive intervals.

More formally, suppose we have a set of $N = n_0$ individuals at the beginning of a study (time t_0), with distinct (ordered) event times $t_1 < t_2 < \ldots < t_N$. For $j \varepsilon \{1,2,\ldots,N\}$, let n_{j-1} represent the number of subjects at risk at time t_{j-1} and d_j represent the number of individuals who have an event in the interval (t_{j-1}, t_j). Then the KM estimator, $\hat{S}(t)$, is defined as

$$\hat{S}(t) = \prod_{j:t_j \le t}\left(1 - \frac{d_j}{n_j}\right) \quad [7]$$

A corresponding estimator for the cumulative hazard function is the Nelson–Aalen (NA) estimator, which literally sums the estimated event hazards for successive intervals (Equation 8, Appendix). The Breslow estimator (6) is an alternative estimator, which is a better method for handling tied event times.

In order to get a sense of the certainty with which our estimate approximates the true value, we need to know the estimator's variance. A common method to estimate the variance of $\hat{S}(t)$ is Greenwood's formula, with its associated confidence interval (Equation 9, Appendix). In practice, these quantities are typically computed using a statistical program, rather than manually. Although alternative estimators are available, their explanation is more complex and beyond the scope of this book. It is useful, however, to discuss in detail the basic formulas used in survival analysis. The reader is encouraged to calculate these estimators manually using a small sample dataset, in order to demystify the process and obtain a more intuitive grasp of the concepts.

CAUSE SPECIFICITY, COMPETING RISKS, AND CUMULATIVE INCIDENCE

Up to now, we have considered event functions and probabilities for only one event of interest. However, investigators are often interested in analyzing multiple events, some of which compete with one another. For example, in clinical oncology, we are often interested in the effects of treatments on cancer-specific events, such as cancer recurrence or cancer-related mortality. However, patients may be subject to competing health events, such as treatment-related mortality, intercurrent mortality due to comorbid disease (or other noncancer-related events), second malignancies, or competing patterns of failure (Figure 16.2) (7). More generally, "competing risks" settings occur whenever a patient is at risk for an event, or a set of events, that precludes or alters the observation of a primary event of interest.

An important quantity in competing risks settings is the cause-specific hazard. It is defined analogously to the hazard function $\lambda(t)$, but specific to failure from event type k. For a parameter δ indicating one of k distinct event types, that is, $\delta \in \{1,2,\ldots,k\}$, we define the cause-specific hazard as $\lambda_k(t;\delta)$ (Equation 10 – Appendix). The cumulative cause-specific hazard, $\Lambda_k(t;\delta)$, is defined analogously to $\Lambda(t)$:

$$\Lambda_k(t;\delta) = \int_0^t \lambda_k(u;\delta)du \quad [11]$$

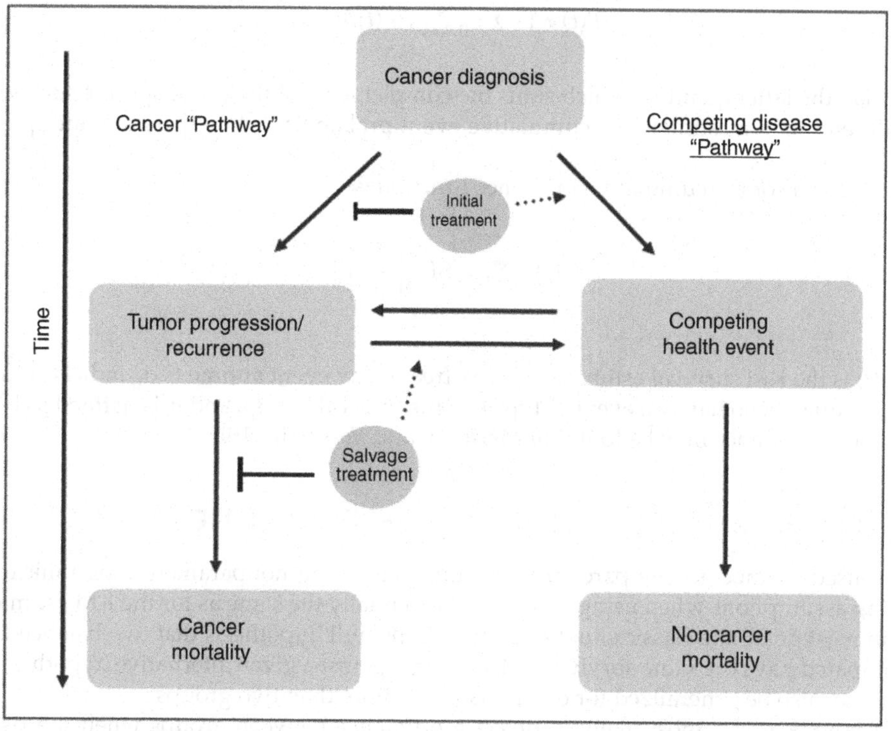

FIGURE 16.2 Schematic representation of clinical event pathways in oncology patients with competing risks.

Source: Reprinted from Mell LK, Dignam JJ, Salama JK, et al. Predictors of competing mortality in advanced head and neck cancer. *J Clin Oncol*. 2010;28(1):15–20. doi:10.1200/JCO.2008.20.9288

The cause-specific cumulative distribution function, $F_k(t;\delta)$, also called the cumulative incidence function, is defined as

$$F_k(t;\delta) = \int_0^t S(u)\lambda_k(u;\delta)du \qquad [12]$$

where $S(u)$ is the survival function describing the probability of not experiencing any of the k event types, at least to time u.

A pair of useful identities describes the hazard for any event, $\lambda(t)$, as the sum of the cause-specific hazards, and the cumulative probability of any event, $F(t)$, as the sum of the cause-specific cumulative incidences:

$$\lambda(t) = \Sigma_{\delta\in\{1,2,\cdots,k\}} \lambda_k(t;\delta) \qquad [13]$$

$$F(t) = \Sigma_{\delta\in\{1,2,\cdots,k\}} F_k(t;\delta) \qquad [14]$$

$F(t)$ represents the cumulative probability of failing from any of the k event types by time t. Finally, we can define the cause-specific survival function as follows:

$$S_k(t;\delta) = \exp(-\Lambda_k(t;\delta)) \qquad [15]$$

It is important to note that while $F(t) = 1 - S(t)$ describes the cumulative probability of an event in the case when there is only one (properly distributed) event of interest, such as mortality, this is not the case for cause-specific events, that is

$$F(t) \neq 1 - \Sigma_{\delta \in \{1,2,\cdots,k\}} S_k(t;\delta) \qquad [16]$$

In particular, the latter quantity, which sums the complements of the cause-specific survival functions, will tend to overestimate the cumulative event probability when there are multiple events (8,9).

An estimator for the cumulative incidence function is

$$\hat{F}_k(t) = \Sigma_{j:t_j \leq t} \hat{S}(t_i)\left(\frac{d_{kj}}{n_j}\right) \qquad [17]$$

where $\hat{S}(t_j)$ is the KM survival estimate of being free of any event at time t_j, d_{kj} indicates the number of individuals who have an event of type k in the interval (t_{j-1}, t_j), and n_j is defined as before. A formula for the variance may be found in Marubini and Valsecchi (10).

TESTING DIFFERENCES IN TIME-TO-EVENT FUNCTIONS

A widely used method to compare survival functions is the nonparametric log-rank test. The underlying assumptions when using this test are essentially the same as for the KM estimator. We discuss in most detail the classic situation in which the null hypothesis that two balanced groups being compared have the same survival distribution (against a given alternative hypothesis). Log-rank tests can also be generalized for comparisons of more than two groups.

The log-rank test is most likely to detect a difference between groups when the risk of an event is consistently greater for one group than another, and is unlikely to detect a difference when survival curves cross (11). A disadvantage of the log-rank test is that it does not provide a direct estimate of effect sizes on the hazard ratio scale; it will tell if a difference exists, but not how big the difference is. Estimating effect sizes requires semi-parametric or parametric statistical methods, such as the Cox proportional hazards model (12) or Fine–Gray model (13), discussed further.

The log-rank test is a chi-square test, comparing the total number of observed versus expected events in two or more groups. For a two-group comparison, we let $t_1 < t_2 < \ldots < t_N$ be a set of distinct ordered event times in either group for the whole dataset. For $j \in \{1,2,\ldots,N\}$ we let n_{1j-1} and n_{2j-1} represent the number of subjects in groups 1 and 2, respectively, who are at risk at time t_{j-1} and we let d_{1j} and d_{2j} represent the number of individuals in groups 1 and 2, respectively, who have an event in the interval (t_{j-1}, t_j). The calculation of the log-rank statistic is given in Equation 18 (Appendix). The expected value of the log-rank statistic (L) is E_j, and its variance is V_j, which can be tested against the critical values of the χ^2 distribution with $N-1$ degrees of freedom.

A test for subdistribution hazards is Gray's test (14). Gray proposed a log-rank type test that can compare subdistribution hazards among groups. Gray's test is a *k*-sample test that can be used to evaluate hypotheses of equality of cumulative incidence functions for cause-specific mortality among *k* groups. Specifically, it tests for differences in the subdistribution hazard underlying cumulative incidence functions.

The test is based on the *k*–1 score statistic:

$$Z_k(T) = \int_{t=0}^{T} W_k(t)\left\{\tilde{\lambda}_k(t) - \tilde{\lambda}_0(t)\right\}dt \qquad [19]$$

where T is the largest observed time in the study and $\tilde{\lambda}(t)$ is the subdistribution hazard that is defined as $\tilde{\lambda}_k(t) = \frac{f_k(t)}{1 - F_k(t)}$. In this equation, $F_k(t)$ is the cumulative incidence function, $f_k(t)$ is the subdensity function in group k for the event of interest, $W_k(t)$ can be regarded as a weight function, and $\tilde{\lambda}_0(t)$ is the subdistribution hazard for all groups together. If we consider the variance–covariance matrix for Z is Σ, then the test statistic is given by $Z'\Sigma^{-1}Z$. In terms of large sample theory, the statistic is approximately distributed as a chi -square distribution with k–1 degrees of freedom.

TESTING EFFECTS ON THE HAZARD FUNCTION: COX PROPORTIONAL HAZARDS MODEL

The Cox proportional hazards model (12) is one of the most widely used statistical models in clinical cancer research. Its utility is due in part to its ability to estimate the magnitude of effects of treatments and covariates on outcomes of interest. The model is particularly useful for estimating the magnitude of effects on hazard functions for events of a given type, and adjusting for confounding effects of covariates.

For the usual case of right-censored data, we observe $Z = min(t, C)$ and $\delta = I(t \leq C)$, where t and C are the failure and censoring times, respectively. Let $\lambda(t \mid X)$ denote the hazard function given by a vector of covariates X. The baseline hazard function at time t, that is, when $X = 0$, is denoted as $\lambda_0(t)$. The baseline hazard function is analogous to the intercept term in a multivariate regression model. Notice that the baseline hazard function is not specified, but must be positive.

The ratio of hazard functions can be considered a ratio of risk functions, so the proportional hazards regression model can be considered as a function of relative risk. Changes in a covariate have a multiplicative effect on the baseline risk. The model in terms of the hazard function at time t is

$$\lambda(t \mid X) = \lambda_0(t)\exp(\beta' X) \qquad \textbf{[20]}$$

In the Cox regression model, we treat the partial likelihood as a regular likelihood for estimating β. The log-partial likelihood and partial likelihood score functions are given in Equations 21–22 (Appendix). The variance of $\hat{\beta}$ can be estimated by inverting the second derivative of the partial likelihood. For hypothesis testing for each covariate of interest, we describe the null hypothesis as H_0: $\beta_i = 0$. A Wald chi-square test of the hypothesis is then built according to Equation 23 (Appendix).

TESTING EFFECTS ON THE CUMULATIVE INCIDENCE FUNCTION: FINE–GRAY MODEL

The Fine–Gray model (13) in some sense can be thought of as an extension of the Cox proportional hazards for modeling subdistribution hazards, defined later. A detailed discussion of competing risks models is beyond the scope of this chapter; for further information, the reader is referred to Pintilie (15).

For the usual right-censored data, considering latent failure times $t_1, t_2, \ldots, t_m$ for competing risks and C for censoring time, we observe $t = min(t_1, t_2, \ldots, t_m)$, $Z = min(t, C)$, and $\delta = I(t \leq C)$, the last being an indicator as to whether the event occurred or not. Let $F_k(t \mid X)$ denote the cumulative incidence function (CIF) for events of type k given a set of covariates X. We treat the complement of the CIF as a "survival" function for event type k, and calculate its underlying hazard. To avoid confusion with the *cause-specific hazard* and *overall hazard* functions, we call this a *subdistribution hazard* for cause k, denoted with a tilde:

$$\tilde{\lambda}_k(t \mid X) = -\frac{d}{dt} log\left(1 - F_k(t \mid X)\right) = \frac{f_k(t)}{1 - F_k(t)} \qquad \textbf{[24]}$$

where $F_k(t)$ and $f_k(t)$ are the cumulative incidence function and its derivative, respectively, for event type k (Equation 25, Appendix).

The Fine–Gray model is a proportional hazards model for the *subdistribution* hazard associated with type k, that is

$$\tilde{\lambda}_k(t \mid X) = \tilde{\lambda}_{k0}(t)\exp(\beta' X) \qquad [26]$$

where $\tilde{\lambda}_{k0}(t)$ is the baseline *subdistribution* hazard for events of type k and $\exp(\beta' X)$ is the relative risk associated with covariates X, with definition given in Equation 27 (Appendix). The model counts events of type k in a small interval $(t, t + dt)$ but treats the risk set as those alive at t and those who failed before t due to causes other than k.

In the Fine–Gray model, we consider a proper partial likelihood to estimate β. The log-partial likelihood and partial likelihood score functions are given in Equations 28–29 (Appendix). Estimation of β and its variance can be performed analogous to standard likelihood theory, with further details given in Equations 30–34 (Appendix).

EVALUATING TIME-TO-EVENT MODELS USING MARTINGALE RESIDUALS

It is often important to assess a regression model's goodness of fit. **Martingale residuals** can be used to provide a graphical assessment of the validity of model predictions. Theoretical results regarding Martingale residuals are based on a counting process. Consider a counting process where $N_i(t) = I\{T_i \le t, \delta_i = 1\}$ indicates whether or not an event occurred for the ith subject in the set over time t, $Y_i(t)$ is a process indicating whether the ith subject is at risk at time t, and $Z_i(t)$ is a vector of covariates. Also let $\hat{\beta}$ be the maximum partial likelihood estimator of β, a vector of Cox regression coefficients, and $\hat{\Lambda}_0$ be the Breslow estimator (6) of the cumulative hazard function, Λ_0. The Martingale residual is then defined as

$$\hat{M}_i(t) = N_i(t) - \int_0^t Y_i(s) e^{\hat{\beta}' z_i(s)} d\hat{\Lambda}_0(s) \qquad [35]$$

The sum of sizes of the individual's residual $\hat{M}_i$ indicates the accuracy of the model, with a large positive value for a subject who has more events than predicted by the model and a large negative value for fewer events than predicted by the model (Figure 16.3A).

EVALUATING THE PROPORTIONAL HAZARDS ASSUMPTION

The proportional hazards assumption is an important assumption to recognize and verify when evaluating time-to-event data. It is a strong assumption, in the sense that it is essential for making valid inferences based on the statistical models described here, and often does not hold true. A simple, qualitative "eyeball" test of the proportional hazards assumption involves looking at plots of the survival functions (or preferably, hazard functions), and verifying that they do not diverge or cross substantially over time (Figure 16.1). However, we generally recommend using quantitative methods described further to test the proportional hazards assumption.

Based on the individual contributions to the derivative of the log-partial likelihood, Schoenfeld (16) proposed the first method for assessing residuals for use with Cox regression. Instead of a single residual for each individual, there is a separate residual for each individual for each covariate. By assessing the proportional hazards assumption, Grambsch and Therneau (17) showed that scaled **Schoenfeld residuals** can be of great use in the diagnostics of Cox regression models. Grambsch and Therneau also suggested that under the assumption that the distribution of the predictors is similar in the various risk sets, it can be adjusted using the covariance matrix of the parameter estimators divided by the number of events in the sample.

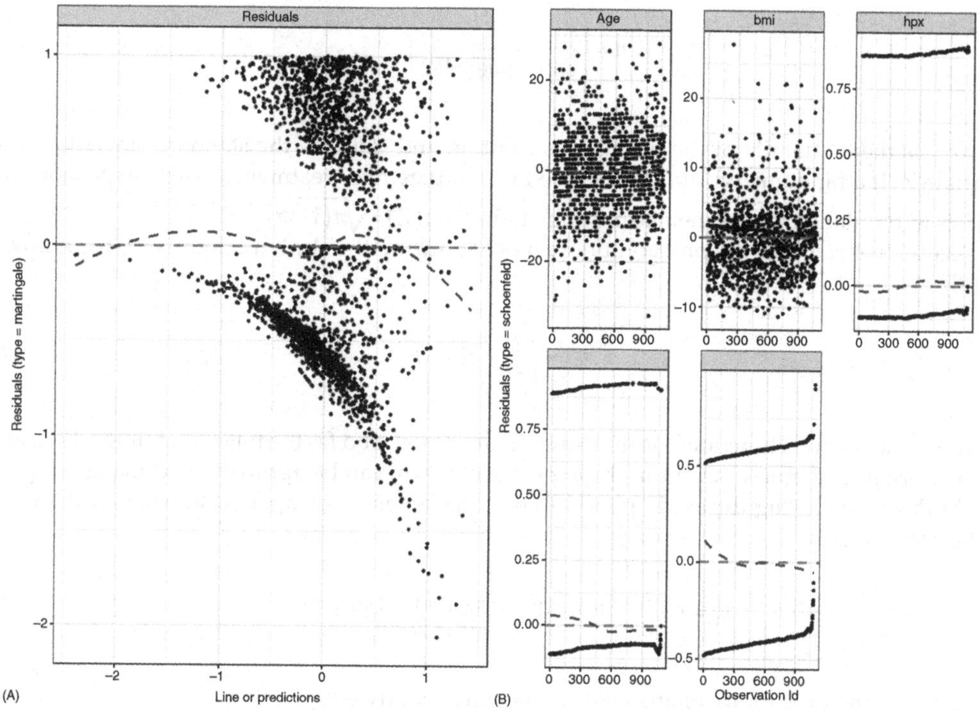

FIGURE 16.3 Martingale plot (A) for a Cox proportional hazards regression model, indicating deviations in the model. The Schoenfeld plot (B) indicates that the proportional hazards assumption holds for several key covariates.

The Schoenfeld residuals test checks whether the slope of scaled residuals across time is zero. In this test, separate residuals exist for each individual for each covariate. The residuals can be regressed against time to further test for independence. If the plot of Schoenfeld residuals against time shows that the slope is not zero, or that another nonrandom pattern exists (Figure 16.3B), then the proportional hazard assumption is violated.

If the proportional hazards assumption is violated, there are several options to consider. First, one can attempt to stratify by the levels of the categorical variable for which the proportionality assumption fails. For example, if the hazards are not proportional with respect to age, either visually based on the survival plots or quantitatively using residual tests, one can perform a stratified model where a separate baseline hazard is assumed within strata (e.g., <50, 50–70, and 70 and over), but all the data are still used to obtain parameter estimates. A second option is to fit a stratified Cox model, which is a modification of the Cox model that allows for control by stratification of a predictor that does not satisfy proportional hazards assumption. A third option is to apply the extended Cox model, which permits time-dependent covariates. A *time-dependent variable* is defined as a variable whose value may differ over time for a given subject. In the Cox model, it is necessary to define a function of time denoted by $z(t)$ (commonly referred as a step function), which is a dummy variable with value 1 if $T \geq t$ and 0 if $T \leq t$, where T is a random variable and t is specific period of observation.

SAMPLE SIZE AND POWER ESTIMATION FOR TIME-TO-EVENT DATA

To calculate the number of patients necessary to detect a hazard ratio (HR) of a given size, for a given significance level α with a power $1 - \beta$, we first need to calculate the number of events (n) required, which is given by

$$n = \left(\frac{z_{1-\alpha/2} + z_{1-\beta}}{std(Z)log(HR)} \right)^2 \quad [36]$$

where z_a is the a quantile of the normal distribution and std(Z) is the standard deviation of the covariate Z. If a randomized study is planned to compare two treatments, with the proportion of subjects in the standard treatment arm being π, then $std(Z) = \sqrt{\pi(1-\pi)}$.

Second, we can find the probability of an event during the study period using the following (15,18):

$$P = 1 - \frac{1}{a}\int_f^{a+f} S(u)du \quad [37]$$

where S is the survival function, a is the duration of accrual, and f is the follow-up time added at the end of accrual. The time-to-event in the experimental arm can be approximated using Simpson's rule. In this case, during the study period in the experimental group, the probability of an event can be computed as

$$P_1 = 1 - \frac{1}{6}\{S_1(f) + 4S_1(0.5a + f) + S_1(a+f)\}. \quad [38]$$

and then the probability of an event for the whole study is

$$P = \pi P_1 + (1-\pi)P_0 \quad [39]$$

Hence, we can calculate the total number of patients needed as $N = \frac{n}{P}$. For the second part, $z_{1-\beta} = \sqrt{n\pi(1-\pi)}log(\theta) - z_{1-\alpha/2}$, where θ represents the ratio of the hazards of the cumulative incidence functions. Also, α and β in Equation 36 define the Types I and II error.

Estimating power in the presence of competing risks is complex. An R-based calculator to use in such applications is given by Pintilie (15) and is reproduced in Rose et al. (19)

COMPOSITE TIME-TO-EVENT ENDPOINTS

Composite time-to-event endpoints quantify the probability of observing any one of a given set of events over time. A particular subclass of composite endpoints, called **event-free survival (EFS) endpoints,** are commonly used in clinical oncology, because they capture a quantity of obvious clinical relevance (i.e., the probability of both being alive and free of a particular event or a set of events). In addition, EFS endpoints are often effective surrogates for overall survival, with higher event rates (which shorten the readout time for trials and can reduce the sample size required).

In general, EFS endpoints combine one or more events of interest (such as cancer recurrence or cancer mortality), with mortality from any cause. Commonly used EFS endpoints in oncology include disease-free survival (DFS), progression-free survival (PFS), or recurrence-free survival (RFS). An interesting point relevant to clinical oncology is that overall survival (OS) can be treated as either a noncomposite endpoint (i.e., mortality from any cause) or a composite EFS endpoint, considering cancer mortality and noncancer mortality as competing events.

In contrast, an endpoint such as time to progression or time to treatment failure is generally considered a cause-specific event, combining various manifestations of treatment failure (local, regional, and/or distant recurrence) into a single event, but excluding mortality from noncancer causes as an event. Although several groups have tried to standardize endpoint nomenclature in clinical oncology, large variations still exist in how endpoints are defined (20), and investigators have often used the same name to refer to different endpoints, leading to much confusion in the literature. Ultimately, it is crucial that investigators describe in detail how a composite endpoint is defined, in terms of the events used in its construction, how the starting point was defined, and which event times were treated as censored and why they were treated as such.

The valid use of composite endpoints relies on several critical assumptions. Composite endpoints are most appropriate to use when (a) the effect of intervention is expected to be relatively homogeneous with respect to the events comprising the composite endpoint, (b) the components of the composite endpoint are of similar importance, and (c) there is biologic plausibility for the effect of intervention on the events of interest. In settings where the risk of competing events is low, such as metastatic disease, using EFS endpoints is often not problematic, as the risk of noncancer mortality is typically negligible. However, in heavy competing risks settings, these criteria are often violated, as many cancer therapies have little or no expected effect on noncancer-related events (though more toxic treatments undoubtedly can, and usually in opposition to the effect on the event of interest).

A key pitfall can occur when investigators wrongly or misleadingly attribute an effect on a composite endpoint as that on a specific component of that endpoint. This is an example of the logical fallacy "*X affects A or B, therefore X affects A.*" First, if there is an effect of treatment on a composite endpoint, it is important to know to what extent the treatment affects the individual components of the endpoint. For example, an observed effect on OS could be attributable entirely or in part to an effect of treatment on competing mortality (i.e., X affecting B). Conversely, if there is a lack of an overall effect, it is critical to distinguish whether this is due to the treatment being completely inert, or due to offsetting of effects on competing events (such as a benefit in cancer mortality reduction being offset by more competing mortality events due to its toxic effects). Second, although it is often assumed that randomization will take care of balancing factors related to nonspecific events, imbalances in critical risk factors for competing events (e.g., age and comorbidity) may still occur by random chance, especially when not included as a stratification factor. When imbalances do occur, inferences may undermined due to **confounding by nonspecificity**, since an observed effect could be due in whole or part to confounders driving risk for the competing event.

There are several such examples in the literature. Consider, for example, the Southwest Oncology Group (SWOG) 8794 study, which randomized patients with locally advanced prostate cancer to either observation or adjuvant radiotherapy following prostatectomy. The investigators reported that radiation therapy reduced the risk of metastasis (21), but what they actually measured was the effect of radiation on metastasis-free survival (MFS)—a different quantity that captures both the probability of being alive and free of metastasis. Subsequent analysis decomposing treatment effects according to cause specificity showed that part of the effect on MFS was attributable to a higher risk of competing death in the control group, due to random imbalances in age, comorbidity, and performance status favoring the radiation group (Table 16.1) (22).

Thus, it is imperative to decompose outcomes and effects on combined endpoints in order to draw proper inferences from competing risks data. The value of treatment effect decomposition is particularly evident when examining highly effective yet toxic therapies. For example, a randomized clinical trial in acute myeloid leukemia concluded that higher radiation doses had no effect on OS, even though radiation reduced disease relapse (23). Higher radiation doses increased treatment-related mortality due to higher toxicity, negating the benefit of improved disease control, suggesting that strategies to reduce radiation toxicity could potentially improve OS. This inference is obviously different from the inference from a trial in which survival is not different because the treatment is inert.

This problem can also occur in analyses of treatment effects in population data. Whereas randomization mitigates the role of selection bias, in real-world settings cancer therapies are usually selectively applied. For example, it has been shown that cancer treatments may be associated with improved OS in population studies, simply because patients who are less likely to die from other causes receive more intensive treatment (Figure 16.4) (24). Decomposing the treatment effect

TABLE 16.1 EFFECTS OF POSTOPERATIVE RADIATION THERAPY ON VARIOUS OUTCOMES IN PATIENTS WITH HIGH-RISK PROSTATE CANCER, FROM THE SOUTHWEST ONCOLOGY GROUP 8794 RANDOMIZED TRIAL. METASTASIS-FREE SURVIVAL IS A COMBINED ENDPOINT COMPRISING EITHER THE OCCURRENCE OF DISTANT METASTASIS OR DEATH FROM ANY CAUSE

Unadjusted and adjusted effects of radiation therapy.

	Unadjusted				Adjusted for metastasis and competing mortality risk*			
	HR† (95%CI)	p	SDHR‡ (95%CI)	p	HR† (95%CI)	p	SDHR‡c (95%CI)	p
Metastasis	0.50 (0.31–0.81)	.005	0.51 (0.31–0.83)	.007	0.49 (0.30–0.81)	.005	0.49 (0.30–0.81)	.005
Competing mortality	0.82 (0.59–1.14)	.24	0.94 (0.68–1.30)	.73	0.94 (0.67–1.31)	.71	1.10 (0.79–1.53)	.56
Metastasis-free survival	0.70 (0.53–0.92)	.01	0.70 (0.53–0.92)	.009	0.76 (0.58–1.00)	.049	0.76 (0.58–1.00)	.05
Overall survival	0.73 (0.55–0.96)	.02	0.73 (0.55–0.96)	.02	0.80 (0.60–1.06)	.12	0.80 (0.60–1.06)	.12

*Only metastasis and competing mortality risk scores were used to estimate adjusted effects.

†Calculated using Cox proportional hazards regression.

‡Calculated using Fine–Gray regression.

CI, confidence interval; HR, hazard ratio; SDHR, subdistribution hazard ratio.

Source: Zakeri K, Rose BS, Gulaya S, et al. Competing event risk stratification may improve the design and efficiency of clinical trials: secondary analysis of SWOG 8794. *Contemp Clin Trials.* 2013;34:74–79. doi:10.1016/j.cct.2012.09.008

into cancer-specific and noncancer-specific components is usually necessary to ensure biologic plausibility.

Heterogeneity of effects on competing events can be checked graphically, using forest plots (Figure 16.5), or statistically, using Cochrane's Q or the I^2 statistic (Chapter 27). Unfortunately, fewer than half of published clinical trials in leading journals report the effects of intervention on both cancer and noncancer events, and far fewer provide statistical analysis on the components of the composite endpoint (25). The problem is worse in studies involving prognostic biomarkers, leading Green et al. (26) to propose a rubric for conducting time-to-event analyses in competing risks settings (Box 16.1).

POWER, COST, AND PERSONALIZED MEDICINE IN COMPETING RISKS SETTINGS

Competing risks can significantly impact the power of clinical trials. The use of composite endpoints is sometimes incorrectly believed to increase power by increasing the overall event rate.

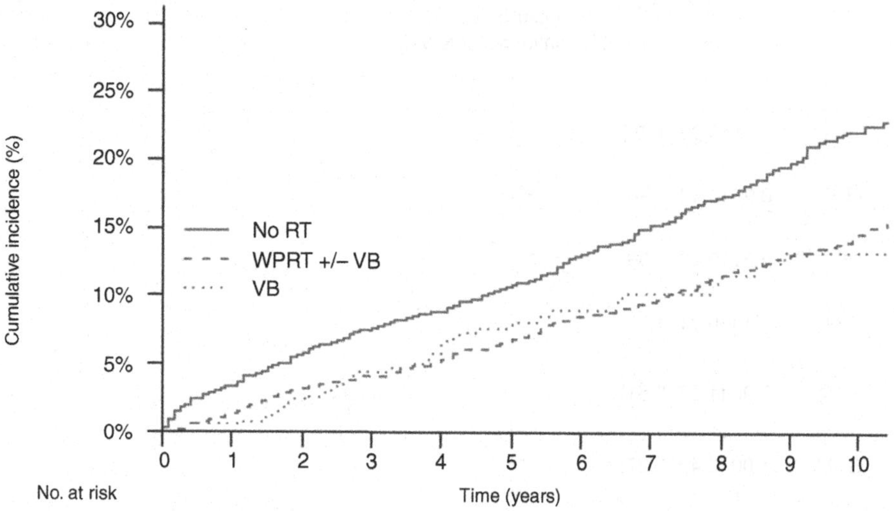

No. at risk

	0	1	2	3	4	5	6	7	8	9	10
No RT	1737	1606	1498	1275	1116	959	802	661	557	450	378
WPRT	1737	1665	1549	1382	1238	1115	969	865	752	657	595
VB	383	375	358	291	225	187	154	121	104	B3	72

(A)

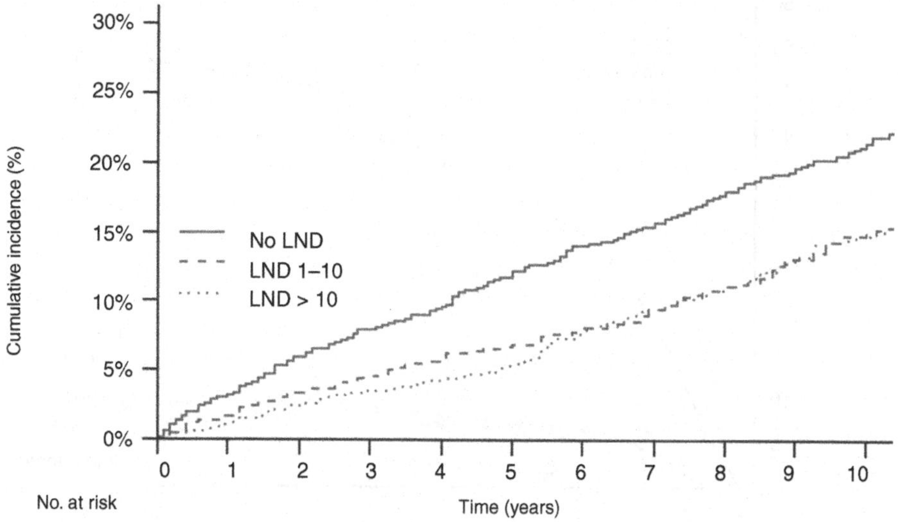

No. at risk

	0	1	2	3	4	5	6	7	8	9	10
No LND	1663	1530	1389	1207	1078	947	820	718	624	536	474
LBD 1–10	916	876	831	725	636	557	481	407	361	311	280
LND >10	1278	1240	1185	1016	865	757	624	522	428	343	291

(B)

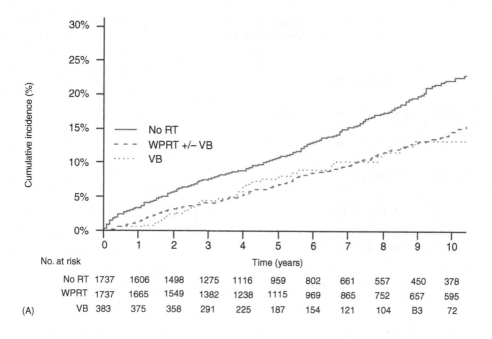

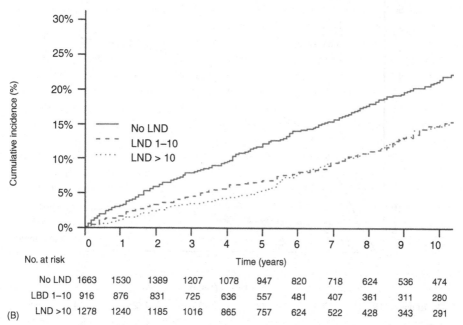

FIGURE 16.4 Cumulative incidence plots showing lower incidences of competing mortality events in early-stage endometrial cancer patients receiving RT (A) or LND (B), indicating the selection of healthier patients for more intensive treatment.

LND, lymph node dissection; LND 1–10, 1–10 nodes dissected; LND >10: >10 nodes dissected; RT, radiation therapy; VB, vaginal brachytherapy; WPRT, whole pelvic.

Source: Reprinted from Mell LK, Carmona R, Gulaya S, et al. Cause-specific effects of radiotherapy and lymphadenectomy in stage I–II endometrial cancer: a population-based study. *J Natl Cancer Inst.* 2013;105(21):1656–1666. doi:10.1093/jnci/djt279

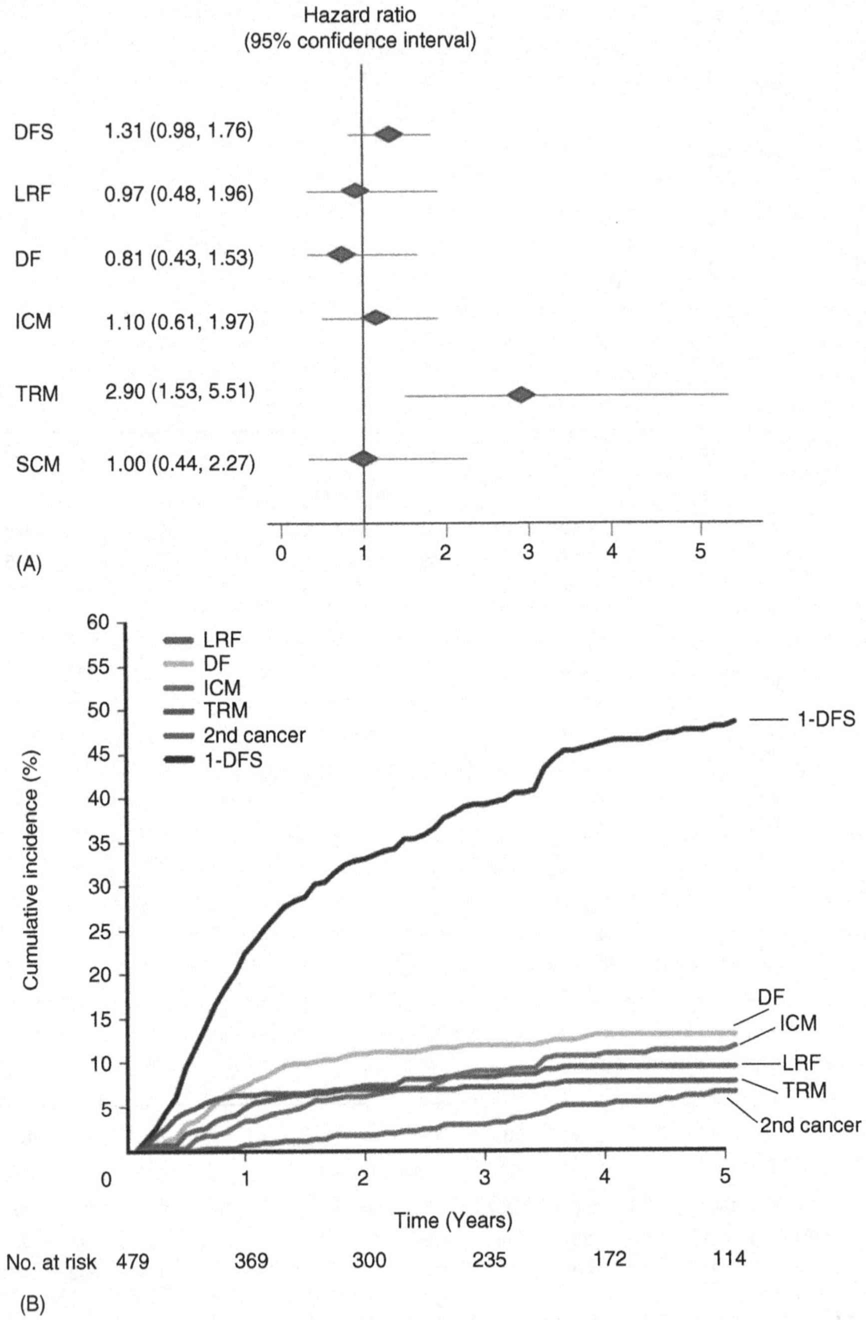

FIGURE 16.5 Schematic forest plot (A) indicating the effect of treatment intensification on various events comprising DFS, including LRF, DF, ICM, TRM, and SCM. Note the adverse effect of intensive therapy on TRM. (B) Cumulative incidence plot showing various competing events in patients with locoregionally advanced head and neck cancer.

DF, distant failure; DFS, disease-free survival; ICM, intercurrent mortality; LRF, locoregional failure; SCM, mortality from second cancers; TRM, treatment-related mortality.

Source: Mell LK, Dignam JJ, Salama JK, et al. Predictors of competing mortality in advanced head and neck cancer. *J Clin Oncol.* 2010;28(1):15–20. doi:10.1200/JCO.2008.20.9288

BOX 16.1

Steps in Conducting Time-to-Event Analyses in Competing Risks Settings

1. Clearly identify the study's primary endpoint(s) (i.e., the endpoint or set of endpoints used for sample size [or power] calculation), and secondary endpoint(s), if any.
2. Clearly identify the starting point for time-to-event calculations (e.g., date of registration, date of diagnosis, and date of treatment completion).
3. For composite endpoints, clearly identify the events comprising the endpoint and criteria used for censoring. In particular, investigators should indicate whether "death from any cause" is treated as an event. Endpoints termed "progression," "recurrence," "failure," "time to progression," "time to recurrence," "time to failure," "distant metastasis," "local control" or "locoregional control," and "cause-specific mortality" or "cancer mortality" are cause specific and should treat deaths from competing causes as censored, whereas endpoints termed "progression-free survival," "disease-free survival," "event-free survival," among others, are not cause specific, and should treat death from any cause as an event.
4. Define the protocol used for assessing time to recurrence/progression, including frequency of clinic visits and imaging, type of imaging used, whether biopsy was required, and indications used to trigger visits, imaging, or biopsy.
5. Clearly and separately distinguish effects on cause-specific events from effects on nonspecific or competing events (particularly competing mortality), along with appropriate tests of statistical significance.
6. Clearly identify the statistical methods and/or models used to test associations, including criteria for significance, how covariates were coded and controlled, how assumptions of the models were checked, and criteria for including/excluding covariates from the model.

This premise only holds, however, if the treatment affects the constituent events similarly—an assumption that does not typically apply to cancer treatments. Competing events tend to attenuate the benefit of cancer therapies on survival, by weighting the overall treatment effect toward the null value. Therefore, ever-higher sample sizes would be needed to compensate for the presence of competing risks in such a case. By treating competing and cause-specific events as interchangeable, one can easily be misled into thinking a smaller sample size is needed than what is actually required (Figure 16.6).

Because the greatest contributor to clinical trial cost tends to be sample size, the reduction in power that accompanies increasing rates of competing events can substantially affect the cost of trials. For many disease sites, a significant portion—or even a majority—of the events comprising the primary endpoint are noncancer events, which, if not taken into proper consideration, can lead to underpowered studies. Failure to account for competing risks may increase the costs of studies by more than twofold (27).

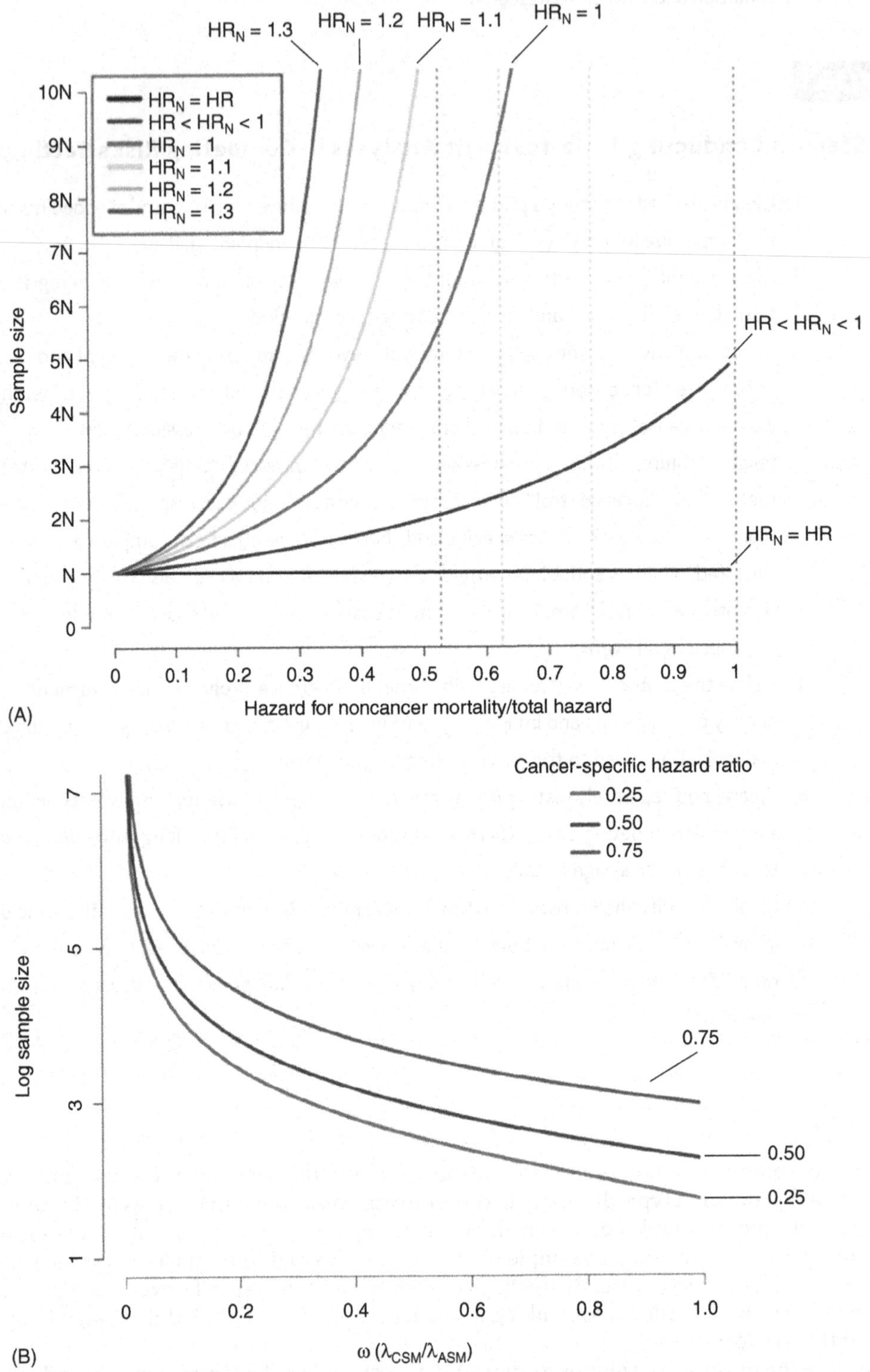

FIGURE 16.6 Asymptotically increasing sample sizes as a function of the relative hazard for cancer mortality (ω). Increasingly toxic therapies with an adverse effect on noncancer mortality (HR_N>1) exacerbate the effect. Note that sample size is invariant to changes in ω under the assumption (either implicit or explicit) of effect homogeneity (A). Optimizing the ratio ω increases a study's power and efficiency (B).

HR, hazard ratio for effect on any event; HR_N, hazard ratio for effect on competing non-cancer events.

Population-based studies, in particular, have shown that many patients with prostate, breast, head/neck, and endometrial cancer are at higher risk for noncancer mortality than cancer-specific mortality (19,28,29). Such patients may be less well served by efforts at intensifying cancer therapy, and better served by interventions aimed at enhancing quality of life or addressing comorbid illnesses and other unmet nononcologic medical and social needs. Personalized medicine here involves tailoring treatment approaches based on the unique qualities of individual patients.

Competing event models can help guide the selection of patients most likely to benefit from treatment intensification by identifying patients with a high relative hazard for cancer events. Although numerous models have been developed to estimate competing mortality in such patients, consensus is lacking and further refinement of these models is needed. For example, an estimation of life expectancy has been advocated as a critical component of decision making in the management of prostate cancer, but the optimal approach is not well defined (30). Comparatively, much less attention has been given to predicting noncancer mortality in disease sites other than prostate cancer. Competing risk models will continue to become increasingly indispensable in the care of cancer patients.

COMPETING EVENT THEORY

Recent studies have focused on the development of competing event models to improve the efficiency of trials and identify personalized treatment approaches by selecting which patients are most at risk for cancer recurrence *relative to competing events*. To achieve this goal, a theoretical framework built on basic principles should be developed.

From Equation 20, we have the following:

$$e^{\beta X} = \frac{\lambda(t)}{\lambda_0(t)} = \Theta \quad [40]$$

and

$$e^{\beta_k X} = \frac{\lambda_k(t)}{\lambda_{k0}(t)} = \Theta_k \quad [41]$$

where Θ and Θ_k represent the treatment effect on a composite event and the cause-specific effect on mutually exclusive events of type k, respectively. From these equations, Mell and Jeong (31) derived the following relationship:

$$\Theta = \frac{\lambda(t)}{\lambda_0(t)} = \frac{\sum_{\delta \in \{1,2,\cdots,k\}} \lambda_k(t;\delta)}{\sum_{\delta \in \{1,2,\cdots,k\}} \lambda_{k0}(t;\delta)} = \frac{\sum_{\delta \in \{1,2,\cdots,k\}} \lambda_{k0}(t;\delta)\ \Theta_k}{\sum_{\delta \in \{1,2,\cdots,k\}} \lambda_{k0}(t;\delta)} \quad [42]$$

That is, the composite treatment effect may be expressed as a weighted average of the cause-specific effects, with the weights given by the ratio of the cause-specific baseline hazard to the overall baseline hazard for any event.

In the special case of two events (event 1 being an event or set of events of interest, and event 2 being a competing event or set of events), Equation 42 simplifies to

$$\Theta = \frac{\Theta_1{}^{*} \lambda_{10}(t) + \Theta_2 \lambda_{20}(t)}{\lambda_0(t)} \quad [43]$$

Rearranging Equation 43 gives us

$$\frac{\lambda_{10}(t)}{\lambda_{20}(t)}=\frac{\Theta-\Theta_2}{\Theta_1-\Theta}=\omega_0^{*}(t) \quad [44]$$

Letting $\omega_0(t)$ represent the ratio of the baseline cause-specific hazard for event 1 to the overall composite baseline hazard yields:

$$\omega_0(t)=\frac{\lambda_{01}(t)}{\lambda_{01}(t)+\lambda_{02}(t)}=\frac{\lambda_{01}(t)}{\lambda_0(t)}=1-\frac{\lambda_{02}(t)}{\lambda_0(t)}=\frac{\Theta-\Theta_2}{\Theta_1-\Theta_2} \quad [45]$$

and

$$\Theta=\omega_0(t)\Theta_1+(1-\omega_0(t))\Theta_2 \quad [46]$$

Here the value $\omega_0(t)$ serves as a quantitative representation of the degree of competing risks, and the value $1-\omega_0(t)$ is called the deadweight factor. The ratio of the cause-specific hazards to each other is represented by $\omega_0^*(t)$. In competing risks settings, $\lambda_{10}(t)$ and $\lambda_{20}(t)$ are both assumed to be nonzero, so $0<\omega_0(t)<1$ and $\omega_0^*(t)>0$. From Equation 46, it is clear that if Θ_1, Θ_2, and Θ are constant, then $\omega_0(t)$ and $\omega_0^*(t)$ must be constant, so $\omega_0(t)=\omega_0$ and $\omega_0^*(t)=\omega_0^*$. If the effect on competing events does not favor therapy (i.e., $\Theta_2 \geq 1$), then it follows that $\Theta \geq \omega_0\,\Theta_1+(1-\omega_0)>1-\omega_0$: that is, the *overall treatment effect is bounded by the deadweight factor*. This is a useful initial check to estimate whether a given treatment effect is feasible. Further derivation is given in the Appendix.

High values of the deadweight factor attenuate the overall benefit of a cancer therapy. To illustrate, consider the case of a cancer therapy that halves the risk for cancer-specific mortality (i.e., $\Theta_1=0.5$) and has no effect on noncancer mortality (i.e., $\Theta_2=1$). As the ratio of noncancer mortality relative to cancer mortality (i.e., the deadweight factor) increases, the effect of the treatment on OS trends toward the null value (regardless of its effectiveness against cancer). In competing event theory, cancer therapies ideally have maximal benefit when the ω_0 value is highest. This is so because, since ω_0 is restricted between 0 and 1, as ω_0 approaches 1 (i.e., ω_0^* approaches ∞), then Θ approaches Θ_1, which is identical to the effect on the primary event, and as ω_0 approaches 0 (i.e., ω_0^* approaches 0), then Θ approaches Θ_2, which is identical to the effect on the competing event, which is usually assumed to be either null or detrimental.

MULTISTATE MODELS

In competing risk research, a **multistate model** can be applied to model a process in which a subject transitions from one state to the next. A classic competing risk problem is that all subjects start on the same state (survival), and each subject can make a single transition to one of multiple terminal states (cause-specific mortality and competing events mortality). The most common multistate models are time-inhomogeneous Markov processes with a finite state space. For further reading on analysis of competing risks data, we refer the reader to several additional papers (32–34).

GENERALIZED COMPETING EVENT REGRESSION

In order to quantify effects of factors and treatment on ω_0 and ω_0^*, and differentiate subgroups of patients according to their ω_0* values, we need to develop regression techniques tailored to this goal. The Cox proportional hazards and Fine–Gray regression methods introduced earlier can be extended to a framework called generalized competing event (GCE) regression.

In the GCE regression model, we seek to estimate effects on the ω_0^* function, rather than the hazard or subdistribution hazard. Therefore, for mutually exclusive events of type *k*, we define

$$\omega_k^*(t \mid X) = \omega_{k0}^*(t)\exp(\beta'_{GCE}X) \qquad [47]$$

where $\omega_{k0}^*(t) = \lambda_{k0}(t)/\Sigma_{j\neq k}\lambda_{j0}(t)$ and X is the covariate matrix. The analogous model for subdistribution hazards is

$$\tilde{\omega}_k^*(t \mid X) = \tilde{\omega}_{k0}^*(t)\ \exp\left(\tilde{\beta}'_{GCE}X\right) \qquad [48]$$

where $\tilde{\omega}_{k0}^*(t) = \tilde{\lambda}_{k0}(t)/\Sigma_{j\neq k}\tilde{\lambda}_{j0}(t)$. From this model, it is easy to show that

$$\beta'_{GCE}X = \beta'_kX - \beta'_{j\neq k}X = (\beta'_k - \beta'_{j\neq k})X \qquad [49]$$

and

$$\tilde{\beta}'_{GCE}\ X = \tilde{\beta}'_k X - \tilde{\beta}'_{j\neq k}X = \left(\tilde{\beta}'_k - \tilde{\beta}'_{j\neq k}\right)X \qquad [50]$$

where β_k and $\beta_{j\neq k}$ represent effects on the baseline hazard for event of interest and all other events, respectively, from the Cox proportional hazard model, and $\tilde{\beta}_k$ and $\tilde{\beta}_{j\neq k}$ represent the analogous effects on the subdistribution hazard from the Fine–Gray model. For a derivation, see Carmona et al. (18,19).

We use $\hat{\omega}_{k0}^*(t) = \hat{\Lambda}_{k0}(t)/\hat{\Lambda}_{j\neq k0}(t)$, where $\hat{\Lambda}_{k0}(t)$ and $\hat{\Lambda}_{j\neq k0}(t)$ represent the Nelson–Aalen estimators for the cumulative hazard for event type k and the set of competing events at time t, respectively. We estimate the predicted value of $\hat{\omega}_k^*(t \mid X)$ for an individual with given data vector X as

$$\hat{\omega}_k^*(t \mid X) = \hat{\omega}_{k0}^*(t)\ \exp\left(\hat{\beta}'_{GCE}\ X\right) \qquad [51]$$

Note then that $\exp\left(\hat{\beta}_{GCE}\right)$ is the estimate of the ω^* ratio, which quantifies how the relative hazards for primary and competing events change in response to changes in covariates. We define the omega value as the ratio of the hazard for an event of type k to the hazard for all events:

$$\omega_k(t) = \frac{\lambda_k(t)}{\Sigma_{j\neq k}\lambda_j(t)} \qquad [52]$$

and we estimate the predicted omega value as

$$\hat{\omega}_k(t \mid \boldsymbol{d}) = \frac{\hat{\omega}_k^*(t)}{(1+\hat{\omega}_k^*(t))} \qquad [53]$$

Note that while $\hat{\omega}_k$ ranges from 0 to 1 inclusive, $\hat{\omega}_k^+$ can range from $-\infty$ to ∞. For $k = 2$, a value of $\hat{\omega}_1^* = 1$ means the hazard for event type 1 equals the hazard for event type 2, and therefore $\hat{\omega}_1 = \hat{\omega}_2 = 0.5$.

An example of output from a Cox model versus a GCE model is given in Table 16.2. GCE model estimates were obtained using the *gcerisk* package in R. This package is designed to develop optimized risk stratification methods for competing risks data based on either the Fine–Gray or Cox proportional hazards model for cause-specific events. Further details on GCE estimation methods are provided in Equation 35 (Appendix). For extended reading on analysis of competing risks data, we refer the reader to several additional papers (35–38).

TABLE 16.2 COMPARISON OF COX PH MODEL FOR OVERALL SURVIVAL VS. GCE REGRESSION OUTPUT IN THE SAME COHORT OF 1043 HEAD AND NECK CANCER PATIENTS. NOTE THE OPPOSING DIRECTION OF EFFECTS FOR SEVERAL COVARIATES SUCH AS AGE, BODY MASS INDEX, PERFORMANCE STATUS, MARITAL STATUS, SMOKING STATUS, AND T CATEGORY

	Cox PH Regression	GCE Regression
Characteristic	HR* (95% CI)	ω+ Ratio† (95% CI)
Age at diagnosis, per 10 years	1.33 (1.21, 1.46)	0.68 (0.53, 0.88)
Sex		
Female vs. Male	0.95 (0.88, 1.04)	0.98 (0.78, 1.23)
Race		
Black	0.98 (0.83, 1.16)	0.96 (0.62, 1.48)
White	0.98 (0.83, 1.16)	0.94 (0.62, 1.42)
Non-Black / Non-White	REF	REF
Body Mass Index		
<20 kg/m² vs. ≥20 kg/m²	1.16 (1.08, 1.25)	0.85 (0.68, 1.06)
ECOG Performance Status		
1-2 vs. 0	1.14 (1.05, 1.25)	0.77 (0.60, 1.00)
Married		
Yes vs. No/Unknown	0.86 (0.78, 0.94)	1.08 (0.84, 1.39)
Education History		
Any College vs. None/Unknown	0.86 (0.79, 0.95)	0.95 (0.74, 1.22)
Anatomic subsite		
Oropharynx	REF	REF
Larynx	0.94 (0.85, 1.03)	1.06 (0.81, 1.39)
Hypopharynx	1.10 (1.01, 1.19)	0.96 (0.76, 1.21)
Oral Cavity	1.07 (0.98, 1.17)	1.24 (0.89, 1.71)

(continued)

TABLE 16.2 COMPARISON OF COX PH MODEL FOR OVERALL SURVIVAL VS. GCE REGRESSION OUTPUT IN THE SAME COHORT OF 1043 HEAD AND NECK CANCER PATIENTS. NOTE THE OPPOSING DIRECTION OF EFFECTS FOR SEVERAL COVARIATES SUCH AS AGE, BODY MASS INDEX, PERFORMANCE STATUS, MARITAL STATUS, SMOKING STATUS, AND T CATEGORY (*continued*)

	Cox PH Regression	GCE Regression
T-Stage		
0–2	REF	REF
3	1.01 (0.90, 1.13)	0.92 (0.67, 1.26)
4	1.21 (1.09, 1.35)	0.92 (0.69, 1.24)
N-Stage		
0	REF	REF
1–2	1.02 (0.91, 1.15)	1.20 (0.86, 1.69)
2b–2c	1.18 (1.04, 1.34)	1.17 (0.82, 1.67)
3	1.24 (1.12, 1.36)	1.00 (0.75, 1.33)
Smoking History, pack-years		
>10 vs. ≤10	0.76 (0.68, 0.84)	1.02 (0.77, 1.37)
P16 Status		
Positive vs. Negative	0.70 (0.63, 0.78)	0.81 (0.61, 1.09)

*>1 indicates increased hazard ratio for overall survival

†>1 indicates increased hazard for cancer recurrence relative to competing mortality

ECOG, Eastern Cooperative Oncology Group; GCE, generalized competing event, HR, hazard ratio; PH, proportional hazards.

CONCLUSION

In this chapter, we reviewed the principal theories underlying the analysis of time-to-event data in clinical cancer research, including methods for estimating outcomes and effects of treatments and covariates. We discussed issues regarding the analysis of multiple events of interest, including competing risks settings, which are of particular importance in clinical oncology. Finally, we included practical examples that will be useful in analyzing time-to-event data and generating publishable results.

GLOSSARY

right-censored: in time-to-event analysis, refers to event times that are only known to be greater than a particular value.

left-censored: in time-to-event analysis, refers to event times that are only known to be less than than a particular value.

noninformative censoring: An assumption underlying the validity of time-to-event data analysis that the processes determining whether data are censored are uncorrelated with event times.

controlled study: a study in which two or more groups are compared who differ only with respect to a key factor or intervention(s) of interest; required to both estimate effects on a given outcome and draw meaningful conclusions regarding treatment effects.

uncontrolled study: a study in which only a single group is analyzed without drawing comparisons; generally appropriate for estimating the probability of a given outcome of interest with high certainty.

Martingale residuals: means of assessing a regression model's goodness of fit; used to provide a graphical assessment of the validity of model predictions.

Schoenfeld residuals: method for assessing residuals for use with Cox regression.

event-free survival (EFS) endpoints: endpoints denoting the probability of both being alive and free of a particular event or a set of events; often used as surrogates for overall survival.

confounding by nonspecificity: occurs when inferences may be undermined by the fact that an observed effect could be due in whole or part to confounders driving risk for the competing event.

multistate model: in competing risk research, applied to model a process in which subjects transition from one state to the next.

REFERENCES

1. Glantz SA. *Primer of Biostatistics*. New York, NY: McGraw-Hill; 2011.
2. Kaplan EL, Meier P. Nonparametric estimation from incomplete observations. *J Am Stat Assoc*. 1958;53(282):457–481. doi:10.1080/01621459.1958.10501452
3. Bonner JA, Harari PM, Giralt J, et al. Radiotherapy plus cetuximab for locoregionally advanced head and neck cancer: 5-year survival data from a phase 3 randomised trial, and relation between cetuximab-induced rash and survival. *Lancet Oncol*. 2010;11(1):21–28. doi:10.1016/S1470-2045(09)70311-0
4. Bernier J, Domenge C, Ozsahin M, et al. Postoperative irradiation with or without concomitant chemotherapy for locally advanced head and neck cancer. *N Engl J Med*. 2004;350(19):1945–1952. doi:10.1056/NEJMoa032641
5. Bland JM, Altman DG. Survival probabilities (the Kaplan-Meier method). *BMJ*. 1998;317:1572–1580. doi:10.1136/bmj.317.7172.1572
6. Breslow, N. Covariance analysis of censored survival data. *Biometrics*. 974;30(1):89–99. doi:10.2307/2529620
7. Mell LK, Dignam JJ, Salama JK, et al. Predictors of competing mortality in advanced head and neck cancer. *J Clin Oncol*. 2010;28(1):15–20. doi:10.1200/JCO.2008.20.9288
8. Satagopan JM, Ben-Porat L, Berwick M, et al. A note on competing risks in survival data analysis. *Br J Cancer*. 2004;91(7):1229–1235. doi:10.1038/sj.bjc.6602102
9. Dignam JJ, Kocherginsky MN. Choice and interpretation of statistical tests used when competing risks are present. *J Clin Oncol*. 2008;26:4027–4034. doi:10.1200/JCO.2007.12.9866
10. Marubini E, Valsecchi MG. *Analysing Survival Data from Clinical Trials and Observational Studies*. Chichester, UK: John Wiley & Sons; 1995.
11. Bland JM, Altman DG. The logrank test. *BMJ*. 2004;328(7447):1073. doi:10.1136/bmj.328.7447.1073
12. Cox DR. Regression models and life tables. *J R Stat Soc Series B Stat Methodol*. 1972;B34:187–220.
13. Fine JP, Gray RJ. A proportional hazards model for the subdistribution of a competing risk. *J Am Stat Assoc*. 1999;94(446):496–509. doi:10.1080/01621459.1999.10474144
14. Gray RJ. A class of K-sample tests for comparing the cumulative incidence of a competing risk. *Ann Stat*. 1988;16(3):1141–1154. doi:10.1214/aos/1176350951
15. Pintilie M. *Competing Risks: A Practical Perspective*. Chichester, UK: John Wiley & Sons; 2006:117.
16. Schoenfeld, D. Partial residuals for the proportzional hazards regression model. *Biometrika*. 1982;69(1):239–241. doi:10.1093/biomet/69.1.239
17. Grambsch PM, Therneau TM. Proportional hazards tests and diagnostics based on weighted residuals. *Biometrika*. 1994;81(3):515–526. doi:10.1093/biomet/81.3.515

18. Collett D. *Modelling Survival Data in Medical Research*. 3rd ed. Boca Raton, FL: Chapman & Hall/CRC; 2015.
19. Rose BS, Jeong JH, Nath SK, et al. Population-based study of competing mortality in head and neck cancer. *J Clin Oncol*. 2011;29:3503–3509. doi:10.1200/JCO.2011.35.7301
20. Mathoulin-Pelissier S, Gourgou-Bourgade S, Bonnetain F, Kramar A. Survival end point reporting in randomized cancer clinical trials: a review of major journals. *J Clin Oncol*. 2008;26(22):3721–3726. doi:10.1200/JCO.2007.14.1192
21. Thompson IM, Tangen CM, Paradelo J, et al. Adjuvant radiotherapy for pathological T3N0M0 prostate cancer significantly reduces risk of metastases and improves survival: long term follow up of a randomized clinical trial. *J Urol*. 2009;181:956–962. doi:10.1016/j.juro.2008.11.032
22. Zakeri K, Rose BS, Gulaya S, et al. Competing event risk stratification may improve the design and efficiency of clinical trials: secondary analysis of SWOG 8794. *Contemp Clin Trials*. 2013;34:74–79. doi:10.1016/j.cct.2012.09.008
23. Clift RA, Buckner CD, Appelbaum FR, et al. Allogeneic marrow transplantation in patients with acute myeloid leukemia in first remission: a randomized trial of two irradiation regimens. *Blood*. 1990;76:1867–1871.
24. Mell LK, Carmona R, Gulaya S, et al. Cause-specific effects of radiotherapy and lymphadenectomy in stage I-II endometrial cancer: a population-based study. *J Natl Cancer Inst*. 2013;105(21):1656–1666. doi:10.1093/jnci/djt279
25. Mell LK, Lau SK, Rose BS, Jeong JH. Reporting of cause-specific treatment effects in cancer clinical trials with competing risks: a systematic review. *Contemp Clin Trials*. 2010;33:920–924. doi:10.1093/jnci/djt279
26. Green G, Carmona R, Zakeri K, et al. Specificity of genetic biomarker studies in cancer research: a systematic review. *PLoS One*. 2016;11(7):e0156489. doi:10.1371/journal.pone.0156489
27. Zakeri K, Rose BS, D'Amico AV, et al. Competing events and costs of clinical trials: analysis of a randomized trial in prostate cancer. *Radiother Oncol*. 2015;115(1):114–119. doi:10.1016/j.radonc.2015.03.018
28. Carmona R, Gulaya S, Murphy JD, et al. Validated competing event model for the stage I-II endometrial cancer population. *Int J Radiat Oncol Biol Phys*. 2014;89:888–898. doi:10.1016/j.ijrobp.2014.03.047
29. Carmona R, Zakeri K, Green G, et al. Improved method to stratify elderly patients with cancer at risk for competing events. *J Clin Oncol*. 2016;34(11):1270–1277. doi:10.1200/JCO.2015.65.0739
30. Mohler JL, Armstrong AJ, Bahnson RR, et al. Prostate Cancer, Version 1.2016. *J Natl Compr Canc Netw*. 2016;14(1):19–30. doi:10.6004/jnccn.2016.0004
31. Mell LK, Jeong JH. Pitfalls of using composite primary end points in the presence of competing risks. *J Clin Oncol*. 2010;28:4297–4299. doi:10.1200/JCO.2010.30.2802
32. Andersen, PK, Abildstrom SZ, Rosthøj S. Competing risks as a multi-state model. *Stat Methods Med Res*. 2002;11(2):203–215. doi:10.1191/0962280202sm281ra
33. Putter H, Marta F, Geskus RB. Tutorial in biostatistics: competing risks and multistate models. *Stat Med*. 2007;26(11):2389–2430. doi:10.1002/sim.2712
34. Beyersmann J, Allignol A, Schumacher M. *Competing Risks and Multistate Models With R*. Berlin, Germany: Springer Science & Business Media; 2011.
35. Kalbfleisch JD, Prentice RL. *The Statistical Analysis of Failure Time Data*. New York, NY: John Wiley & Sons; 1980.
36. Korn EL, Dorey FJ. Applications of crude incidence curves. *Stat Med*. 1992;11:813–829. doi:10.1002/sim.4780110611
37. Dignam JJ, Zhang Q, Kocherginsky M. The use and interpretation of competing risks regression models. *Clin Cancer Res*. 2012;18(8):2301–2308. doi:10.1158/1078-0432.CCR-11-2097
38. Mell LK, Zakeri K, Rose BS. On lumping, splitting, and the nosology of clinical trial populations and end points. *J Clin Oncol*. 2014;32:1089–1090. doi:10.1200/JCO.2013.54.4429

APPENDIX

Equation 4. *Definition of the hazard function.*

$$\lambda(t) = f(t)/S(t) = -S'(t)/S(t) = \lim (\Delta t \to 0)\ Pr(t < T < t + \Delta t | T \geq t)/\Delta t$$

Equation 8. *Nelson–Aalen estimator.*

$$H(t) = \prod_{j:t_j \leq t} \frac{d_j}{n_j} \approx -\ln(S(t))$$

Equation 9. *Greenwood's formula for the variance of $\hat{S}(t)$.*

$$\hat{V}(t) = \hat{S}(t) \Sigma_{j:t_j \leq t} \frac{d_j}{n_j(n_j - d_j)}$$

Equation 10. *Definition of the cause-specific hazard function.*

$$\lambda_k(t;\delta) = \lim (\Delta t \to 0)\ \Pr(t < T < t + \Delta t; \delta = k | T \geq t)/\Delta t$$

Equation 18. *Calculation of the log-rank statistic.*

$$L = \sum_{j \in \{1,2,\cdots,N\}} \frac{d_{1j} - E_j}{(\Sigma_{j \in \{1,2,\cdots,N\}} V_j)^{1/2}}$$

where

$$E_j = (d_{1j} + d_{2j}) * n_{1j}/(n_{1j} + n_{2j})$$

and

$$V_j = [E_j * (1 - n_{1j}/(n_{1j} + n_{2j})) * ((n_{1j} + n_{2j}) - (d_{1j} + d_{2j}))]/((n_{1j} + n_{2j}) - 1)$$

Equation 21. *The log-partial likelihood function.*

$$l(\beta) = log\left[\prod_{i=1}^{n} \frac{e^{\beta' X_i}}{\sum_{l \in R_i} e^{\beta' X_l}}\right]^{\delta_i} = \sum_{i=1}^{n} \delta_i \left[\beta' X_i - log\left\{\sum_{l \in R_i} e^{\beta' X_l}\right\}\right] = \sum_{i=1}^{n} l_i(\beta)$$

where l_i is the log-partial likelihood contribution from individual i and R_i is the risk set of individual i.

Equation 22. *The partial likelihood score function.*

$$U(\beta) = \frac{\partial l(\beta)}{\partial \beta} = \sum_{i=1}^{n} \delta_i \left[X_i - \frac{\Sigma_{l \in R_i} X_l e^{\beta' X_l}}{\Sigma_{l \in R_i} e^{\beta' X_l}}\right]$$

The maximum partial likelihood estimation can be calculated by solving $U(\beta) = 0$. Analogous to the standard likelihood theory, the asymptotical results can be shown as $\frac{\hat{\beta} - \beta}{se(\hat{\beta})} \sim N(0,1)$.

Equation 23. *Wald-chi square test used in partial likelihood hypothesis testing.*

$$Z = \frac{\hat{\beta}_i}{se(\hat{\beta}_i)} \text{ or } \chi^2 = \left(\frac{\hat{\beta}_i}{se(\hat{\beta}_i)} \right)^2$$

Note that if we have a factor D with d levels, then we would need to build a χ^2 test with degree of freedom $(d-1)$, using a test statistic $\chi^2_{(d-1)} = \breve{\beta}_D' Var(\breve{\beta}_D) \breve{\beta}_D$, where $\beta_D = (\beta_1, \ldots, \beta_{d-1})'$ are the $(d-1)$ coefficients related to the binary variables $X_1, \ldots X_{d-1}$.

Equation 25. *Cumulative incidence function and its derivative.*

$$f_k(t) = \lim_{dt \downarrow 0} \frac{P\{T \in (t, t+dt) \, and \, K = k\}}{dt}$$

$$F_k(t) = \int_0^t f_k(u) du = P(T \le t \, and \, K = k)$$

Equation 27. *Definition of the subdistribution hazard function.*

$$\tilde{\lambda}_k(t \mid Z) = \lim_{dt \downarrow 0} \frac{P\{T \in (t, t+dt) \, and \, K = k \mid T > t \text{ or } T \le t \, and \, K \ne k\}}{dt}$$

Equation 28. *Partial likelihood equation for the Fine–Gray estimator.*

$$l(\beta) = log \left[\prod_{i=1}^{n} \frac{e^{\beta' X_i}}{\sum_{l \in R_i} e^{\beta' X_l}} \right]^{\delta_i} = \sum_{i=1}^{n} \delta_i \times \left(\beta' X_i(T_i) - log \left[\sum_{j \in R_i} e^{\beta' X_i(T_i)} \right] \right)$$

where R_i is the risk set of individual i.

Equation 29. *Partial likelihood score function for the Fine–Gray estimator.*

$$U(\beta) = \frac{\partial l(\beta)}{\partial \beta} = \Sigma_{i=1}^{n} \delta_i \times \left(X_i(T_i) - \frac{\Sigma_{j \in R_i} X_i(T_i) e^{\beta' X_i(T_i)}}{\Sigma_{j \in R_i} e^{\beta' X_i(T_i)}} \right).$$

Equations 30–34. *Maximum partial likelihood estimation and hypothesis testing for the Fine–Gray estimator.*

Letting $N_i(t) = I(T_i \le t, \delta_i)$ and $Y_i(t) = \; - N_i(t-)$,

$$U(\beta) = \sum_{i=1}^{n} \int_0^{\infty} \left[X_i(s) - \frac{\Sigma_{j \in R_i} Y_j(s) X_i(T_i) e^{\beta' X_i(T_i)}}{\Sigma_{j \in R_i} Y_j(s) e^{\beta' X_i(T_i)}} \right] dN_i(s)$$

The maximum partial likelihood estimation can be calculated by solving $U(\beta) = 0$. Analogous to standard likelihood theory, it can be shown that $n^{1/2}(\hat{\beta} - \beta)$ is asymptotically normal with limiting covariance matrix Ω^{-1}. Estimation of β can be made by normal distribution with covariance matrix $\hat{\Omega}^{-1}$, a consistent estimate for the asymptotic variance, which can be calculated from

$$\hat{\Omega} = \frac{1}{n}\sum_{i=1}^{n}\left\{\frac{S_1^{(2)}\left(\hat{\beta},T_i\right)}{S_1^{(0)}\left(\hat{\beta},T_i\right)} - \bar{Z}\left(\hat{\beta},T_i\right)^{\otimes 2}\right\}\delta_i,$$

$$\bar{Z}(\beta,u) = \frac{S_1^{(1)}(\beta,u)}{S_1^{(0)}(\beta,u)}$$

and

$$S_1^{(p)}(\beta,u) = \frac{1}{n}\sum_{i=1}^{n} Y_i(u)X_i(u)^{\otimes p}\, e^{\beta' X_i(u)}$$

A Wald test of the above hypothesis is built as

$$Z = \frac{\hat{\beta}_i}{se\left(\hat{\beta}_i\right)} \text{ or } \chi^2 = \left(\frac{\hat{\beta}_i}{se\left(\hat{\beta}_i\right)}\right)^2$$

Note that if we have a factor D with d levels, then we would need to build a χ^2 test with degree of freedom $(d-1)$, using a test statistic $\chi^2_{(d-1)} = \hat{\beta}_D' Var\left(\hat{\beta}_D\right)\hat{\beta}_D$, where $\beta_D = \left(\beta_1,\ldots,\beta_{d-1}\right)'$ are the $(d-1)$ coefficients related to the binary variables $X_1, \ldots, X_{d-1}$.

Equation 54. *Likelihood function and variance of GCE coefficients based on Cox regression.*

Considering the situation with two events of interest (e.g., cancer mortality and competing event mortality), the Cox PH model can be written as

$$\lambda_{11}(t \mid X) = \lambda_{01}\exp(\beta_1 X)$$

$$\lambda_{12}(t \mid X) = \lambda_{02}\exp(\beta_2 X)$$

Hence, $\beta^*_{GCE} = \beta_1 - \beta_2$.

Assume a Cox regression model with covariates x, δx stratifying by event type, $\delta = 1$ or 0 (1 represents cancer mortality and 0 represents competing event mortality). Hence, the partial likelihood function can be found by

$$L(\beta_1,\beta_2) = \prod_{t_i,\delta_i=1}\left(\frac{e^{\beta_1' x_i}}{\sum_{R_i} e^{\beta_1' x_i}}\right)\prod_{t_i,\delta_i=0}\left(\frac{e^{\beta_2' x_i}}{\sum_{R_i} e^{\beta_2' x_i}}\right)$$

$$= \prod_{t_i,\delta_i=1}\left(\frac{e^{\beta_2' x_i + \beta_{GCE}^{*\prime} x_i}}{\sum_{R_i} e^{\beta_2' x_i + \beta_{GCE}^{*\prime} x_i}}\right)\prod_{t_i,\delta_i=0}\left(\frac{e^{\beta_2' x_i}}{\sum_{R_i} e^{\beta_2' x_i}}\right) = L(\beta^*_{GCE},\beta_2)$$

where R_i is the risk set at failure time t_i. A main assumption for this approach is that there is no relationship between two baseline hazards λ_{01} and λ_{02}. Further, the log-partial likelihood function can be calculated as

$$l(\beta^*_{GCE}, \beta_2) = log\{L(\beta^*_{GCE}, \beta_2)\}$$
$$= \sum_{t_i,\delta_i=1} \left\{ \beta_2' x_i + \beta^{*'}_{GCE} x_i - log\left(\sum_{R_i} e^{\beta_2' x_i + \beta^{*'}_{GCE} x_i} \right) \right\}$$
$$+ \sum_{t_i,\delta_i=0} \left\{ \beta_2' x_i - log\left(\sum_{R_i} e^{\beta_2' x_i} \right) \right\}$$

Hence, the maximum likelihood estimator $\widehat{\beta^*_{GCE}}$ and $\widehat{\beta_2}$ can be calculated by solving

$$\begin{cases} \dfrac{\partial l(\beta^*_{GCE}, \beta_2)}{\partial \beta^*_{GCE}} = \sum_{t_i,\delta_i=1} \left\{ x_i - \dfrac{\sum_{R_i} x_i e^{\beta_2' x_i + \beta^{*'}_{GCE} x_i}}{\sum_{R_i} e^{\beta_2' x_i + \beta^{*'}_{GCE} x_i}} \right\} = 0 \\ \dfrac{\partial l(\beta^*_{GCE}, \beta_2)}{\partial \beta_2} = \sum_{t_i,\delta_i=1} \left\{ x_i - \dfrac{\sum_{R_i} x_i e^{\beta_2' x_i + \beta^{*'}_{GCE} x_i}}{\sum_{R_i} e^{\beta_2' x_i + \beta^{*'}_{GCE} x_i}} \right\} + \sum_{t_i,\delta_i=0} \left\{ x_i - \dfrac{\sum_{R_i} x_i e^{\beta_2' x_i}}{\sum_{R_i} e^{\beta_2' x_i}} \right\} = 0 \end{cases}$$

The standard likelihood theory can show that

$$\frac{\widehat{\beta^*_{GCE}} - \beta^*_{GCE}}{s.e.(\beta^*_{GCE})} \sim N(0,1)$$

The variance of $\widehat{\beta^*_{GCE}}$ can be estimated by inverting the second derivative of the partial likelihood,

$$\widehat{Var(\beta^*_{GCE})} = \left[-\frac{\partial^2 l(\beta^*_{GCE}, \beta_2)}{\partial {\beta^*_{GCE}}^2} \right]^{-1}$$

16–1. Derivation: *Under proportional hazards, the omega function is equal to the relative cumulative incidences of primary and all-cause events.*

Let the function ω_0 be defined as in Equation 45, and let the composite treatment effect (Θ) be expressed as a weighted average of the cause-specific effects, as in Equation 46. Let us further assume ω_0 is constant, such that

$$\Theta = \omega^*\Theta_1 + (1 - \omega)^*\Theta_2 > \omega^*\Theta_1 + (1 - \omega) > 1 - \omega$$

Thus, the overall treatment effect is bounded by the deadweight factor. Note also that ω is constant if and only if the ratio of the baseline cause-specific hazard functions is constant (i.e., both have the same basic form), since

$$\frac{\lambda_{01}(t)}{\lambda_{02}(t)} = \frac{\omega\, \lambda_0(t)}{(1-\omega)\lambda_0(t)} = \frac{\omega}{(1-\omega)}$$

(By definition, if competing risks are present, then $\omega \neq 1$.)

In practice, it is usually assumed (due to proportional hazards) that both Θ and Θ_1 are fixed constants, and ω is not increasing (i.e., $\frac{d}{dt}[\omega] \leq 0$). In this case

$$\omega = \frac{\Theta_2 - \Theta}{\Theta_2 - \Theta_1}$$

and

$$\frac{d}{dt}[\omega] = \frac{\Theta_2'(\Theta_2 - \Theta_1) - \Theta_2'(\Theta_2 - \Theta)}{(\Theta_2 - \Theta_1)^2} = \frac{\Theta_2'(\Theta - \Theta_1)}{(\Theta_2 - \Theta_1)^2}$$

which implies that Θ_2 is not increasing (since $\Theta > \Theta_1$). However, typically adverse effects of therapy on competing events, when present, manifest over time, implying that Θ_2 is not decreasing either. Hence, treating ω as constant is reasonable (and verifiable).

Here we show that when ω is constant, it is identical to the ratio of the cumulative incidence of primary events to the cumulative incidence of all-cause events. Let $F_1(t)$, $F_2(t)$, and $F(t)$ define the (baseline) cumulative incidence functions for the primary event(s), competing event(s), and all events, respectively. By definition

$$F_1(t) = \int_0^t \lambda_{01}(u)*S(u)\, du$$

where $S(t)$ represents the survival function for all events. Also, by definition

$$F(t) = \int_0^t \lambda_0(u)*S(u)\, du$$

Replacing $\lambda_{01}(t) = \omega\lambda_0(t)$, we get

$$F_1(t) = \int_0^t \omega*\lambda_0(u)*S(u)\, du = \omega\int_0^t \lambda_0(u)*S(u)\, du = \omega F(t)$$

Therefore

$$\omega = \frac{F_1(t)}{F(t)}$$

because cumulative cause-specific incidences are additive to the total

$$1 - \omega = \frac{F(t) - F_1(t)}{F(t)} = \frac{F_2(t)}{F(t)}$$

17

Machine Learning and High-Dimensional Data Analysis

SANJAY ANEJA ■ JAMES B. YU

In previous chapters, we discussed statistical methods for analyzing structured datasets within clinical oncology. **Structured data** is loosely defined as data that have been curated by researchers per a specific study design within a database for statistical analysis. With the advent of electronic health records (EHRs), regulated clinical trials, and tumor registries, we are fortunate that within clinical oncology there are a plethora of structured datasets that are freely available to researchers. However, as clinical oncology research continues to evolve, there is an increasing desire to analyze new and interesting data sources.

The obvious disadvantage of structured data sources is the considerable amount of effort and resources required to curate a database. This is an often time-intensive and expensive process and limits the continuous creation of new interesting data sources. Because of the time lag that exists as one compiles and curates data, the majority of healthcare data remains trapped in an unstructured format. Moreover, even with curated datasets, we often do not have the foresight or technology to collect relevant data until years later. For example, despite tumor registry data dating back to the 1970s, we do not have structured data of known prognostic mutations for a number of cancers. This means that these older data have less utility for today's clinical cancer research.

Ideally, we could identify ways to continually collect and analyze unstructured data such that we could dynamically pivot our research questions to adapt to the changing research landscape. Examples of unstructured data within oncology are radiologic images, raw text from clinician notes, digitized pathology images, and sequenced genetic information. These data are particularly difficult because they are often high dimensional in nature and not suited to analysis using traditional statistical techniques. **Machine learning techniques** are mathematical techniques that are well suited to analyze high-dimensional, noisy data and can make sense of unstructured high-dimensional datasets.

Machine learning is a field that has formed from a marriage between computer science and mathematics. In this chapter, we first provide an introduction to the field of machine learning, then discuss common machine learning algorithms that are most frequently employed in clinical oncology research today. A comprehensive understanding of machine learning methods merits a much more involved discussion, which is beyond the scope of this textbook. This chapter is meant to act as a simple primer on important aspects of machine learning, terminology, and current applications. For those interested in a more detailed discussion, we have provided a list of more advanced texts for reference at the end of the chapter.

WHAT IS MACHINE LEARNING?

Machine learning is a field that attempts to make sense of complex, noisy data sets. It is defined in part by the process in which a predictive algorithm is developed. Machine learning algorithms are created using an iterative process, wherein a computer builds a provisional model to describe data and continually modifies the model as it is exposed to more data (1). Typically, machine learning algorithms attempt to optimize accuracy or minimize some predefined error function. The nuances of optimization are often what delineate different machine learning algorithms and the applicability of the algorithm to different types of data.

Machine learning methods are typically divided into two categories: supervised and unsupervised learning methods. **Supervised learning methods** consist of labeled data where variables are paired with a known outcome of interest (2). **Labeled data** can be thought of as examples that a machine learning algorithm can use to build a model. Therefore, regression methods described in Chapter 16 are technically considered supervised learning algorithms, because they use labeled datasets with known outcomes to create their model. In contrast, unsupervised methods are unlabeled and merely attempt to understand similarities, correlations, interactions, and patterns that exist among the variables. To illustrate the differences between unsupervised and supervised learning methods, we first describe a clinical data source. We describe both a supervised research question and an unsupervised question that can be answered using the data.

Imagine we were given all the data within a hospital's EHRs. An example of a supervised learning problem with this dataset would be one where researchers predict which patients will be diagnosed with cancer. The labeled data would include variables from the EHRs and the label would be the presence of a cancer diagnosis. A supervised machine learning algorithm would attempt to find a pattern between the variables and the presence of a cancer diagnosis. The algorithm would first develop a provisional model for the data using a small sample of patients. The provisional model would be able to generate a prediction of whether a patient has a cancer diagnosis given the variables within the EHRs. Then, as the algorithm saw data from more patients, it could generate a prediction on the presence of a cancer diagnosis. This prediction would be compared to the true presence of a cancer diagnosis and the model would be adjusted to reduce inaccuracies.

An unsupervised problem using the EHR data would not directly be interested in finding variables that predict cancer; instead, it would be interested in discovering general similarities that exist among patients using all variables. Rather than focusing on a singular outcome such as cancer, unsupervised learning tasks often do not have an *a priori* outcome in mind. That said, when evaluating the similarities among patients, we might discover that one group of patients exhibiting significant similarities are patients who are also diagnosed with cancer. As you can see, despite the differences between unsupervised and supervised learning methods, we can often discover similar insights.

MACHINE LEARNING VERSUS TRADITIONAL STATISTICAL MODELS

Before we begin describing specific supervised and unsupervised machine learning algorithms, it is important to understand why unstructured data may be better suited for a machine learning process compared to the regression techniques discussed in the previous chapters. We can use our example of a hospital's EHRs to illustrate the utility of machine learning methods. Within the EHRs, there exist thousands of variables. In addition to demographic variables such as age, sex, race, geographic location, there are also variables that correspond to all the unique types of treatments and diagnostic procedures that patients underwent at some point in their lives. If we had a user-curated form of the data that identified important variables, then the previously described statistical approaches would be ideal. However, suppose we were not sure which data were important for our particular question and we are interested in exploring potential relationships among these variables. This means we wanted to be sure that our own biases regarding the causal factors of our outcome did not ignore a more important discovery. In this situation, it would be most prudent to utilize all available data at our disposal.

Given the large number of variables within our data, it is likely that using the entire dataset violates a number of the assumptions for the models we discussed in the previous chapters. In contrast, one of the major benefits to certain machine learning techniques is the lack of strict constraints with respect to data. For example, machine learning methods may have fewer assumptions regarding data distributions and are able to process high-dimensional data, allowing us to place all available data within one model.

It is important to formalize some major differences between machine learning and the modeling techniques described in the previous chapters. The first difference is largely based on the motivation behind each field. Whereas traditional statistics entails deriving or **fitting** an equation to model a process, machine learning often is focused more on building a program or algorithm to automate a process. This difference has significant implications in the benefits and disadvantages of both fields.

The benefit of formalizing an equation using a method like regression is the increased interpretability that is afforded to researchers. We learned in Chapter 16 that coefficients from regression models are often useful in identifying the nature of relationships between different independent variables and an outcome of interest. Although machine learning is still an emerging area of research, most would agree that traditional regression models are considerably easier to interpret than a machine learning algorithm. Machine learning algorithms, which are focused more on automation than on interpretation, often sacrifice interpretability for accuracy (1). Traditional statistical models, in contrast, are more rigidly constrained to fit predefined distributions in order to create interpretable equations. This increased interpretability, however, often comes at the cost of accuracy and discriminatory ability (3).

The second difference between machine learning and traditional statistics is their academic origins. Statistics has traditionally been thought of as a field that emerged from applied mathematics. In contrast, given the computational skill needed to perform machine learning algorithms, many who practice machine learning come from backgrounds in computer science as well as applied mathematics.

As previously mentioned, there are notable differences in the assumptions associated with regression models and machine learning algorithms. In general, machine learning algorithms attempt to limit the assumptions in lieu of increased applicability across different data types. We previously described the numerous assumptions associated with regression models that allow for increased interpretability when fitting data to regression equations. In general, regression requires the dependent variable of interest to fit a predefined distribution.

For example, linear regression assumes a normally distributed outcome and logistic regression assumes a binary outcome distribution. Many machine learning methods do not require any specific distribution of outcome data, but do require that the data be a relatively robust representation of how the data appear in the real world. Linear regression models also frequently assume a linear and/or monotonic relationship between dependent and independent variables. In a *linear relationship*, as one of the independent variables increases or decreases, the dependent variables will change in a linear fashion; *monotonic* implies that as the independent variable changes, the dependent variable changes in the same "direction." Machine learning methods do not assume a linear or even monotonic relationship between dependent and independent variables (4,5). This allows them to have increased flexibility to model data from complex heterogeneous data sources, such as a complex electronic medical record.

One might wonder, then, why we still rely on traditional statistical methods for the majority of clinical oncology research? In addition to machine learning being a relatively nascent field, there are a number of reasons why traditional modeling techniques continue to have utility. The first is when dealing with smaller datasets. Although machine learning methods can be used for small datasets in certain cases, employing them is computationally expensive and requires a large amount of high-performance computing power, which might not be necessary. In contrast, traditional statistical methods are well suited to the analysis of smaller datasets, and they can be done with readily available computing power. Moreover, machine learning algorithms often require larger amounts of data to generate accurate predictions and may not be well suited for small datasets. Additionally, although regression methods are restrictive in their assumptions, there is a similarly restrictive quality inherent in accurate machine learning algorithms. Given the ability for machine learning methods to effectively model data, and high probability of multicollinearity, there is a risk of **overfitting** the model to the data used to create the algorithm (i.e., identifying spurious relationships between model inputs and the outcome).

Overfitting is problematic because it makes the model less generalizable. In our previous example of using EHRs to predict cancer diagnosis, a machine learning algorithm may generate a less accurate prediction for a different patient population. Similarly, machine learning algorithms are increasingly dependent on large amounts of labeled data to improve the algorithm and identify underlying patterns within the data. This, in many ways, limits the utility of machine learning algorithms to study research questions on small subpopulations of patients for whom there is no wealth of data.

The data requirements associated with machine learning algorithms become increasingly important when handling missing data. Missing data is a problem in all aspects of clinical research; models generated using traditional statistics are affected by missing data just like machine learning methods. When dealing with machine learning algorithms, it is often more beneficial to impute missing data rather than exclude cases (1). As mentioned earlier, the other major disadvantage to machine learning methods is the relative lack of interpretability compared to traditional statistical modeling. For example, the coefficients from a regression model to predict cancer diagnosis for patients within an EHR would allow us to identify potential risk factors and the magnitude and direction of their association. Conversely, a machine learning algorithm would likely be able to predict cancer diagnosis from EHR data with high accuracy, but would have considerably more difficulty locating specific risk factors associated with a cancer diagnosis. Practically, the lack of interpretability limits the utility of machine learning algorithms to addressing specific drivers of a given outcome. This has been described as the **"black box" problem** of machine learning (6).

Overall, when dealing with complex high-dimensional, noisy data, many would argue that machine learning methods are often better at accurately modeling data and predicting outcomes compared to regression methods. However, regression methods are usually better for revealing potential drivers associated with a particular outcome in a typical well-designed research setting.

METRICS FOR EVALUATING MACHINE LEARNING ALGORITHMS

Prior to our discussion of specific machine learning algorithms, it is worth providing a framework for algorithm development. The majority of this chapter focuses on supervised machine learning methods. At the end of the chapter, we briefly discuss methods in unsupervised machine learning. Supervised machine learning algorithms are typically developed using a training-test-validation method. Prior to developing a machine learning algorithm, the data are segregated into three parts: **training**, **test**, and **validation**. Conventionally, the training data consist of approximately 80% of the samples, and constitute the primary source for developing the algorithm (7). Because machine learning algorithms have different configurations that could affect accuracy, the test set is used to compare different algorithm configurations during the development process. The validation set is a blinded set, which is only used when the algorithm has been finalized. It is critical that the algorithm not be changed after evaluation with the validation set in order to truly assure algorithm performance.

When evaluating machine learning models, we often utilize the same metrics that are typically employed in traditional statistics and clinical medicine. The most common metrics for evaluating

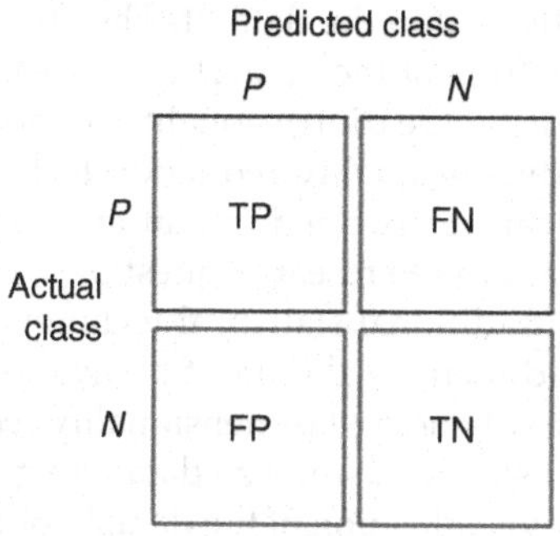

FIGURE 17.1 Confusion matrix.

FN, false negatives; FP, false positives; TN, true negatives; TP, true positives.

the effectiveness of a machine learning algorithm are framed by creating a **confusion matrix**. A confusion matrix (Figure 17.1) allows one to quickly identify the specificity, sensitivity, positive predictive value (PPV), and negative predictive value (NPV) of a machine learning algorithm (also see Chapters 7, 13, and 24). As the machine learning algorithm is refined, it is helpful to compare the confusion matrix to assess performance.

The second most common metric for evaluating machine learning algorithms is the **receiver operating characteristic (ROC) curve** (see also Chapters 7 and 24). An ROC curve is an important tool that assesses the relative sensitivity and specificity of a particular algorithm. An important metric from the ROC is the **area under the curve (AUC)**. The AUC is a common metric to evaluate the discriminatory ability of a possible machine learning algorithm. Although the AUC is often the most reported metric by machine learning enthusiasts, it is important to remember that the best model may not be the one with the highest AUC.

Suppose we compared two machine learning algorithms, one model with a very high AUC and the second with a lower AUC, but a higher sensitivity at a particular cutoff point. If this algorithm were meant to screen for an outcome, we would rather sacrifice discriminatory ability seen in the higher AUC model in favor of increased sensitivity. There are a number of other metrics that are used by data scientists to compare machine learning algorithms; discussing them all is beyond the scope of this chapter (8). Nevertheless, most would agree that the cornerstone for evaluation would always be the confusion matrix and ROC curves.

COMMON MACHINE LEARNING ALGORITHMS FOR DIMENSIONALITY REDUCTION

In this section, we briefly discuss different types of machine learning algorithms that are commonly used in cancer research. After each algorithm is discussed, we have a table with papers that employ these algorithms for more in-depth review.

An advantage of machine learning techniques is the ability to analyze high-dimensional datasets not suited for traditional modeling techniques like regression. A common way in which researchers leverage machine learning is to reduce high-dimensional datasets, in order to better evaluate them using traditional statistical modeling techniques. **Dimensionality reduction techniques** aim to reduce the number of variables necessary to analyze an outcome without compromising the overall integrity of the data and the underlying relationships that potentially exist.

For example, suppose we had a dataset of tumor samples with three variables of interest: (1) tumor location, (2) size in millimeters (mm) of the tumor, and (3) size in centimeters (cm) of the tumor. A less effective data reduction technique would not remove tumor location because that information is not represented anywhere else within the two remaining variables. In contrast, an effective data reduction algorithm would remove one of the size components, given that the same information is present redundantly within the dataset. The effect of data reduction on our hypothetical dataset would be the reduction of the dataset to two variables (tumor site and one of the size components), effectively reducing the dimensionality of the data by 1.

There are many benefits to dimensionality reduction techniques. By reducing the collinear variables within the dataset, we can remove redundant and/or less important information and focus on the data that are important to the research questions. This can also prevent violations of the assumptions associated with traditional statistical techniques. Therefore, reducing the number of dimensions within a high-dimensional dataset allows us to employ traditional modeling techniques more easily. A secondary benefit of dimensionality reduction is that it limits the size of the dataset and makes it easier to store and analyze data using limited computational resources. Another potential benefit is easier visualization of the data. In our earlier example, we initially had three variables that would have been visualized in a 3-D space. However, after data reduction, we could view the same information in a 2-D space. Imagine if we had 60 variables (nearly impossible to visualize), but were able to reduce this to a simple 2-D scatterplot. It is important to note that often it is difficult to reduce the dimensionality of a large dataset to a simple 2-D scatterplot, but there are emerging techniques in dimensionality reduction, notably **t-Distributed Stochastic Neighbor Embedding** (**t-SNE**), that allow for the visualization of high-dimensional data using dimensionality reduction (9).

Lastly, dimensionality reduction can help us reduce noise within messy datasets. By reducing our data to the most essential components, which describe the process we are studying, we objectively eliminate unrelated parts of the dataset. Imagine that in our example we were given data detailing patients' home addresses. Intuitively, we know that a patient's address is likely unrelated to tumor size or tumor location and can ignore it in our analysis. We in essence have performed a dimensionality reduction algorithm ourselves. However, imagine if we had a large dataset, like the EHRs for an entire hospital. Such a judgment would be difficult and impractical, given the number of potentially useless variables. Also, just because we intuitively believe something is not important does not mean it truly is unrelated. Dimensionality reduction techniques can help us avoid subjectively dismissing possible relationships that exist within the data.

PRINCIPAL COMPONENT ANALYSIS

One of the most common dimensionality reduction techniques is **principal component analysis** (**PCA**). With PCA, variables in a dataset are transformed into a new set of variables representing linear combinations of the original variables (i.e., represented in a new basis). The transformed variables are known as *principal components* (PCs). The nuance to this algorithm is that the principal components are ordered such that the first principal component accounts for the greatest variance in the original dataset. The second (orthogonal) principal component then is derived by capture variance within the data that is not explained by the first principal component. If one is able to reduce the dimensionality of a dataset to a smaller number of principal components, then one could effectively enter them into a regression for analysis (10).

PCA is an unsupervised machine learning technique, as it does not rely on a labeled target or response variable. Thus, a disadvantage of PCA is the limited interpretability of the analysis with respect to the individual PCs. The coefficients of the regression using principal components generally provide details regarding effects of changes in the PCs themselves, rather than the variables within the original data. Nevertheless, if one found a principal component to be highly correlated to a desired outcome, then it is possible to study what aspects of the data contributed to that principal component. For example, Liang et al. (11) used a supervised application of PCA called principal components regression to generate heat maps of pelvic regions in which radiation dose accumulation was most strongly correlated with acute bone marrow toxicity (Figure 17.2).

With this method, each patient's 3-D dose distribution is represented by a high-dimensional vector corresponding to dose within a set of tiny voxels spanning the pelvic space (Figure 17.2A). Applying PCA to the dose distribution data, one can see from the **scree plot** (which displays the

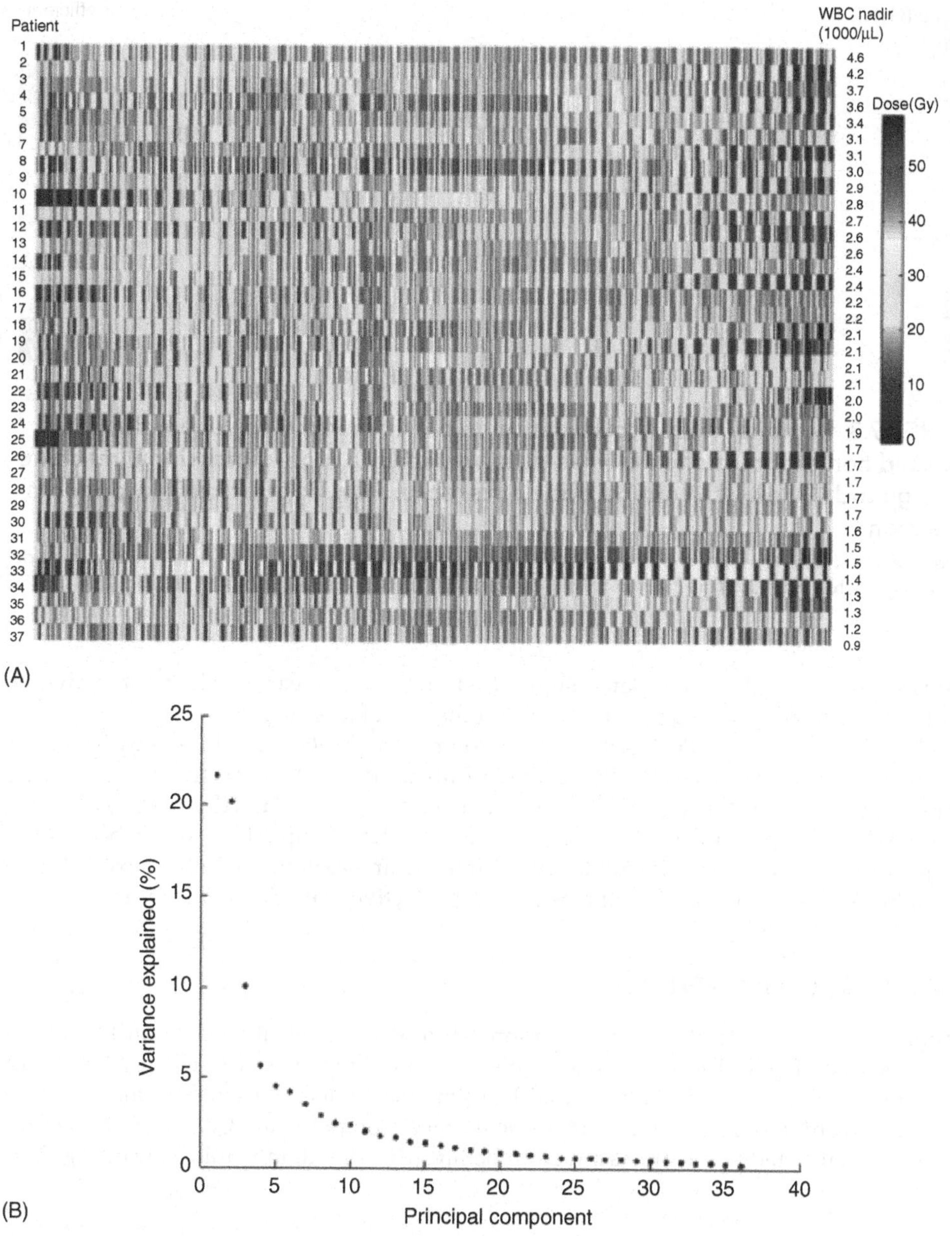

FIGURE 17.2 (A) Heat map of a three-dimensional dose array in patients with pelvic cancers, with rows representing dose vectors for each patient and columns representing corresponding voxels in 3-D space after deformable image registration. The goal is to reduce dimensionality of this set to correlate key (principal) components of its variation that correlate with observed toxicity. (B) Scree plot indicating the percentage of variation in the dose array explained by each principal component.

principal components in decreasing order) that more than half of variation in dose was explained by only three principal components (Figure 17.2B). When toxicity values were regressed on these PCs, the coefficients can be mapped in 3-D space, generating an image of "critical" regions where dose accumulation most highly corresponds to increased toxicity, namely, the ilium and posterior

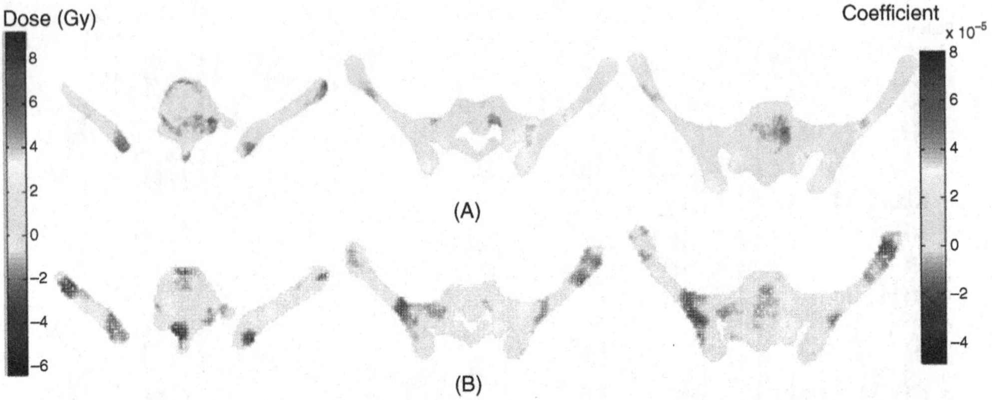

FIGURE 17.3 Regional dose accumulation in pelvic marrow corresponding to increased hematopoietic toxicity, as determined by a high-dimensional machine learning model. Row A: Average dose difference. Row B: principal components regression.

Source: Liang M, Li Z, Chen T, Zeng J. Integrative data analysis of multi-platform cancer data with a multimodal deep learning approach. *IEEE/ACM Trans Comput Biol Bioinform.* 2015;12(4):928–937. doi:10.1109/TCBB.2014.2377729

sacrum (Figure 17.3). Another related supervised method is linear discriminant analysis (LDA); for further information, consult sources listed at the end of this chapter.

A key disadvantage of PCA is its inability to preserve *local* connections between data points. The common theoretical dataset, which remains difficult for PCA to effectively reduce, is a spatial rotation (Figure 17.4). Intuitively, we see that each letter can be explained by a size component and rotation. When we apply PCA, it is difficult to see that relationship. This is partly because the rotation and size of the letter are difficult to reduce into linear components. In the next section, we see that nonlinear dimensionality techniques are more effective at modeling this process.

MANIFOLD LEARNING

Manifold learning is a relatively newer approach to dimensionality reduction for high-dimensional datasets. Manifold learning algorithms are very complex, but in essence can be thought of as nonlinear versions of PCA. Manifold learning allows one to appreciate the connectivity of data points in order to find a lower-dimensional space. Compared to PCA, where the components for dimensionality reduction are assumed to be linearly related, in manifold learning there is no

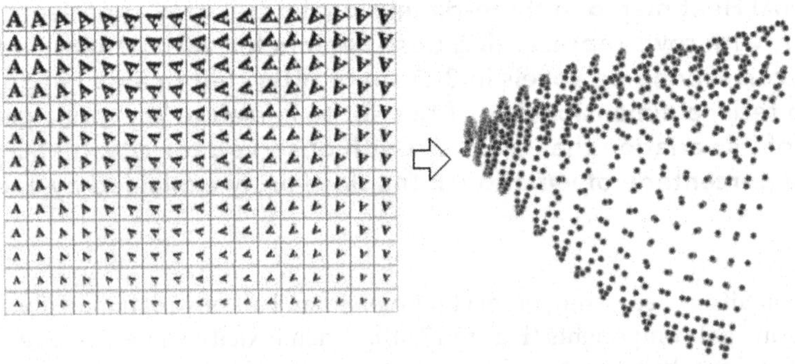

FIGURE 17.4 Principal component analysis applied to a spatial rotation.

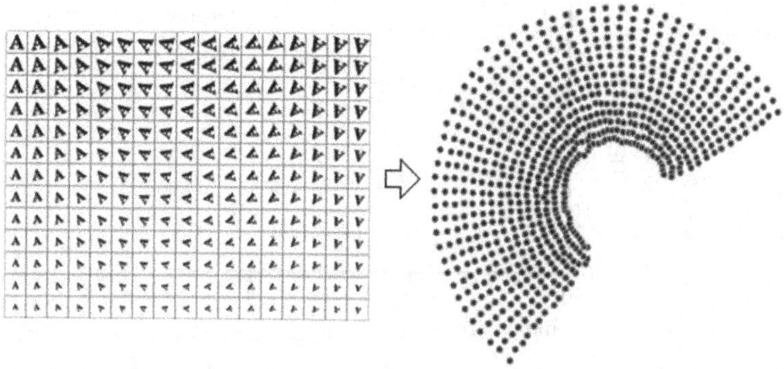

FIGURE 17.5 Nonlinear dimensionality reduction using manifold learning.

assumption about the linearity of components. As we can see in Figure 17.5, manifold learning is better able to represent spatial rotation datasets. Table 17.1 presents studies that have employed PCA and manifold learning for dimensionality reduction.

SUPPORT VECTOR MACHINES

An important machine learning algorithm that is often used in the setting of binary classification problems is the **support vector machine (SVM)**. SVMs are algorithms that find the optimal

TABLE 17.1 STUDIES EMPLOYING MANIFOLD LEARNING AND PCA

Author	Data Type	Method	PMID
Hira et al.	Genetic	Manifold Learning	24595155 (12)
Yang et al.	MR Spectroscopy	Manifold Learning	25199640 (13)
Huang et al.	Genetic	Manifold Learning	22442131 (14)
Park et al.	CT Images	Manifold Learning	25370629 (15)
Lin et al.	CT Images	Manifold Learning	19229098 (16)
Perrier et al.	Health Costs	PCA	25399725 (17)
Sun et al.	Genetic	PCA	26405977 (18)
Ahmadi et al.	Clinical Data	PCA	23035696 (19)
Taguchi et al.	Genetic	PCA	23874370 (20)
Navarro et al.	Survey Data	PCA	21435900 (21)
Liang et al.	Clinical Data	PCA	20472344 (11)

PCA, principal components analysis.

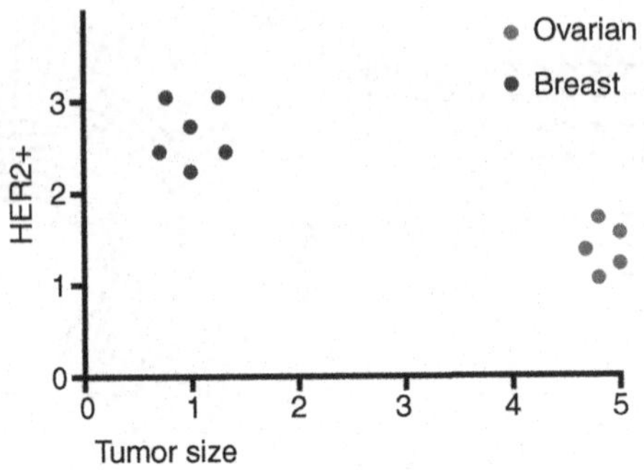

FIGURE 17.6 HER2+ versus tumor size for breast and ovarian cancer patients.

boundary to separate two classes of data. They are useful for high-dimensional data and the boundary created, known as a **hyperplane**, can be essentially of any shape and span multiple dimensions. To better understand how the SVM describes the boundary, we review a simple two-dimensional example describing how an SVM solves a classification task. Imagine we had a set of breast and ovarian cancer samples along with data regarding tumor size and HER2 expression. We hope to build a model that would use size and HER2 expression to predict if the tumor was from a breast cancer or ovarian cancer primary. If we plotted the hypothetical dataset, it might look like Figure 17.6.

Visually, there is a clear boundary between the breast and ovarian cancers. The SVM tests multiply different hyperplanes in order to find the one that effectively separates the two classes of tumors. Figure 17.7 shows that there are multiple possible hyperplanes for which the two classes of tumors are easily separated such that we achieve 100% accurate classification. SVMs attempt to identify the optimal hyperplane such that the hyperplane will be generalizable for any data (1,22).

The optimal hyperplane identified by the SVM is the boundary that maximizes the distance between the points and the hyperplane boundary (known as the *margin*). The margin is calculated for all the points and the hyperplane is chosen in order to maximize the overall margin between the two groups. In our example, the SVM would choose hyperplane B. The optimization of the margin size is part of the reason why the SVM is felt to be particularly robust and generalizable. In our example, we had the ideal dataset for an SVM problem. However, oftentimes, real clinical data are not as simple. Imagine if we had a more complex distribution of data, as seen in Figure 17.8.

One might believe that the SVM would choose hyperplane A as optimal because it maximizes margin. However, because the hyperplane A does not classify the data as well as hyperplane B, the algorithm would choose hyperplane B as optimal. The margin is only used to determine the

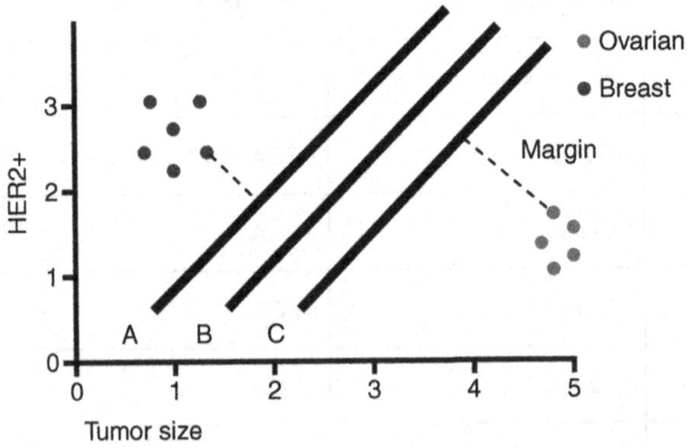

FIGURE 17.7 Possible hyperplanes classifying breast and ovarian cancer patients by HER2+ and tumor size.

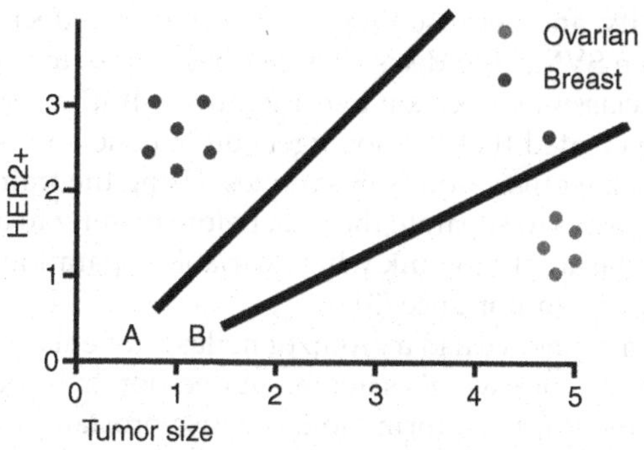

FIGURE 17.8 HER2+ versus tumor size for breast and ovarian cancer patients.

optimal hyperplane among hyperplanes with the highest classification accuracy. This represents one of the drawbacks of machine learning algorithms, namely, overfitting, and provides an example of a different solution if we were to solve this classification problem using a regression technique described in Chapter 16, given it is permitted by the dimensionality.

On a related note, because the SVM optimizes margin, it is less influenced by **outliers** compared to regression techniques. For this reason, SVMs are often preferred to regression for particularly noisy data, which may be inappropriately influenced by outliers (22,23). SVMs have been used in a variety of classification tasks within oncology. They have had particular success in classifying medical imaging and predicting clinical outcomes. Table 17.2 lists studies that have employed SVMs for clinical oncology problems.

DECISION TREES AND RANDOM FOREST MODELS

Another common algorithm used in machine learning is the **decision tree**. Decision trees are among the most popular machine learning algorithms. Decision trees have grown in popularity

TABLE 17.2 STUDIES EMPLOYING SVMs

Author	Data Type	Method	PMID
Hajiloo et al.	Genetic	SVM	24266942 (24)
Larroza et al.	MRI	SVM	25865833 (25)
Upstill-Goddard et al.	Genetic	SVM	23894323 (26)
Klement et al.	Clinical Data	SVM	24411630 (27)
Ni et al.	CBC Data	SVM	23930813 (28)
Hazai et al.	Pathology Slides	SVM	23586520 (29)
Liu	Genetic	SVM	15554662 (23)
Fehr et al.	MRI	SVM	26578786 (30)

SVM, support vector machine.

partly due to their simplicity, and because they have been quite effective when applied correctly to complex datasets. Unlike SVMs, the decision tree does not require a binary outcome and can classify data into multiple classes. A decision tree attempts to find separation within the data such that groups of data can be created that are homogeneous to one another, but have high levels of heterogeneity compared to the other groups of samples. Using the training data, the decision tree attempts to study multiple ways to separate the data before coming to a final solution. One added benefit of decision trees is the ability to rank which variable separations are of higher importance and which are of relatively less importance (31).

To demonstrate, let us assume we had a group of males and females who were diagnosed with prostate cancer, ovarian cancer, or Ewing's sarcoma. A decision tree could be useful in classifying these patients based on demographic information. Because prostate cancer predominantly affects older males and Ewing's sarcoma predominantly affects younger males, a decision tree would likely rely heavily on both age and gender to initially separate the data. The decision tree would also identify an age cutoff that allows the data to most easily separate.

The benefits of a decision tree are the interpretability of the model, the fact that it is considered nonparametric, and that it can analyze multiple types of data. The disadvantage of the decision tree is overfitting of the training data. In our earlier example, the relative importance of gender and age is largely dependent on the sample of patients used to train the decision tree. To mitigate this disadvantage, data scientists often employ a modified version of the decision tree known as a **random forest model**. Compared to a single decision tree, a random forest model is composed of multiple decision trees, each of which is composed of a random subset of all variables. Similarly, each individual tree is built on a random subset of samples within the data such that the configuration of each tree differs from others within the random forest. The ultimate classification for a case is based on a majority vote or the average of all the predictions from the different decision trees. This "voting" technique is also known as an **ensemble technique** (32,33).

Among the most significant benefits of a random forest model is the ability to determine the subset of variables that are of relative importance for a given classification task. This also can be used as a form of dimensionality reduction where the variables that are of the highest importance are used for a statistical regression problem. Despite the benefits of a random forest model, it does still have a tendency to overfit data, which is one of its major disadvantages. Table 17.3 lists studies that have employed decision trees and random forests for clinical oncology problems.

TABLE 17.3 STUDIES EMPLOYING DECISION TREES OR RANDOM FORESTS

Author	Data Type	Method	PMID
Anaissi et al.	Genetic	Random Forest	23981907 (34)
Tsuji et al.	Clinical Data	Random Forest	22095227 (35)
Ospina et al.	Dosimetric	Random Forest	25035205 (36)
Chu et al.	Bone Scans	Random Forest	25333168 (37)
Chen et al.	Clinical Data	Random Forest	26054335 (38)
Tartar et al.	CT Images	Decision Tree	24111444 (39)
Tabakov et al.	Pathology Slides	Decision Tree	24709057 (40)
Abe et al.	Clinical Data	Decision Tree	26374088 (41)

DEEP LEARNING MODELS

In this section, we discuss **deep learning,** one of the most exciting areas of machine learning. Deep learning is a rapidly emerging machine learning technique that has recently gained prominence within healthcare. Deep learning is the basis for many of the innovative technologies that will impact society, including **facial recognition**, self-driving cars, and natural language processing. We previously discussed how machine learning techniques can save us considerable resources and time by limiting our need to curate and structure high-dimensional data. However, imagine if the data were so unstructured that they were beyond human perception, meaning researchers would be unable to curate the data even if given unlimited time and resources. For example, if we were given a dataset of intensities of pixels within an image, it would be impossible for a human to classify the image. Deep learning has emerged as one of the most effective techniques for the analysis of unstructured data (4). Unlike the previously described techniques, deep learning algorithms do not require user-defined variables like age and tumor size to be engineered by researchers and instead can extract features from the most unstructured data sources.

A common application of deep learning is in image analysis. As you remember from Chapter 16, we discussed an example problem of estimating pathologic breast tumor size from mammographic breast tumor size. This problem required us to have a dataset with mammographic tumor size as measured by a trained radiologist. However, supposed we only had the mammogram images from our EHR and were unable to have a radiologist measure the lesions prior to completing our study. Using deep learning, we could still build a model that predicted pathologic tumor size by instead analyzing the raw pixel-level data, obviating the need for any radiologist measurement.

Deep learning algorithms attempt to learn representations of data employing **neural network** architectures, which attempt to mimic the human brain (Figure 17.9). A neural network consists of multiple layers of nodes representing different levels of data abstraction. Each node is connected to the nodes of the previous layer via numerous parameters known as "**weights.**" Traditionally employing a form of supervised learning, training occurs through an iterative process in which the neural network is given training examples and calculates predicted outcomes. The predicted outcomes are compared to the actual outcomes and the weights throughout the neural network are adjusted. As the neural network analyzes more training examples, the weights are optimized to best model the data. In our example, the neural network would analyze pixel-level data and attempt to predict the pathologic tumor size. As more examples were shown to the neural network, the weights connecting the layers of the neural network would be optimized to improve the prediction.

As mentioned earlier, each layer of the network would represent different levels of data abstraction. Intuitively, the initial layers often identify features that are very simple (overall

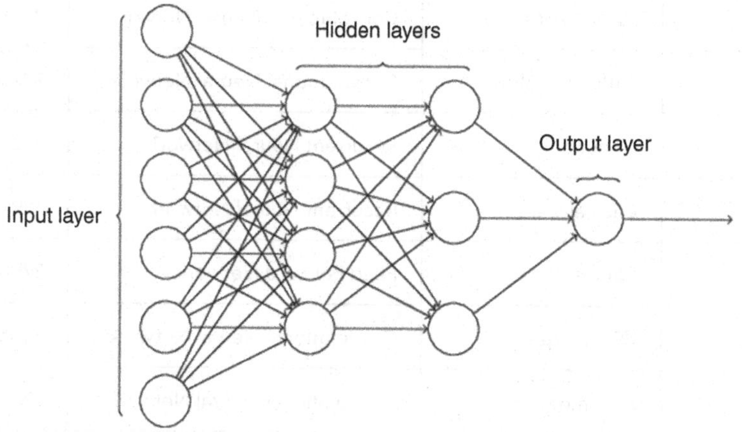

FIGURE 17.9 Example of artificial neural network.

hyper-/hypo-intensity of an image), whereas with the later layers the network would likely learn more nuanced aspects of the image, such as curved borders of the lesion. In reality, deep learning is significantly more complex and each layer may represent features that are increasingly difficult to describe or even see with the naked eye. The benefits of deep learning are the ability to analyze the most unstructured data in healthcare, which in effect allows us to construct potentially end-to-end algorithms that are able to analyze data as they are generated within the clinical setting.

There is significant interest in employing deep learning to power artificially intelligent machines, which can help in diagnosis and treatment within oncology. Another advantage to deep learning techniques is the relative flexibility in analyzing different types of data sources and tailoring neural network architectures for a given data type. Depending on the type of data we wished to analyze, we may employ a different type of neural network. For more information on different types of neural networks, we recommend consulting the additional readings associated with this chapter. The main disadvantage to a deep learning algorithm is the amount of data that is required to produce an accurate algorithm. In addition, a significant amount of computational power is required to effectively train a neural network. Lastly, like all machine learning algorithms, deep learning is subject to overfitting of the training data. Table 17.4 lists studies that have employed deep learning for clinical oncology problems.

UNSUPERVISED LEARNING METHODS

Most of the previous algorithms we have discussed are considered supervised machine learning techniques. Supervised machine learning techniques are those for which we use training data that are labeled with our desired outcome in order to build our machine learning algorithm. However, suppose we were given data for which we did not have a specific outcome and wished instead to understand if there was a natural grouping of the data. Unsupervised machine learning techniques allow us to divide a set of data into a number of groups such that the data in each group possess

TABLE 17.4 STUDIES EMPLOYING DEEP LEARNING

Author	Data Type	Method	PMID
Ertosun et al.	Pathology Slides	Convolutional Neural Network	26958289 (42)
Liang et al.	Genetic	Feed Forward Network	26357333 (43)
Esteva et al.	Skin Lesions	Convolutional Neural Network	28117445 (44)
Ehteshami et al.	Pathology Slides	Convolutional Neural Network	29234806 (45)
Vineetha et al.	Genetic	Recurrent Neural Network	23266630 (46)
Ravdin et al.	Clinical Data	Recurrent Neural Network	1391994 (47)
Peng et al.	Clinical Data	Feed Forward Network	27008710 (48)
Ypsilantis et al.	PET Images	Convolutional Neural Network	26355298 (49)
Samala et al.	Mammogram	Convolutional Neural Network	27908154 (50)

TABLE 17.5 STUDIES EMPLOYING UNSUPERVISED MACHINE LEARNING ALGORITHMS

Author	Data Type	Method	PMID
Nguyen et al.	MRI	K-Means Clustering	24943272 (51)
Oghabian et al.	Genetic	Biclustering	24651574 (52)
Mahata et al.	Genetic	Hierarchical Clustering	20150676 (53)
Landau et al.	Genetic	K-Means Clustering	26466571 (54)
Shen et al.	Genetic	Hierarchical Clustering	18003927 (55)
Huo et al.	Survey Data	Hierarchical Clustering	19704069 (56)

similar traits. The most common unsupervised learning technique is **clustering**. Imagine we had a group of patients for whom we have sequenced their entire genetic makeup. Clustering would allow us to group the patients based on similarities within their genomic sequences. Clustering is useful when one has a large amount of data, but one is unsure about its overall relevance. Often clustering is used as a precursor to isolate a unique group for which to perform additional statistical analysis. In our example, if we found one cluster with similar genetic sequences to all have a particular cancer type, we could then explore further what it is about this cluster that differs from the rest of the population.

One of the most common clustering techniques is **k-means clustering**. The first step to k-means clustering is assigning the potential number of groups into which we wish to divide our data. Each data point within the data set is assigned randomly to one of the k clusters and a centroid of the clusters is computed. After the centroids of the random clusters have been computed, the data points are reassigned to the centroids based on closeness and then the centroids are recalculated. This process of reassigning to clusters and recalculating centroids is carried out for multiple iterations until there are no more improvements to the centroid distance. The disadvantage of k-means clustering is that one must define *a priori* the number of clusters into which one will divide the data. With that said, often researchers attempt different numbers of clusters in order to find a suitable grouping.

Another disadvantage of k-means clustering is reproducibility. Because the data are initially randomly assigned to a cluster, one might find different results if the clustering is repeated. Although k-means clustering is an unsupervised learning task, it can often be completed on labeled data in conjunction with a supervised learning technique. For example, one can create clusters of data and then build a supervised learning model (random forest, SVM, deep learning model) for each individual cluster, which is more personalized to that cluster of data. Table 17.5 lists studies that have employed unsupervised learning for clinical oncology problems.

CONCLUSION

In this chapter, we briefly introduced machine learning techniques employed in clinical oncology research. This chapter is by no means an exhaustive treatment of machine learning, but does cover much of the basic terminology and many of the common techniques. For further reading on specific applications of machine learning algorithms discussed in this chapter and other more complex machine learning algorithms, please refer to the suggested readings (4,7,57).

GLOSSARY

structured data: data that have been curated by researchers per a specific study design within a database for statistical analysis.

machine learning techniques: mathematical techniques that are well suited to analyze high-dimensional, noisy data and can make sense of unstructured high-dimensional datasets.

supervised learning methods: consist of labeled data where variables are paired with a known outcome of interest.

labeled data: examples that a machine learning algorithm can use to build a model.

fitting: creating or manipulating equations, programs, or data for use in modeling.

overfitting: manipulation of a model to accommodate the data used to create the algorithm that ends up identifying spurious relationships between model inputs and the outcome.

"black box" problem: fact that the lack of interpretability limits the utility of machine learning algorithms to addressing specific drivers of a given outcome.

training data: primary data source for developing a machine learning algorithm.

test data: a dataset used to compare different algorithm configurations during the development process of a machine learning algorithm.

validation data: a blinded dataset used only when a machine learning algorithm has been finalized.

confusion matrix: a construct that allows one to quickly identify the specificity, sensitivity, positive predictive value, and negative predictive value of a machine learning algorithm.

receiver operating characteristic (ROC) curve: a tool that assesses the relative sensitivity and specificity of a particular algorithm.

area under the curve (AUC): a common metric (derived from the receiver operating characteristic curve) to evaluate the discriminatory ability of a possible machine learning algorithm.

dimensionality reduction techniques: methods that aim to reduce the number of variables necessary to analyze an outcome without compromising the overall integrity of the data and the underlying relationships that potentially exist.

t-Distributed Stochastic Neighbor Embedding (t-SNE): technique that allows for the visualization of high-dimensional data using dimensionality reduction.

principal component analysis (PCA): a common dimensionality reduction technique.

scree plot: graph that displays the principal components in decreasing order.

support vector machine (SVM): algorithm that finds the optimal boundary to separate two classes of data; useful for high-dimensional data.

hyperplane: the boundary created by a support vector machine.

outliers: a data point that diverges significantly from the overall data pattern.

decision tree: a popular machine learning algorithm that does not require a binary outcome and can classify data into multiple classes.

random forest model: an algorithm composed of multiple decision trees, each of which is composed of a random subset of all variables; each individual tree is built on a random subset of samples within the data such that the configuration of each tree differs from others within the random forest.

ensemble technique: A "voting" technique in which the ultimate classification for a case is based on a majority vote or the average of all the predictions from the different decision trees in a random forest model.

deep learning: a subset of machine learning that develops networks capable of learning from unsupervised data that is unstructured or unlabeled.

neural network: deep learning algorithm that attempts to learn representations of data employing architectures that attempt to mimic the human brain.

weights: parameters governing the connection of nodes in a neural network.

clustering: a common unsupervised learning technique useful when one has a large amount of data, but is unsure about its overall relevance.

k-means clustering: a common clustering technique in which one must define a priori the number of clusters into which to divide the data.

REFERENCES

1. Marsland S. *Machine Learning : An Algorithmic Perspective.* 2nd ed. Boca Raton, FL: CRC Press; 2015:437.
2. Cleophas TJ, Zwinderman AH. *Machine Learning in Medicine—a Complete Overview.* New York, NY: Springer Berlin Heidelberg; 2015.
3. Cleophas TJ. *Machine Learning in Medicine.* New York, NY: Springer; 2013.
4. Goodfellow I, Bengio Y, Courville A. *Deep Learning.* Cambridge, MA: The MIT Press; 2016:775.
5. Buyya R, Calheiros RN, Dastjerdi AV. *Big Data : Principles and Paradigms.* Cambridge, MA: Elsevier/Morgan Kaufmann; 2016:468.
6. Ranganath R, Gerrish S, Blei D. *Black Box Variational Inference: Artificial Intelligence and Statistics.* Princeton, NJ: Princeton University; 2014.
7. Cleophas TJ, Zwinderman AH. *Machine Learning In Medicine—Cookbook.* New York, NY: Springer; 2013.
8. Spiliopoulou M, Schmidt-Thieme L, Janning R, eds. *Data Analysis, Machine Learning and Knowledge Discovery.* New York, NY: Springer Berlin Heidelberg; 2013.
9. Van Der Maaten L, Hinton G. Visualizing high-dimensional data using t-sne. *J Mach Learn Res.* 2008;9:26.
10. Abdi H, Williams LJ. Principal component analysis. *Wiley Interdiscip Rev Comput Stat.* 2010;2(4):433–459. doi:10.1002/wics.101
11. Liang Y, Messer K, Rose BS, et al. Impact of bone marrow radiation dose on acute hematologic toxicity in cervical cancer: principal component analysis on high dimensional data. *Int J Radiat Oncol Biol Phys.* 2010;78(3):912–919. doi:10.1016/j.ijrobp.2009.11.062
12. Hira ZM, Trigeorgis G, Gillies DF. An algorithm for finding biologically significant features in microarray data based on *a priori* manifold learning. *PLoS One.* 2014;9(3):e90562. doi:10.1371/journal.pone.0090562
13. Yang G, Raschke F, Barrick TR, Howe FA. Manifold learning in MR spectroscopy using nonlinear dimensionality reduction and unsupervised clustering. *Magn Reson Med.* 2015;74(3):868–878. doi:10.1002/mrm.25447
14. Huang H, Feng H. Gene classification using parameter-free semi-supervised manifold learning. *IEEE/ACM Trans Comput Biol Bioinform.* 2012;9(3):818–827. doi:10.1109/tcbb.2011.152
15. Park SH, Gao Y, Shi Y, Shen D. Interactive prostate segmentation using atlas-guided semi-supervised learning and adaptive feature selection. *Med Phys.* 2014;41(11):111715. doi:10.1118/1.4898200
16. Lin T, Li R, Tang X, et al. Markerless gating for lung cancer radiotherapy based on machine learning techniques. *Phys Med Biol.* 2009;54(6):1555–1563. doi:10.1088/0031-9155/54/6/010
17. Perrier L, Buja A, Mastrangelo G, et al. Transferability of health cost evaluation across locations in oncology: cluster and principal component analysis as an explorative tool. *BMC Health Serv Res.* 2014;14:537. doi:10.1186/s12913-014-0537-x
18. Sun L, Xu J, Yin Y. Principal component-based feature selection for tumor classification. *Biomed Mater Eng.* 2015;26(Suppl 1):S2011–S2017. doi:10.3233/BME-151505
19. Ahmadi H, Mitra AP, Abdelsayed GA, et al. Principal component analysis based pre-cystectomy model to predict pathological stage in patients with clinical organ-confined bladder cancer. *BJU Int.* 2013;111(4 Pt B):E167–E172. doi:10.1111/j.1464-410x.2012.11502.x
20. Taguchi YH, Murakami Y. Principal component analysis based feature extraction approach to identify circulating microRNA biomarkers. *PLoS One.* 2013;8(6):e66714. doi:10.1371/journal.pone.0066714

21. Navarro Silvera SA, Mayne ST, Risch HA, et al. Principal component analysis of dietary and lifestyle patterns in relation to risk of subtypes of esophageal and gastric cancer. *Ann Epidemiol.* 2011;21(7):543–550. doi:10.1016/j.annepidem.2010.11.019
22. Adankon MM, Cheriet M. Support vector machine. In: *Encyclopedia of Biometrics*. New York, NY: Springer; 2009; 1303–1308. doi:10.1007/978-0-387-73003-5_299
23. Liu Y. Active learning with support vector machine applied to gene expression data for cancer classification. *J Chem Inf Comput Sci.* 2004;44(6):1936–1941. doi:10.1021/ci049810a
24. Hajiloo M, Rabiee HR, Anooshahpour M. Fuzzy support vector machine: an efficient rule-based classification technique for microarrays. *BMC Bioinformatics.* 2013;14(Suppl 13):S4. doi:10.1186/1471-2105-14-S13-S4
25. Larroza A, Moratal D, Paredes-Sanchez A, et al. Support vector machine classification of brain metastasis and radiation necrosis based on texture analysis in MRI. *J Magn Reson Imaging.* 2015;42(5):1362–1368. doi:10.1002/jmri.24913
26. Upstill-Goddard R, Eccles D, Ennis S, et al. Support vector machine classifier for estrogen receptor positive and negative early-onset breast cancer. *PLoS One.* 2013;8(7):e68606. doi:10.1371/journal.pone.0068606
27. Klement RJ, Allgauer M, Appold S, et al. Support vector machine-based prediction of local tumor control after stereotactic body radiation therapy for early-stage non-small cell lung cancer. *Int J Radiat Oncol Biol Phys.* 2014;88(3):732–738. doi:10.1016/j.ijrobp.2013.11.216
28. Ni W, Tong X, Qian W, et al. Discrimination of malignant neutrophils of chronic myelogenous leukemia from normal neutrophils by support vector machine. *Comput Biol Med.* 2013;43(9):1192–1195. doi:10.1016/j.compbiomed.2013.06.004
29. Hazai E, Hazai I, Ragueneau-Majlessi I, et al. Predicting substrates of the human breast cancer resistance protein using a support vector machine method. *BMC Bioinformatics.* 2013;14:130. doi:10.1186/1471-2105-14-130
30. Fehr D, Veeraraghavan H, Wibmer A, et al. Automatic classification of prostate cancer Gleason scores from multiparametric magnetic resonance images. *Proc Natl Acad Sci U S A.* 2015;112(46):E6265–E6273. doi:10.1073/pnas.1505935112
31. Magerman DM. Statistical decision-tree models for parsing. Proceedings of the 33rd annual meeting on Association for Computational Linguistics, 1995; Association for Computational Linguistics.
32. Liaw A, Wiener M. Classification and regression by randomForest. *R news.* 2002;2(3):18–22.
33. Reddy D, Lingras P, Kuppili V, eds. *Advances in Machine Learning and Data Science.* New York, NY: Springer Berlin Heidelberg; 2018.
34. Anaissi A, Kennedy PJ, Goyal M, Catchpoole DR. A balanced iterative random forest for gene selection from microarray data. *BMC Bioinformatics.* 2013;14:261. doi:10.1186/1471-2105-14-261
35. Tsuji S, Midorikawa Y, Takahashi T, et al. Potential responders to FOLFOX therapy for colorectal cancer by random forests analysis. *Br J Cancer.* 2012;106(1):126–132. doi:10.1038/bjc.2011.505
36. Ospina JD, Zhu J, Chira C, et al. Random forests to predict rectal toxicity following prostate cancer radiation therapy. *Int J Radiat Oncol Biol Phys.* 2014;89(5):1024–1031. doi:10.1016/j.ijrobp.2014.04.027
37. Chu G, Lo P, Ramakrishna B, et al. Bone tumor segmentation on bone scans using context information and random forests. *Med Image Comput Comput Assist Interv.* 2014;17(Pt 1):601–608. doi:10.1007/978-3-319-10404-1_75
38. Chen Y, Cao W, Gao X, et al. Predicting postoperative complications of head and neck squamous cell carcinoma in elderly patients using random forest algorithm model. *BMC Med Inform Decis Mak.* 2015;15:44. doi:10.1186/s12911-015-0165-3
39. Tartar A, Kilic N, Akan A. A new method for pulmonary nodule detection using decision trees. *Conf Proc IEEE Eng Med Biol Soc.* 2013;2013:7355–7359. doi:10.1109/embc.2013.6611257
40. Tabakov M, Kozak P. Segmentation of histopathology HER2/neu images with fuzzy decision tree and Takagi-Sugeno reasoning. *Comput Biol Med.* 2014;49:19–29. doi:10.1016/j.compbiomed.2014.03.001
41. Abe SE, Hill JS, Han Y, et al. Margin re-excision and local recurrence in invasive breast cancer: a cost analysis using a decision tree model. *J Surg Oncol.* 2015;112(4):443–448. doi:10.1002/jso.23990
42. Ertosun MG, Rubin DL. Automated grading of gliomas using deep learning in digital pathology images: a modular approach with ensemble of convolutional neural networks. *AMIA Annu Symp Proc.* 2015;2015:1899–1908.
43. Liang M, Li Z, Chen T, Zeng J. Integrative data analysis of multi-platform cancer data with a multimodal deep learning approach. *IEEE/ACM Trans Comput Biol Bioinform.* 2015;12(4):928–937. doi:10.1109/TCBB.2014.2377729
44. Esteva A, Kuprel B, Novoa RA, et al. Dermatologist-level classification of skin cancer with deep neural networks. *Nature.* 2017;542(7639):115–118. doi:10.1038/nature21056
45. Ehteshami Bejnordi B, Veta M, Johannes van Diest P, et al. Diagnostic assessment of deep learning algorithms for detection of lymph node metastases in women with breast cancer. *JAMA.* 2017;318(22):2199–2210. doi:10.1001/jama.2017.14585
46. Vineetha S, Chandra Shekara Bhat C, Idicula SM. MicroRNA-mRNA interaction network using TSK-type recurrent neural fuzzy network. *Gene.* 2013;515(2):385–390. doi:10.1016/j.gene.2012.12.063
47. Ravdin PM, Clark GM. A practical application of neural network analysis for predicting outcome of individual breast cancer patients. *Breast Cancer Res Treat.* 1992;22(3):285–293. doi:10.1007/BF01840841
48. Peng JH, Fang YJ, Li CX, et al. A scoring system based on artificial neural network for predicting 10-year survival in stage II A colon cancer patients after radical surgery. *Oncotarget.* 2016;7(16):22939–22947. doi:10.18632/oncotarget.8217
49. Ypsilantis PP, Siddique M, Sohn HM, et al. Predicting response to neoadjuvant chemotherapy with pet imaging using convolutional neural networks. *PLoS One.* 2015;10(9):e0137036. doi:10.1371/journal.pone.0137036
50. Samala RK, Chan HP, Hadjiiski L, et al. Mass detection in digital breast tomosynthesis: deep convolutional neural network with transfer learning from mammography. *Med Phys.* 2016;43(12):6654. doi:10.1118/1.4967345
51. Nguyen HT, Jia G, Shah ZK, et al. Prediction of chemotherapeutic response in bladder cancer using K-means clustering of dynamic contrast-enhanced (DCE)-MRI pharmacokinetic parameters. *J Magn Reson Imaging.* 2015;41:1374–1382. doi:10.1002/jmri.24663
52. Oghabian A, Kilpinen S, Hautaniemi S, Czeizler E. Biclustering methods: biological relevance and application in gene expression analysis. *PLoS One.* 2014;9(3):e90801. doi:10.1371/journal.pone.0090801
53. Mahata P. Exploratory consensus of hierarchical clusterings for melanoma and breast cancer. *IEEE/ACM Trans Comput Biol Bioinform.* 2010;7(1):138–152. doi:10.1109/tcbb.2008.33

54. Landau DA, Tausch E, Taylor-Weiner AN, et al. Mutations driving CLL and their evolution in progression and relapse. *Nature*. 2015;526(7574):525–530. doi:10.1038/nature15395
55. Shen L, Toyota M, Kondo Y, et al. Integrated genetic and epigenetic analysis identifies three different subclasses of colon cancer. *Proc Natl Acad Sci U S A*. 2007;104(47):18654–18659. doi:10.1073/pnas.0704652104
56. Huo D, Ikpatt F, Khramtsov A, et al. Population differences in breast cancer: survey in indigenous African women reveals over-representation of triple-negative breast cancer. *J Clin Oncol*. 2009;27(27):4515–4521. doi:10.1200/JCO.2008.19.6873
57. Cleophas TJM, Zwinderman AH. *Machine Learning in Medicine*. New York, NY: Springer; 2013; vol 3.

18

Health Outcomes and Disparities Research

PAIGE SHERIDAN ■ JAMES MURPHY

Health outcomes research represents research that focuses on studying the impact of healthcare delivery on real-world patient outcomes. In general, this branch of research focuses on safety, efficacy, and health equity while striving to improve the quality and value of healthcare for patients. Given the complexities of delivering healthcare in the real world, this area of research often engages researchers from multiple disciplines, including clinicians, epidemiologists, biostatisticians, psychologists, and sociologists, as well as experts in health economics, health policy, and law. Furthermore, the field of health services research will often employ both qualitative and quantitative research methodology depending on the question at hand. The field of health outcomes research brings a broad array of research methodologies together with the singular focus of studying real-world patient outcomes.

This chapter provides an overview of the fundamental concepts behind health outcomes research. We begin by providing an overview of health outcomes research, then describe the types of data and study designs unique to this type of research. Finally, we provide general examples of common research questions and limitations within health outcomes research. This chapter introduces concepts developed further in future chapters in this book.

OVERVIEW OF HEALTH OUTCOMES RESEARCH

Health outcomes research stands apart from the more conventional field of biomedical research (Figure 18.1). In general, biomedical research encompasses basic science research as well as conventional clinical research, whereas health outcomes research focuses on the real-world implementation of clinical research or healthcare delivery outside the context of a clinical trial. Clinical trials represent the gold standard approach to defining efficacy in healthcare; however, clinical trials have limitations that impair their direct translation into effective real-world clinical practice. Health outcomes research, if done well, can help fill important knowledge gaps in conventional clinical research.

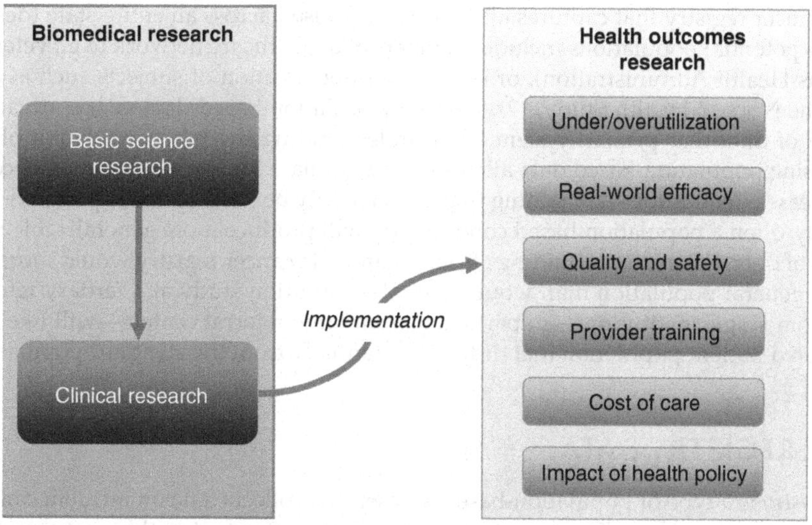

FIGURE 18.1 Relationship between biomedical research and health outcomes research.

In addressing the real-world application of healthcare delivery, the field of health outcomes research tackles an array of different endpoints. While conventional clinical research focuses largely on the individual patient, health outcomes research will often consider outcomes from a variety of stakeholders: the patient, the patient's family members or caregivers, the clinic, hospital, healthcare system, payer, and society.

The endpoints measured in health outcomes research will depend on the stakeholder of interest. Patient-related endpoints can include disease-related symptoms, toxicities, quality of life, and survival. For example, health outcomes research might evaluate the long-term risks of pelvic radiation therapy among Medicare beneficiaries with cancer (1). Examples of caregiver endpoints include the number of hours spent and corresponding wages lost for taking care of a loved one. Hospital endpoints can include systemwide quality metrics such as survival rates after surgery, in-hospital complication rates, and patient satisfaction scores. Example endpoints from a societal perspective include measures of the population-level burden of disease, or measures of national healthcare expenditure. Considering the societal perspective allows researchers to address broad questions that often verge on the subject of public health given the scope of the research question.

TYPES OF DATA USED IN HEALTH OUTCOMES RESEARCH

The types of data commonly used in oncology health outcomes research have unique characteristics that warrant further discussion. Health outcomes research can involve primary or secondary data. **Primary datasets** include data collected specifically for research purposes, whereas **secondary datasets** refer to data collected for reasons other than research. **Cancer registry data** represent an example of primary data because these data were collected intentionally for research purposes. Insurance claims data represent an example of secondary data because, though commonly used for research, they were initially collected for billing purposes. Both primary and secondary datasets are commonly used in health outcomes research, and both datasets have positive and negative features. Detailed examples of different types of data used in health outcomes research are provided subsequently.

POPULATION-BASED DATASETS

Population-based data refers to a group of patients under study in a well-defined population. The definition of a population varies, but often will refer to a geographically defined region such as a statewide cancer registry that captures all cancers diagnosed across an entire state (described further). Other potential populations include members of a healthcare network (e.g., veterans within the Veterans Health Administration), or some other demarcation of subjects such as by occupation (e.g., the Nurses' Health Study) (2). Using a population-based dataset has advantages over other types of data that primarily stem from understanding the base population of study. For example, using population-based data allows one to estimate the incidence, prevalence, and mortality of diseases in question—something that cannot easily be done in nonpopulation-based data. Additionally, often a population-based cohort study will produce more generalizable results than other types of data. For example, findings from a statewide cancer registry would more likely generalize to a general population than would a single-institution study at a tertiary referral center. Research from single institutions—in particular from large referral centers—will likely include a highly selected patient population that differs substantially from the standard population.

CANCER REGISTRY DATA

A *cancer registry* is a type of population-based dataset that collects data on incident cancer cases in a defined geographic region. These datasets are critically important within cancer epidemiology when estimating trends in the national cancer burden, though these datasets also play a large role in health outcomes research given the real-world nature of the data they collect.

Within the United States, individual cancer registries are primarily run at the state level. The National Cancer Institute (NCI) oversees a collection of individual state and regional cancer registries within the **Surveillance, Epidemiology, and End Results (SEER) program**. The SEER program started in 1973, and it has grown to include registries that cover 28% of the U.S. population. Data within cancer registries come from cancer *registrars* who are individuals specially trained to collect data on incident cancer cases. The data collected include basic demographic information, workup details, staging, tumor histology, treatment delivered, and cause-specific survival data. A similar program run by the Centers for Disease Control and Prevention (CDC), called the **National Program of Cancer Registries (NPCR),** includes cancer registries for non-SEER states, and together the NPCR and SEER cover the entire United States.

Aside from state-run cancer registries, another registry worth mentioning is the **National Cancer Database (NCDB)**. The NCDB is jointly sponsored by the American College of Surgeons and the American Cancer Society. NCDB differs from SEER in that incident cancer cases are collected from hospitals or treatment facilities accredited by the American College of Surgeons Commission on Cancer. NCDB collects data on more than 70% of incident cancer cases, and has important distinctions from SEER. For example, NCDB collects more detailed treatment information with respect to details of chemotherapy and radiation, but does not include cause-specific survival. NCDB data are generally considered insufficient to calculate incidence, prevalence, and mortality rates because the catchment area is hospital based as opposed to geographically based like SEER. Overall, NCDB and SEER complement each other, and the research question of interest and data required will ideally drive the choice of whether to use NCDB or SEER.

CLAIMS DATA

Insurance claims data are used for billing purposes, though claims indirectly collect information about a patient's medical history, which make them attractive for use in health outcomes research. Each time a patient touches the healthcare system in an outpatient setting, emergency department, or in a hospital, a billing claim is generated. Billing claims contain information about diagnoses and procedures performed, which are captured in ICD-9/10 codes, HCPCS codes, and BETOS codes. Along with information about diagnoses and procedures, billing claims incorporate data about the provider and hospital, as well as reimbursement information. Together, these claims allow one to indirectly follow the patient's medical course longitudinally over time. Claims data represent a valuable resource for research, and stand-alone claims databases used in cancer research include public datasets from Medicare and Medicaid, and commercial data such as **MarketScan**, which contains pooled private and public insurance claims data.

In addition to these stand-alone claims databases, researchers often use claims data linked to cancer registry data, such as **SEER-Medicare linked data**. These linked datasets can be useful with certain research questions because of the complementary nature of these datasets. Claims data often contain comorbidity data, or long-term patient outcome data missing in cancer registry data. Registry data often contain information missing in claims data such as direct information about tumor stage and histology.

Despite the attractive nature of using claims in research, these data do have limitations worth mentioning. Claims are collected for billing purposes; therefore, errors in billing could lead to **misclassification**. In general, both providers and payers have incentives to bill accurately, though the possibility of misclassification remains. Another limitation relates to the issue of underreporting. For example, diagnoses of serious conditions (e.g., myocardial infarction) are more likely to be accurately documented and reported in claims data, whereas minor conditions (e.g., mild radiation dermatitis) are more likely to be underreported. Finally, the question of data integrity is often difficult to assess in claims data. Most research datasets come in a deidentified form and do not include actual medical records; therefore, validating individual claims by referencing against a medical record may not be possible.

ELECTRONIC HEALTH RECORD DATA

The increased adoption of **electronic health record (EHR)** systems provides exciting opportunities for research. EHR data can come from individual clinics, single institutions, or large health-care networks (e.g., Kaiser-Permanente). A simple retrospective cohort study done by manually reviewing electronic medical records would be considered an example of EHR research; in this section of the chapter, however, we focus on research with larger datasets for which manual chart review would not be considered feasible.

When working with large amounts of EHR data for research purposes, one must consider the logistics of data processing, which can be formidable. First, extracting data for multiple patients from a single system is often not straightforward, given the confidentiality and security protections built into most EHR systems. Second, the data extracted will often require substantial post-processing to allow analysis.

From a research perspective, data within an EHR comes in both structured and unstructured formats. **Structured data** refers to data within an EHR organized in such a format that it can be extracted and used easily for research purposes. For example, laboratory data such as serum potassium levels often come in a standardized format or table that allows relatively easy extraction. Depending on the interface with the EHR, one could automatically extract thousands or hundreds of thousands of potassium measurements and use these data for research purposes. **Unstructured data** refers to data within an EHR buried in an unorganized format such as a clinical note. For example, a researcher interested in surgical margin status would need to find these data within the free text of a pathology note or a clinic note. Extracting margin status for thousands of patients might not be feasible manually; therefore, one may have to devise a strategy to automate the process.

Extracting surgical margin status from unstructured medical text notes could require, for example, a text mining approach. The goal of **text mining** is to devise an algorithm that will search through text notes, find margin status, and transfer this information into a structured data element. Often this sort of study will draw from methods within the domain of **natural language processing**, which stems from the intersection of computer science and linguistics. In selected cases, teasing out margin status from notes could be quite difficult.

Table 18.1 shows an example of hypothetical text in a pathology report, and the ideal structured data element returned by a text mining approach. Text mining approaches require validation in a gold-standard dataset, where one measures the accuracy of the automated algorithm against known outcomes. For example, a natural language processing approach with prostate cancer margin status can accurately ascertain margin status in 97% of cases (3).

TABLE 18.1 EXAMPLE OF HOW SURGICAL MARGIN STATUS COULD BE REPORTED IN A SERIES OF UNSTRUCTURED PATHOLOGY REPORTS

Text Note	Text Mining (Ideally) Would Return the Following Value for Surgical Margin Status
. . .in assessing **margin** status it appears all surgical **margins** were **not involved** with tumor, but the posterior inked margin was **close** (1 mm). . .	Close
. . .**margins negative**. . .	Negative
. . .after dissection we found the surgical **margins** to be grossly **positive**. . .	Positive
. . .the surgical specimen as sent to pathology was difficult to assess, therefore we are **not clear** about the surgical **margin** status. . .	Not assessable
. . .the **margins** on the right anterolateral and left posterolateral aspects of the tumor were **not positive**, but the tumor came **within 2 mm** of ink. . .	Close

Extracting data from an EHR requires careful **validation**, and one must also consider questions about the validity of the data itself. A substantial portion of EHR data is entered by healthcare providers including medical assistants, nurses, residents, and physicians. The quality of the data extracted from an EHR is only as good as what is entered into the EHR. Issues such as misclassification and **underreporting** must be considered (4), though despite these concerns we will likely continue to see increased use of EHR data in research in the future.

HEALTH OUTCOMES RESEARCH STUDY DESIGNS

Health outcomes research utilizes study designs that come from classic research within the fields of epidemiology and other areas within clinical research. This section discusses several study designs specifically applicable to health outcomes research. The more general topic of study designs is covered in Chapter 10.

OBSERVATIONAL RESEARCH

Given the focus on real-world patient outcomes, the field of health outcomes research often relies on observational study designs. The classic observational study designs defined in Table 18.2 are frequently used in health outcomes research. In the following paragraphs, we illustrate different types of study designs with an example question that seeks to understand how insurance coverage affects outcomes among breast cancer patients.

A **cohort study** follows a disease-free group of patients over time and counts incident cases of disease in exposed and nonexposed groups. For example, researchers could follow individuals with differing levels of insurance coverage (e.g., uninsured, Medicaid, private insurance, or Medicare) and analyze the occurrence of breast cancer diagnoses over time. A cohort study would allow one to determine whether uninsured patients have an increased risk of developing breast cancer, whether they receive the same treatment, or whether they have the same long-term outcomes as their insured counterparts.

TABLE 18.2 OBSERVATIONAL STUDY DESIGNS IN HEALTH OUTCOMES RESEARCH

Study Design	Definition	Optimal For	Example
Cohort Study	Patients in different groups are followed from a fixed time point, comparing the occurrence of events over time.	Assessing differences in common events that develop rapidly over a short period of time.	Comparing breast cancer incidence rates for uninsured vs. insured patients.
Case–Control Study	Patients with different event occurrences are compared retrospectively for group assignment.	Assessing differences in rare events that develop slowly over a long period of time.	Estimating the odds of neuroblastoma diagnosis in uninsured vs. insured children.
Cross-Sectional Study	Patients in different groups are assessed for an event at a fixed time point or period.	Assessing differences in events when risk groups are not changing significantly over time.	Comparing the compliance with cancer screening in U.S. vs. Canadian adults for a specific time period.

A **case–control study** (see also Chapters 10 and 13) selects diseased (cases) and nondiseased (controls) groups and determines their respective exposure status. For example, researchers could analyze a group of children diagnosed with neuroblastoma and compare their insurance coverage rates to a group of cancer-free controls. Case–control studies often include some form of **matching algorithm**, whereby researchers "match" patients based on key characteristics such as race, age, geography, or other potentially modifying factors in order to make groups more comparable with respect to all factors besides the exposure of interest. The matching strategy and ratio of cases to controls (1:1, 1:2, etc.) is a function of both feasibility and sample size requirements for statistical analysis. In general, a case–control study will include substantially fewer patients than a conventional cohort study. This can be an advantage in situations where resources are limited or when the outcome of interest is relatively rare.

Finally, a **cross-sectional study** looks at a group of patients at a single, fixed time period. For example, a researcher could analyze a group of individuals from different countries at the same time to determine the prevalence of compliance with cancer screening recommendations. Cross-sectional studies often focus on large populations of patients, and by doing so can estimate prevalence of different outcomes of interest. A cross-sectional study could estimate the prevalence of uninsured breast cancer survivors in order to determine the magnitude of resources needed to better care for this at-risk population. Cross-sectional study designs offer advantages in terms of breadth over other study designs, though they focus on a single point in time that may limit the types of analytic questions that can be asked.

INTERVENTION STUDIES

Health outcomes research strives to study real-world healthcare outcomes and, in doing so, will often study different healthcare interventions. Within conventional clinical research, the term **intervention** most often refers to a treatment, surgery, procedure, or other management strategy that directly involves the *individual* patient. Health outcomes research uses a broader definition of the term, which could refer to factors outside of the individual patient. With health outcomes research, an *intervention* could refer to any of the patient-directed interventions with clinical research, but could also include interventions directed at the clinic, hospital, healthcare

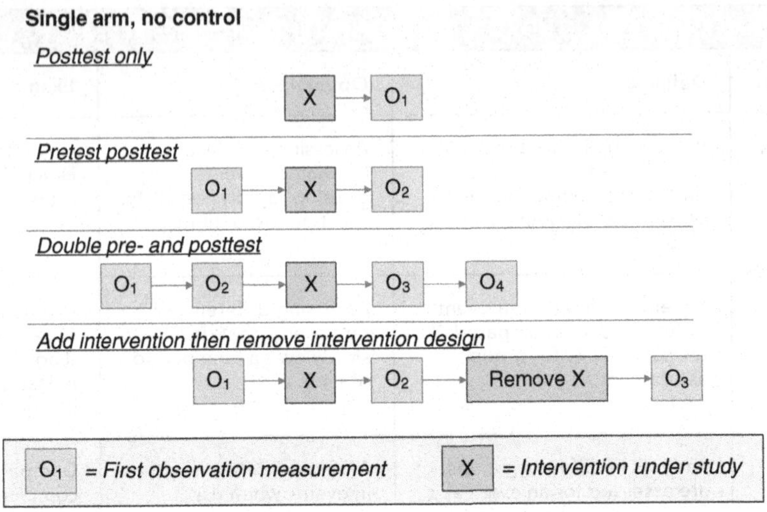

FIGURE 18.2 Single-arm quasi-experimental study designs.

system, or government. While cancer-directed treatment represents a central theme, other potential interventions could include a clinical education tool for patients, a novel training approach for practicing physicians, an institution cost-reduction strategy, or a national healthcare coverage policy change.

When considering intervention study designs, one can roughly classify studies as either **randomized** or **nonrandomized**. *Randomization* refers to the gold-standard study design in which the random allocation of treatment or exposure is among a group of participants. The term *quasi-experimental* is sometimes used to describe nonrandomized study designs in fields such as public health, social sciences, and other related fields. **Quasi-experimental studies** are undertaken to determine the impact of an intervention on a population when randomization is not feasible. Many different quasi-experimental study designs exist, including single-arm studies with no control group (Figure 18.2), controlled studies (Figure 18.3), and interrupted time series (Figure 18.4).

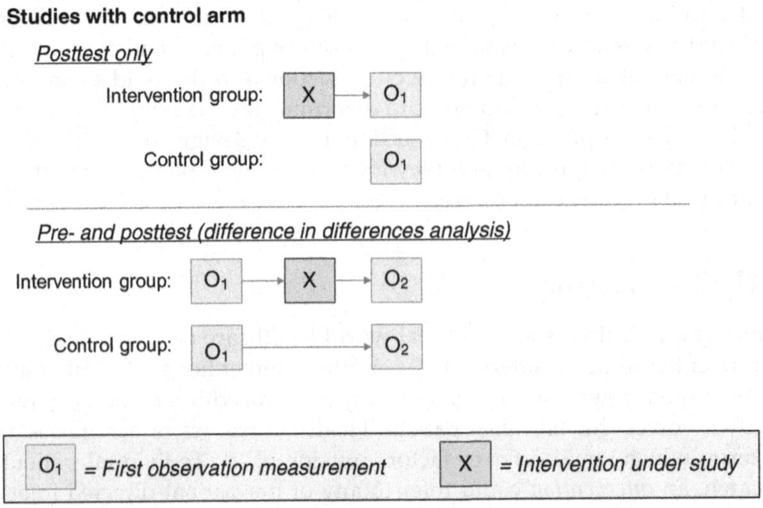

FIGURE 18.3 Controlled quasi-experimental study designs.

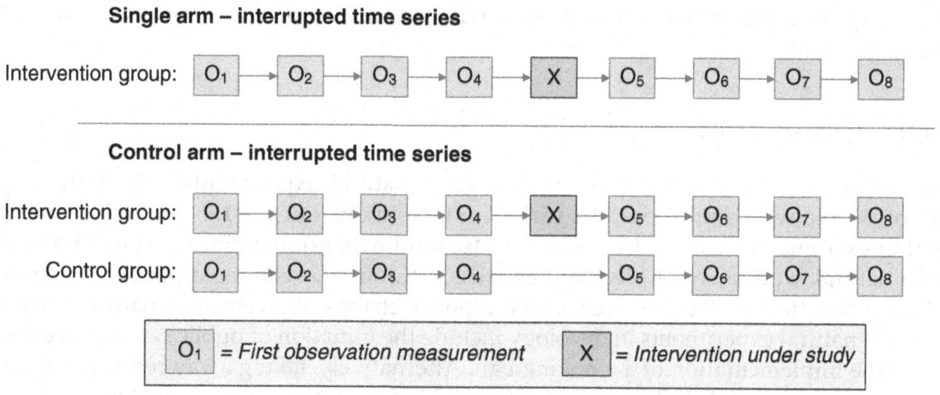

FIGURE 18.4 Interrupted time series quasi-experimental study designs.

For example, suppose a researcher wished to test the hypothesis that Medicaid expansion with the Affordable Care Act would decrease the frequency of late-stage breast cancer diagnoses. The researchers plan to study the distribution of breast cancer stage at diagnosis using state cancer registry data. With this goal in mind, the investigator could use a single-arm **pretest/posttest** study design (Figure 18.2) that would measure the incidence of late-stage breast cancer before and after a state-expanded Medicaid. An **interrupted time series study design** (Figure 18.4) would study the trends in incidence annually both before and after implementation of Medicaid expansion.

However, one must consider potential sources of bias in single-arm studies without a control arm. In this example, if one were to find a decrease in late-stage breast cancer incidence with Medicaid expansion, one would need to consider other potential explanations that could confound these results. For example, if Medicaid expansion occurred concurrently with advances in cancer screening, a decrease in late-stage breast cancer might reflect improved screening as opposed to expanded Medicaid coverage.

Single-arm studies suffer from limitations that can be partially reduced by using controls. Studies that use control groups (Figure 18.3), or multiple measurement or observations (Figure 18.4), generally have more robust results. There are several controlling methods one can use in such settings, including cohort controls, intervention controls, and outcome controls.. A **cohort control** compares results across different cohorts, which ensures that the effect of the intervention and the outcome are specific to the group of interest. For example, one could conduct a pretest/posttest study design to analyze the incidence of lung cancer before and after Medicaid expansion in states that opted to undergo Medicaid expansion (exposure group) and in states that did not (cohort control). An **intervention control** refers to comparing the same outcome measure within the same cohort(s) but studying a different intervention, which one expects may also result in an observed difference. For example, one could analyze the incidence of lung cancer under other changes in the law that may have occurred during the same time, such as a new cigarette tax. Sometimes analyzing a **nuisance exposure**, that is, an exposure that one expects should have no relation to the outcome, such as a farm subsidy, is useful to consider as a negative control. This method helps ensure specificity of the effect of the exposure of interest. An **outcome control** refers to comparing the same intervention of interest within the cohort(s), using an alternate outcome that may or may not be specific to the effect under study. For example, studying the effect of Medicaid expansion on the incidence of other types of cancer or chronic obstructive pulmonary disease, rates of smoking cessation, or prevalence of motor vehicle accidents could help elucidate whether the effect was specific to preventing lung cancer or applies to risky behaviors in general. Such approaches can help mitigate (but not eliminate) potential biases.

Quasi-experimental study designs have limitations that come from their nonrandomized nature. Specifically, the issue of **selection bias** (discussed subsequently) remains a persistent threat to study validity. Despite these limitations, pure randomized controlled trials are not always feasible, so quasi-experimental study designs will continue to play an important role in health outcomes research.

NATURAL EXPERIMENTS

Health outcomes research often takes advantage of **natural experiments**, which are empirical studies of people who are exposed to various interventions outside the control of researchers. The earlier example evaluating the impact of Medicaid expansion on breast cancer takes advantage of a natural experiment of Medicaid expansion through government policy (the Affordable Care Act). In health outcomes research, a health policy change often creates a natural experiment. Examples of natural experiments in oncology include the initiation of public cancer screening programs, or the implementation of a smoking ban. Alternatively, taking away resources also represents a natural experiment. A classic example outside of oncology is a study looking at the impact of defunding Planned Parenthood on pregnancy rates among low-income women (5). Different study designs can be applied to natural experiments, and the optimal study design will depend on the question of interest.

QUANTITATIVE VERSUS QUALITATIVE RESEARCH

Health outcomes research often employs both quantitative and qualitative methods (Figure 18.5). **Quantitative research** in general focuses on hard, discretely measurable endpoints, such as disease progression or survival. **Qualitative research** by nature includes more descriptive methods, including interviews, focus groups, or case studies. In general, qualitative and quantitative research will tackle problems from opposite but complementary angles. For example, let us suppose a research project aimed to understand the impact of multidisciplinary disease teams (MDTs) on patient care. A quantitative study could assess the impact of MDTs on disease-specific survival. Trying to understand the influence of MDTs on clinic operations and workflow might require a qualitative approach, wherein a researcher would interview administrators, physicians, nurses, or patients. **Mixed methods research** represents an increasingly used and comprehensive research strategy that combines both quantitative and qualitative research methodologies.

OUTCOMES RESEARCH VERSUS CLINICAL RESEARCH

The diversity of research methodologies and study designs within the field of "outcomes research" can make it difficult to succinctly define what constitutes outcomes research and what does not. Older definitions of *health outcomes research* strictly excluded clinical trials evaluating efficacy (6). However, more modern hybrid study designs contain elements of both conventional clinical trials and health outcomes research.

For example, **pragmatic clinical trials** attempt to evaluate effectiveness in real-world settings (7). Pragmatic clinical trials often involve some form of clustering in which different clinics or treatment centers receive different interventions. A **stepped-wedge trial** design represents a type of

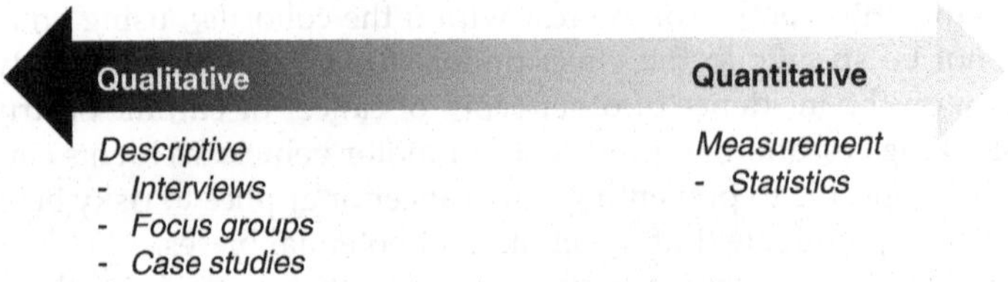

FIGURE 18.5 Spectrum of qualitative and quantitative methods in health outcomes research.

pragmatic trial design that is becoming increasingly popular (8). The stepped-wedge trial includes a sequential crossover of clusters until all clusters receive the intended intervention. **Randomized registry trials** (9) represent another example of a pragmatic trial design unique to oncology. This design encompasses aspects of prospective clinical research using population-based cancer registries to collect information about patients, treatments, and outcomes. Registry-based trials have a clear economic advantage in that they rely on existing frameworks (cancer registries) to track patient outcomes, which would cost substantially less than long-term follow-up in a conventional clinical trial.

PATTERNS OF CARE RESEARCH

Defining **patterns of care** of various healthcare interventions represents a central goal within health outcomes research. As noted earlier, the term *intervention* most often refers to a cancer-directed treatment, though it could represent any aspect of healthcare delivery. Common themes of patterns of care questions are illustrated in Table 18.3. Understanding deficiencies in patterns of healthcare delivery can help inform education and outreach priorities, influence reimbursement, or impact healthcare policy. While multiple parties within the healthcare system have interest in patterns of care, this research also sparks attention from external stakeholders such as patients and advocacy groups.

HEALTH DISPARITIES RESEARCH

Health disparities research involves the study of differences in quality of health and healthcare across a variety of populations (14). Within oncology, this includes the study of differences in the incidence, prevalence, mortality, and burden of cancer and related adverse health conditions that exist among specific populations (15). Within health disparities research, the term **priority population** refers to a population that is at higher risk of experiencing a health disparity. This nonexhaustive list includes racial and ethnic minorities, low-income groups, women, children, older adults, residents of rural regions, individuals with special healthcare needs, disabled, people at the end of life, and lesbian, gay, bisexual, or transgender (LGBT) individuals.

Health disparities research is a critical subdiscipline of clinical cancer research, affecting patients across the disease spectrum. Although cancer health disparities may go unnoticed by many practitioners, they represent a major public health issue that impacts a large proportion of the United States and countries around the world. Disparities can occur in cancer risk factors, rates of screening, access to care, probability of early or correct diagnosis, delivery and compliance with treatment, and adverse treatment effects that affect survivorship (16). The overall impact of health disparities is significant. For example, black women face a 17% increased risk of death from

TABLE 18.3 COMMON THEMES IN PATTERNS OF CARE RESEARCH

Theme	Example Research
Receipt of guideline-concordant care	The use of BRCA testing in women with a family history of breast or ovarian cancer (10)
Diffusion of technology	The use and attitudes of tumor sequencing in breast cancer (11)
Impact of health policy	The impact of reimbursement policy on androgen deprivation therapy use in men with prostate cancer (12)
Overutilization	The use of long-course radiation for bone metastases (13)

cancer compared to white women, and black men face a 33% increased risk of death from cancer compared to white men (17). To put this number in perspective, one must consider that most oncology drugs approved for treatment do not confer a survival advantage (18), and among those that improve survival, the median improvement in overall survival is only 2.7 months.

The multifactorial nature of health disparities creates a need for a comprehensive research strategy. The overarching goal of health disparities research is to improve health equity and reduce disparity. The process of reducing health disparities requires multiple distinct steps, illustrated in Figure 18.6. The first step—identifying the health disparity—is most often achieved with a larger population-based or epidemiologic study. For example, a study looking at racial disparities in colorectal cancer might analyze race-based incidence, prevalence, and mortality rates within a population-based cancer registry.

Once a relevant disparity has been identified, the next step seeks to define the underlying cause. During this step, researchers must consider multiple interconnected factors when trying to deduce the mechanism of disparity. With a study considering racial disparities in colorectal cancer, one could examine disparities in screening, behavioral risk factors (tobacco, obesity, diet), environmental risk factors, socioeconomic status, genetic differences in disease, disparities in treatment, or disparities in survivorship care. Seeking to understanding the root of health disparities often necessitates the use of both quantitative and qualitative research methods.

After identifying a mechanism of disparity, a researcher should seek to define an intervention to reduce this disparity. For example, research demonstrates substantial disparities in the use of colonoscopy among racial and ethnic minorities. Potential interventions to improve screening among minorities include multimedia computer programs, telephone education, telephone reminders, mailed brochures, patient educational videos, patient navigators, transportation assistance, multimodal interventions, physician education, and/or physician financial rewards (19). A randomized trial or other study design can be used to determine the efficacy of the intervention.

The final step in health disparities research is to implement the intervention and study the implementation. Defining efficacy in a trial is important, though frequently its practical implementation does not replicate the successes observed in randomized trials, because the artificial conditions of a clinical trial and selected patient population may not generalize to a real-world setting. The field of **implementation science** studies the barriers and facilitators of implementing interventions in the real world. A successful example of implementation comes from the state of Delaware, which in the 1990s had very low rates of colon cancer screening, particularly among the black population. In the early 2000s, the governor of Delaware helped initiate a screening program for the uninsured, a screening nurse navigator, and a cancer treatment program for the uninsured. To determine the efficacy of this intervention, the study evaluated statewide colonoscopy rates, colorectal cancer incidence, and colorectal cancer mortality before and after implementation of the intervention (20). The researchers found that the intervention was associated with increased rates of colon cancer screening, as well as decreased incidence and decreased mortality. Assessing the efficacy of interventions in the real world represents a key step to confirm that interventions generalize to a population outside of a clinical trial.

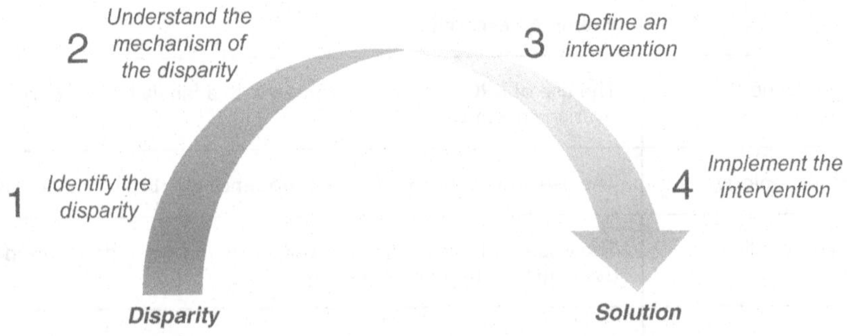

FIGURE 18.6 Framework for health disparity research.

SAFETY AND QUALITY RESEARCH

Quality and safety are often overlooked aspects of healthcare delivery, but have the potential to impact the lives of thousands of patients. It is estimated that one in seven hospitalized patients will experience a **medical error** (21), costing the United States an estimated $17 billion a year (22). Furthermore, experts estimate that between 134,000 and 400,000 patients per year will die in the United States alone due to medical errors (23), making them the third leading cause of death behind heart disease and cancer.

When considering causes of medical errors, three major themes arise: competency of providers, the complicated nature of treatments, and fragmentation of healthcare delivery. Similar to health disparities research, improving quality and safety requires a stepwise process starting with identifying the "medical error" and ideally ending with a "solution" to reduce the frequency of or eliminate the error (Figure 18.7).

The first step in identifying the error can come from a variety of sources, ranging from large epidemiologic studies down to a single (often catastrophic) event at a single institution. Medical errors are, by definition, human errors: either a provider *chooses* an inappropriate course of care, or there is improper *execution* of an appropriate course of care. Medical *errors* differ from medical *complications*. A **complication** comes as a natural side effect from therapy. A retained surgical instrument leading to a bowel obstruction would be an error, whereas a bowel obstruction from surgical adhesions would be a complication. In medicine and oncology specifically, distinguishing a medical error from a normal complication is sometimes difficult.

Once an error has been isolated, the next phase focuses on identifying the cause of the error, which relies on relatively specific approaches unique to quality and safety research. **Root cause analysis** represents one approach, which is a reactive method that retrospectively and systematically evaluates how an error occurred. Another approach is called **failure mode and effect analysis (FMEA)**, which is a proactive method for evaluating processes to identify how and where an error might occur. These approaches fall outside the scope of this chapter, and we refer the reader to the following textbooks for further education on these topics: *Root Cause Analysis in Health Care: Tools and Techniques* (6th ed., Joint Commission Resources and Jim Parker, 2017), and *Effective FMEAs: Achieving Safe, Reliable, and Economical Products and Processes Using Failure Mode and Effects Analysis* (1st ed., Carl Carlson, 2012).

Once an error has been identified, the next phase involves defining and testing an intervention, which often occurs in a single institution within the context of a conventional clinical trial. The last phase includes implementation and research to show that the intervention generalizes to a broader population. A classic example of large-scale implementation in quality and safety research comes from a multi-institutional project that aimed to decrease central catheter bloodstream

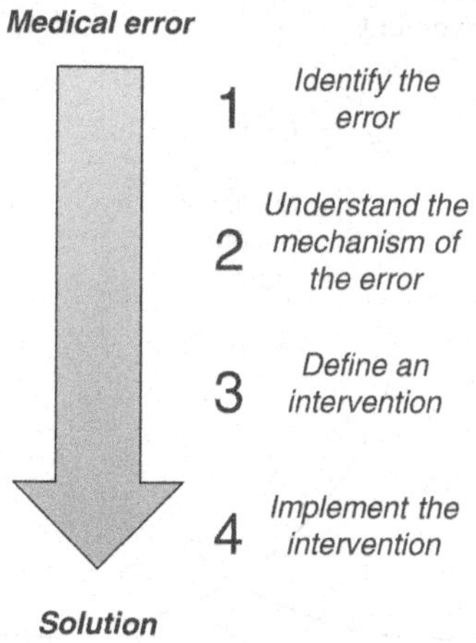

FIGURE 18.7 Framework for quality and safety research.

infections in the intensive care unit (ICU) setting. Bloodstream infections represent a preventable error that costs the United States up to $2.3 billion and results in 28,000 deaths annually (24). In this study involving 108 ICUs across the state of Michigan, an evidence-based intervention was used to reduce the incidence of catheter-related bloodstream infections (24). This study found that the intervention led to a 66% sustainable reduction in catheter infections, which has a substantial impact on healthcare costs and patient-related outcomes.

Stakeholders across the medical spectrum have incentives to reduce medical errors. Patients and physicians have clear incentives, and furthermore hospitals and healthcare systems are incentivized through reimbursement tied to quality of care. Hospitals and healthcare systems all undertake **quality improvement** efforts, which strive to improve quality of patient care through systematic improvements. In general, "quality and safety research" and "quality improvement" share the common goal to improve quality. These two domains have important distinctions, however, including the fact that quality improvement activities generally fall outside of research and thus do not require approval from an internal review board (IRB) (Figure 18.8). Individuals who work in the field of quality improvement most often do not work in the field of quality and safety research, though merging these two efforts presents a clear opportunity given the common goal of improving patient outcomes.

COMPARATIVE EFFECTIVENESS RESEARCH

According to the Institute of Medicine, **comparative effectiveness** is defined as research that "compares the benefits and harms of alternative methods to prevent, diagnose, treat, and monitor a clinical condition or to improve the delivery of care" (25). Simply put, comparative effectiveness seeks to identify the best of two or more interventions. Comparative effectiveness research includes study designs that range from prospective randomized clinical trials to retrospective observational research. Although prospective research represents the gold-standard approach to defining clinical efficacy, one must consider the limitations inherent in conventional clinical research.

First, clinical trials typically occur in highly selected patient populations, which raises important questions about their generalizability (i.e., will the treatment have the same effect in a real-world population?). Second, the time and effort required to conduct clinical research coupled with limited funding creates a situation where many important clinical research questions go unanswered. Within the realm of cancer, oncologists prescribe up to 30% of cancer drugs off label (26). Additionally, the disciplines of radiation oncology and surgery lack the same level of backing from

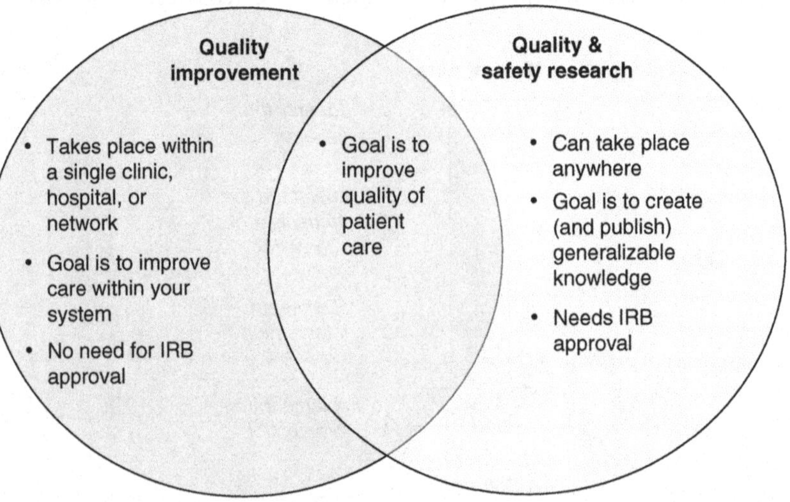

FIGURE 18.8 Overlap between quality improvement and quality and safety research.

pharmaceutical companies and FDA requirements that drive clinical research in medical oncology. This lack of prospective clinical research leads to national treatment guidelines that frequently must draw from nonrandomized data (27).

The limitations of prospective research create the need to use observational study designs for assessing comparative effectiveness. Furthermore, researchers often can easily ask comprehensive questions given the mass amount of readily available data. Datasets mentioned earlier, including cancer registries (SEER or NCDB), claims data (Medicare), or EHR data, all provide large patient numbers to compare different treatment modalities across the landscape of oncology. Despite the promise of using these data for comparative effectiveness research, one must consider important limitations that influence the validity of observational research. The following paragraphs include examples of some common types of bias to consider in comparative effectiveness research.

MISCLASSIFICATION BIAS

Misclassification bias results from measurement or classification errors. Problems with data collection in large datasets could lead to incomplete or erroneous recording of study variables or endpoints. For example, with cancer registries, registrars collect information about the staging and treatment of individual cancer patients. Given the fragmented nature of cancer care delivery, patients will often receive different aspects of treatment (chemotherapy, radiation, and surgery) at different institutions and facilities. This treatment paradigm creates a situation in which different aspects of treatment may go uncaptured, particularly for treatments delivered in clinical outpatient settings outside of the diagnosing facility. A study of the SEER cancer registry found that among women who received radiation for breast cancer, nearly 20% were recorded in the SEER as having *not* received radiation (28). This sizable degree of underascertainment has the potential to influence analyses, thus leading to misclassification bias.

SELECTION BIAS

Selection bias represents a critical primary limitation with comparative effectiveness research using observational data. Selection bias arises from innate differences in nonrandomized comparisons of two or more selected groups of patients that lead to biased results. Let us illustrate the concept with the story of hormone replacement therapy in postmenopausal women. In the 1990s, large-scale observational cohort studies found that hormone replacement therapy reduced the risk of cardiovascular disease among postmenopausal women (29). These observational studies were not randomized, and the methodological approaches in these studies compared rates of cardiovascular events among women taking hormone replacement therapy to those not taking hormone replacement therapy. The observational studies used multivariable approaches to control for known confounders of cardiovascular disease, and overall found that hormone replacement therapy *reduced* the risk of cardiovascular disease. Following these observational studies, however, large-scale randomized trials were conducted and subsequently found that hormone therapy *increased* the risk of cardiovascular disease (30).

It is important to consider potential explanations for the divergent results between the observational studies and randomized trials. While numerous potential explanations have been debated (31), selection bias represents a likely factor that skewed the results in the observational studies. Women taking hormone replacement therapy in the observational studies were likely "healthier" than women not taking hormone replacement therapy. This selection bias skewed the results of the observational study toward the hormone replacement therapy group. The observational studies used multivariable statistical approaches to reduce the effect of known confounding factors, but these techniques do not readily address unmeasured or unknown confounders, which could influence the patients' risk of cardiovascular disease. A central theme that all researchers should take to heart is that all observational research is at risk of bias from unmeasured, or unmeasurable, confounders (sometimes called **residual confounding**). Although statistical techniques such as **instrumental variable analyses** can, in theory, reduce the influence of unmeasured confounding (32), applying these methods effectively in clinical research is a challenge.

Selection bias has the potential to influence any nonrandomized study, though the potential for selection bias to influence results is more pronounced when using observational data. Within oncology specifically, the potential for bias creeps into multiple scenarios, and the impact of selection bias can work in multiple directions. For example, let us look at a hypothetical observational nonrandomized study interested in understanding the survival difference between low-dose and high-dose radiation in lung cancer. Selection bias could influence results in multiple ways. On the one hand, the patients receiving high-dose radiation may have received a higher dose because they had more aggressive disease than the patients receiving low-dose radiation, which would tend to bias survival analyses in favor of the low-dose radiation group. On the other hand, patients receiving low-dose radiation may have received this lower dose because they were less "fit" or had a decreased **performance status** at baseline, which would bias survival analyses in favor of the high-dose radiation group. As one can see with this example, the influence of selection bias on research results is complex, often nuanced, and can sway results in different directions (potentially both simultaneously). It is possible that the study biases could negate each other and the results could reflect the true reality; or one bias could dominate, and the study would be biased in favor of one treatment or another. Interestingly, a randomized trial comparing low- to higher-dose radiation dose surprisingly found worse survival in the high-dose cohort (33). These issues with selection bias in observational research raise important issues surrounding study validity, and also create a persistent need for randomized clinical trials to test research hypotheses.

IMMORTAL TIME BIAS

A final source of bias that is particularly important to consider with observational comparative effectiveness research is **immortal time bias**. We illustrate the concept of immortal time bias in a hypothetical study evaluating the survival impact of adjuvant chemotherapy compared to observation after surgery for stage II/III esophageal cancer. This fictitious analysis generated a survival curve indicating that survival is significantly improved in the surgery plus adjuvant chemotherapy group (Figure 18.9). The survival curve for the "surgery plus adjuvant chemotherapy" group has a

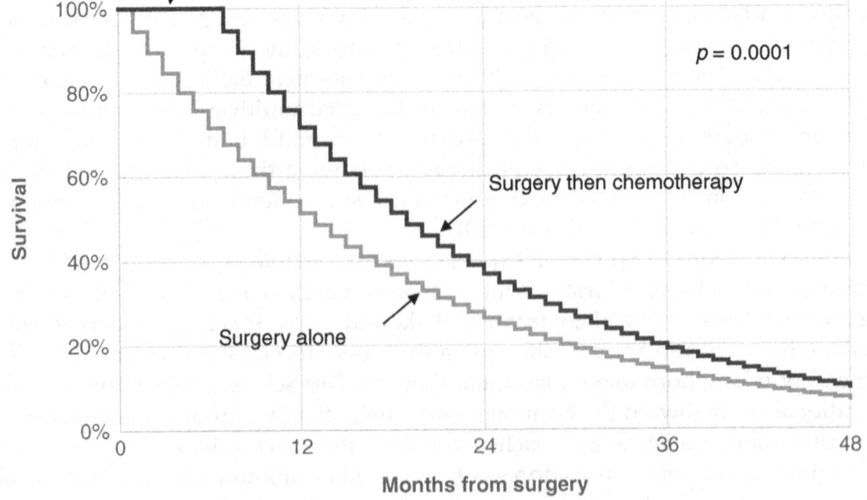

FIGURE 18.9 Immortal time bias example.

flat section initially where no patient dies (survival stays at 100%), whereas the survival curve for the "surgery alone" group trends down immediately with patients dying soon after surgery. This flat section in the survival curve arises during the time when patients receive chemotherapy after surgery. During this "immortal time," it was not possible for the patients in the chemotherapy group to die, because they had to survive to the point that they received chemotherapy.

This scenario introduces immortal time bias into the analysis, which biases the analysis in favor of the adjuvant chemotherapy group. Immortal time bias creeps into other research scenarios in oncology. In particular, any research question comparing survival between cohorts where treatment duration differs in length will encounter the risk of immortal time bias. Different analytic methodologies can help assess and control for this bias, including **landmark analyses** (34) or **time-dependent analytic approaches**. Unfortunately, researchers often do not account for immortal time bias, which occurs regularly in clinical cancer research, in their analyses (35).

CONCLUSION

This chapter introduces health outcomes research and highlights core concepts within this branch of research. Health outcomes research has many advantages and limitations, and when conducted appropriately, forms a crucial branch of cancer research by revealing insights that complement the findings from preclinical studies and clinical trials.

GLOSSARY

health outcomes research: research focused on studying the impact of healthcare delivery on real-world patient outcomes.

primary datasets: data collected specifically for research purposes.

secondary datasets: data collected for reasons other than research.

cancer registry data: an example of primary data were collected intentionally for research purposes.

Surveillance, Epidemiology, and End Results (SEER) program: a National Cancer Institute collection of individual state and regional cancer registries within the United States.

National Program of Cancer Registries (NPCR): A program similar to SEER, run by the Centers for Disease Control and Prevention (CDC), which includes cancer registries for non-SEER states.

National Cancer Database (NCDB): a registry jointly sponsored by the American College of Surgeons and the American Cancer Society.

MarketScan: a commercial data source that contains pooled private and public insurance claims data.

SEER-Medicare linked data: health insurance claims data linked to cancer registry data.

misclassification: error possibility that limits use of health insurance claims data for research purposes.

electronic health record (EHR): health and healthcare data accumulated and preserved electronically.

structured data: data within an EHR organized in such a format that it can be extracted and used easily for research purposes.

unstructured data: data within an EHR buried in an unorganized format such as a clinical note.

text mining: algorithmic means of creating structured data from unstructured data.

natural language processing: type of algorithm, stemming from the intersection of computer science and linguistics, that is often useful in extracting data from unstructured sources.

validation: process for checking data, particularly data extracted from an EHR.

cohort study: research type that follows a disease-free group of patients over time and counts incident cases of disease in exposed and nonexposed groups.

case–control study: research type that selects diseased (cases) and nondiseased (controls) groups and determines their respective exposure status.

matching algorithm: means whereby researchers "match" patients based on key characteristics and potentially modifying factors so as to make groups more comparable with respect to all factors besides the exposure of interest.

cross-sectional study: research type that looks at a group of patients at a single, fixed time period.

intervention: usually, a treatment, surgery, procedure, or other management strategy that directly involves an individual patient; may also include such strategies directed at a clinic, hospital, healthcare system, or government.

randomized: describes the gold-standard study design in which the random allocation of treatment or exposure is among a group of participants.

quasi-experimental studies: undertaken to determine the impact of an intervention on a population when randomization is not feasible.

pretest/posttest: study design that investigates outcomes before and after a change in conditions.

interrupted time series study design: investigates the trends in incidence both before and after implementation of a change in conditions.

cohort control: control method that compares results across different cohorts, which ensures that the effect of the intervention and the outcome are specific to the group of interest.

intervention control: control method that compares the same outcome measure within the same cohort(s) but studies a different intervention, which one expects may also result in an observed difference.

nuisance exposure: an exposure that one expects should have no relation to the outcome; useful to consider as a negative control.

outcome control: control method in which one compares the same intervention of interest within the cohort(s), using an alternate outcome that may or may not be specific to the effect under study.

selection bias: bias introduced by the selection of individuals, groups, or data for analysis in such a way that proper balance is not achieved, resulting in a sample that is not representative of the population intended to be analyzed.

natural experiments: empirical studies of people who are exposed to various interventions outside the control of researchers.

quantitative research: generally focuses on hard, discretely measurable endpoints, such as disease progression or survival.

qualitative research: uses descriptive methods of gathering data, such as interviews, focus groups, or case studies.

mixed methods research: an increasingly used and comprehensive research strategy that combines both quantitative and qualitative research methodologies.

pragmatic clinical trial: research that attempts to evaluate effectiveness in real-world settings; often involves some form of clustering.

stepped-wedge trial design: a type of pragmatic trial design that includes a sequential crossover of clusters until all clusters receive the intended intervention.

randomized registry trial: a pragmatic trial design unique to oncology, which encompasses aspects of prospective clinical research using population-based cancer registries to collect information about patients, treatments, and outcomes.

patterns of care: describes a research type that investigates various healthcare interventions around a central goal or theme.

health disparities research: the study of differences in quality of health and healthcare across a variety of populations.

priority population: a population that is at higher risk of experiencing a health disparity.

implementation science: field that studies the barriers and facilitators of implementing interventions in the real world.

medical error: human mistake usually caused by competency of providers, the complicated nature of treatments, and/or fragmentation of healthcare delivery.

complication: problem that arises as a natural side effect from therapy.

root cause analysis: a reactive method that retrospectively and systematically evaluates how an error occurred.

failure mode and effect analysis (FMEA): a proactive method for evaluating processes to identify how and where an error might occur.

quality improvement: describes efforts that strive to improve quality of patient care through systematic improvements.

comparative effectiveness: research that "compares the benefits and harms of alternative methods to prevent, diagnose, treat, and monitor a clinical condition or to improve the delivery of care"; seeks to identify the best of two or more interventions.

residual confounding: a risk of all observational research from unmeasured, or unmeasurable, confounders.

instrumental variable analyses: statistical techniques that can, in theory, reduce the influence of unmeasured confounding.

performance status: a type of selection bias that arises in survival analyses.

immortal time bias: a type of bias that arises from improper measurement of survival time.

landmark analyses: analytic methodologies that can help assess and control for immortal time bias.

time-dependent analytic approaches: analytic methodologies that can help assess and control for immortal time bias.

REFERENCES

1. Baxter NN, Habermann EB, Tepper JE, et al. Risk of pelvic fractures in older women following pelvic irradiation. *JAMA*. 2005;294(20);2587–2593. doi:10.1001/jama.294.20.2587
2. Brigham and Women's Hospital, Harvard Medical School, Harvard T.H. Chan School of Public Health. Nurses' Health Study. http://www.nurseshealthstudy.org
3. Kim BJ, Merchant M, Zheng C, et al. A natural language processing program effectively extracts key pathologic findings from radical prostatectomy reports. *J Endourol*. 2014;28(12):1474–1478. doi:10.1089/end.2014.0221
4. Hubbard RA, Johnson E, Chubak J, et al. Accounting for misclassification in electronic health records-derived exposures using generalized linear finite mixture models. *Health Serv Outcomes Res Methodol*. 2017;17(2):101–112. doi:10.1007/s10742-016-0149-5
5. Stevenson AJ, Flores-Vazquez IM, Allgeyer RL, et al. Effect of removal of planned parenthood from the Texas Women's Health Program. *N Engl J Med*. 2016;374(9):853–860. doi:10.1056/NEJMsa1511902
6. Lee SJ, Earle CC, Weeks JC. Outcomes research in oncology: history, conceptual framework, and trends in the literature. *J Natl Cancer Inst*. 2000;92(3):195–204. doi:10.1093/jnci/92.3.195
7. Ford I, Norrie J. Pragmatic trials. *N Engl J Med*. 2016;375(5):454–463. doi:10.1056/NEJMra1510059
8. Hemming K, Haines TP, Chilton PJ, et al. The stepped wedge cluster randomised trial: rationale, design, analysis, and reporting. *BMJ*. 2015;350:h391. doi:10.1136/bmj.h391
9. Booth CM, Tannock IF. Randomised controlled trials and population-based observational research: partners in the evolution of medical evidence. *Br J Cancer*. 2014;110(3):551–555. doi:10.1038/bjc.2013.725
10. Childers CP, Childers KK, Maggard-Gibbons M, Macinko J. National estimates of genetic testing in women with a history of breast or ovarian cancer. *J Clin Oncol*. 2017;35(34):3800–3806. doi:10.1200/jco.2017.73.6314
11. Gingras I, Sonnenblick A, de Azambuja E, et al. The current use and attitudes towards tumor genome sequencing in breast cancer. *Sci Rep*. 2016;6:22517. doi:10.1038/srep22517
12. Wagle DG. Reimbursement policy and androgen-deprivation therapy for prostate cancer. *N Engl J Med*. 2011;364(6);579–580. doi:10.1056/nejmc1013967
13. Bekelman JE, Epstein AJ, Emanuel EJ. Single- vs multiple-fraction radiotherapy for bone metastases from prostate cancer. *JAMA*. 2013;310(14):1501–1502. doi:10.1001/jama.2013.277081
14. Riley WJ. Health disparities: gaps in access, quality and affordability of medical care. *Trans Am Clin Climatol Assoc*. 2012;123:167–174.
15. U.S. Department of Health and Human Services. NCI Center to Reduce Cancer Health Disparities (CRCHD). https://www.cancer.gov/about-nci/organization/crchd
16. Koh HK. *Toward the Elimination of Cancer Disparities*. New York, NY: Springer; 2009.
17. O'Keefe EB, Meltzer JP, Bethea TN. Health disparities and cancer: racial disparities in cancer mortality in the United States, 2000–2010. *Front Public Health*. 2015;3:51. doi:10.3389/fpubh.2015.00051
18. Davis C, Naci H, Gurpinar E, et al. Availability of evidence of benefits on overall survival and quality of life of cancer drugs approved by European Medicines Agency: retrospective cohort study of drug approvals 2009–13. *BMJ*. 2017;359:j4530. doi:10.1136/bmj.j4530
19. Naylor K, Ward J, Polite BN. Interventions to improve care related to colorectal cancer among racial and ethnic minorities: a systematic review. *J Gen Intern Med*. 2012;27(8):1033–1046. doi:10.1007/s11606-012-2044-2
20. Grubbs SS, Polite BN, Carney J, et al. Eliminating racial disparities in colorectal cancer in the real world: it took a village. *J Clin Oncol*. 2013;31(16):1928–1930. doi:10.1200/jco.2012.47.8412
21. U.S. Department of Health and Human Services. Agency for Healthcare Research and Quality. https://www.ahrq.gov/research/findings/factsheets/errors-safety/index.htm
22. Van Den Bos J, Rustagi K, Gray T, et al. The $17.1 billion problem: the annual cost of measurable medical errors. *Health Aff (Millwood)*. 2011;30(4):596–603. doi:10.1377/hlthaff.2011.0084
23. Makary MA, Daniel M. Medical error—the third leading cause of death in the US. *BMJ*. 2016;353:i2139. doi:10.1136/bmj.i2139
24. Pronovost P, Needham D, Berenholtz S, et al. An intervention to decrease catheter-related bloodstream infections in the ICU. *N Engl J Med*. 2006;355(26):2725–2732. doi:10.1056/NEJMoa061115
25. Institute of Medicine. *Initial national priorities for comparative effectiveness research*. Washington, DC: The National Academies Press; 2009. doi:10.17226/12648
26. Conti RM, Bernstein AC, Villaflor VM, et al. Prevalence of off-label use and spending in 2010 among patent-protected chemotherapies in a population-based cohort of medical oncologists. *J Clin Oncol*. 2013;31(9):1134–1139. doi:10.1200/jco.2012.42.7252
27. Poonacha TK, Go RS. Level of scientific evidence underlying recommendations arising from the National Comprehensive Cancer Network clinical practice guidelines. *J Clin Oncol*. 2011;29(2):186–191. doi:10.1200/jco.2010.31.6414
28. Jagsi R, Abrahamse P, Hawley ST, et al. Underascertainment of radiotherapy receipt in Surveillance, Epidemiology, and End Results registry data. *Cancer*. 2012;118(2):333–341. doi:10.1002/cncr.26295
29. Grodstein F, Stampfer MJ, Manson JE, et al. Postmenopausal estrogen and progestin use and the risk of cardiovascular disease. *N Engl J Med*. 1996;335(7):453–461. doi:10.1056/nejm199608153350701
30. Rossouw JE, Anderson GL, Prentice RL, et al. Risks and benefits of estrogen plus progestin in healthy postmenopausal women: principal results from the Women's Health Initiative randomized controlled trial. *JAMA*. 2002;288(3):321–333. doi:10.1001/jama.288.3.321
31. Grodstein F, Clarkson TB, Manson JE. Understanding the divergent data on postmenopausal hormone therapy. *N Engl J Med*. 2003;348(7):645–650. doi:10.1056/NEJMsb022365

32. Hadley J, Yabroff KR, Barrett MJ, et al. Comparative effectiveness of prostate cancer treatments: evaluating statistical adjustments for confounding in observational data. *J Natl Cancer Inst*. 2010;102(23):1780–1793. doi:10.1093/jnci/djq393
33. Bradley JD, Paulus R, Komaki R, et al. Standard-dose versus high-dose conformal radiotherapy with concurrent and consolidation carboplatin plus paclitaxel with or without cetuximab for patients with stage IIIA or IIIB non-small-cell lung cancer (RTOG 0617): a randomised, two-by-two factorial phase 3 study. *Lancet Oncol*. 2015;16(2):187–199. doi:10.1016/s1470-2045(14)71207-0
34. Park HS, Gross CP, Makarov DV, Yu JB. Immortal time bias: a frequently unrecognized threat to validity in the evaluation of postoperative radiotherapy. *Int J Radiat Oncol Biol Phys*. 2012;83(5):1365–1373. doi:10.1016/j.ijrobp.2011.10.025
35. Lash TL, Cole SR. Immortal person-time in studies of cancer outcomes. *J Clin Oncol*. 2009;27(23): e55–e56. doi:10.1200/jco.2009.24.1877

19

Cost-Effectiveness Analysis

REITH ROY SARKAR ■ JAMES MURPHY

Cost-effectiveness of healthcare represents an important, yet highly charged topic in the United States and around the world. U.S. expenditure on cancer care has rapidly increased over the past several decades. In 1990, the United States spent an estimated $27 billion on cancer care, which by 2008 increased to $100 billion (1). Current projections estimate that the cost of cancer care could reach $158 billion by 2020, making it a central driver of the rise in U.S. healthcare spending (2).

Cost-effectiveness research aims to compare the cost and health benefits of different treatments or healthcare interventions. In other words, cost-effectiveness research strives to measure the *value* of different components of healthcare. In societies with limited resources, cost-effectiveness analyses can help to inform decision makers on how to allocate healthcare dollars to maximize the health of their constituents. Despite the need to introduce cost into the discourse of healthcare, people understandably feel uncomfortable when discussing health and human lives in parallel with dollars and cents. The general concept of cost-effectiveness research in the United States has long been a highly politicized issue. The idea of considering costs in healthcare evokes fears of rationing, death panels, and government interference in patient choice. Along these lines, the U.S. government currently prevents the use of cost-effectiveness research to influence reimbursement policy (3).

Despite the political undertones, the need to inject cost into the discourse of cancer care has become increasingly apparent. Novel noncurative cancer drugs routinely cost hundreds of thousands of dollars (4). Newly constructed proton therapy centers provide questionable incremental clinical benefit, yet cost substantially more than the existing radiation therapy techniques (5). These costly therapies lead to "financial toxicity" for our patients who shoulder an increasing burden of the cost of cancer care (6). Financial toxicity leads to treatment nonadherence, reduced quality of life (QOL), and increased morbidity and mortality (7). Professional organizations such as the American Society of Clinical Oncology (ASCO) and the National Comprehensive Cancer Network (NCCN) recently acknowledged the critical need to consider value in cancer care (8). The importance of evaluating cost and value of cancer treatment will become increasingly important in years to come.

This chapter provides an overview of the core concepts behind cost-effectiveness research. We start by describing the general components of cost-effectiveness research, followed by a discussion of the analytic approaches used to conduct cost-effectiveness research.

OVERVIEW OF COST-EFFECTIVENESS RESEARCH

Cost-effectiveness research defines the value of different approaches to delivering healthcare. Cost-effectiveness research addresses questions that span the continuum of cancer care: prevention, screening, diagnosis, treatment, and survivorship. Examples of classic cost-effectiveness research questions are provided in Table 19.1.

Cost-effectiveness research depends on three main factors: cost, survival, and QOL. For example, when considering the cost-effectiveness of a new cancer treatment, our perception of its value depends on how much this treatment costs, what survival benefit it provides, and how this treatment affects patients' QOL. Incorporating cost, survival, and QOL into a single framework requires specific analytic techniques such as decision analytic modeling, Markov modeling, or microsimulation modeling. These analytic approaches stand apart from other areas of clinical research and the terminology involved in cost-effectiveness research is relatively unique. This chapter provides a general framework of cost-effectiveness for people involved in healthcare and outlines the core concepts involved. Conducting in-depth cost-effectiveness research requires skills and techniques beyond the scope of this single chapter, though we point out resources for readers interested in pursuing this line of research throughout the text.

MEASURING COST

Measuring cost in healthcare can be deceptively challenging due to the complexity of healthcare delivery. Let us consider an example of the cost of a simple chest x-ray. When considering the cost of a chest x-ray, one needs to consider the cost of the chest x-ray itself, as well as the cost of the time and transportation required for the patient to travel to and undergo the x-ray. In this example, the cost of the x-ray itself would be considered a **direct cost**, whereas the cost of transportation and lost patient wages would be considered an **indirect cost**.

TABLE 19.1 EXAMPLE COST-EFFECTIVENESS RESEARCH QUESTIONS IN ONCOLOGY

Cost-effectiveness question	Comparison arms
Screening for lung cancer (9)	1. No screening 2. Chest x-ray 3. Chest CT
PET/CT screening versus planned neck dissection in head-and-neck cancer (10)	1. PET/CT scan screening 2. Planned neck dissection
Using molecular profiling for adjuvant therapy decision making in breast cancer (11)	1. Chemotherapy for all patients 2. Decision based on clinical factors 3. Decision based on molecular profiling
Adding bevacizumab to standard chemotherapy in metastatic colorectal cancer (12)	1. FOLFOX 2. FOLFOX with bevacizumab
Fracture prevention in breast cancer patients receiving aromatase inhibitors (13)	1. No intervention 2. Bone mineral density screening 3. Selective bisphosphonate therapy

CT, computed tomography; FOLFOX, folinic acid, fluorouracil, and oxaliplatin; PET, positron emission tomography.

When measuring the direct cost of the chest x-ray itself, one needs to consider the cost of the x-ray machine, room for the x-ray machine, service contract for the machine, radiologist's time to read the images, the computer system to store the images, x-ray technician's time, scheduler's time, waiting room staff time, utilities, as well as support for the health center administration. In reality, a single x-ray will consume only a fraction of each of these resources, which you would need to factor into the calculations. This detailed approach of ascertaining cost is called **micro-costing**. On the one hand, micro-costing can provide precise measurements of the cost of delivering healthcare. However, the complexity involved in measuring the components of cost can be daunting; in addition, the estimations of cost will vary between different locations. These inherent limitations in micro-costing often lead researchers to search for surrogate measures of cost in cost-effectiveness research.

Many methods exist to estimate the cost of healthcare services, and the best method will often depend on the individual study. One relatively crude but simple approach is to use healthcare **charge** information, or the price that a hospital sets for a given service. Unfortunately, healthcare charges represent a poor surrogate for cost, because hospitals most often charge multiple times what a service actually costs to deliver. Furthermore, the amount charged varies substantially between hospitals, without clear patterns (14). One solution to help overcome this issue is to pool charge data across multiple hospitals or healthcare networks, and then use a cost-to-charge ratio to convert charge numbers into estimates of healthcare costs. This approach of using charge data to estimate cost is used by the Healthcare Cost and Utilization Project (HCUP) sponsored by the Agency for Healthcare Research and Quality (AHRQ) (15).

Another approach to estimating cost of healthcare is to use Medicare reimbursement data. In general, Medicare seeks to reimburse providers at a rate commensurate with the cost of providing services. This approach of using Medicare reimbursement data as a proxy for cost has limitations worth discussing. First, Medicare reimbursement policy tends to better compensate specialists and more procedurally oriented fields (like radiation oncology). This inflated compensation would lead researchers to overestimate the costs of these aspects of healthcare. Second, Medicare primarily provides healthcare for patient populations 65 years or older; therefore, these cost estimates may not generalize to younger populations. Despite these limitations, Medicare reimbursement schedules are freely available, thus this approach is widely used and has the advantage of leading to consistency across studies (16).

Activity-based costing represents an additional technique to estimate the cost of different elements of healthcare increasingly used in the past several years. Activity-based costing estimates the costs of healthcare procedures or services based on direct measurement or estimation of the resources they consume. Activity-based costing will consider factors such as hospital space, provider time, supervision, information technology, and energy costs (17). While activity-based costing can in theory increase the accuracy of cost measurement, one must consider that the cost estimates derived from this activity often arise from a single institution, and therefore may not generalize to other scenarios or locations. When considering what costs to include in a cost-effectiveness project, one must consider the viewpoint or *perspective* from which one is asking the question. Table 19.2 demonstrates the wide range of perspectives in cost-effectiveness research.

To illustrate the concept of perspective, let us consider an example of a child with cancer who received cranial radiation for treatment of leukemia. The *payer perspective* would include all costs related to treatment, including the consultation, radiation, prescription medications, follow-up visits, imaging studies, and long-term health-related direct medical costs. The *healthcare perspective* would include all the costs in the payer perspective, but would also include patient out-of-pocket expenditures, costs for patient and family time, as well as missed school and work, and travel to and from the clinic or hospital. If the patient suffered cognitive dysfunction later in life, then the healthcare perspective would also include the costs associated with lost productivity, and long-term care costs associated with the cognitive dysfunction. The *societal perspective* not only encompasses all costs listed in the payer and healthcare perspectives, but also considers the cost borne by society. For example, if the patient suffered cognitive dysfunction, then the societal perspective would include the publicly provided costs of special education, and other services for

TABLE 19.2 DIFFERENT PERSPECTIVES IN COST-EFFECTIVENESS RESEARCH

Perspective	Definition
Payer	The payer could include a private insurer or a public entity (e.g., Medicare). The payer perspective would consider only direct medical costs paid for by the insurer, and would not consider indirect costs paid for by the patient.
Healthcare	The healthcare perspective includes all direct medical costs paid for by the payer, and indirect medical costs paid for by the patient. This includes out-of-pocket costs, patient time lost because of the illness/treatment, transportation costs, and caregiver time.
Societal	The societal viewpoint captures all costs related to the illness, as well as all non-health-related costs as a result of the illness.

disabled people. Although the societal perspective is the most comprehensive, measuring costs to society with any degree of accuracy poses challenges. Ultimately, the best perspective for a cost-effectiveness research study depends on the audience, and often researchers will present results from more than one perspective.

One final consideration with cost relates to the concept of inflation. *Inflation* refers to the increase in the price of goods and services across the economy over time. Cost-effectiveness research will often include costs for different aspects of healthcare spread across different years. For example, if you undertook a project where you measured the cost of a chest x-ray in 2004, and your study occurs in 2017, you would need to adjust the 2004 cost into 2017 dollars. In other words, the chest x-ray that cost $100 in 2004 would cost $131.12 in 2017. Inflation rates come from the Consumer Price Index from the U.S. Bureau of Labor Statistics (18). It is a standard practice to inflation-adjust all costs to present-day dollars in cost-effectiveness research.

MEASURING EFFECTIVENESS

"Effectiveness" in cost-effectiveness research depends on both QOL and survival. For example, chemotherapy may improve survival, but this treatment also comes with toxicity. When evaluating the effectiveness of chemotherapy, a patient considers both the survival benefit and the impact on QOL. Along these lines, the standard measure of effectiveness that researchers use is the **quality-adjusted life year (QALY)**, which represents the product of QOL and the years lived with that QOL (19). Although the QALY represents the most commonly used metric to quantify effectiveness, another related measure is the **disability adjusted life year (DALY)**, which is commonly used by the World Health Organization and lower-income countries. The DALY represents a standardized measure of disease burden that incorporates disability and life years lost. Readers interested in DALYs should consider the papers by Murray et al. (20) and Sassi (21).

Cost-effective researchers most commonly use the **health utility** score as a measure of QOL. Health utility is a continuous number that represents the "preference" for being in a desired health state bounded by the anchors of zero (death) and one (perfect health). Health utility is a type of QOL measurement, though it has some fundamental differences from more commonly used QOL measures. Additionally, most general QOL measurements do not easily translate into health utility scores.

To better understand the concept of health utility, we consider an example of a patient with a shoulder injury (rotator cuff tear) that causes mild pain, but limits the patient's ability to move the shoulder. If we ask that patient arbitrarily to rate her QOL with this shoulder injury on a scale from 0 (bad) to 100 (great), we might expect scores in the 30, 40, and 50 range. A QOL score of 30 out of 100 does not translate to a health utility score of 30/100 (or 0.3). A health utility score of 0.3 would mean that the patient would be indifferent to the choice of living with the shoulder injury or undergoing surgery with a 30% chance ($p = .3$) of fixing the injury and a 70% chance of immediate

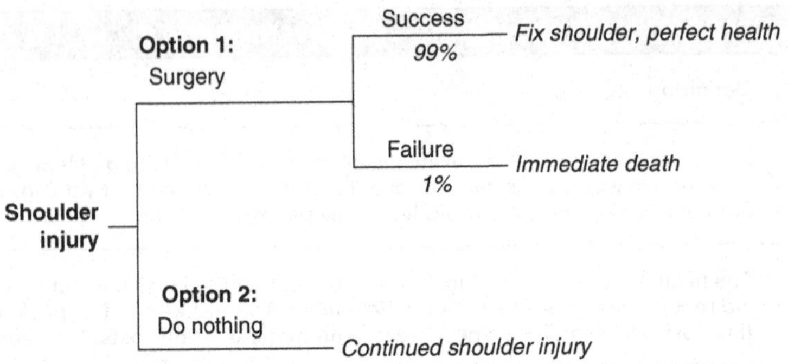

FIGURE 19.1 Example of a standard gamble to determine the health utility of a shoulder injury.

death. With a shoulder injury, most people would not accept surgery with a 70% chance of immediate death. Most people would rank the health utility of this shoulder injury at 0.99 or higher, which means that they would be indifferent to surgery (with a 99% chance of success, and a 1% chance of immediate death) or living with the shoulder injury. This technique for defining health utility is referred to as a **standard gamble** (22). The actual practice of obtaining health utility scores through the standard gamble approach typically involves interviewing individual subjects and presenting different scenarios where subjects are asked to choose one "preferred" outcome over another (as in the previous example). A researcher would obtain a health utility score for a group of individuals, and the average health utility scores to help estimate a societal score for a given medical condition. The concept of the standard gamble is demonstrated in Figure 19.1.

This figure shows the general concept of a standard gamble. In this scenario, the patient would be indifferent to choosing option 1, which includes surgery (with a 99% chance of success and a 1% chance of failure), as opposed to option 2, where the patient lives with the shoulder injury. The health utility of a shoulder injury in this scenario would be 0.99.

The standard gamble is the primary approach used to ascertain health utility scores, though a secondary method called the **time trade-off** is often employed as well (22). Both the standard gamble and time trade-off are instruments specifically designed to capture health utilities. Alternatively, a handful of validated QOL questionnaires exist, including the EQ-5D and SF-6D, that can be mapped to health utility scores. As noted earlier, the QALY represents the standard measure of "effectiveness" in cost-effectiveness research. The QALY is the product of health utility and time. For example, Figure 19.2 demonstrates the health utility score of a patient with cancer,

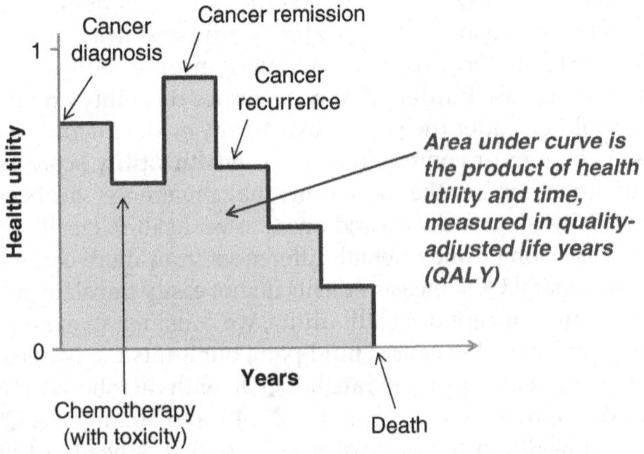

FIGURE 19.2 Graphical demonstration of QALY for a cancer patient.

QALY, quality-adjusted life years.

which will vary during different phases of the patient's disease. In this example, the health utility changes with treatment, remission, cancer recurrence, and finally death. The area under the curve in Figure 19.2 represents the total QALY for this example patient.

COST-EFFECTIVENESS ANALYSIS

Now that readers are armed with knowledge of the concepts of "cost" and "effectiveness," this next section gives an overview of the different analytic techniques used to conduct a cost-effectiveness analysis. We illustrate the analytic techniques used in a cost-effectiveness project with a simple example. Suppose a patient recently diagnosed with cancer faces a choice between two treatments. "Treatment A" represents an experimental treatment, which if successful results in the patient living an average of 8 years, but if Treatment A fails the patient lives an average of only 2 years. Let us assume a 50% probability that Treatment A will be successful, and a 50% probability of failure. "Treatment B," in contrast, is more consistent and all patients will live an average of 4 years. Let us assume that Treatment A and Treatment B have different health utility scores, and different costs. Table 19.3 shows hypothetical values for the costs, utilities, and survival for both Treatment A and Treatment B.

When considering the question of cost-effectiveness of Treatment A compared to Treatment B, it helps to construct a **decision tree** that maps out the different options, outcomes, and costs for the two treatment options. Figure 19.3 shows a decision tree for this example case. A decision tree node should lead to states that are mutually exclusive and collectively exhaustive.

The decision tree in this figure depicts a patient with cancer who has two treatment options, Treatment A and Treatment B. The blue square represents a **decision node** indicating that the patient is free to choose between the two options. The green circle represents a **chance node,** which in this example indicates that there is a defined probability that Treatment A will succeed or fail. Finally, the red triangles are **terminal nodes,** which represent the end of that particular path.

To determine the cost-effectiveness of Treatment A compared to Treatment B, we must solve the decision tree. The first step to solve the tree is to determine the effectiveness or number of QALYs associated with each possible outcome. This involves a simple calculation in which we multiply the survival in years by the health utility score. The following shows the total number of QALYs for each of the possible outcomes for this decision tree.

QALY when Treatment A succeeds = (8 years) * (utility of 0.5) = 4.0 QALY

QALY when Treatment A fails =(2 years) * (utility of 0.2) = 0.4 QALY

QALY when Treatment B fails = (4 years) * (utility of 0.5) = 2.0 QALY

TABLE 19.3 SURVIVAL, HEALTH UTILITY, AND COST VALUES FOR TWO HYPOTHETICAL CANCER TREATMENTS

Treatment	Survival	Health utility	Cost
Treatment A			
Success	8 years	0.5	$150,000
Failure	2 years	0.2	$50,000
Treatment B	4 years	0.5	$80,000

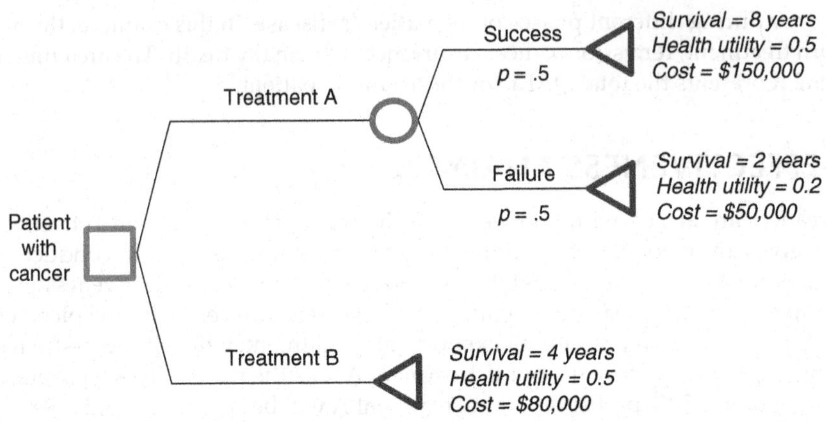

FIGURE 19.3 Basic decision tree.

Figure 19.4 shows the decision tree incorporating these effectiveness calculations.

The next step in solving the decision tree includes summarizing the two outcomes of Treatment A (success and failure) into a single outcome. This entails determining the expected value for effectiveness and the expected value for cost. These expected values come from the following simple calculations:

Treatment A effectiveness = (QALY of success) * (probability of success) + (QALY of failure) * (probability of failure)

= (4 QALY) * 0.5 + (0.4 QALY) * 0.5

= 2.2 QALY

Treatment A cost = (cost of success) * (probability of success) + (cost of failure) * (probability of failure)

= ($150,000) * 0.5 + ($50,000) * 0.5

= $100,000

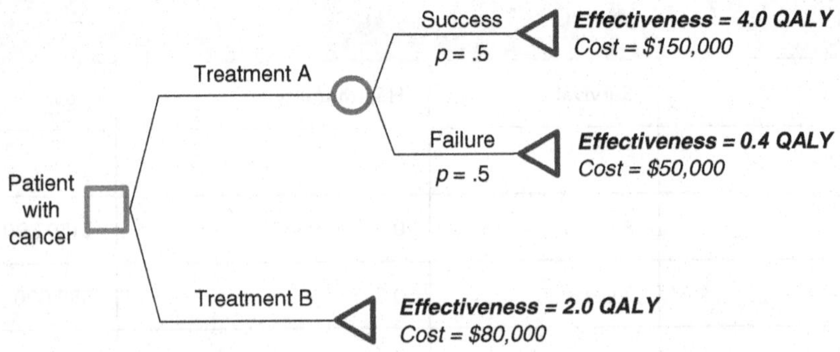

FIGURE 19.4 Decision tree including effectiveness calculations.

These summarized outcomes show that, on average, Treatment A will produce 2.2 QALY at a cost of $100,000. In general, the formula to calculate the expected value is:

$$\text{Expected value} = x_1p_1 + x_2p_2 + \ldots + x_np_n,$$

where $x_1, x_2, \ldots, x_n$ represent n different outcomes (i.e., QALYs or costs) with probabilities $p_1, p_2, \ldots, p_n$. Figure 19.5 shows the final decision tree with the summarized outcomes. Here we can see that Treatment A is slightly costlier and slightly more effective than Treatment B.

The final step in this analysis is to determine cost-effectiveness, which is measured by the **incremental cost-effectiveness ratio (ICER)**. The ICER represents the incremental costs divided by the incremental effectiveness, denoted as follows:

$$\text{ICER} = \frac{(\text{Cost}_{\text{Treatment A}} - \text{Cost}_{\text{Treatment B}})}{(\text{QALY}_{\text{Treatment A}} - \text{QALY}_{\text{Treatment B}})}$$

$$\text{ICER} = \frac{(\$100{,}000 - \$80{,}000)}{(2.2\text{QALY} - 2.0\text{QALY})} = \$100{,}000 / \text{QALY}$$

In this example, the ICER for Treatment A compared to Treatment B was $100,000 per QALY. This means that if you choose Treatment A, on average you will gain one QALY at a cost of $100,000.

In this example, the ICER of $100,000/QALY defines the value of Treatment A compared to Treatment B, though one can go further and ask whether this $100,000/QALY number would be considered cost-effective. To address this question, one must consider a concept called **willingness to pay**, which represents a dollar-per-QALY threshold above which treatments would not be considered cost-effective.

The concept of willingness to pay can be controversial, because it asks how much one would pay for human life. How much an individual would pay for healthcare by nature varies depending on the perspective of the stakeholder. Patients, payers, government, and society all view costs differently. Despite this controversy surrounding willingness to pay, several numbers frequently arise within the literature. One of the more common thresholds is $50,000/QALY. The origin of the $50,000/QALY threshold is not entirely clear, though some argue that it dates back to the 1970s when Medicare decided to cover hemodialysis for patients with end-stage renal disease (23). It was estimated that dialysis would provide one QALY for $50,000, thus a $50,000/QALY threshold. However, this $50,000/QALY threshold does not reflect what people actually pay for healthcare in the United States, which more realistically ranges from $200,000 to $300,000/QALY (23–25). Regardless, willingness-to-pay thresholds of $50,000/QALY and $100,000/QALY are commonly used in cost-effectiveness studies despite the lack of evidence to support these numbers.

The cost-effectiveness analyses presented as examples in this chapter thus far are overly simplified. More realistic analyses within cancer would independently include acute toxicity from

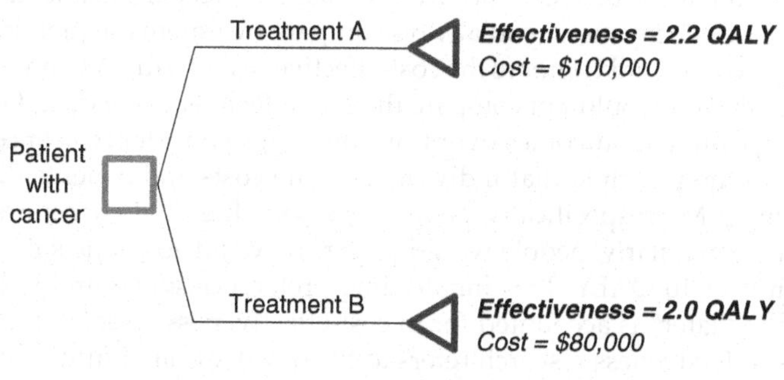

FIGURE 19.5 Summarized decision tree.

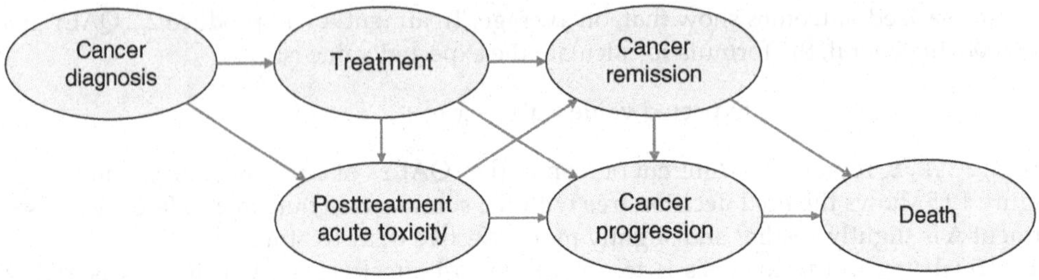

FIGURE 19.6 Sample state transition diagram.

treatment, disease progression, second-line treatments, long-term complications, and death from noncancer causes. When constructing these more complex decision trees that extend over multiple years, researchers will often use a **Markov model** which incorporates decision trees as presented earlier, in addition to allowing patients to transition between different **health disease states** as they progress through their disease over time (26). If the model is a Markov model, then the tree is "solved" similar to how we solved the earlier example model (but more computationally rigorous than can easily be done by hand). For microsimulation models (discussed further), the ICER is derived by running individual patients through a simulated model and averaging costs and QALYs to determine an ICER.

Figure 19.6 shows a sample **state transition diagram** for a patient with cancer. Markov models can address very complex cost-effectiveness analyses, and the general principles of solving a Markov model parallel the approach used to solve the decision trees mentioned earlier. Aside from decision analysis trees and Markov models, other modeling approaches used in cost-effectiveness research include **microsimulation models** and other simulation techniques (26). The optimal modeling approach depends on the structure and complexity of the cost-effectiveness research question. Markov models require that researchers define all the potential health states that a hypothetical patient could experience, and thus can become exponentially more complex with greater numbers of potential outcomes. Additionally, Markov models lack "memory" of the prior events a patient has experienced. In contrast, microsimulation models can track the outcomes for individual patients (i.e., they have "memory") and can thus account for the influence that prior events have on future outcomes (e.g., prior toxicity influencing the risk of future toxicity) (27). Microsimulation models often have more flexibility than a conventional Markov model, though it requires more technical expertise to practically implement the model. The figure shows an example of a state transition diagram. The shaded ovals represent potential health states and the arrows represent potential transitions between health states.

When comparing more than two treatment options in cost-effectiveness research, it helps to graphically present data on a **cost-effectiveness frontier**, which is a simple plot showing the cost on the y-axis, and effectiveness (QALY) on the x-axis. Figure 19.7 shows an example of a cost-effectiveness frontier used to compare four different drugs to a "no treatment" option. In this figure the lines connecting the treatment options represents the cost-effectiveness frontier, and the slope of the line represents the ICER between the two options. The steeper the line, the higher the ICER. When considering cost-effectiveness, you always compare treatments sequentially by cost, which, in Figure 19.7, means you would compare the cost-effectiveness of drug A to no treatment, and drug B to drug A, and so on. You would not compare the cost-effectiveness of drug D to no treatment.

When modeling different outcomes over time, one must consider the concept of **time preference,** which refers to the principle that individuals value costs and benefits differently at different times in their lives. More specifically, people tend to value $100 now more than they would value $100 in 10 years. Similarly, people would prefer to extend someone's life from 0 to 1 QALY more so than from 9 to 10 QALY. This innate time preference where individuals prefer things "now" as opposed to "later" is accounted for in cost-effectiveness research through **discounting.** Discounting in cost-effectiveness research refers to the devaluation of future costs and QALYs by a set amount. The equation to determine discounted costs and discounted QALYs is as follows:

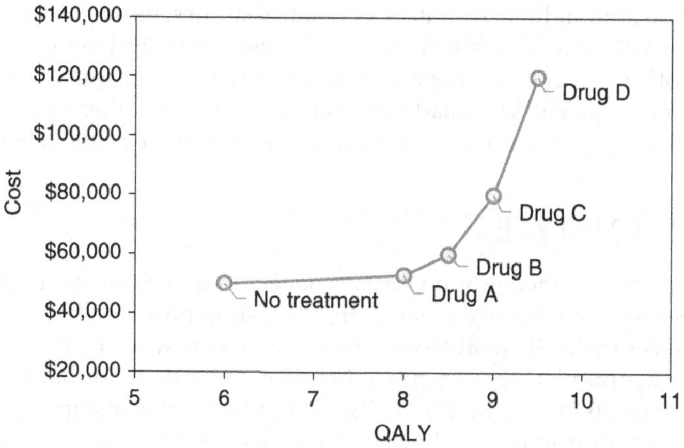

FIGURE 19.7 Sample cost-effectiveness frontier.

$$\text{Present} - \text{day cost} = \frac{\text{Cost in future}}{(1+r)^t}$$

$$\text{Present day} - \text{QALY} = \frac{\text{QALY in future}}{(1+r)^t}$$

where r is the discount rate and t is the future time in years (26). Let us look at an example situation where a patient has a complication from radiation that costs $1,000 per year for 5 years. The undiscounted and discounted costs (assuming a 3% discount rate) would be as follows:

$$\text{Undiscounted cost} = \$1{,}000 + \$1{,}000 + \$1{,}000 + \$1{,}000 + \$1{,}000 = \$5{,}000$$

$$\text{Discounted cost} = \$1{,}000 + \frac{\$1{,}000}{(1+0.03)^1} + \frac{\$1{,}000}{(1+0.03)^2} + \frac{\$1{,}000}{(1+0.03)^3} + \frac{\$1{,}000}{(1+0.03)^4}$$

$$= \$1{,}000 + \$970 + 943 + \$915 + \$888 = \$4{,}717$$

Note that, in this example with a discount rate of 3% per year, after 5 years the discounted cost of $4,717 was only moderately less than the undiscounted cost of $5,000. On the other hand, if you assume the same $1,000 annual cost over 50 years, the undiscounted cost of $50,000 would differ substantially from the discounted cost of $26,502. In general, discounting affects costs and QALYs more in cost-effectiveness models that stretch over longer periods of time. The ideal discount rate remains a subject of debate among health economists, though in general researchers will use a discount rate of 3% for both costs and QALYs (28).

One final note about cost-effectiveness research relates to validity of the individual models. As one could imagine, the cost-effectiveness models depend exclusively on the actual data used to inform the models. If you were comparing the cost-effectiveness of two chemotherapy agents, the analysis and resulting ICER would depend on rates, costs, and health utilities of toxicity, disease control, and survival, as well as on long-term side effects. The validity of the cost-effectiveness analysis will depend completely on the quality of the model inputs. In general, researchers should strive to use the highest levels of evidence as model inputs with cost-effectiveness modeling. Ideally, one would inform a cost-effectiveness model with data from a randomized trial comparing these two chemotherapy agents. If these were not available, then one could use lower-quality data including prospective nonrandomized data, case-control studies, retrospective cohort studies, and lastly expert opinion where good-quality data do not exist. Cost-effectiveness research follows the same paradigm as other branches of research—best summarized by a quote from the poet Edward Thomas: "You cannot make chicken salad out of chicken s***." In other words, if you have poor data informing your model, then confidence in your resultant ICER will likely be low.

SENSITIVITY ANALYSES

Cost-effectiveness research inherently involves models or simulations that depend on a variety of data. A key aspect of cost-effectiveness research is testing how *sensitive* one's model is to different assumptions. A **sensitivity analysis** refers to the process whereby one tests how the model responds when the assumptions are changed. Let us assume that you have a cost-effectiveness analysis that found drug B to have an ICER of $75,000/QALY when compared to drug A. In your model, you assumed that drug B would reduce the risk of death by 10% compared to drug A. A **one-way sensitivity analysis** for survival would vary the risk of death in the model across a range and determine how this affects the ICER. The results for this hypothetical one-way sensitivity analysis are presented in Figure 19.8. This figure demonstrates the results of a cost-effectiveness analysis when one varies the estimated survival advantage of drug B over drug A.

As the survival advantage of drug B diminishes, the ICER becomes higher and drug B becomes less cost-effective. As the survival advantage of drug B increases, the ICER becomes lower and drug B becomes more cost-effective. The results of this one-way sensitivity analysis show that this cost-effectiveness analysis is moderately sensitive to assumptions about survival. In practice, researchers would vary all model parameters to determine which parameters have the greatest effect on the model output. This exercise can help provide researchers an understanding of the key parameters that drive a cost-effectiveness analysis.

The one-way sensitivity analysis represents the standard approach to determine how a cost-effectiveness model changes with uncertainty around a single variable. However, in real life, researchers will have some degree of uncertainty surrounding all model inputs. In cost-effectiveness research, the **probabilistic sensitivity analysis** represents the standard tool to assess how a model performs when varying all parameters simultaneously. Though the specifics of a probabilistic sensitivity analysis are beyond the scope of this chapter, a brief overview of the steps involved is warranted.

First, probability distributions are fit to individual parameters in the cost-effectiveness models. Commonly used probability distributions include gamma or log-normal distributions for costs, and beta distributions for health utility and probabilities. The probability distributions ideally have means and standard deviations that reflect estimates of the parameter in question. Sampling

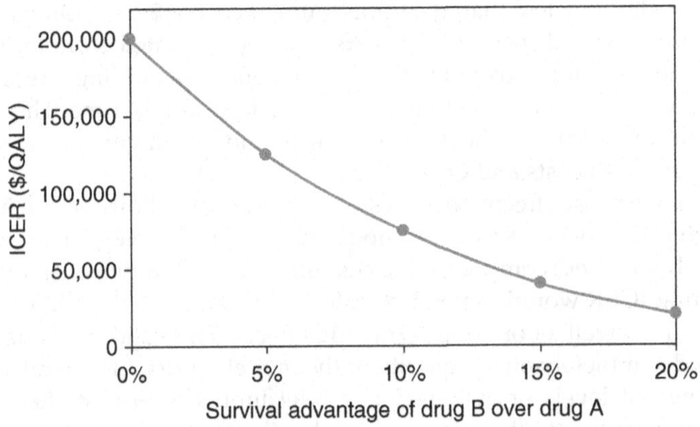

FIGURE 19.8 One-way sensitivity analysis example.

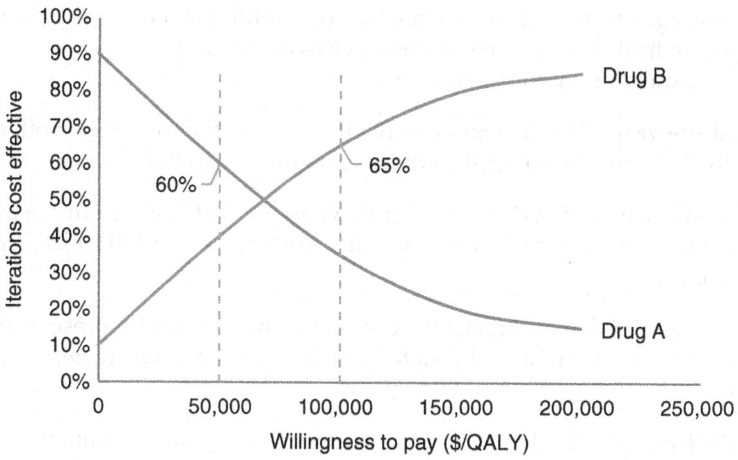

FIGURE 19.9 Acceptability curve from a probabilistic sensitivity analysis.

from these distributions introduces a degree of variability into each parameter estimate when running the cost-effectiveness model. A Monte Carlo simulation is conducted with thousands or millions of trials, with each trial representing an independent cost-effectiveness analysis using a set of parameters according to the probability distributions. The results of the Monte Carlo simulation are summarized to demonstrate the uncertainty inherent in the entire analysis.

The **acceptability curve** in Figure 19.9 shows the results from a probabilistic sensitivity analysis for a cost-effectiveness analysis comparing drug A to drug B. An attractive feature of the acceptability curve is that it allows the reader to select different willingness-to-pay thresholds and see how likely each drug would be considered cost-effective. In Figure 19.9, at a willingness-to-pay threshold of $50,000/QALY, drug A would be the cost-effective option 60% of the time. However, at a willingness to pay of $100,000/QALY, drug B would be the cost-effective option 65% of the time. As the willingness-to-pay threshold increases further, drug B becomes even more likely to be the cost-effective treatment option.

CONCLUSION

This chapter provided an overview of cost-effectiveness research and highlighted the key components involved to help a reader better understand this area of research. For additional information about cost-effectiveness research, we recommend the texts *Decision Making in Health and Medicine*, *Cost-Effectiveness in Health and Medicine*, and *Methods for the Economic Evaluation of Health Care Programmes* (26,29,30).

GLOSSARY

direct cost: expense of a procedure or treatment.

indirect cost: expense incurred in the course of obtaining a healthcare procedure or treatment that is not specifically for that procedure/treatment.

micro-costing: detailed approach to ascertaining cost; can provide precise measurements of the cost of delivering healthcare.

charge: the price that a healthcare provider sets for a given service.

activity-based costing: a technique to estimate the cost of different elements of healthcare; estimates the costs of healthcare procedures or services based on direct measurement or estimation of the resources they consume.

quality-adjusted life year (QALY): a measure of effectiveness that considers both quality of life (QOL) and survival; the product of QOL and the years lived with that QOL.

disability-adjusted life year (DALY): a standardized measure of disease burden that incorporates disability and life years lost; commonly used by the World Health Organization and lower-income countries.

health utility: a type of QOL measurement; a continuous number that represents the "preference" for being in a desired health state bounded by the anchors of zero (death) and one (perfect health).

standard gamble: technique for defining health utility; typically involves interviewing individual subjects and presenting different scenarios where subjects are asked to choose one "preferred" outcome over another.

time trade-off: secondary technique designed to capture health utilities information.

decision tree: means of determining cost-effectiveness that maps out the different options, outcomes, and costs for two treatment options. A decision tree node should lead to states that are mutually exclusive and collectively exhaustive.

decision node: decision-tree point indicating that a patient is free to choose between the two options.

chance node: decision-tree choice indicating a defined probability.

terminal node: decision-tree choice representing the end of a particular path.

incremental cost-effectiveness ratio (ICER): means of determining cost-effectiveness; represents the incremental costs divided by the incremental effectiveness.

willingness to pay: a dollar-per-QALY threshold above which treatments would not be considered cost-effective.

Markov model: a complex type of decision tree for cost-effectiveness analysis that incorporates the passage of time and transitions between different health states. This type of model is typically solved by a computer.

health disease state: a predefined condition that represents an individuals health status at any one point in time. These health states are mutually exclusive and hypothetical individuals in the model can move between different health states (for example from Healthy to Disease Recurrence). Each health state will typically have an effectiveness value assigned to it.

state transition diagram: a diagram that depicts how individuals in a model can transition between different health states.

microsimulation model: one type of modeling approach used in cost-effectiveness research.

cost-effectiveness frontier: a simple plot showing the cost on the *y*-axis, and effectiveness (QALY) on the *x*-axis.

time preference: name for the principle that individuals value costs and benefits differently at different times in their lives.

discounting: in cost-effectiveness research, the devaluation of future costs and QALYs by a set amount.

sensitivity analysis: in cost-effectiveness research, a process whereby one tests how a model responds when the assumptions are changed.

one-way sensitivity analysis: in cost-effectiveness research, a process whereby one tests how a risk in the model varies across a range and determines how this affects the ICER.model.

probabilistic sensitivity analysis: in cost-effectiveness research, the standard tool to assess how a model performs when varying all parameters simultaneously.

acceptability curve: shows the results from a probabilistic sensitivity analysis for a cost-effectiveness analysis.

REFERENCES

1. Elkin EB, Bach PB. Cancer's next frontier: addressing high and increasing costs. *JAMA*. 2010;303:1086–1087. doi:10.1001/jama.2010.283
2. Mariotto AB, Yabroff KR, Shao Y, et al. Projections of the cost of cancer care in the United States: 2010–2020. *J Natl Cancer Inst*. 2011;103:117–128. doi:10.1093/jnci/djq495
3. Social Security Administration. *Limitations on Certain Uses of Comparative Clinical Effectiveness Research*. Washington, DC: Social Security Administration; 2017.
4. Prasad V, De Jesús K, Mailankody S. The high price of anticancer drugs: origins, implications, barriers, solutions. *Nat Rev Clin Oncol*. 2017;14:381–390. doi:10.1038/nrclinonc.2017.31
5. Amin NP, Sher DJ, Konski AA. Systematic review of the cost effectiveness of radiation therapy for prostate cancer from 2003 to 2013. *Appl Health Econ Health Policy*. 2014;12:391–408. doi:10.1007/s40258-014-0106-9
6. Ramsey SD, Bansal A, Fedorenko CR, et al. Financial insolvency as a risk factor for early mortality among patients with cancer. *J Clin Oncol*. 2016;34:980–986. doi:10.1200/JCO.2015.64.6620
7. Khera N. Reporting and grading financial toxicity. *J Clin Oncol*. 2014;32:3337–3338. doi:10.1200/JCO.2014.57.8740
8. Schnipper LE, Davidson NE, Wollins DS, et al. American Society of Clinical Oncology statement: a conceptual framework to assess the value of cancer treatment options. *J Clin Oncol*. 2015;33:2563–2577. doi:10.1200/JCO.2015.61.6706
9. Black WC, Gareen IF, Soneji SS, et al. Cost-effectiveness of CT screening in the National Lung Screening Trial. *N Engl J Med*. 2014;371:1793–1802. doi:10.1056/NEJMoa1312547
10. Mehanna H, Wong WL, McConkey CC, et al. PET-CT surveillance versus neck dissection in advanced head and neck cancer. *N Engl J Med*. 2016;374:1444–1454. doi:10.1056/NEJMoa1514493
11. Bonastre J, Marguet S, Lueza B, et al. Cost effectiveness of molecular profiling for adjuvant decision making in patients with node-negative breast cancer. *J Clin Oncol*. 2014;32:3513–3519. doi:10.1200/JCO.2013.54.9931
12. Goldstein DA, Chen Q, Ayer T, et al. First- and second-line bevacizumab in addition to chemotherapy for metastatic colorectal cancer: a United States-based cost-effectiveness analysis. *J Clin Oncol*. 2015;33:1112–1118. doi:10.1200/JCO.2014.58.4904
13. Ito K, Blinder VS, Elkin EB. Cost effectiveness of fracture prevention in postmenopausal women who receive aromatase inhibitors for early breast cancer. *J Clin Oncol*. 2012;30:1468–1475. doi:10.1200/JCO.2011.38.7001
14. Park JD, Kim E, Werner RM. Inpatient hospital charge variability of U.S. hospitals. *J Gen Intern Med*. 2015;30:1627–1632. doi:10.1007/s11606-015-3352-0
15. Agency for Healthcare Research and Quality. National inpatient sample (NIS) user guide. Healthcare Cost and Utilization Project; 2014. https://www.hcup-us.ahrq.gov/db/nation/nis/NIS_Introduction_2014.jsp
16. Schousboe JT, Paudel ML, Taylor BC, et al. Estimation of standardized hospital costs from Medicare claims that reflect resource requirements for care: impact for cohort studies linked to Medicare claims. *Health Serv Res*. 2014;49:929–949. doi:10.1111/1475-6773.12151
17. Kaplan RS, Witkowski M, Abbott M, et al. Using time-driven activity-based costing to identify value improvement opportunities in healthcare. *J Healthc Manag*. 2014;59:399–412. doi:10.1097/00115514-201411000-00005
18. U.S. Department of Labor. Consumer Price Index. 2017. https://www.bls.gov/data/inflation_calculator.htm/
19. Torrance GW, Thomas WH, Sackett DL. A utility maximization model for evaluation of health care programs. *Health Serv Res*. 1972;7:118–133. https://www.ncbi.nlm.nih.gov/pmc/articles/PMC1067402/
20. Murray CJ. Quantifying the burden of disease: the technical basis for disability-adjusted life years. *Bull World Health Organ*. 1994;72:429–445. https://www.ncbi.nlm.nih.gov/pmc/articles/PMC2486718/
21. Sassi F. Calculating QALYs, comparing QALY and DALY calculations. *Health Policy Plan*. 2006;21:402–408. doi:10.1093/heapol/czl018
22. Torrance GW. Measurement of health state utilities for economic appraisal. *J Health Econ*. 1986;5:1–30. doi:10.1016/0167-6296(86)90020-2
23. Neumann PJ, Cohen JT, Weinstein MC. Updating cost-effectiveness—the curious resilience of the $50,000-per-QALY threshold. *N Engl J Med*. 2014;371:796–797. doi:10.1056/NEJMp1405158

24. Braithwaite RS, Meltzer DO, King JT, et al. What does the value of modern medicine say about the $50,000 per quality-adjusted life-year decision rule? *Med Care.* 2008;46:349–356. doi:10.1097/MLR.0b013e31815c31a7
25. Hirth RA, Chernew ME, Miller E, et al. Willingness to pay for a quality-adjusted life year: in search of a standard. *Med Decis Making.* 2000;20:332–342. doi:10.1177/0272989X0002000310
26. Hunink MGM. *Decision Making in Health and Medicine: Integrating Evidence and Values.* New York, NY: Cambridge University Press; 2001.
27. Hiligsmann M, Ethgen O, Bruyère O, et al. Development and validation of a Markov microsimulation model for the economic evaluation of treatments in osteoporosis. *Value Health.* 2009;12:687–696. doi:10.1111/j.1524-4733.2008.00497.x
28. Sanders GD, Neumann PJ, Basu A, et al. Recommendations for conduct, methodological practices, and reporting of cost-effectiveness analyses: second panel on cost-effectiveness in health and medicine. *JAMA.* 2016;316:1093–1103. doi:10.1001/jama.2016.12195
29. Neumann P, Gillian DS, Russell LS, et al. *Cost-Effectiveness in Health and Medicine.* 2nd ed. New York, NY: Oxford University Press; 2016.
30. Drummond M, Sculpher M, Claxton K, et al. *Methods for the Economic Evaluation of Health Care Programmes.* 4th ed. New York, NY: Oxford University Press; 2015.

20 Introduction to Clinical Trials

LOREN K. MELL

The National Institutes of Health (NIH) defines a **clinical trial** as:

> *"a research study in which one or more human subjects are prospectively assigned to one or more interventions (which may include placebo or other control) to evaluate the effects of those interventions on health-related biomedical or behavioral outcomes"* (1)

This is a broad definition that encompasses most forms of prospective human subjects research. As a result, clinical trials come in many sizes, shapes, and forms, with a variety of different goals. However, cancer clinical trials generally follow a hierarchy involving several phases.

Broadly speaking, clinical trials are categorized as early or late phase. The primary role of early phase clinical trials is to pilot novel therapeutic approaches, whereas the role of late phase trials is to establish the effectiveness of these therapies in specific populations. The overall goal of this hierarchy is to develop, in a stepwise manner, new approaches that can alter standards of care in the field of oncology, as safely and efficiently as possible. Canonically, **phase I** trials are for testing the safety, **phase II** trials are for testing the potential for efficacy, and **phase III** trials are for testing the benefit of novel therapies. Because they are so common, these trial designs receive the greatest emphasis, with introductory discussion of early and late phase trials in Chapter 21 and Chapter 22, respectively, which cover many basic concepts in clinical trials, as well as some technical details related to the implementation of more sophisticated clinical trial designs. Later chapters cover the applications of clinical trial designs to particular settings.

Early phase clinical trials typically involve fewer than 100 total study subjects, and include **phase 0**, **lead-in**, and **feasibility studies**, phase I and **phase IB** trials, and small phase II trials. The most common primary aim of early phase trials is to define a safe dose for subsequent testing, which is typically achieved using phase I designs. However, in certain contexts, streamlined designs are used to gather very preliminary assessments, usually with fast readout times in trials with limited sample sizes. Phase 0 trials (sometimes termed "window of opportunity" trials) are a special type of early phase trial reserved for collecting basic preliminary data in human subjects, such as pharmacokinetic (PK) and pharmacodynamic (PD) information, for highly novel therapies. Often these involve first-in-human testing and are geared toward patients with cancers that are refractory to multiple standard therapies. Phase 0 studies typically come with little expectation that the patient will directly benefit from the intervention. In addition to novel drugs, early radiopharmaceuticals, such as those used in novel imaging applications (Chapter 24), may undergo phase 0 testing.

Phase I designs play the dominant role in the initial formal testing of new treatments, and thus warrant the most attention. Although the classic 3 + 3 phase I trial design continues to be among the most common trial designs in oncology, it is known to be inefficient and suboptimal in most cases for finding the **maximum tolerated dose** (**MTD**) for subsequent phase II testing. Though it has a salient advantage of conceptual simplicity, the inefficient operating characteristics of the 3 + 3 design often sacrifice precious time needed to identify the best phase II regimen. Thus, it is strongly recommended to become acquainted with alternative phase I designs (see Chapter 21) and consider implementing them when embarking on such trials. The implementation of complicated trial designs should be approached with early input from statisticians with expertise in this area.

Phase IB trials typically are designed as extensions of a phase I trial for additional safety testing in a particular cohort, and often (though ostensibly designed to test for toxicity) to gain preliminary data on treatment response. Feasibility studies are often used in the setting when dose finding is not the primary objective, but rather, there may be questions about the ability to accrue patients belonging to rarer or more challenging populations, or in technology implementation with a highly technical and exclusive modality (e.g., novel MRI or PET applications specific to a given vendor's platform, and unconventional particle therapy delivery). The statistical plan may be loosely described for such preliminary designs, and based on achieving a fixed number of accruals (e.g., 8–12 patients) for initial analysis. In some cases, feasibility may be formally defined with a strict goal of meeting a specific **go/no-go threshold** for the next phase of testing.

Late phase clinical trials typically involve larger (>100 patient) sample sizes, and include single-arm and randomized phase II trials, randomized phase III, and **phase IV** trials, with randomized phase II and III trials being the most critical. Randomized phase II trials are frequently designed with a **surrogate endpoint** for efficacy, such as response, tumor control, or progression-free survival (PFS), which is meant to serve as a proxy marker for effects to be tested in phase III. Although sometimes criticized as an "underpowered" phase III trial, phase II designs play a central role in oncology trials, particularly when comparing novel regimens to test against the standard of care in a future phase III trial, or when background data from historical controls are considered unreliable for obtaining an unbiased efficacy estimate for a novel regimen. Further discussion of various randomized phase II designs is presented by Rubinstein et al. (2).

Often, investigators may choose to combine one or more phases into a single-trial protocol, which has the advantage of consolidating several steps and avoiding regulatory delays and administrative costs associated with opening multiple protocols. However, such designs typically involve a greater commitment of time and resources as well. Common examples of combined-phase designs include phase I/II and phase II/III trials and phase II or III trials with safety lead-ins. Phase IV trials are designed to test the integration of a new drug into widespread public use. These are generally designed by companies for postmarketing surveillance to evaluate the long-term effects of new drugs in the broader population. The so-called **phase V** trials may refer to comparative effectiveness or community-based prospective studies (Chapter 18) that do not involve monitoring of individuals (such as registry randomized trials). These latter trial designs at the extremes of the spectrum are less common and consequently receive less emphasis; for further discussion, see Mahan (3).

Choosing the primary endpoint(s) for a trial takes care and consideration. Many oncology trials will use time-to-event endpoints to evaluate effects on patient outcomes (see Chapter 16). Other times, the primary endpoint could be an incidence rate, such as for cancer screening and prevention (Chapter 24); quality of life (Chapter 23); or imaging endpoints, such as response, and positive predictive value (Chapter 25). Adaptive trial designs, including Bayesian adaptive designs, have been applied more in the areas of early phase trials or medical devices in general. The advantage and disadvantages of adaptive designs have been discussed recently

(4). Assessing noninferiority (Chapter 26) in oncology settings is also challenging, as many studies are not blinded, and the current standards for trial design may differ under Food and Drug Administration (FDA) versus NCI guidelines. For example, Zhang and colleagues designed the RTOG 1016 trial as a phase III noninferiority trial to compare radiotherapy (RT) with cisplatin versus cetuximab for patients with locoregionally advanced oropharyngeal cancer (5). The trial was designed with a 9 percentage point lower boundary (inferiority margin) at 5 years to determine whether the experimental regimen (RT/cetuximab) could be considered noninferior to the standard (RT/cisplatin) in this population. Lastly, meta-analyses of randomized trials allow the assessment of treatment effects in a more general setting, which provide additional evidence for designing future studies (6).

REGULATORY ASPECTS OF CLINICAL TRIALS

The role of **principal investigator** (**PI**) of a clinical trial is a tremendous responsibility. A **protocol PI** is the primary individual responsible for the conduct and oversight of a research project and is generally charged with protecting the rights, safety, and welfare of any human subjects that fall under the care involved in the protocol. For multicenter clinical trials, a **site PI** is usually designated as the individual responsible for research activities pertaining to the trial at a specific institution. The criteria for being eligible to serve as a PI can vary across institutions, but typically any faculty member and often research staff members as well, including postdoctoral fellows, can be PI eligible. A PI does not have to hold a medical degree; many clinical trials are overseen by nonphysician faculty members, such as clinical psychologists, medical physicists, or epidemiologists.

Many other individuals play key roles in the process of conducting a clinical trial, including (but not limited to) co-investigators, project managers, trial coordinators, research nurses, investigational pharmacists, biostatisticians, regulatory associates, protocol and data managers, data analysts, laboratory technicians, medical monitors, and auditors. These and other individuals involved with a study should be identified on the trial's **delegation log**. Many of these personnel are hired through an institution's **clinical trials office** (**CTO**), which often serves to negotiate the conduct of trials with sponsors on behalf of their affiliated PIs. If a trial is conducted through a cooperative group, the organization's headquarters will also provide additional personnel and expertise necessary for managing multicenter trials, including contracting, protocol and data management, statistical support, coverage analysts, and regulatory staff.

All study personnel, including and under the supervision of the PI, are expected to adhere to the principle of **Good Clinical Practice** (**GCP**) in human subjects research. PIs must have federal approval to serve in the role, which involves filing an FDA 1572 form, and they are expected to conduct all required training programs, such as those offered through the **Collaborative Institutional Training Initiative** (**CITI**). The PI is responsible, among other things, for reporting adverse events, ensuring the acquisition of informed consent, adhering to requirements of the protocol, guaranteeing that staff are properly trained, and supervising any third parties or subcontractors who are working on the study. Many tasks, such as informed consent and trial monitoring, however, may be delegated to approved personnel. The PI must also ensure that proper regulatory documents, including **Investigational New Drug** (**IND**) applications (or exemptions), are on file and current (see also Chapter 9).

Often, the conduct of clinical trials is carried out with the aid of a **contract research organization** (**CRO**). These are professional trial management organizations serving indispensable roles, especially in the conduct of larger multicenter and international trials. CROs can also help in developing **Standard Operating Procedures** (**SOPs**) to ensure that trials are adequately monitored for safety and adhere to Good Manufacturing Practice (GMP) and Good Laboratory Practice (GLP) guidelines. CROs also help ensure fulfillment of regulatory requirements in other countries or large federations, such as the European Union.

The FDA has broad authority to regulate U.S. investigators and any IND or device seeking regulatory approval in the United States. It holds the power to halt clinical trials and bring legal action against GCP violators, such as those that have resulted in cases of falsified trial documents and improper handling of investigational drugs. In addition, many local governing bodies regulate the conduct of clinical trials within individual institutions and organizations, such as **Institutional Review Boards (IRBs)**, **Protocol Review and Monitoring Committees (PRMCs)**, and Data Safety and Monitoring Boards (DSMBs).

An often underappreciated additional regulatory step is contracting and insurance coverage, usually overseen by the equivalent of an **Office of Contracts and Grants Administration (OCGA)** or **Office of Coverage Analysis Administration (OCAA)**, or both. These offices are empowered to delineate study-related expenditures, which are billable to the trial sponsor, and standard-of-care expenditures, which may be lawfully passed to insurers/third-party payers. In addition, contracting offices are required to approve language pertaining to intellectual property resulting from research collaborations, and ensure that institutions are properly indemnified against any risks associated with participating in clinical research, including liability resulting from harm to patients.

PRACTICAL ELEMENTS OF DESIGNING CLINICAL TRIALS

GETTING STARTED

In Chapter 9, we discussed several approaches to funding clinical trials. At the outset of a trial, there is often much excitement, but clinical trials frequently can take much longer than expected to complete due to various issues, including regulatory startup, contracting delays, protocol clarifications and amendments, slow recruitment, and waiting for primary events to occur long after recruitment is complete. Because personnel costs are a large component of the expense of a trial, as long as the trial stays active, it can quickly exceed the constraints of a standard research budget. Depending on the design, clinical trials may cost anywhere from several thousand to tens of thousands of dollars *per patient*. A reasonable starting point for trial budgeting in 2018 is an average cost of around $10,000 per patient, with higher average costs for more complex data collection and handling, and lower average costs for more streamlined study designs.

Financing a trial is a key portion of trial planning that frequently involves many iterative steps. The first step is to identify a prospective sponsor, through industry, cooperative groups, federal grants, or nonprofit foundations such as the Patient-Centered Outcomes Research Institute (PCORI). The second step is to clearly delineate your specific aims. Usually it is a good idea to draft a one-page summary that briefly describes the background motivating the project, the general outline of what you intend to accomplish, and the principal aim(s) you will specifically try to achieve (including how you will quantify your main endpoints). This can help when circulating your concept for initial review. A third initial step is to understand a brief statistical plan to test your primary hypothesis, as this is often critical for defining your sample size, and thus your budget. A last initial step is to delineate your **schedule of assessments**. This is usually presented in a tabular format that shows what items you plan to collect (rows) and when you plan to collect them (columns). It can also be helpful to flag those assessments that are standard of care (and thus should be covered by an insurer) versus those that are study related (and thus must be factored into your budget).

Once the aims, sample size, and schedule of assessments are defined, a budget for your project can be sketched or drafted. Often the personnel/staffing for your project can be supported through a CTO, which helps efficiency because it spreads out the fixed costs of hiring, training, and managing turnover of personnel across many trials. Budgeting for the costs of investigators' effort is also important, though many PIs and co-investigators end up donating a large proportion of their time to such trials to defray expenses. At some institutions, the use of large equipment or shared resources, such as biorepositories and specimen processing cores, can be effectively budgeted per usage based on a recharge system. Many biostatistics offices function this way as well, such as on an hourly rate. These systems help buffer investigators against having to make large purchases or hires for an individual use, which can be inefficient. Finally, identifying work that must be subcontracted or can be more efficiently done by a contractor with expertise (such as specialized laboratory tests) is important in the early budgeting stages.

The next step is to draft a protocol. Various templates are available online, such as through osp.od.nih.gov/clinical-research/clinical-trials or e-protocol.od.nih.gov. Also, many CTOs have protocol and **informed consent form** (**ICF**) templates that can be used to facilitate initial drafting of both key documents. Often, trainees and junior faculty have opportunities to participate in grant-writing or protocol-writing workshops sponsored through professional organizations or private foundations, such as the Vail Workshop (vailworkshop.org). Sometimes admission to such programs can be competitive, however. Another helpful do-it-yourself approach is to pick out a protocol with a similar design to what you intend to accomplish to use as a model. This can be an efficient way to design a protocol document and ensure that key elements that are pertinent to your chosen design are covered.

ANATOMY OF A PROTOCOL

The contents and organization of a **protocol** can vary substantially depending on the aims and scope of the study. However, there are several core elements in common to most protocol documents. First, the protocol face page should identify the title of the study, PI, and key co-investigators, along with their contact information and the version number and date of the protocol. The background section is an introductory section that explains the rationale for the study and its particular design, and should describe what new information the study will provide. Because many nonexperts will be reviewing your protocol and deciding whether or not it gets approved, it is wise to explain concepts simply for a more general audience, without assuming esoteric levels of expertise. This section should also clearly explain the rationale for the choice of intervention and the choice of primary, secondary, and exploratory endpoints.

Early in the protocol, one should present an overall picture of the study design, including general eligibility criteria, design, and randomization procedures. A graphical **schema** should be provided as well, especially for randomized trials; see the schema for the KEYCHAIN randomized trial in head/neck cancer (Figures 20.1 and 20.2), for example. If blinding is to be used, the specific approach (single-blinding, double-blinding, placebo, or sham (7,8) control) should be described here along with the specific processes used to guarantee concealment of the treatment assignment, as applicable. Randomized trials that do not use blinding processes, because it is either infeasible or considered unnecessary to conceal the treatment assignment, are considered **open label**. In open-label trials, especially when the primary endpoint is qualitative or subjective, the procedures used to control observer bias (such as blinding reviewers of outcomes to the treatment assignment) should be specified.

The next section should delineate and describe the primary, secondary, and exploratory aim(s), hypothesis(es), and/or **endpoints** related to the project, including how each endpoint will be defined. A primary endpoint(s) is (are) what is used to drive the sample size estimate, whereas secondary (or correlative) endpoint(s) usually correspond to nested hypotheses that can be tested with the given or smaller sample size. Exploratory endpoints are usually considered hypothesis generating and thus do not depend heavily on the existence of preliminary data, though some rationale should still be provided to justify the collection of these data.

Next follows a detailed description of the **population** and **sampling methods**, including how and where patients will be recruited and screened and what specific **inclusion** and **exclusion criteria** will be used to determine eligibility. A note on terminology: patients who are potential candidates for a trial (such as may be identified at the time of consultation or in a tumor board conference) are considered in a **prescreening** stage. Often a **waiver of consent** is provided (and required) by IRBs in order to access a patient's medical record for the

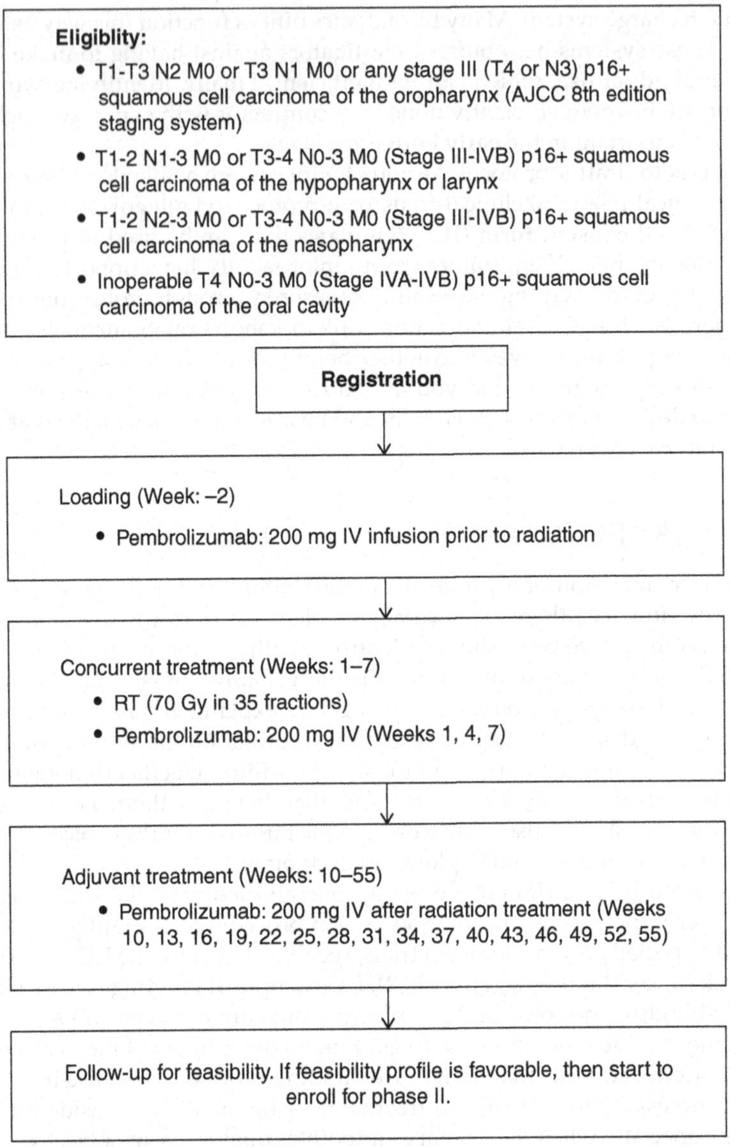
Eligiblity:
• T1-T3 N2 M0 or T3 N1 M0 or any stage III (T4 or N3) p16+ squamous cell carcinoma of the oropharynx (AJCC 8th edition staging system)
• T1-2 N1-3 M0 or T3-4 N0-3 M0 (Stage III-IVB) p16+ squamous cell carcinoma of the hypopharynx or larynx
• T1-2 N2-3 M0 or T3-4 N0-3 M0 (Stage III-IVB) p16+ squamous cell carcinoma of the nasopharynx
• Inoperable T4 N0-3 M0 (Stage IVA-IVB) p16+ squamous cell carcinoma of the oral cavity
Registration
Loading (Week: –2)
• Pembrolizumab: 200 mg IV infusion prior to radiation
Concurrent treatment (Weeks: 1–7)
• RT (70 Gy in 35 fractions)
• Pembrolizumab: 200 mg IV (Weeks 1, 4, 7)
Adjuvant treatment (Weeks: 10–55)
• Pembrolizumab: 200 mg IV after radiation treatment (Weeks 10, 13, 16, 19, 22, 25, 28, 31, 34, 37, 40, 43, 46, 49, 52, 55)
Follow-up for feasibility. If feasibility profile is favorable, then start to enroll for phase II.

FIGURE 20.1 Schema for lead-in phase of a trial of radiotherapy with concurrent and adjuvant pembrolizumab versus concurrent chemotherapy in patients with advanced/intermediate-risk p16+ head and neck squamous cell carcinoma (KEYCHAIN trial)

RT, radiotherapy.

purpose of identifying and approaching potential candidates who have not yet consented to participation. Once patients have consented to participation, they are considered to be in the **screening** stage, during which additional testing (including laboratory or pathology tests and imaging) may be required by the protocol to determine eligibility; those patients who consent to a trial but do not pass screening are considered to have **screen failed**. It is helpful to track screen failures in addition to eligible enrollees for documentation. Once a patient passes screening, she or he is considered eligible and should be **registered** to the

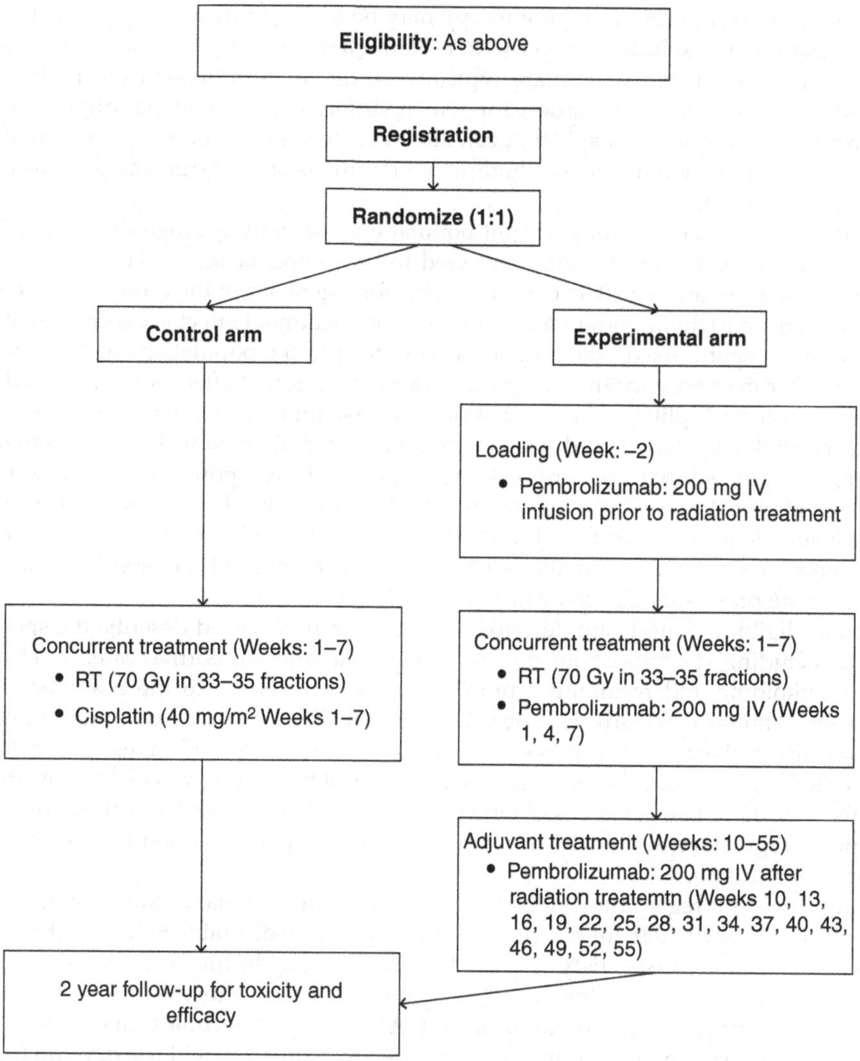

FIGURE 20.2 Schema for phase II portion of the KEYCHAIN trial.
RT, radiotherapy.

trial with a specific index date. The index or registration date is often used as the starting point for measuring key outcomes for the trial, such as survival time. Finally, patients who actively withdraw from the trial by retracting consent are considered **withdrawals**, whereas those who passively withdraw by failing to make scheduled follow-up appointments or comply with subsequent study procedures without withdrawing consent are considered **lost to follow-up**.

One important factor to consider in a trial design, particularly with respect to eligibility criteria, is the **lumping versus splitting dichotomy** (9). *Lumping* refers to the inclusion of two or more distinct groups in the study population, whereas *splitting* refers to separate handling of two or more distinct groups to comprise different study populations. In every clinical trial, some degree of lumping is necessary, because it is impossible to have every individual subject have identical characteristics. For example, often patients with both intermediate- and high-risk factors may be included in the same chemotherapy trial, or patients receiving both preoperative and postoperative chemotherapy may be included in a surgical trial. Conversely, it is often desirable to exclude patients with certain characteristics to ensure similarity in the study population; for instance, men are typically excluded from breast cancer trials, because they constitute an atypical population for which different treatment paradigms are considered appropriate. Lumping and splitting can also refer to aspects about the treatment (such as combining two or more elements of a therapeutic regimen) or to endpoints (such as combined endpoints [see Chapter 16]).

In general, the decision to lump or split populations for analysis hinges on two critical questions: (1) Are the outcome probabilities expected to be homogeneous in the groups being combined? and (2) Is the treatment effect expected to be homogeneous in the groups being combined? The latter is a particularly important assumption. If the treatment effect is expected to differ (i.e., an **interaction** is hypothesized), then it makes sense to split the populations. If the outcomes are expected to differ markedly for the two groups, but the treatment effect is not expected to differ, then either lumping or splitting the population could be appropriate, depending on the desired power for the trial (Chapter 22) and which subpopulation is dominant. The subpopulation with the higher event rate will have the greatest impact on the study's power, but if this is a rare subgroup, then it may make sense to combine them with a more abundant subpopulation in order to guarantee a sufficient rate of accrual. If both the outcome probabilities and treatment effects for the two groups are similar, then it makes sense to combine them in a trial for analysis, as the study will thus be more powerful and accrue faster.

Once the eligibility criteria are described, the next section should describe the specific treatment plan, including specifics about dosing, scheduling, and supportive care. In addition, the rules for withholding and resuming protocol therapy in response to the observed toxicity or adverse events should be clearly laid out. This also includes criteria for handling and storing any investigational therapies and processing medical waste or unused investigational drugs. In addition, criteria used to ensure compliance with protocol therapy and to define deviations from protocol therapy should be demarcated. Often, criteria for recording and reporting adverse events to appropriate regulatory authorities are established in a separate section that is specific to the investigator's institution.

In many trials, preregistration steps to ensure protocol compliance are specified, often in a separate section. In particular, for multicenter trials, it may be desirable to have a checklist of criteria that an institution must satisfy in order to participate, including any special equipment or specific imaging platforms/vendors, as well as an established history of prior protocol participation and experience with **quality assurance (QA)**. For highly technical interventions such as those used in radiology and radiation oncology, often investigators will use **dry-run** (or **dummy run**) and **wet-run** checkpoints to ensure quality control of the data (10). Dry-run steps consist of passing a series of checkpoints before any patient is enrolled, such as verification of central data transfer, whereas a wet run consists of active quality control in the initial subjects enrolled from a site, while holding accrual to ensure the QA processes and workflow are functioning properly. This may be crucial, for example, for primary endpoints like PFS that may rely heavily on a radiologist's interpretation of imaging findings, to ensure that the radiologist is familiar with the protocol guidelines.

A detailed statistical plan should be provided later in the protocol as well, which describes how the analysis on primary and secondary endpoints will be performed; the basis for the hypothesized primary treatment effect; the process used to arrive at the proposed sample size; the type I and type II errors associated with the primary and often secondary hypothesis tests; and the processes for data collection, storage, and secure handling, particularly as these pertain to **protected health information (PHI)**. Interim monitoring of safety and efficacy is also clearly described in the statistical section, for further details; see Chapter 22 on late phase trials. Lastly, the protocol should clearly identify processes used to acquire informed consent, criteria for disenrolling or withdrawing patients from the study, and procedures to ensure confidentiality and protocol compliance.

Separate from the protocol document, an ICF is required and it must explain the risks of both the investigational and standard therapy associated with the protocol, using simple (8th-grade) language. The ICF must also explain the expected outcomes with standard therapy and describe what the patient will receive if he or she opts not to participate in the trial. Any optional correlative studies should also be described, along with contact information should the patient have questions or concerns about the study. The ICF also should describe any benefits to participation, including remuneration that may offset costs or encourage participation, and general benefits to future patients from the knowledge gained by the study.

RUNNING TRIALS: THE BIG PICTURE

Conducting a clinical trial requires exceptional patience. To set realistic expectations, sometimes it is helpful to remember the PI's (unofficial) rule of 4: (1) however many patients you think you can feasibly enroll per year, divide by 4; (2) however long you think it will take to complete your study, multiply by 4; (3) for every center you need to help accrue to your study, contact 4; (4) there are 4 phases of running a trial: *denial, anger, grief,* and *acceptance*. More helpful still is to keep the larger focus on the intent of trials, which is to help advance the care of cancer patients and eventually lead us to cure(s). Occasionally, adhering to the letter of a protocol is at odds with the best interest of the patient, or what a treating physician may perceive this to be. For example, according to how a protocol is written, an adverse event could trigger withholding therapy that a physician believes should still be given, or the protocol could mandate that therapy be given even if the patient's clinical situation changes in a way not predicted in the document. As a scientist, one has a duty to adhere to the protocol, but as a physician, one's duty is to the patient. Discriminating between what constitutes a **treatment modification** (allowed) versus a **protocol deviation** (not allowed) is sometimes challenging.

Traditionally, clinical trials have been at the vanguard of defining new cancer treatments, in striving to cure historically incurable diseases. One definition of a cure is a therapy that returns the patient to her or his original, prediagnosis condition, free from both malignancy and morbidity of therapy. In this classic framework, mortality and survival are respectively equated with therapeutic failure or success. Staging systems and nomograms to predict survival are used to differentiate natural histories of cancers and match the intensity of therapy to the intensity of the disease. This is reflected in standard approaches to phase III trials that pit new against old therapies in the quest to improve overall survival. For the most recalcitrant and refractory cancers, the nature of this quest has hardly changed over many decades.

However, as patients are surviving longer, in the context of ever more effective treatments for some cancers (and other diseases), the approach to clinical trials is evolving as well. An alternative, if more cynical, definition of *cure* is a therapy that allows patients to die from something other than cancer or its treatment. Newer treatments that can suppress tumor growth and hold it in check for extended periods of time, even without completely eradicating the disease, are functionally curative therapies in this context, and mortality from noncancer causes (also called **competing mortality**, or **intercurrent mortality**, in contrast to cancer mortality and treatment-related mortality) is paradoxically viewed as a treatment *success*. Increasingly, considerations about the context of the whole patient are being implemented to risk-stratify cancer patients according to not only the severity of their cancer, but their competing risks as well (Figure 20.3) (11).

James Lind is generally credited with having conducted the first randomized trial, when he randomly subjected British sailors alternatively to citrus fruits, sulfuric acid, vinegar, cider, seawater, or nutmeg paste, in order to determine the best treatment for scurvy (12). As you will see in the coming chapters, clinical trial designs have evolved considerably in the ensuing 271 years. But the basic mission has remained constant: to subject both new and old therapies to impartial testing, on the grounds that the best medicine for patients is objective truth. Continuing along this thalassic theme, conducting clinical trials has been likened to setting sail: occasionally one encounters obstacles, and may even capsize, but to never attempt a trial is to *never set sail at all*. So happy sailing! And don't forget your vitamin C! (13)

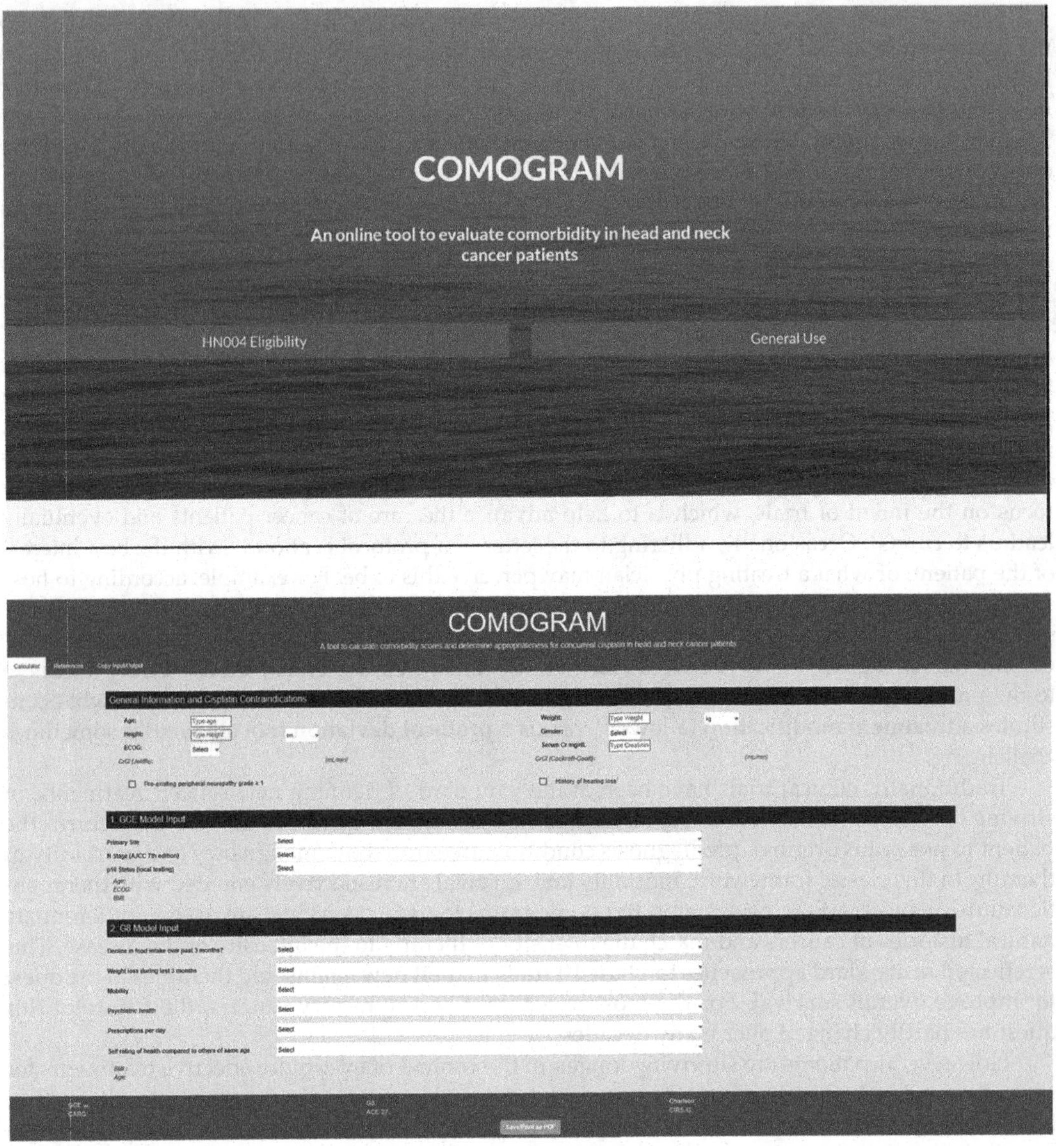

FIGURE 20.3 Website (comogram.org) to help determine a patient's likelihood to benefit from intensive therapy based on both disease-related factors that predict the risk of cancer recurrence and demographic and health characteristics that predict the risk of competing (noncancer) mortality events.

GLOSSARY

clinical trial: a research study in which one or more human subjects are prospectively assigned to one or more interventions (which may include placebo or other control) to evaluate the effects of those interventions on health-related biomedical or behavioral outcomes.

phase I trials: clinical trials for testing the safety of novel therapies.

phase II trials: clinical trials for testing the potential for efficacy of novel therapies.

phase III trials: clinical trials for testing the benefit of novel therapies.

phase 0 trial: sometimes termed "window of opportunity" trials; a special type of early phase trial reserved for collecting basic preliminary data in human subjects, such as pharmacokinetic and pharmacodynamic information, for highly novel therapies.

lead-in study: introductory study that is part of a larger phase II or phase III trial protocol, in which a fixed dose or regimen is tested initially to assure tolerability and feasibility.

feasibility study: often used when dose finding is not the primary objective, but there may be questions about the ability to accrue patients belonging to rarer or more challenging populations, or in technology implementation with a highly technical and exclusive modality.

phase IB trial: typically designed as an extension of a phase I trial for additional safety testing in a particular cohort, and often to gain preliminary data on treatment response.

maximum tolerated dose (MTD): the maximum dose at which a prespecified safety or toxicity level is assured, usually defined in order to determine a recommended phase 2 dosing schedule.

go/no-go threshold: a trial or study objective that indicates whether to proceed to the next phase of testing.

phase IV trial: a trial designed to test the integration of a new drug into widespread public use.

surrogate endpoint: a proxy marker for effects to be tested in later trials.

phase V trial: a trial that does not involve monitoring of individuals; often a comparative effectiveness or community-based prospective study.

principal investigator (PI): the individual primarily responsible for a clinical trial.

protocol PI: the primary individual responsible for the conduct and oversight of a research project; generally charged with protecting the rights, safety, and welfare of any human subjects that fall under the care involved in the protocol.

site PI: in multicenter clinical trials, the individual responsible for research activities pertaining to the trial at a specific institution.

delegation log: identifies those performing key roles in conducting a clinical trial.

clinical trials office (CTO): body that hires personnel and negotiates the conduct of trials with sponsors on behalf of affiliated PIs.

Good Clinical Practice (GCP): an international ethical and scientific quality standard for designing, conducting, recording, and reporting trials that involve the participation of human subjects.

Collaborative Institutional Training Initiative (CITI): a body that offers required training programs in GCP.

Investigational New Drug (IND): a drug or device for which U.S. regulatory approval is being sought.

contract research organization (CRO): a professional trial management organization that serves many roles, especially in the conduct of larger multicenter and international trials.

Standard Operating Procedures (SOPs): guidelines established to ensure that trials are adequately monitored for safety and adhere to GMP and GLP guidelines.

institutional review board (IRB): a local governing body that regulates the conduct of clinical trials within an individual institution or organization.

protocol review and monitoring committee (PRMC): a local governing body that regulates the scientific aspects of conducting clinical trials within an individual institution or organization.

office of contracts and grants administration (OCGA): body that oversees the regulatory step of contracting and insurance coverage for a clinical trial.

office of coverage analysis administration (OCAA): body that oversees the regulatory step of contracting and insurance coverage for a clinical trial.

schedule of assessments: part of a clinical trial protocol that shows what items investigators plan to collect and when they plan to collect those data.

informed consent form (ICF): participant document critical to a clinical trial.

protocol: the plan for conduct of a clinical trial.

schema: a graphic depiction of the study design of a clinical trial.

open label: describes a randomized trial that does not use blinding processes.

endpoint: a defined stopping point in a study/trial design.

population: the group of individuals from which study subjects is sampled and to which the results of a study are intended to apply.

sampling method: way in which a trial or study population is selected.

inclusion and exclusion criteria: rules governing who will be considered eligible for participation in a trial or study.

prescreening: stage of a trial or study at which potential candidates are considered.

waiver of consent: document needed to access a patient's medical record for the purpose of identifying potential study or trial candidates.

screening: study/trial protocol stage at which testing for eligibility is done.

screen failed: describes a patient who does not pass screening for a study/trial.

registered: enrolled in a study/trial.

withdrawal: patient who actively leaves a trial/study by retracting consent.

lost to follow-up: describes a patient who passively withdraws from a study/trial by failing to continue participation.

lumping versus splitting dichotomy: trial-design problem regarding eligibility criteria that concerns grouping of participants.

interaction: when a treatment effect differs according to the presence of a given factor or variable.

treatment plan: portion of a trial/study protocol that includes specifics about dosing, scheduling, and supportive care.

preregistration steps: portion of a trial/study protocol that includes specifics about institutional participation to ensure protocol compliance.

quality assurance (QA): trial/study requirements for ensuring proper protocol adherence and valid data gathering.

dry run: test of checkpoints to ensure quality control done before any patient is enrolled.

wet run: active quality control testing, done with the initial subjects in a trial/study while holding accrual to ensure that the QA processes and workflow are functioning properly.

protected health information (PHI): confidential patient data.

treatment modification: permissible variation from a trial protocol for a particular patient/participant.

protocol deviation: impermissible variation from a trial protocol for a particular patient/participant.

competing mortality (intercurrent mortality): death from a cause not related to the disease or treatment at issue in a trial/study.

REFERENCES

1. National Institute of Health. NIH's definition of a clinical trial. https://grants.nih.gov/policy/clinical-trials/definition.htm. Updated August 8, 2017.
2. Rubinstein L, Crowley J, Ivy P, et al. Randomized phase II designs. *Clin Cancer Res.* 2009;15(6):1883–1890. doi:10.1158/1078-0432.CCR-08-2031
3. Mahan VL. Clinical trial phases. *Int J Clin Exp Med.* 2014;5:1374–1383. doi:10.4236/ijcm.2014.521175
4. Korn EL, Freidlin B. Adaptive clinical trials: advantages and disadvantages of various adaptive design elements. *J Natl Cancer Inst.* 2017;109(6). doi:10.1093/jnci/djx013
5. Radiation Therapy Oncology Group. https://www.rtog.org/ClinicalTrials/ProtocolTable/StudyDetails.aspx?action=openFile&FileID=8629. 2018.
6. Lacas B, Bourhis J, Overgaard J, et al. Role of radiotherapy fractionation in head and neck cancers (MARCH): an updated meta-analysis. *Lancet Oncol.* 2017;18(9):1221–1237. doi:10.1016/s1470-2045(17)30458-8
7. Lu W, Wayne PM, Davis RB, et al. Acupuncture for chemoradiation therapy-related dysphagia in head and neck cancer: a pilot randomized sham-controlled trial. *Oncologist.* 2016;21(12):1522–1529. doi:10.1634/theoncologist.2015-0538
8. Greenlee H, Crew KD, Capodice J, et al. Randomized sham-controlled pilot trial of weekly electro-acupuncture for the prevention of taxane-induced peripheral neuropathy in women with early stage breast cancer. *Breast Cancer Res Treat.* 2016;156(3):453–464. doi:10.1007/s10549-016-3759-2
9. Mell LK, Zakeri K, Rose BS. On lumping, splitting, and the nosology of clinical trial populations and end points. *J Clin Oncol.* 2014;32(10):1089–1090. doi:10.1200/JCO.2013.54.4429
10. Davis JB, Reiner B, Dusserre A, et al. EORTC. Quality assurance of the EORTC trial 22911. A phase III study of post-operative external radiotherapy in pathological stage T3N0 prostatic carcinoma: the dummy run. *Radiother Oncol.* 2002;64(1):65–73. doi:10.1016/S0167-8140(02)00143-3
11. Vitzthum L, Noticewala SS, Hines P, et al. A web-based tool to compare comorbidity models and geriatric risk-assessment in head and neck cancer patients (abstr.). *Int J Radiat Oncol Biol Phys.* 2017;99(2):E379. doi:10.1016/j.ijrobp.2017.06.1508
12. Chalmers I. The development of fair tests of treatments. *Lancet.* 2014;383(9930):1713–1714. doi:10.1016/S0140-6736(14)60821-7
13. Bjelakovic G, Nikolova D, Gluud LL, et al. Antioxidant supplements for prevention of mortality in healthy participants and patients with various diseases. *Cochrane Database Syst Rev.* 2012;(3):CD007176. doi:10.1002/14651858.cd007176

21

Early Phase Clinical Trials

YING YUAN ■ YANHONG ZHOU ■ JACK J. LEE

SINGLE-AGENT PHASE I STUDY DESIGNS

The objective of most phase I oncology trials is to find the **maximum tolerated dose** (**MTD**), which is defined as the dose with the **dose-limiting toxicity** (**DLT**) probability closest to the target DLT rate. Phase I trials are critically important for determining the MTD for further investigation in subsequent phase II or III trials. Misidentification of the MTD could result in treating a large number of patients at excessively toxic doses in later phase trials, or discarding a treatment that actually is effective by incorrectly deeming it to be too toxic. Numerous phase I trial designs have been proposed to find the MTD. These designs are generally classified into algorithm-based designs, model-based designs, and **model-assisted designs** (1–3).

ALGORITHM-BASED DESIGNS

Algorithm-based designs use a set of simple, prespecified rules (an algorithm) to determine the dose escalation and de-escalation, without assuming any model on the dose–toxicity curve. The most widely used algorithm-based design is the **3 + 3 design**. The so-called 3 + 3 design actually is a family of designs, including numerous variations. Figure 21.1 shows two commonly used versions of the 3 + 3 design: one targeting the MTD with the DLT rate ≤1/6, and the other targeting the MTD with the DLT rate ≤2/6.

A key consideration in selecting a phase I trial design is its **operating characteristics**. This term refers to several key aspects of the chosen design, such as the probability of correctly selecting the MTD, the probability of dose escalation and de-escalation, and the probability of overdosing patients. It has long been widely known that the 3 + 3 design has relatively poor operating characteristics (e.g., no specific target toxicity rate, poor accuracy to identify the MTD, and a greater tendency to underdose patients). Nonetheless, the 3 + 3 design is still widely used in practice, primarily because it is easy to implement. As we show later, however, model-assisted designs (e.g., the Bayesian optimal interval [BOIN] design) can be implemented as simply and easily as the 3 + 3 design. Therefore, the classic 3 + 3 design has been falling out of favor compared to more novel phase I designs.

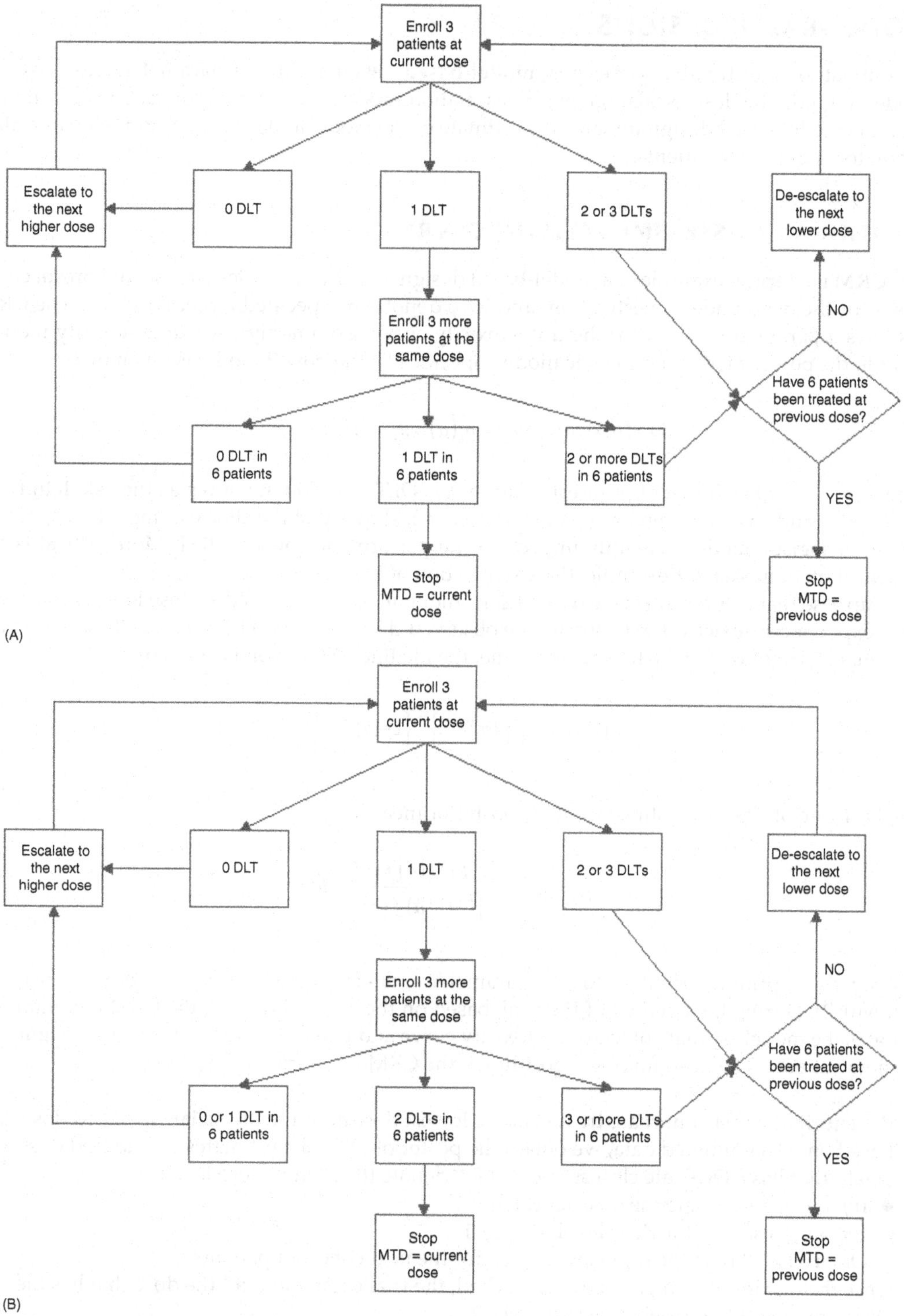

FIGURE 21.1 Two different versions of the 3 + 3 design: (A) a 3 + 3 design targeting the MTD with the DLT rate ≤1/6; (B) a 3 + 3 design targeting the MTD with the DLT rate ≤2/6.

DLT, dose-limiting toxicity; MTD, maximum tolerated dose.

MODEL-BASED DESIGNS

In contrast to algorithm-based designs, **model-based designs** utilize a **parametric** dose–toxicity model to guide the dose escalation and de-escalation process. As information accrues during the trial, the model-based design updates the estimate of the model and uses it to guide the dose allocation for subsequent patients.

CONTINUAL REASSESSMENT METHOD (CRM)

The **CRM** is a typical example of a model-based design. Let $(d_1, \ldots, d_J)$ denote a set of J prespecified doses for the drug under investigation, and let ϕ denote the specified target DLT rate. The CRM assumes a parametric model for the dose–toxicity curve. Commonly used dose–toxicity models include the power model and logistic model. Specifically, the power model is given by

$$Pr\left(\text{toxicity at}\, d_j\right) = p_j(a) = \pi_j^{exp(a)}, j = 1, \cdots J \tag{1}$$

where $(\pi_1, \ldots, \pi_J)$ is the set of prior estimates of the DLT rates (often known as the "**skeleton**") at the J doses, and a is an unknown parameter. Research shows that the choice of model (e.g., power model or logistic model) has little impact on the performance of the CRM. More critical is the specification of model, for example, the specification of the skeleton.

Suppose that at a certain stage of the trial, among n_j patients treated at dose level j, y_j patients have experienced toxicity. Let D denote the observed data, $D = \{(n_j, y_j), j = 1, \ldots, J\}$. Based on the binomial distribution for the toxicity outcome, the likelihood function is given by

$$L(D \mid a) = \prod_{j=1}^{J} \left\{\pi_j^{\exp(a)}\right\}^{y_j} \left\{1 - \pi_j^{\exp(a)}\right\}^{n_j - y_j}$$

The DLT rate of dose d_j is estimated by its posterior mean

$$\hat{p}_j = \int \pi_j^{\exp(a)} \frac{L(D \mid a) f(a)}{\int L(D \mid a) f(a) da} da$$

where $f(a)$ is a prior distribution for the parameter a, often assumed to follow a normal distribution $N(0; 2)$. During the conduct of the trial, based on the accrued data D, the CRM continuously updates the model estimate of the dose–toxicity curve and makes the decision of dose assignment for new patients. The dose-finding algorithm of the CRM is described as follows:

1. Patients in the first cohort are treated at the lowest dose d_1 or the physician-specified dose.
2. Based on the cumulated data, we obtain the posterior DLT rate estimates $\hat{p}_j$, and find dose level j^* that has a DLT rate closest to ϕ. Let j^{curr} denote the current dose level:
   - If $j^* < j^{curr}$, de-escalate the dose level to $j^{curr} - 1$
   - If $j^* > j^{curr}$, escalate the dose level to $j^{curr} + 1$
   - Otherwise, stay at the same level as j^{curr} for the next cohort of patients
3. Once the maximum sample size N is reached, the trial completes and the dose that has the DLT rate closest to ϕ is selected as the MTD.

In practice, for patient safety, we often impose an early stopping rule such that if $Pr(\text{toxicity at } d_1 > \phi \mid D) > 0.9$, the trial is terminated.

Numerous studies show that the CRM has a substantially better performance than the 3 + 3 design; however, the use of the CRM remains limited due to several reasons. Because of statistical and computational complexity of the CRM, it remains a challenge to communicate to clinical investigators how the design works, leading them to perceive dose allocations as coming from a "black box." In addition, from the methodological viewpoint, as a model-based approach, although generally robust, the CRM is still subject to the influence of model misspecification.

To obtain good operating characteristics, the CRM model (e.g., the skeleton) must be appropriately calibrated, which is challenging and requires extensive statistical expertise. To simplify the model calibration, Lee and Cheung (4) proposed a systematic method to generate a "default" skeleton for the CRM. Their method requires users to specify only a half width of **indifference interval** and the prior location of the MTD, and can be easily done using the "getprior()" function in the R package "dfcrm." Note that the indifference interval for a given dose level is defined as an interval of DLT rates associated with the neighboring doses, such that these neighboring doses may be selected instead of the true MTD.

Lee and Cheung's method simplifies the specification of the skeleton, but does not resolve the sensitivity issue of the CRM pertaining to model misspecification. Table 21.1 shows the simulation results of the CRM with two different skeletons, skeleton 1 = (0.070, 0.127, 0.200, 0.286, 0.377, 0.468) and skeleton 2 = (0.012, 0.069, 0.200, 0.380, 0.560, 0.706), generated by using the method of Lee and Cheung with a half width of indifference intervals of 0.04 and 0.08, respectively. We can see that skeleton 1 substantially outperforms skeleton 2 in scenario 1, whereas the result is opposite in scenario 2. In other words, a skeleton works well in one scenario but it may not work that well in another scenario, and there does not exist a single "best" skeleton that dominates all others.

BAYESIAN MODEL-AVERAGING CRM (BMA-CRM)

The **BMA-CRM** proposed by Yin and Yuan (5) provides a novel approach to improve the robustness of the CRM to the choice of skeleton. The BMA-CRM prespecifies multiple skeletons, each of which leads to a CRM model of the form in **(1)** with a different set of π_j's. The idea is to let the data tell which skeleton or model fits the data better and automatically favor that model as the basis for making the decision to escalate or de-escalate dose. The details of BMA-CRM are provided in the Appendix.

Yin and Yuan (5) also described a closely related approach that uses the Bayesian model selection to pick the best fitted skeleton to guide the dose escalation and de-escalation, described further in the Appendix. As shown in Table 21.1, the BMA-CRM is more reliable than the CRM. The performance of the BMA-CRM is close to that of the CRM with the better skeleton in both scenarios 1 and 2. Such robustness and reliability are important because in practice we often prefer a method that yields reliable performance to a method that has high variability (i.e., performs well in one scenario but not in another scenario).

MODEL-ASSISTED DESIGNS

Recently, there has been increasing interest in a new class of designs that combine the simplicity of algorithm-based designs and the performance of model-based designs. Following Yan et al. (3) and Zhou et al. (6), we refer to this new class of designs as the **model-assisted designs**. Similar to a model-based design, a model-assisted design utilizes a statistical model (e.g., mostly the binomial model) to derive the design. Like an algorithm-based design, the model-assisted design's rule of dose escalation and de-escalation can be pretabulated before the onset of the trial. Examples of model-assisted designs include the **modified toxicity probability interval (mTPI)** design (7), **BOIN** design (8,9), and **Keyboard** design (3). In what follows, we introduce these three mode-assisted designs, and the comparison of their performance is provided later in the chapter.

TABLE 21.1 THE PERFORMANCE OF THE CRM AND BMA-CRM WITH TWO DIFFERENT SKELETONS GENERATED WITH HALF INDIFFERENCE INTERVALS OF 0.04 AND 0.08. THE TARGET TOXICITY RATE Φ = 0.2 AND SAMPLE SIZE *N* = 36

Scenario 1							
True DLT rate		0.03	0.04	0.05	0.06	0.07	0.20
CRM with skeleton 1	% sel	0	0.10	1.25	3.85	21.05	73.20
	#pts	1.5	1.7	2.2	3.5	8.0	18.8
CRM with skeleton 2	% sel	0.05	1.35	5.70	8.10	28.25	56.40
	#pts	1.5	2.2	3.4	5.2	10.1	13.4
BMA-CRM	% sel	0	0.25	2.45	5.65	21.8	69.6
	#pts	1.5	1.9	2.7	3.9	8.6	17.4
Scenario 2							
True DLT rate		0.12	0.24	0.33	0.60	0.70	0.80
CRM with skeleton 1	% sel	35.15	43.50	10.45	0.25	0	0
	#pts	13.9	12.2	5.2	1.2	0.3	0.1
CRM with skeleton 2	% sel	30.6	53.1	11.15	0	0	0
	#pts	12.3	15.1	6.1	1.0	0.1	0
BMA-CRM	% sel	32.3	49.85	10.05	0	0	0
	#pts	12.7	14.3	5.5	1.0	0.3	0.1

% sel, the selection percentage at each dose; #pts, the average number of patients treated at each dose level; BMA-CRM, Bayesian model-averaging CRM; CRM, continual reassessment method; DLT, dose-limiting toxicity.

mTPI DESIGN

The mTPI design starts by defining three dosing intervals: the underdosing interval $(0, \delta_1)$, proper dosing interval (δ_1, δ_2), and overdosing interval $(\delta_2, 1)$. For example, given the target DLT rate of 0.2, the three intervals may be respectively defined as (0, 0.15), (0.15, 0.25), and (0.25, 1) in terms of the DLT rate. Suppose that at the current dose level j, y_j of n_j patients have experienced toxicity. The mTPI design assumes that y_j follows a beta-binomial model:

$$y_j \mid n_j, p_j \sim \text{Binom}(n_j, p_j) \qquad (2)$$
$$p_j \sim \text{Beta}(a, b).$$

Then, the posterior distribution of p_j is given by

$$p_j \mid (y_j, n_j) \sim \text{Beta}\ (y_j + a, n_j - y_j + b), \text{ for } j = 1, \ldots, J \tag{3}$$

Let $D_j = (y_j, n_j)$ denote the "local" data observed at dose level j. The mTPI design makes decisions on dose escalation and de-escalation based on the unit probability mass (UPM) of the three intervals, defined as

$$\text{UPM}_{(0,\delta_1)} = \Pr\left(p_j \in (0,\delta_1) \mid D_j\right) / \delta_1$$

$$\text{UPM}_{(\delta_1,\delta_2)} = \Pr\left(p_j \in (\delta_1,\delta_2) \mid D_j\right) / (\delta_2 - \delta_1)$$

$$\text{UPM}_{(\delta_2,1)} = \Pr\left(p_j \in (\delta_2,1) \mid D_j\right) / (1 - \delta_2).$$

That is, given a specific dosing interval, the UPM is defined as the posterior probability of an interval, for which the DLT rate falls, divided by the length of the interval.

For treating the next patient, the dose escalation and de-escalation rules of the mTPI design are given in the following:

- Escalate the dose if $\text{UPM}_{(0,\delta_1)}$ (i.e., the UPM of the underdosing interval) is the largest.
- De-escalate the dose if $\text{UPM}_{(\delta_2,1)}$ (i.e., the UPM of the overdosing interval) is the largest.
- Stay at the same dose if $\text{UPM}_{(\delta_1,\delta_2)}$ (i.e., the UPM of the proper dosing interval) is the largest.

The mTPI design stops the trial when the maximum sample size N is reached. The MTD is selected based on $\tilde{p}_j$, the isotonically (i.e., nondecreasing) transformed values of the observed DLT rates $\hat{p}_j$'s. Specifically, we select the MTD as dose j^*, for which the isotonic estimate of DLT rate $\tilde{p}_{j^*}$ is closest to the target DLT rate ϕ. If there are ties for $\tilde{p}_{j^*}$, we select from the ties the highest dose level when $\tilde{p}_{j^*} < \phi$ or the lowest dose level when $\tilde{p}_{j^*} > \phi$. The isotonic estimates $\tilde{p}_j$ can be obtained by applying the pool adjacent violators algorithm (PAVA) (10) to $\hat{p}_j$. Operatively, the PAVA replaces any adjacent $\hat{p}_j$ that violates the nondecreasing order by their (weighted) average so that the resulting estimates $\tilde{p}_j$ become monotonic. In the case in which the observed DLT rates are monotonic, $\tilde{p}_j$ and $\hat{p}_j$ are equivalent.

Because the decision as to dose escalation and de-escalation is made using only the local data at the current dose, the mTPI design may oscillate between two adjacent doses for which one is safe and the other is toxic. To avoid such undesirable behavior, a dose exclusion/safety stopping rule is included in the mTPI design:

If $Pr(p_j > \phi \mid D_j) > 0.95$, d_j and higher doses are excluded from the trial, and the trial is terminated if the lowest dose level is excluded.

One attractive feature of the mTPI design is that its decision rule can be precalculated for each possible $n_j = 1, \ldots, N$. This feature makes the mTPI design easy to implement in practice. However, one serious deficiency of the mTPI design is that it has a high risk of overdosing patients. For example, given the target DLT rate of 0.3, even when we observe that DLT rate is $3/6 = 0.5$ (50% of patients experienced toxicity), the mTPI design will continue to treat the next cohort of patients at the same dose, which is intuitively excessively risky. The aggressiveness of the mTPI design stems from its use of the UPM as the criterion to determine dose escalation. To see this problem, consider a trial for which the target DLT rate is 0.2, and the underdosing, proper dosing, and overdosing intervals are (0, 0.17), (0.17, 0.23), and (0.23,1), respectively. Suppose that at a certain stage of the trial, the observed data indicate that the posterior probabilities of the underdosing interval, proper dosing interval, and overdosing interval are 0.01, 0.09, and 0.9, respectively. That is, there is 90%

chance that the current dose is overdosing patients and only 9% chance that the current dose provides proper dosing. Despite such dominant evidence of overdosing, the mTPI design retains the same dose for treating the next new patient because the UPM for the proper dosing interval is the largest. Specifically, the UPM for the proper dosing interval is 0.09/(0.23–0.17) = 1.5, and the UPM for the overdosing interval is 0.9/(1–0.23) = 1.17. This example demonstrates that the UPM cannot appropriately quantify the evidence of overdosing.

KEYBOARD DESIGN

Yan et al. (3) proposed the Keyboard design to address the overdosing issue of the mTPI design. Unlike the mTPI design, which divides the DLT rates into three intervals (i.e., underdosing, proper dosing, and overdosing), the Keyboard design defines a series of equal-width dosing intervals (referred to as "keys") that correspond to all potential locations of the true toxicity of a particular dose, and using the key with the highest posterior probability to guide dose escalation and de-escalation. Figure 21.2 contrasts the Keyboard design with the mTPI design. Guo et al. (11) proposed a modified mTPI design called mTPI-2. Although taking a different theoretical viewpoint, the mTPI-2 is virtually the same as the Keyboard design. Nevertheless, the Keyboard design is more transparent and easier to understand.

Specifically, the Keyboard design starts by specifying a proper dosing interval $I^* = (\delta_1, \delta_2)$, referred to as the "target key," and then populates this interval toward both sides of the target key, forming a series of keys of equal width. The keys span the range of 0 to 1. For example, given the proper dosing interval or target key of (0.25, 0.35), on its left side, we form two keys of width 0.1, that is, (0.15, 0.25) and (0.05, 0.15); and on its right side, we form six keys of width 0.1, that is, (0.35, 0.45), (0.45, 0.55), (0.55, 0.65), (0.65, 0.75), (0.75, 0.85), and (0.85, 0.95). We denote the resulting intervals/keys as $I_1, \ldots, I_K$. As all keys have equal width and must be within [0, 1], some DLT rate values at the two ends (e.g., <0.05 or >0.95 in the example) may not be covered by keys because the two ends are not long enough to form a key. As explained in Yan et al. (3), ignoring these "residual" DLT rates at the two ends does not pose any issue for decision making regarding dose escalation and de-escalation.

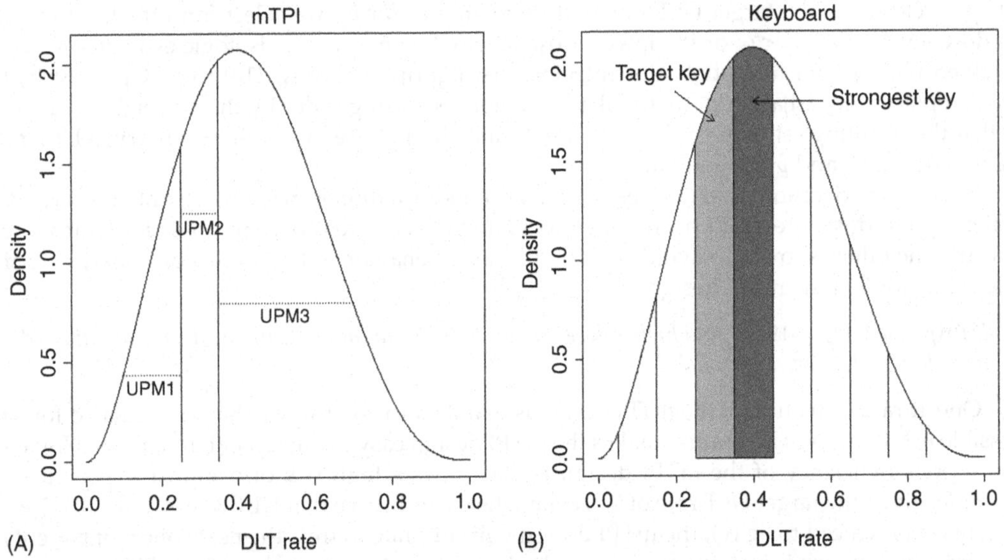

FIGURE 21.2 Contrast between (A) the mTPI design and (B) the Keyboard design. The curves are the posterior distributions of p_j. To determine the next dose, the mTPI design compares the values of the three UPMs, whereas the Keyboard design compares the location of the strongest key with respect to the target key.

mTPI, modified toxicity probability interval; UPM, unit probability mass.

To make the decision of dose escalation and de-escalation, given the observed data $D_j = (n_j, y_j)$ at the current dose level j, the Keyboard design identifies the interval I_{max} that has the largest posterior probability, that is,

$$\underset{I_1,\cdots,I_k}{\operatorname{argmax}}\left\{\Pr\left(p_j \in I_k \mid D_j\right);k=1,\cdots,K\right\}$$

which can easily be evaluated based on p_j's posterior distribution given by equation (3), assuming that p_j follows a beta-binomial model (equation [2]).

I_{max} represents the interval in which the true value of p_j is most likely to be located; this is referred to as the "strongest" key by Yan et al. (3). Graphically, the strongest key is the one with the largest area under the posterior distribution curve of p_j (see Figure 21.2B). If the strongest key is on the left (or right) side of the target key, that means that the observed data suggest that the current dose is most likely to represent underdosing (or overdosing), and thus dose escalation (or de-escalation) is needed. If the strongest key is the target key, the observed data support that the current dose is most likely to be in the proper dosing interval, and thus it is desirable to retain the current dose for treating the next patient. In contrast, the UPM used by the mTPI design does not have such an intuitive interpretation and tends to distort the evidence for overdosing, as described previously.

Suppose j^{curr} is the current dose level. The Keyboard design determines the next dose as follows:

- If the strongest key is on the left side of the target key, escalate the dose to level $j^{curr} + 1$.
- If the strongest key is the target key, retain the current dose level j^{curr}.
- If the strongest key is on the right side of the target key, de-escalate the dose to level $j^{curr} - 1$.

The trial continues until the prespecified sample size is exhausted. The MTD is selected based on $\tilde{p}_j$, the isotonically transformed values of the observed DLT rate ($\hat{p}_j$). In the Keyboard design, the dose exclusion/safety stopping rule, as described for mTPI design, is also used to prevent the dose finding from oscillating between two adjacent doses, and to stop the trial if the lowest dose is toxic.

Similar to the mTPI design, the Keyboard design pretabulates the decision rule for each possible $n_j = 1, \ldots, N$, making it easy to implement in practice. As the location of the strongest key approximately indicates the mode of the posterior distribution of p_j, the Keyboard design can be viewed as a posterior-mode-based Bayesian dose-finding method. This makes the Keyboard design a new method different from the UPM-based mTPI design, despite some structural similarity (e.g., partitioning the DLT rates into intervals and pretabulating the decision rule) between two designs.

Berger (12) showed that decision making based on the mode of the posterior distribution is optimal under the 0-1 loss, providing the statistical justification for the Keyboard design. Yan et al. (3) showed that the Keyboard design substantially outperforms the mTPI, especially in terms of overdose control, thereby providing a useful upgrade to the mTPI design.

BOIN DESIGN

Compared to the mTPI and Keyboard designs, which require specifying the prior distribution of p_j and calculating p_j's posterior for each possible data pattern of (n_j, y_j), the BOIN design is more transparent and straightforward. Under the BOIN design, the dose escalation/de-escalation decision involves only a simple comparison of the DLT rate at the current dose with a pair of fixed, prespecified dose **escalation and de-escalation boundaries**. Specifically, let $\hat{p}_j = y_j / n_j$ denote the observed DLT rate at the current dose, and λ_e and λ_d denote prespecified dose escalation and de-escalation boundaries. The BOIN design is illustrated in Figure 21.3 and described as follows:

1. Patients in the first cohort are treated at the lowest dose d_1, or the physician-specified dose.

2. Assuming that the current dose level for treating the latest cohort of patients is j^{curr}, to assign a dose to the next cohort of patients:
   - Escalate the dose to level $j^{curr} + 1$ if $\hat{p}_j \leq \lambda_e$.
   - De-escalate the dose to level $j^{curr} - 1$ if $\hat{p}_j \geq \lambda_d$.
   - Otherwise, retain the current dose.
3. Repeat step 2 until the maximum sample size N is reached. At that point, select the MTD based on the isotonic estimates of DLT rates as described previously for the mTPI design.

During the trial conduct, the BOIN design imposes a dose elimination (or overdose control) rule as follows: if $\Pr(p_j > \phi \mid D_j) > 0.95$ and $n_j \geq 3$, dose level j and higher are eliminated from the trial, and the trial is terminated if the lowest dose level is eliminated, where $\Pr(p_j > \phi \mid D_j)$ is evaluated based on the posterior distribution (3). The model-assisted component of the BOIN design is reflected by how the escalation and de-escalation boundaries (λ_e, λ_d) are derived. Specifically, the BOIN assumes that at the current dose level j, the number of patients experiencing the DLT (y_j) follows a binomial model:

$$y_j \mid n_j, p_j \sim \text{Binom}(n_j, p_j)$$

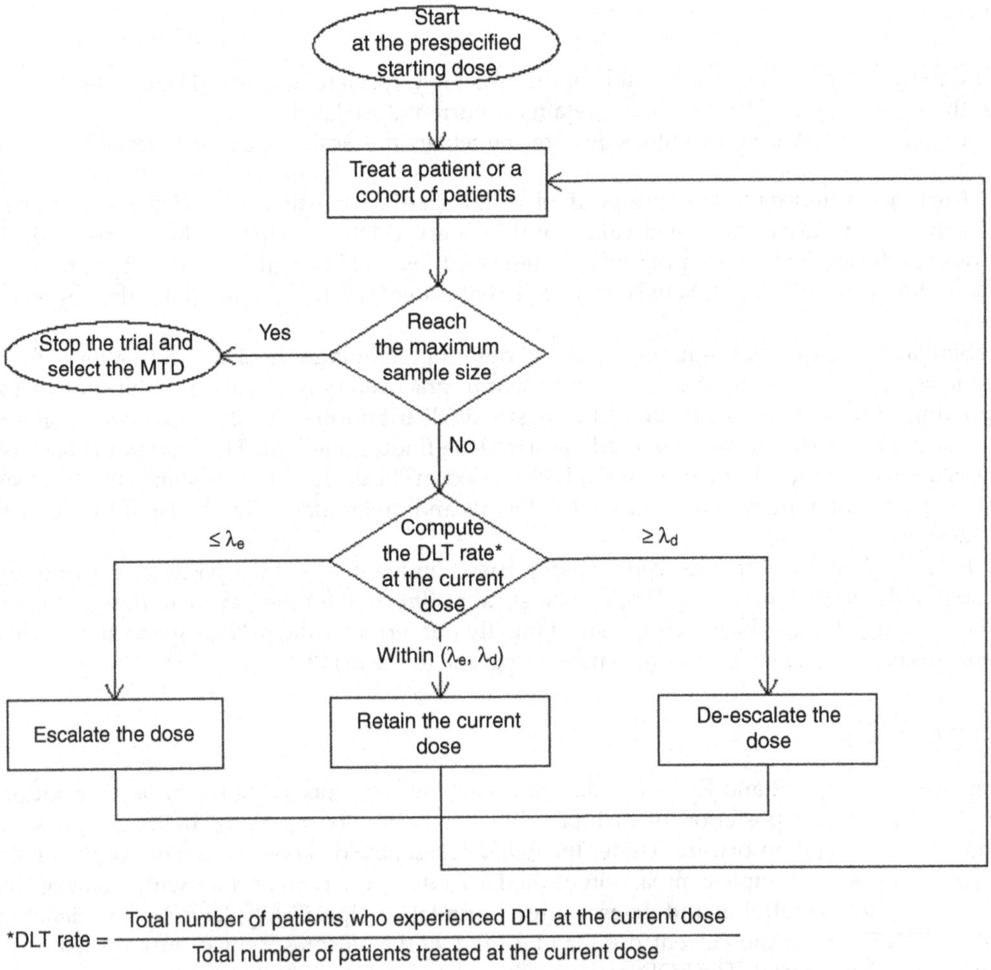

FIGURE 21.3 The flowchart of the BOIN design.

BOIN, Bayesian optimal interval; DLT, dose-limiting toxicity; MTD, maximum tolerated dose.

Under this model assumption, the BOIN minimizes the incorrect decision of dose escalation and de-escalation based on three point hypotheses: H_1: $p_j = \phi$; H_2: $p_j = \phi_1$; H_3: $p_j = \phi_2$, where ϕ_1 denotes the highest DLT rate that is deemed subtherapeutic (i.e., underdosing) such that dose escalation should be made, and ϕ_2 denotes the lowest DLT rate that is deemed overly toxic (i.e., overdosing) such that dose de-escalation is required.

Liu and Yuan (8) recommend that the default values be used as $\phi_1 = 0.6\phi$, $\phi_2 = 1.4\phi$, which generally yield a design with good operating characteristics. Alternatively, the values of ϕ_1 and ϕ_2 can be calibrated to achieve a particular requirement of the trial at hand. For example, if a more conservative dose escalation is required, then setting $\phi_2 = 1.2\phi$ may be adequate. In general, the optimal escalation and de-escalation boundaries (λ_e, λ_d) arise as

$$\lambda_e = \frac{\log\left(\dfrac{1-\phi_1}{1-\phi}\right)}{\log\left\{\dfrac{\phi(1-\phi_1)}{\phi_1(1-\phi)}\right\}}, \quad \lambda_d = \frac{\log\left(\dfrac{1-\phi}{1-\phi_2}\right)}{\log\left\{\dfrac{\phi_2(1-\phi)}{\phi(1-\phi_2)}\right\}},$$

which minimize the decision error of dose escalation and de-escalation.

Table 21.2 provides the dose escalation and de-escalation boundaries (λ_e, λ_d) for commonly used target DLT rate ϕ with the recommended default values $\phi_1 = 0.6\phi$, and $\phi_2 = 1.4\phi$. For example, given $\phi = 0.3$, the corresponding escalation and de-escalation boundaries are $\lambda_e = 0.236$ and $\lambda_d = 0.358$, respectively. Interestingly, in this case, the 3 + 3 rule is nested within the BOIN design. That is, escalate/de-escalate/retain the current dose if 0/3 or 2/3 or 1/3 patients have DLT. This feature of the BOIN design links it to established phase I approaches, and thus also facilitates the communication with clinicians.

Operatively and conceptually, the BOIN design is simpler and more transparent than the mTPI and Keyboard designs. To make the decision of dose escalation and de-escalation, the BOIN design simply compares the observed DLT rate $\hat{p}_j$ with a pair of fixed escalation and de-escalation boundaries (λ_e, λ_d), whereas the Keyboard and mTPI designs require calculating the posterior distribution and identifying the "strongest" key and UPM, respectively, for each possible outcome data (n_j, y_j), though these evaluations and corresponding decision boundaries can be calculated prior to the onset of the trial. In addition, thanks to the feature through which the BOIN design guarantees de-escalating the dose when the observed toxicity rate $\hat{p}_j$ is higher than the de-escalation boundary λ_d, it is particularly easy for clinicians and regulatory agents to assess the safety of a trial using the BOIN design. For example, given a target DLT rate $\phi = 0.25$, we know a priori that a phase I trial using the BOIN design guarantees de-escalating the dose if the observed DLT rate is higher than 0.298. Accordingly, the BOIN design also allows users to easily calibrate the design to satisfy a specific safety requirement mandated by regulatory agents by choosing an appropriate target DLT rate ϕ.

TABLE 21.2 THE ESCALATION/DE-ESCALATION BOUNDARIES (λ_e, λ_d) UNDER THE BOIN DESIGN FOR DIFFERENT TARGET TOXICITY RATES (Φ) WITH DEFAULT UNDERDOSING TOXICITY RATE $\Phi_1 = 0.6\Phi$ AND OVERDOSING TOXICITY RATE $\Phi_2 = 1.4\Phi$

	Target toxicity rate ϕ					
Boundaries	0.15	0.20	0.25	0.30	0.35	0.40
λ_e	0.118	0.157	0.197	0.236	0.276	0.316
λ_d	0.179	0.238	0.298	0.359	0.419	0.480

Suppose for a phase I trial with a new compound, the regulatory agent mandates that if the observed toxicity rate is higher than 0.25, the dose must be de-escalated. We can easily fulfill that requirement by setting the target DLT rate $\phi = 0.2$, under which the BOIN automatically guarantees de-escalating the dose if the observed toxicity rate $\hat{p}_j > 0.238$. If needed, the de-escalation boundary λ_d can be further fine-tuned by calibrating the value of ϕ_2. Such flexibility and transparency indicates the important advantage of the BOIN design over the mTPI and Keyboard designs in practice.

The BOIN design has similar flexibility as the CRM design. It can target any prespecified DLT rate. For instance, for some cancer populations for whom there is no effective treatment, a target DLT rate higher than 0.3 may be an acceptable trade-off to achieve higher treatment efficacy; whereas for other cancer populations, a lower target DLT rate, for example, 0.15 or 0.2, may be more appropriate. In addition, unlike the 3 + 3 design, for which the dose escalation and de-escalation decisions can be made only when we have three or six evaluable patients, the BOIN design does not require a fixed cohort size and allows for decision making at any time during the trial by comparing the observed DLT rate at the current dose with the escalation and de-escalation boundaries.

Decisions regarding dose escalation and de-escalation can be made at any time as long as we can calculate the DLT rate at the current dose. Such flexibility has important practical utility and implications. It allows clinicians to "adaptively" change the cohort size during the course of the trial to achieve certain design goals. For example, to shorten the trial duration and reduce the sample size, clinicians often prefer to use a cohort size of 1 for the initial dose escalation, and then switch to a cohort size of 3 after observing the first DLT, as with the commonly used accelerated titration design (ATD) (13). Such an accelerated titration can be easily and seamlessly performed using the BOIN design by simply switching the cohort size from 1 to 3 when the first DLT is observed. Unlike the ATD, which combines two independent empirical rules (the accelerated titration rule and the 3 + 3 rule) in an ad hoc way, the BOIN design achieves the same design goal under a single, coherent framework with assured statistical properties.

COMPARISON OF PHASE I DESIGNS

SIMULATION SETTINGS

We considered target toxicity rates of $\phi = 0.2$ and $\phi = 0.3$ with $J = 6$ dose levels. Under each setting, 1,000 dose–toxicity scenarios were randomly generated using the method of Clertant and O'Quigley (14). Under each scenario, we simulated 2,000 trials. Figure 21.4 displays 50 randomly selected scenarios with $\phi = 0.2$ with $J = 6$. These exhibit a variety of dose–toxicity curve shapes and spacing. We compared the CRM, mTPI, Keyboard, and BOIN designs. For the CRM, we used (0.032, 0.095, 0.200, 0.332, 0.470, 0.596) as the skeleton. For the mTPI and Keyboard designs, we set $\delta_1 = \phi - 0.05$ and $\delta_2 = \phi + 0.05$, which are the recommended default values. For the BOIN design, we set $\phi_1 = 0.6\phi$ and $\phi_2 = 1.4\phi$, which are the recommended default values. We set the cohort size equal to 1, and the maximum sample size equal to 36. More comprehensive and complete comparison of these designs are provided by Zhou et al. (6,15).

PERFORMANCE METRICS

For each of the 1,000 scenarios, we calculated the following metrics.

MTD selection:

- The percentage of correct selection (PCS), which we defined as the percentage of simulated trials in which the correct dose is selected as the MTD

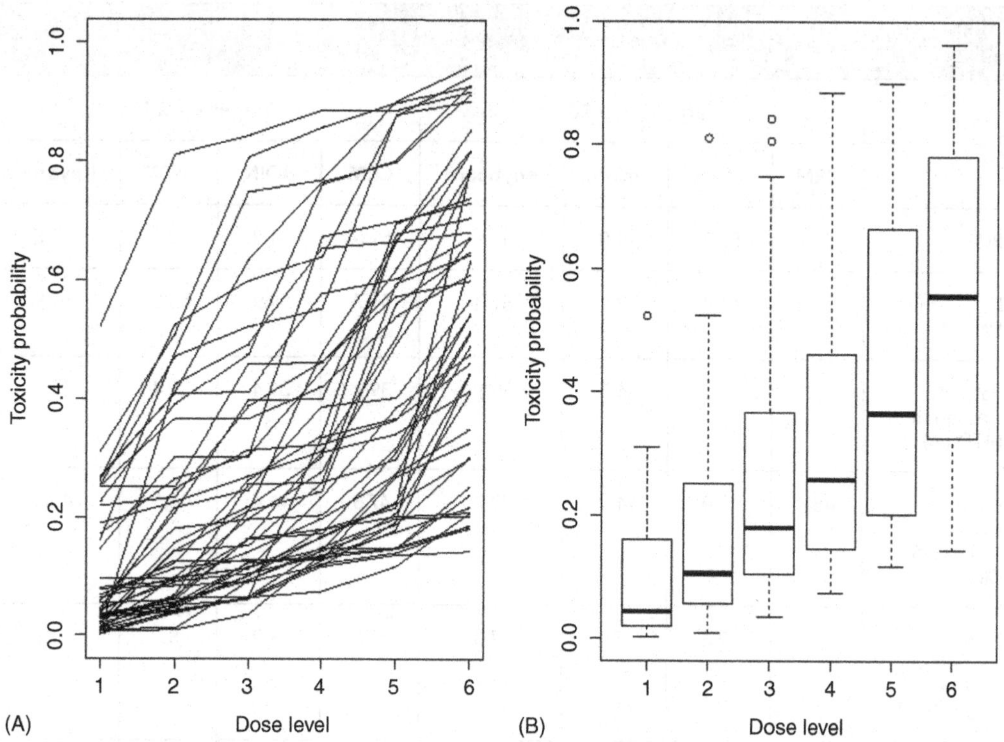

FIGURE 21.4 Panel (A) shows 50 randomly selected dose–toxicity curves, and panel (B) shows the distribution of the toxicity probabilities by dose level from the 1,000 scenarios with six dose levels.

- The PCS within a 5% acceptable region, which we defined as the percentage of simulated trials in which the dose selected as the MTD has a DLT rate that lies in the interval [$\phi - 0.05$; $\phi + 0.05$]

Patient allocation:

- The average percentage of patients assigned to the MTD in the simulated trials
- The average percentage of patients assigned to a dose with a DLT rate that lies in the interval [$\phi - 0.05$; $\phi + 0.05$] in the simulated trials

Overdose control:

- The average number of patients assigned to a dose that is above the MTD in the simulated trials.
- The risk of overdosing, which we define as the percentage of simulated trials in which a large percentage of patients (e.g., 80%) are assigned to a dose that is above the MTD (this metric quantifies how likely a particular design is to overdose a large percentage of patients)

RESULTS

Table 21.3 summarizes the average performance of the CRM, mTPI, BOIN, and Keyboard designs. In general, the CRM, BOIN, and Keyboard designs provide comparable, excellent operating characteristics. Each outperforms the mTPI design, with higher probabilities to correctly select the MTD and less likely to overdose patients.

TABLE 21.3 AVERAGE PERFORMANCE OF THE CRM, BOIN, MTPI, AND KEYBOARD DESIGNS ACROSS 1,000 SCENARIOS WITH SIX DOSE LEVELS

	Target $\phi = 0.20$				Target $\phi = 0.30$			
	CRM	BOIN	mTPI	Keyboard	CRM	BOIN	mTPI	Keyboard
PCS (%)	50.2	51.9	44.0	51.4	51.0	51.8	49.0	51.8
PCS within 5% (%)	61.3	61.8	52.1	61.3	59.7	59.9	56.8	59.9
Patients treated at MTD (%)	39.1	39.3	36.7	39.1	39.9	39.4	39.4	39.3
Patients treated within 5% (%)	48.6	48.0	44.2	47.9	47.3	46.4	46.3	46.3
Number of patients treated above MTD	6.2	7.6	7.4	7.3	7.5	7.9	8.9	7.8
Risk of overdosing 80% (%)	6.6	7.4	15.6	7.2	9.0	8.4	16.0	8.0

BOIN, Bayesian optimal interval; CRM, continual reassessment method; MTD, maximum tolerated dose; mTPI, modified toxicity probability interval; PCS, percentage of correct selection.

MTD Selection

Figure 21.5 shows the results for PCS and PCS within a 5% acceptable region for the mTPI, BOIN, and Keyboard designs, with respect to the CRM. Each boxplot reflects the distribution of the corresponding metric across the 1,000 scenarios, and the "X" mark reflects the average. As an example, the top-left panel of Figure 21.5 shows a boxplot of the PCS difference between mTPI and CRM, between BOIN and CRM, and between Keyboard and CRM when $\phi = 0.2$. For mTPI versus CRM, most of the data points are negative, which indicates that the CRM tends to outperform mTPI. For BOIN and Keyboard versus CRM respectively, most of the data points are close to zero, which indicates that the BOIN and Keyboard tend to perform similarly to the CRM. For PCS within 5% (bottom panels), we see a similar pattern. As evidenced by the right panels of Figure 21.5, when $\phi = 0.3$ the CRM, BOIN, and Keyboard have comparable PCS and PCS within 5%, and all outperform mTPI, though to a lesser extent than when $\phi = 0.2$.

Patient Allocation

Figure 21.6 shows the results for the average percentage of patients who are assigned to the MTD, and the average percentage of patients treated at the doses within 5% acceptable region of target DLT rate, respectively, for $\phi = 0.20$ and $\phi = 0.30$ with $J = 6$ doses. When $\phi = 0.20$, CRM, BOIN, and Keyboard are comparable, and all tend to outperform mTPI. When $\phi = 0.30$, all four designs are comparable with respect to these metrics.

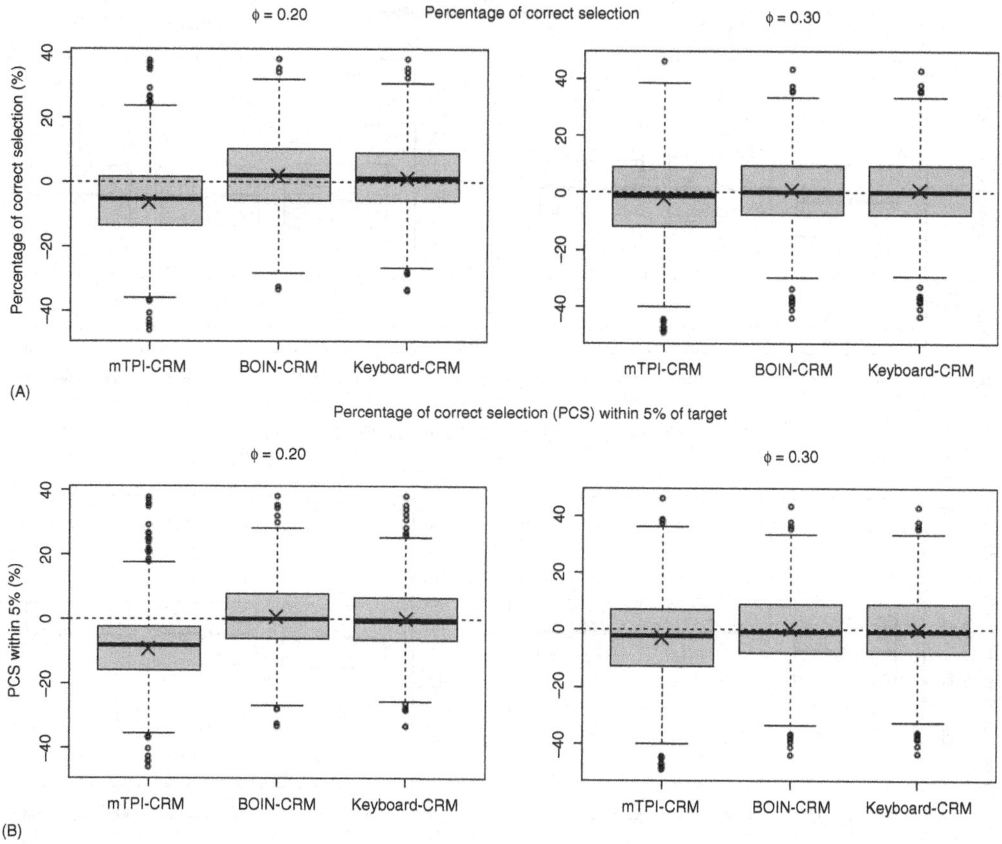

FIGURE 21.5 Boxplot of the difference in the PCS of the MTD and the PCS of the doses within 5% of the target for mTPI vs. CRM, BOIN vs. CRM, and Keyboard vs. CRM under 1,000 scenarios with six dose levels. The X in the center of the boxes reflects the average difference.

BOIN, Bayesian optimal interval; CRM, continual reassessment method; MTD, maximum tolerated dose; mTPI, modified toxicity probability interval; PCS, percentage of correct selection.

Overdose Control

Overdose control is important for protecting patients from overly toxic doses. The upper panel of Figure 21.7 shows our results for the number of patients treated above MTD in each simulated trial under the 1,000 scenarios. Generally speaking, the four designs have comparable performance. Table 21.3 shows that, compared with BOIN, mTPI, and Keyboard, the CRM tends to assign fewer patients to doses that are above the MTD when $\phi = 0.20$. When $\phi = 0.30$, the CRM, BOIN, and Keyboard perform similarly and tend to assign fewer patients to doses that are above the MTD than the mTPI.

The lower panel of Figure 21.7 shows the results for the risk of overdosing at least 80% of the patients. The difference between the designs for this safety metric is more striking than the other metrics. For instance, the difference between mTPI and the CRM in the risk of overdosing at least 80% of the patients is greater than zero in every scenario, which indicates that the CRM is always safer than the mTPI design. In contrast, CRM, BOIN, and Keyboard are comparable in the risk of overdosing at least 80% of the patients. When $\phi = 0.20$, the CRM is slightly safer than BOIN and Keyboard, whereas when $\phi = 0.30$, BOIN and Keyboard are slightly safer than the CRM. Figure 21.7 shows that the average risk of overdosing at least 80% of the patients is substantially lower for the CRM, BOIN, and Keyboard than for mTPI.

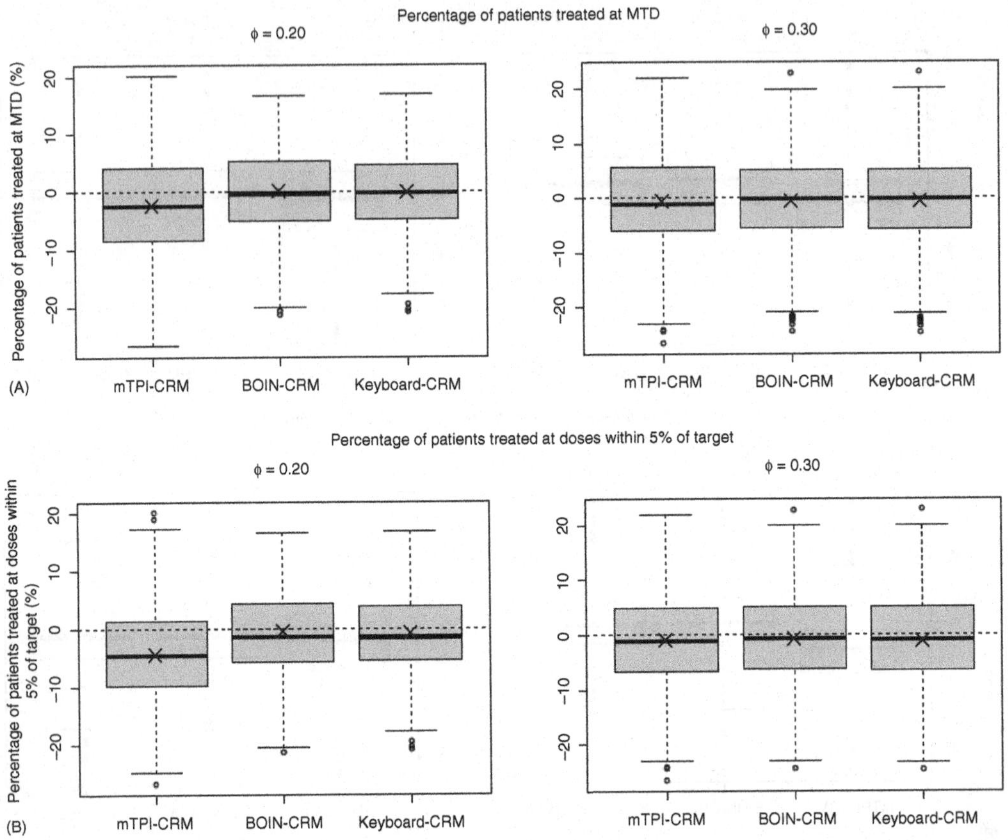

FIGURE 21.6 Boxplot of the difference in the percentage of patients treated at the MTD and the percentage of patients treated at doses within 5% of the target for mTPI vs. CRM, BOIN vs. CRM, and Keyboard vs. CRM under 1,000 scenarios with six dose levels. The X in the center of the boxes reflects the average difference.

BOIN, Bayesian optimal interval; CRM, continual reassessment method; MTD, maximum tolerated dose; mTPI, modified toxicity probability interval; PCS, percentage of correct selection.

CONCLUSION

The CRM, BOIN, and Keyboard designs provide comparable, excellent operating characteristics, and each outperforms the mTPI design. These three designs are more likely to correctly select the MTD and less likely to overdose a large percentage of patients in comparison to the mTPI design. The CRM has good performance, but it is complicated to implement and difficult to communicate to clinical investigators how the design works. In addition, sensitivity to the model misspecification is also a potential concern that affects the performance of the CRM in practice (5,15).

The BOIN and Keyboard designs have extremely similar performance metrics, although they are based on different statistical frameworks: the Keyboard design uses the posterior distribution of p_j for dose escalation and de-escalation, whereas the BOIN design does not require the calculation of posterior distribution and directly uses the observed toxicity rate $\hat{p}_j$ for dose escalation and de-escalation. Operatively and conceptually, the BOIN design is simpler and more transparent than the mTPI and Keyboard designs. The BOIN design compares the $\hat{p}_j$ with a pair of fixed prespecified escalation and de-escalation boundaries (λ_e, λ_d) to direct the dose escalation and de-escalation. The Keyboard and mTPI designs require calculating the posterior distribution and identifying the "strongest" key and UPM, respectively, for each possible outcome data (n_j, y_j),

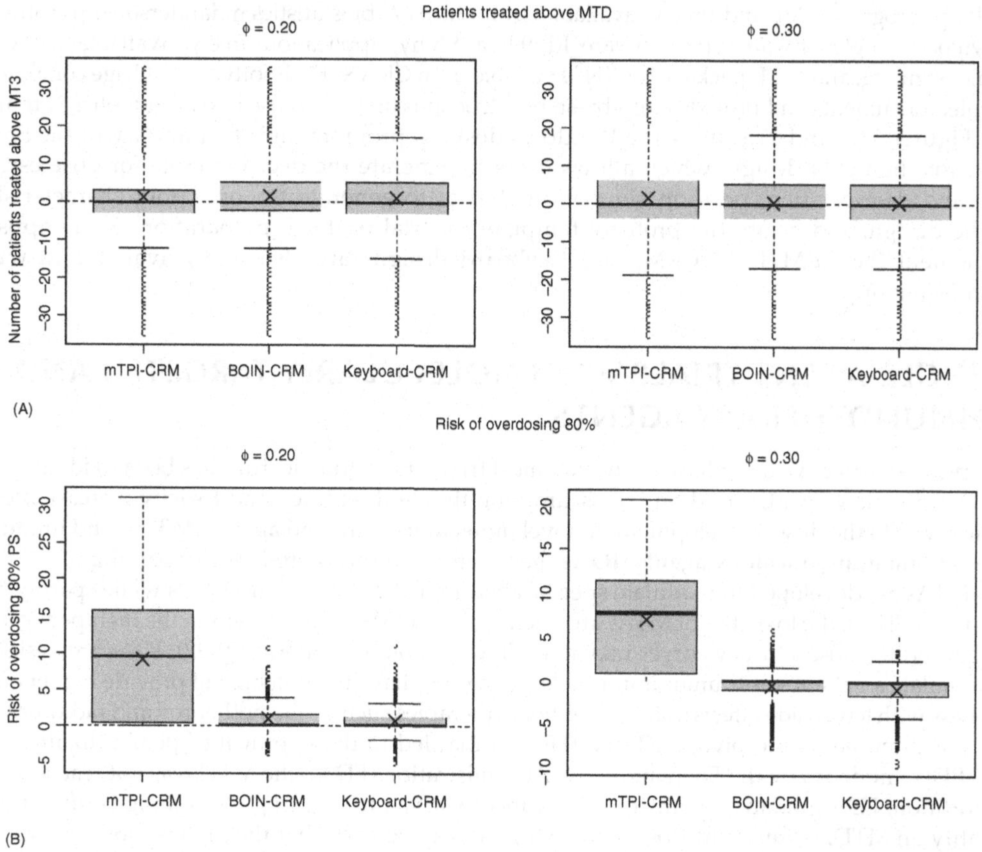

FIGURE 21.7 Boxplot of the difference in the number of patients treated above MTD and the risk of overdosing at least 80% of patients for mTPI vs. CRM, BOIN vs. CRM, and Keyboard vs. CRM under 1,000 scenarios with six dose levels. The "X" mark reflects the average difference.

BOIN, Bayesian optimal interval; CRM, continual reassessment method; MTD, maximum tolerated dose; mTPI, modified toxicity probability interval; PCS, percentage of correct selection.

though these evaluations and corresponding decision boundaries can be calculated prior to the onset of the trial.

In addition, as described previously, the BOIN design allows clinicians and regulatory agents to easily assess the safety of the trial design, and enables users to easily calibrate their trials to satisfy the safety requirement mandated by the regulatory agents. This gives the BOIN an important practical advantage over the mTPI and Keyboard designs. Also, the BOIN design is a more versatile method that has been extended to find the MTD or MTD contour for drug-combination trials (16,17) and late-onset toxicity (18), and to account for toxicity grade and continuous toxicity outcome (19). Recently, Zhou et al. (15) compared the BOIN with the dose escalation with overdose control (EWOC) and Bayesian logistic regression model (BLRM), and also showed the favorable performance of the BOIN. Considering overall performance, implementation simplicity, and flexibility, the BOIN design is recommended for practical use.

SOFTWARE

Several software packages have been developed to facilitate the use of novel phase I designs. For example, the BOIN design is available in three easy-to-use forms, including a stand-alone Windows desktop program (20) and freely available from https://biostatistics.mdanderson.org/software download/SingleSoftware.aspx?Software_Id=99, a Shiny application freely available at www.trialdesign.org, and the R package "BOIN" available from CRAN. Each software package comes with detailed documents and provides step-by-step instructions on how to use it to design phase I trials.

Figures 21.8 and 21.9 show the Windows desktop program and the interface of the Shiny apps for the BOIN design, which allows users to generate the decision table for dose escalation and de-escalation, perform simulation studies to generate the operating characteristics of the design, and create the protocol template for trial protocol preparation. Shiny apps to implement the CRM/BMA-CRM, and Keyboard designs are also freely available at www.trialdesign.org.

SINGLE-AGENT TRIALS WITH MOLECULARLY TARGETED AND IMMUNOTHERAPY AGENTS

The primary objective of a phase I cancer clinical trial for a cytotoxic drug has been to identify the MTD of the new agent, based on the assumption that both efficacy and toxicity increase monotonically with the dose. Development of novel **molecularly targeted agents (MTAs)** and immunotherapy/**immuno-oncology agents (IOAs)** has challenged this more-is-better paradigm.

MTAs are developed to modulate specific aberrant pathways in cancer cells while sparing normal tissue. Thus, the toxicities of MTAs are often expected to be minimal within the therapeutic dose range, and the dose–efficacy curves may not follow monotonic patterns (21,22). IOAs are designed to stimulate a patient's antitumor immune response, and have the potential to provide higher effectiveness with fewer side effects than conventional therapies such as chemotherapy and radiotherapy.

For example, in the pivotal KEYNOTE trial that led to the approval of pembrolizumab (an anti-PD-1 antibody) by the Food and Drug Administration (FDA), the MTD was not reached (23). In addition, FDA guidance points out that cancer vaccine trials using 3 + 3 designs often fail to identify an MTD, because the dose–toxicity curve may be such that the highest dose that can be administered is limited by manufacturing or anatomic issues, rather than by toxicity (24).

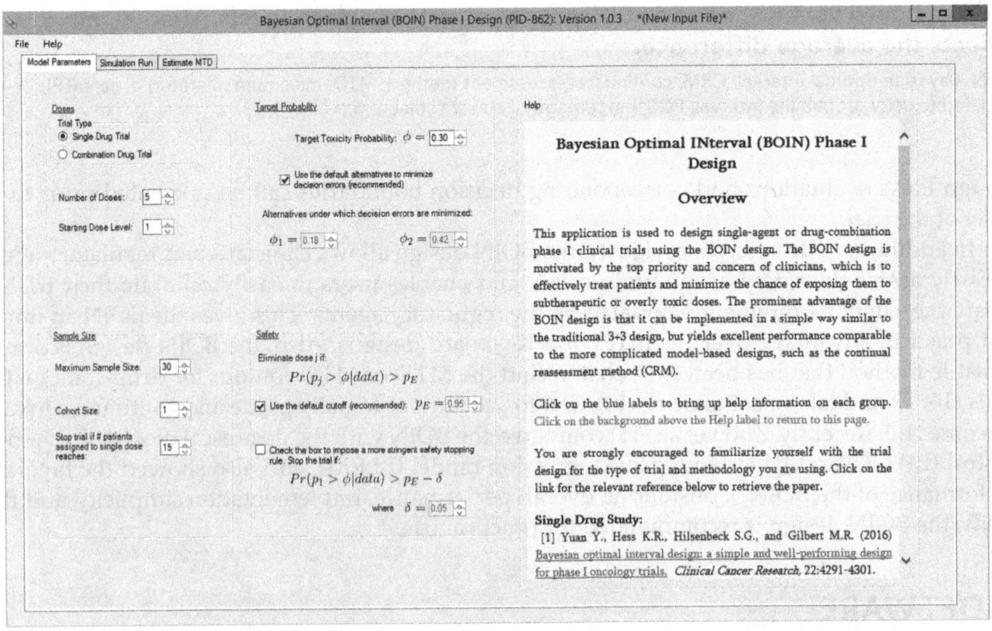

FIGURE 21.8 Windows desktop program for the BOIN design.

BOIN, Bayesian optimal interval.

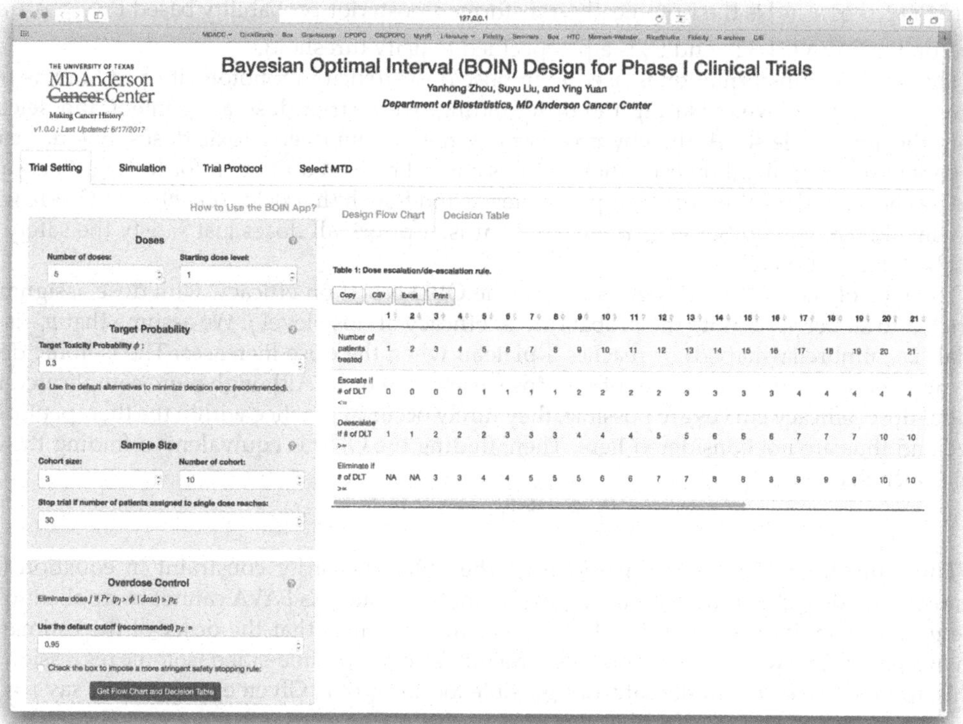

FIGURE 21.9 Shiny app for implementing the BOIN design for single-agent trials.
BOIN, Bayesian optimal interval.

The primary objective of a dose-finding trial for MTAs and IOAs is not to find the MTD, but to find the optimal biological dose (OBD), which can be defined as the lowest dose that has the highest efficacy rate while simultaneously safeguarding patients, that is, the dose at the beginning of the plateau of the dose–efficacy curve. Depending on the goal of the clinical trial, the other definition of OBD is also possible, for example, the dose with the highest utility in terms of efficacy–toxicity trade-off (25).

A number of designs have been proposed to find the OBD (26–30). In what follows, we introduce an isotonic design, which is simple, robust (i.e., does not make any parametric assumption on the dose–efficacy curve), and performs well. Because MTAs and IOAs are often expected to have minimal toxicity, dose-finding trials in this setting should be primarily driven by efficacy, while simultaneously safeguarding patients by monitoring the toxicity of each dose.

Let ϕ denote the target DLT rate; the safety of dose level j can be monitored by the posterior probability $\Pr(p_j > \phi \mid n_j, y_j)$, assuming a beta-binomial model:

$$y_j \mid n_j, p_j \sim \text{Binom}(n_j, p_j)$$

$$p_j \sim \text{Beta}(a, b)$$

where Binom(·) and Beta(·) denote binomial and beta distributions, respectively, and a and b are hyperparameters. For the purpose of safeguarding patients during the dose escalation, we define the admissible set A as a set of doses satisfying the following safety rule:

$$A = \left\{ j : \widetilde{\Pr}\left(p_j > \phi \mid n_j, y_j\right) < C_T, j = 1, \cdots, J \right\} \quad (4)$$

where $\widetilde{\Pr}\left(p_j > \phi \mid n_j, y_j\right)$ is the isotonically transformed posterior probability based $\Pr(p_j > \phi \mid n_j, y_j)$ based on the PAVA (31,32), and C_T is a prespecified toxicity threshold.

The isotonic transformation is used to impose dose–toxicity monotonicity and borrow information across dose levels. During the dose finding, we restrict dose assignment and selection within the admissible set A, thereby protecting patients from overly toxic doses. Before treating any patient in the trial, all investigational doses should be in A and open for testing. This can be done by choosing the values of hyperparameters a and b such that Beta (ϕ; a; b) = $1 - C_T + \delta$, where b is a small positive number (e.g., $\delta = 0.05$). That is, a priori, all doses just satisfy the safety rule described in equation (4).

The idea of the isotonic design is to find the OBD based on efficacy, with dose assignments restricted to A. Let $p_{E,j}$ denote the probability of efficacy at dose level j. We assume that $p_{E,j}$ is unimodal (i.e., umbrella-shaped) or reaches a plateau when the dose increases. The isotonic design also can handle a conventional monotonic dose–response curve. Although more complicated multimodal dose–efficacy curves are possible, they rarely occur in practice within the therapeutic dose range and thus are not considered here. Then, finding the OBD is equivalent to finding the dose level j^* such that

$$p_{1,j} \leq \cdots \leq p_{E,j^*} \geq \cdots \geq p_{E,J} \tag{5}$$

The difficulty is that, before we identify the OBD, the order constraint in equation (5) is unknown and thus standard isotonic regression methods such as PAVA cannot be applied to estimate $p_{E,j}$ and identify the OBD. The PAVA algorithm assumes that the order of the estimates is known a priori. One way to overcome this difficulty is to use double-sided isotonic regression (33). In this approach, we first enumerate all J possible locations of j^*. Given each location, say $j^* = r, r = 1, \ldots, J$, the isotonic estimates $\left\{\tilde{p}_{E,j}^{(r)}\right\}$ can be obtained by fitting the following two separate standard isotonic regressions to the interim data:

1. $\hat{p}_{E,1}, \cdots, \hat{p}_{E,j^*}$ with the known constraints $p_{E,1} \leq \cdots \leq p_{E,j^*}$
2. $p_{E,j^*+1}, \cdots, \hat{p}_{E,j}$ with the known constraints $p_{E,j^*+1} \geq \cdots \geq \hat{p}_{E,J}$

where $\hat{p}_{E,j} = x_j / n_j$ is the observed efficacy rate (x_j is the number of patients having response out of the n_j patients treated at dose level j). Each of these two isotonic regressions can be done using the PAVA algorithm. After applying this procedure to each of the J possible locations of j^*, we obtain J sets of possible isotonic estimates $\left\{\tilde{p}_{E,j}^{(r)}\right\}$, $r = 1, \ldots, J$. We select as the final isotonic estimates $\left\{\tilde{p}_{E,j}\right\} = \left\{\tilde{p}_{E,j}^{(r^*)}\right\}$ that have theh smallest sum of square error, that is,

$$r^* = \underset{r \in (1, \cdots, J)}{\operatorname{argmin}} \sum_{j=1}^{J} \left(\tilde{p}_{E,j}^{(r)} - \frac{x_j}{n_j} \right)^2$$

The isotonic design is carried out as follows.

1. Treat the first cohort of patients at the lowest dose d_1 or at the physician-specified starting dose.
2. Determine the admissible set A.
3. Identify the dose level j^* having the largest $\tilde{p}_{E,j}$ among the tried doses in A. If there are ties, select j^* as the lowest dose level among the ties. Let j^{curr} denote the current dose level, and j^h denote the highest dose level tried thus far:
   - If $j^* > j^{curr}$, escalate to $j^{curr} + 1$;
     If $j^* < j^{curr}$ de-escalate to $j^{curr} - 1$;
     If $j^* > j^{curr} = j^h$, escalate to $j^{curr} + 1$ given that $j^{curr} + 1$ is in A.
   - Otherwise, remain at dose level j^{curr}.

4. Once the maximum sample size N is reached, select the lowest dose having the highest $\tilde{p}_{E,j}$ in A as the OBD.

One limitation of isotonic regression is that it cannot estimate the $p_{E,j}$ for any untried doses, at which no patients have been treated. Therefore, during trial conduct, when the dose with the highest estimate of efficacy is the highest tried dose (i.e., $j^* = j^{curr} = j^h$), there may be insufficient information to determine whether the maximum of the dose–efficacy curve has been identified. To overcome this limitation, in the aforementioned dose-finding algorithm step 3, when $j^* = j^{curr} = j^h$, we escalate the dose level to further explore the dose–efficacy curve and search for the maximum, given that the next higher dose level is safe (i.e., within the admissible set A).

SOFTWARE

A Shiny application to implement the isotonic design is freely available at www.trialdesign.org. Figure 21.10 shows the interface of the Shiny application for the design, which allows users to perform simulation study to generate the operating characteristics of the design, create the protocol template for trial protocol preparation, and conduct the trial in real time based on accrued data.

DRUG-COMBINATION TRIALS

Combining drugs or agents while treating patients has become commonplace in cancer clinical trials. The objectives of using drug combinations are to induce a synergistic treatment effect, increase the joint dose intensity with nonoverlapping toxicities, and target various tumor cell susceptibilities and disease pathways.

A major challenge in designing combination trials is that combinations are only partially ordered in their toxicity probabilities. Consider a trial combining J doses of agent A, denoted as $A_1 < A_2 < \ldots A_J$, and K doses of agent B, denoted as $B_1 < B_2 < \ldots B_K$. Let A_jB_k denote the combination of A_j and B_k, and p_{jk} denote the probability of DLT rate for A_jB_k. It is typically reasonable to assume that when the dose of one agent (e.g., agent A) is fixed, the toxicity of the combination

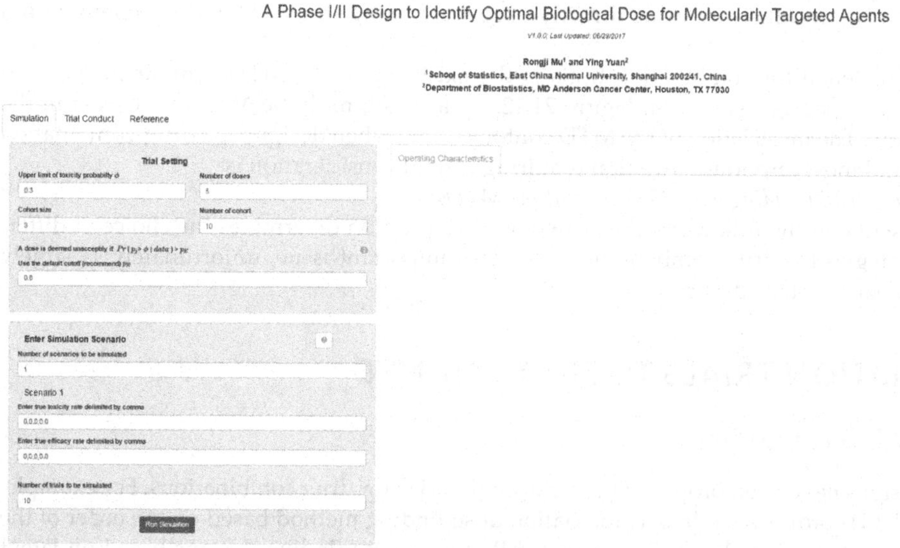

FIGURE 21.10 Shiny app for implementing the isotonic design for molecularly targeted agents and immunotherapy agents.

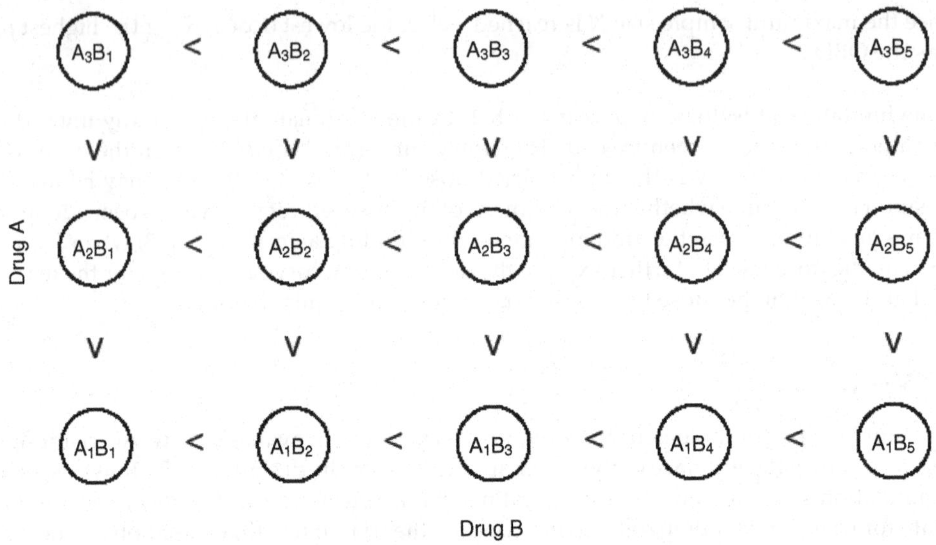

FIGURE 21.11 Partial order in toxicity for drug combinations.

increases as the dose of the other agent increases (i.e., agent B). In other words, as shown in Figure 21.11, in the dose matrix, the rows and columns are ordered, with the DLT rate increasing along with the dose. However, in other directions of the dose matrix (e.g., along the diagonals from the upper left corner to the lower right corner) the toxicity order is unknown due to unknown drug–drug interactions. For example, between A_2B_2 and A_1B_3, we do not know which one is more toxic, because the first combination has a higher dose of agent A whereas the second combination has a higher dose of agent B. Thus, we cannot fully rank $J \times K$ combinations from low to high in terms of their DLT rates. This is distinctly different from single-agent trials, for which the dose can be unambiguously ranked assuming that higher dosage yields higher probability of toxicity. The implication of such a partial ranking is that conventional single-agent dose-finding designs cannot be directly used for finding the MTD in drug-combination trials.

Another challenge for combination trials is the existence of the MTD contour in the two-dimensional dose space, as shown in Figure 21.12. As a result, multiple MTDs may exist in the $J \times K$ dose matrix. The implication of the MTD contour is that when designing a drug-combination trial, the first and most important question requiring careful consideration is:

Are we interested in finding one MTD or multiple MTDs?

As we describe in the following, the answer to this question determines the choice of different design strategies for drug-combination trials. This important issue, unfortunately, is largely overlooked by existing trial designs.

COMBINATION TRIALS TO FIND ONE MTD

MODEL-BASED DESIGNS

Numerous designs have been proposed to find a single MTD for drug combinations. For example, Conaway et al. (34) proposed a drug-combination dose-finding method based on the order of the restricted inference. Yin and Yuan (35) proposed Bayesian dose-finding designs based on latent contingency tables and Yin and Yuan (36) proposed a copula-type model for drug-combination trials. Braun and Wang (37) developed a dose-finding method based on a Bayesian hierarchical

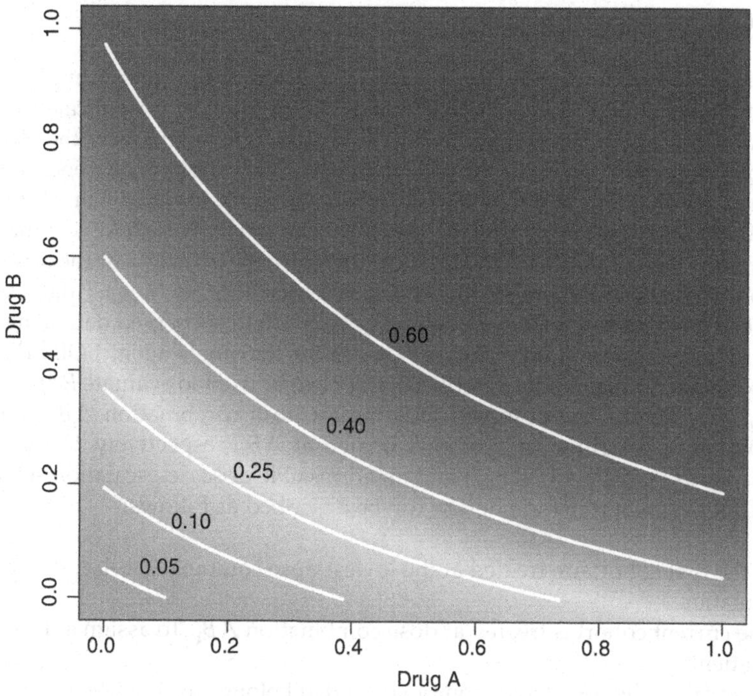

FIGURE 21.12 The maximum tolerated dose (MTD) contour for drug combinations. The combinations located on a curve have the same DLT rate, as indicated by the numbers.

model. Wages et al. (38) extended the CRM (39) based on partial ordering of the dose combinations. Braun and Jia (40) generalized the CRM to handle drug-combination trials. Riviere et al. (41) proposed a Bayesian dose-finding design based on the logistic model. Cai et al. (42,43) and Riviere et al. (44) proposed Bayesian adaptive designs for drug-combination trials involving MTAs. Albeit very different, most of these designs adopt a common dose-finding strategy similar to the CRM: devise a model to describe the dose–toxicity surface and then, based on the accumulating data, continuously update the model estimate and make the decision of dose assignment for the new patient, typically by assigning the new patient to the dose for which the estimated toxicity is closest to the MTD.

Although these designs perform reasonably well, they are rarely used in practice, for several reasons. First, these designs are statistically and computationally complicated. Lack of easy-to-use software further hinders the adoption of these designs in practice. Robustness is another potential issue for model-based drug-combination trial designs. As the models used in the drug-combination designs are more complicated than the CRM, the designs are more vulnerable to model misspecification, and the dose-finding scheme is more likely to become stuck at local "suboptimal" doses. Some strategies (e.g., giving high priority to exploring new doses (43) and randomization (44)) have been proposed to alleviate this issue, but given the small sample size of early phase trials, this remains an issue that affects the robustness of drug-combination trial designs. The robustness of the model-based drug-combination trial designs warrants further research. Because of the aforementioned issues, we will not discuss these model-based approaches further. Instead, in what follows, we focus on a model-assisted design that can be easily implemented using the existing Shiny application or Windows desktop program, and thus is more likely to be used in practice.

MODEL-ASSISTED DESIGN

The BOIN drug-combination design (16) is a model-assisted design that provides a simple, well-performing method to find a single MTD. It makes the decision of dose escalation/de-escalation based on the same rule as the single-agent BOIN design described previously, thereby inheriting the latter's desirable properties, including simplicity, transparency, design coherence, and consistence. The only difference is that, in combination trials, when we decide to escalate or de-escalate the dose, there is more than one neighboring dose to which we can move. For example, when we escalate/de-escalate the dose, we can escalate/de-escalate either the dose of drug A or the dose of drug B. The BOIN drug-combination design makes this choice based on $Pr\{p_{jk} \in (\lambda_e, \lambda_d) \mid \text{data}\}$ which measure how likely a dose combination is located within (λ_e, λ_d) given the observed data, where λ_e and λ_d are the escalation and de-escalation boundaries, same as for the single-agent BOIN design described previously. The beta-binomial model described earlier can be used to evaluate $Pr\{p_{jk} \in (\lambda_e, \lambda_d) \mid \text{data}\}$.

Let $\hat{p}_{jk} = y_{jk} / n_{jk}$ denote the observed DLT rate at dose combination A_jB_k, where y_{jk} and n_{jk} denote the number of toxicities and patients treated at A_jB_k, respectively. Define an admissible dose escalation set as $A_E = \{A_{j+1}B_k, A_jB_{k+1}\}$ and an admissible dose de-escalation set as $A_D = \{A_{j-1}B_k, A_jB_{k-1}\}$. The BOIN drug-combination design can be described as follows:

1. Patients in the first cohort are treated at the lowest dose combination A_1B_1 or a prespecified dose combination.
2. Suppose the current cohort is treated at dose combination A_jB_k. To assign a dose to the next cohort of patients:
   - If $\hat{p}_{jk} \le \lambda_e$, escalate the dose to the combination that belongs to A_E and has the largest value of $Pr\{p_{j'k'} \in (\lambda_e, \lambda_d) \mid \text{data}\}$.
   - If $\hat{p}_{jk} \ge \lambda_d$, de-escalate the dose to the combination that belongs to A_D and has the largest value of $Pr\{p_{j'k'} \in (\lambda_e, \lambda_d) \mid \text{data}\}$.
   - Otherwise, if $\lambda_e < \hat{p}_{jk} < \lambda_d$, then the dose stays at the same combination A_jB_k.
3. This process is continued until the maximum sample size is reached or the trial is terminated because of excessive toxicity.

During dose escalation and de-escalation, if the two combinations in A_E or A_D have the same value of $Pr\{p_{j'k'} \in (\lambda_e, \lambda_d) \mid \text{data}\}$, we randomly choose one with equal probability. If no dose combinations exist in the sets of A_E or A_D (i.e., we are at the boundaries of the dose matrix), we retain the current dose combination. After the trial is completed, the MTD is selected as the dose combination with the estimated DLT rate closest to ϕ. The estimates of DLT rates are obtained using isotonic regression as described previously, but in a matrix form. More details on the BOIN drug-combination design can be found in Lin and Yin (16).

COMBINATION TRIALS TO FIND MULTIPLE MTDS

Because of the existence of the MTD contour and the fact that doses on the MTD contour may have different efficacy due to drug–drug interactions, for many drug-combination trials it is of intrinsic interest to find multiple MTDs. The MTDs can be further evaluated in subsequent phase II trials to identify the one with the highest efficacy. Given a prespecified $J \times K$ dose matrix, finding the MTD contour is equivalent to finding an MTD, if it exists, in each row of the dose matrix. Without loss of generality, we assume that $J \le K$. That is, drug B has more dose levels than drug A.

Finding the MTD contour is substantially more challenging than finding a single MTD. This is because, in order to find all MTDs in the dose matrix, we must explore the whole dose matrix using the limited sample size that is typical for phase I trials. Otherwise, we risk missing some MTDs. In contrast to numerous drug-combination designs for finding a single MTD, a very limited number of designs have been proposed to find the MTD contour. Thall et al. (45) proposed a drug-combination design to find three MTDs, but that design assumes that the doses are continuous and can be freely changed during the trial, which is not common in practice. Wang and Ivanova (46) proposed a design to find the MTD contour based on a parametric model, assuming that the logarithm of the DLT rate of a drug combination is a linear function of the doses of the two drugs. Yuan and Yin (47) proposed a sequential dose-finding method that converts the task of finding the MTD contour into a series of easier one-dimensional dose-finding problem. Mander and Sweeting (48) proposed a product of independent beta probabilities escalation (PIPE) design to find the MTD contour based on Bayesian model averaging, without assuming a parametric form on the dose–toxicity curve. Zhang and Yuan (18) extended the approach of Yuan and Yin (47) and proposed a so-called **waterfall design** to incorporate some practical considerations. The waterfall design is easy to implement, has good performance, and also has easy-to-use software available. Here we describe the design in detail.

The basic idea of the waterfall design is straightforward: divide the two-dimensional dose-finding problem into a series of simpler one-dimensional dose-finding problems that can be easily solved by existing single-agent dose-finding methods, where each one-dimensional dose finding is known as a "subtrial." As illustrated in Figure 21.13, the waterfall design partitions the $J \times K$ dose matrix into J subtrials, within which the doses are fully ordered. These subtrials are conducted sequentially from the top of the matrix to the bottom, which is why we refer to the design as the waterfall design. The goal of the design is to find the MTD contour, which is equivalent to finding the MTD, if it exists, in each row of the dose matrix.

The waterfall design can be described as follows:

1. Divide the $J \times K$ dose matrix into J subtrials $S_J, \ldots, S_1$, according to the dose level of drug A:

$$S_J = \{A_1B_1, \ldots, A_JB_1, A_JB_2, \ldots, A_JB_K\}$$
$$S_{J-1} = \{A_{J-1}B_2, \ldots, A_{J-1}B_k\}$$
$$S_{J-2} = \{A_{J-2}B_2, \ldots, A_{J-2}B_k\}$$
$$\ldots$$
$$S_1 = \{A_1B_2, \ldots, A_1B_K\}$$

Note that subtrial S_J also includes lead-in doses $A_1B_1, A_2B_1, \ldots, A_JB_1$ (the first column of the dose matrix) to impose the practical consideration that the trial starts at the lowest dose. Within each subtrial, the doses are fully ordered with monotonically increasing toxicity.

2. Conduct the subtrials sequentially using the BOIN design (or another single-agent dose-finding method) as follows:
   - **(i)** Conduct subtrial S_J, starting from the lowest dose combination A_1B_1, to find the MTD. We call the dose selected by the subtrial the "candidate MTD" to highlight that the dose selected by the individual subtrial may not be the "final" MTD that we will select at the end of the trial. The final MTD selection will be based on the data collected from all the subtrials. The objective of finding the candidate MTD is to determine which subtrial will be conducted next and the corresponding starting dose.
   - **(ii)** Assuming that subtrial S_J selects dose $A_{j^*}B_{k^*}$ as the candidate MTD, next, conduct subtrial S_{j^*-1} with the starting dose $A_{j^*-1}B_{k^*+1}$. That is, the next subtrial to be conducted is the one with drug A's dose one level lower than that of the candidate MTD found in the previous subtrial but drug B's dose one level higher. After identifying the candidate MTD of subtrial S_{j^*-1}, the same rule is used to determine the next subtrial and its starting dose. See Figure 21.13 for an example.
   - **(iii)** Repeat step (ii) until subtrial S_1 is completed.
3. Estimate the DLT rate p_{jk} based on the toxicity data collected from all the subtrials using matrix isotonic regression (49). For each row of the dose matrix, select the MTD as the dose

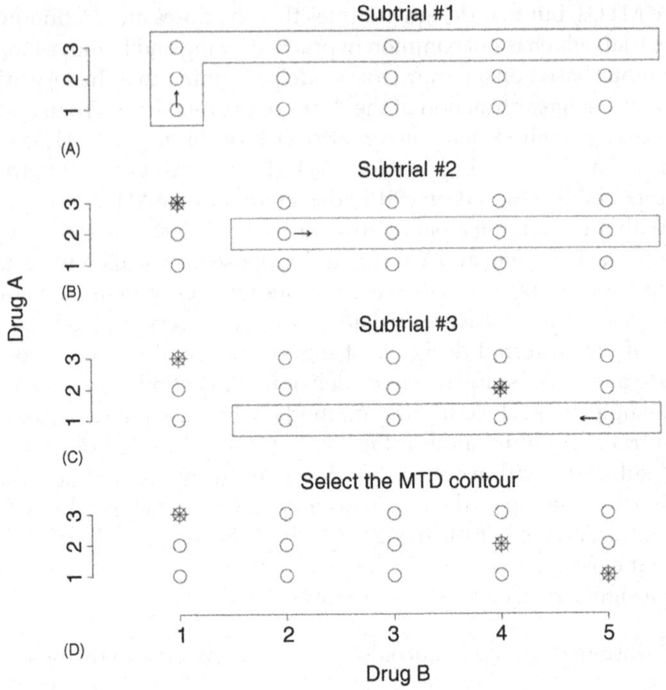

FIGURE 21.13 Illustration of the waterfall design for a 3 × 5 combination trial. The doses in the box form a subtrial, and the asterisk denotes the candidate MTD. As shown in panel (A), the trial starts by conducting the first subtrial with the starting dose A_1B_1. After the first subtrial identified A_3B_1 as the candidate MTD, we then conduct the second subtrial with the starting dose A_2B_2; see panel (B). After the second subtrial identified A_2B_4 as the candidate MTD, we conduct the third subtrial with the starting dose A_1B_5; see panel (C). After all subtrials are completed, we select the MTD contour based on the data from all subtrials, as shown in panel (D).

MTD, maximum tolerated dose.

combination that has the estimate of DLT rate closest to the target toxicity rate ϕ unless all combinations in that row are overly toxic.

The waterfall design conducts the subtrials sequentially such that the results of each subtrial will be used to inform the design (e.g., the dose range and the starting dose) of subsequent subtrials. Such information borrowing allows the design to explore the two-dimensional dose space efficiently using a limited sample size, and decreases the chance of overdosing and underdosing patients. For example, in step 2, the reason that subtrial S_{j^*-1} starts with dose $A_{j^*-1}B_{k^*+1}$ rather than the lowest dose in that subtrial (i.e., $A_{j^*-1}B_2$) is that $A_{j^*-1}B_{k^*+1}$ is the lowest dose that is potentially located at the MTD contour. Starting from $A_{j^*-1}B_{k^*+1}$ allows us to quickly reach the MTD.

SOFTWARE

The BOIN drug-combination and waterfall designs can be easily implemented using the Windows desktop program (Figure 21.8) or Shiny application (Figure 21.14). Each software package has an

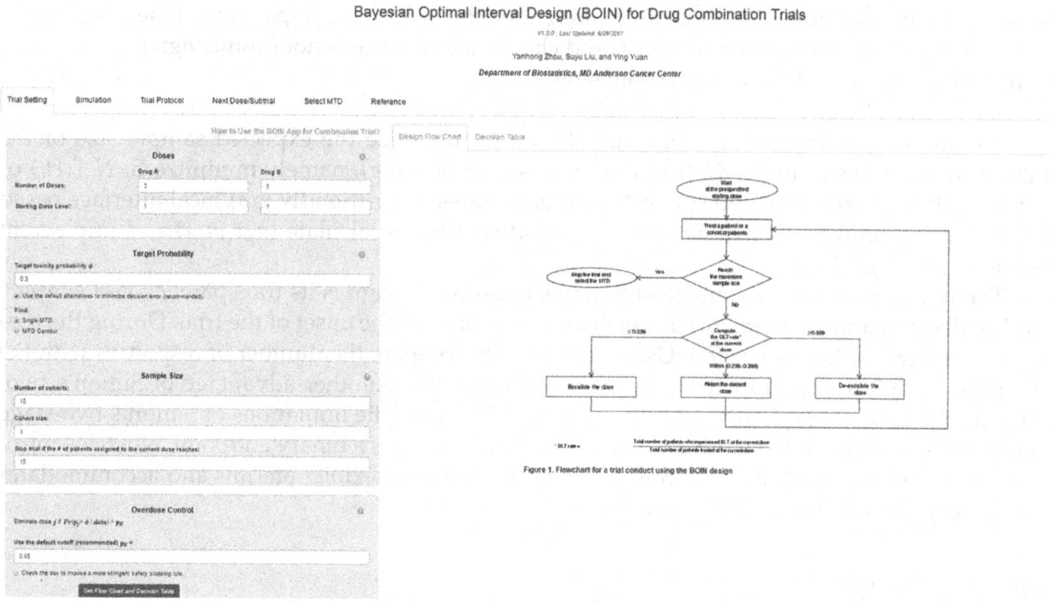

FIGURE 21.14 Shiny app for implementing the BOIN design for drug-combination trials.

BOIN, Bayesian optimal interval.

intuitive graphical user interface and rich documents to help users navigate through the process. The software can be used to perform simulations to obtain the operating characteristics of the design, generate the protocol template, and conduct the trial in real time.

PHASE II CLINICAL TRIAL DESIGNS

The objective of a phase II clinical trial is to evaluate the preliminary efficacy of a new treatment and to determine whether an efficacious treatment warrants further investigation in a large-scale randomized phase III trial. A fundamental design feature for these phase II clinical trials is the early stopping rule to prevent the exposure of an excessive number of patients to a possibly futile treatment. In what follows, we introduce a well-known, frequentist phase II design and a novel, flexible Bayesian phase II design.

SIMON'S TWO-STAGE DESIGN

The most well-known frequentist phase II design is Simon's optimal two-stage design (50). The design assumes a binary endpoint (e.g., tumor response). Let p denote the true response rate of the drug under investigation, and p_0 and p_1 denote the response rates that are deemed futile and efficacious, respectively, where $p_0 < p_1$. Given the null hypothesis H_0 and the alternative hypothesis H_1

$$H_0\colon p \le p_0 \text{ versus } H_1\colon p \ge p_1$$

Simon's optimal two-stage design is described as follows:

- *Stage I*: enroll n_1 patients, if there are r_1 or fewer responses, terminate the trial and accept H_0 that the drug is not promising; otherwise, move to stage II.

- *Stage II*: enroll additional n_2 patients. Among the total of $N = n_1 + n_2$ patients, if the total number of response is r or fewer, accept H_0 and claim that the drug is not promising; otherwise, reject H_0 to claim that the drug is promising.

The design parameters (n_1, r_1, n_2, r) are chosen to minimize the expected sample size or the maximum sample size under H_0 (i.e., the drug is unpromising), namely minimize E $(N \mid H_0)$ or max(N), given prespecified type I and type II error rates. User-friendly graphical interface based Shiny application is freely available at *www.trialdesign.org* to calculate (n_1, r_1, n_2, r) and implement Simon's two-stage design.

The most prominent advantage of Simon's two-stage design is its transparency and simplicity. The design parameters (n_1, r_1, n_2, r) are determined prior to the onset of the trial. During the trial conduct, no calculation is needed. Users only have to compare the number of responses with the stopping boundaries r_1 and r to make go/no-go decisions. Another advantage of Simon's two-stage design is that it explicitly controls type I and II errors. The limitations of Simon's two-stage design include that it only allows one interim and only handles a binary endpoint. Next, we introduce a Bayesian optimal phase II (BOP2) design that allows flexible interims and accommodates both binary and more complicated endpoints.

BOP2 DESIGN

Traditionally, phase II clinical trials have focused on binary efficacy endpoints (e.g., tumor response), but they have become much more complicated with the advent of novel molecular targeted agents and immunotherapy. The endpoints for such treatments may be ordinal or multivariate, and the investigators are often interested in simultaneously monitoring multiple types of events in the trial. Table 21.4 provides four trial examples with different types of endpoint (51–53). The BOP2 provides a novel unified framework to handle all these different types of phase II trials.

Example 1 considers a binary efficacy endpoint, namely objective response, to evaluate the efficacy of pembrolizumab in treating patients with small bowel adenocarcinoma. The treatment is considered futile if the objective response rate (ORR) ≤ 0.2 and efficacious if the ORR ≥ 0.4.

Example 2 considers a nested efficacy endpoint to evaluate the efficacy of nivolumab in patients with Hodgkin lymphoma. The efficacy endpoint is ordinal: complete remission (CR), partial remission (PR), progressive disease (PD), and stable disease (SD). The treatment is deemed efficacious if $\Pr(CR + PR) \geq 0.3$ *or* $\Pr(CR) > 0.15$. The endpoints are nested here because the endpoint of the second condition (i.e., CR) is nested in that of the first condition (i.e., CR + PR).

Example 3 considers coprimary endpoints to evaluate the efficacy of trebananib administered at 15 mg/kg intravenous (IV) per week in patients with persistent or recurrent carcinoma of the endometrium. The two coprimary efficacy endpoints are ORR and event-free survival at 6 months (EFS6). The treatment is regarded as efficacious if $\Pr(ORR) \geq 0.3$ or $\Pr(EFS6) > 0.35$.

Example 4 jointly monitors efficacy and toxicity of lenalidomide in combination with rituximab. The treatments are regarded as promising if ORR ≥ 0.45 and toxicity rate ≤0.3.

STATISTICAL MODEL

Although the endpoints of the aforementioned trials take different forms, they can be unified and represented by a random variable Y that follows a multinomial distribution,

$$Y \mid \theta \sim \text{Multinomial}\,(\theta_1, \ldots, \theta_k)$$

with $\theta = (\theta_1, \ldots, \theta_k)^T$ where θ_k is the probability that Y belongs to the kth category, $k = 1, \ldots, K$. The K categories can be the actual levels of a single endpoint or the combinational levels of multiple categorical endpoints. For example, in trial example 2, Y is the ordinal outcome, with $Y = 1, 2, 3$, and 4 denoting CR, PR, SD, and PD, respectively. In trial example 3, Y is a multinomial variable with four categories where 1 = (OR, EFS6), 2 = (OR, no EFS6), 3 = (no OR, EFS6), and 4 = (no OR, no EFS6).

TABLE 21.4 THE FOUR EXAMPLES CONSIDERED BY THE BOP2 DESIGN

Endpoint type	Outcome	Study setting	Decision criterion
Example 1: **binary**	ORR defined using RECIST, version 1.1.	Evaluate the efficacy of pembrolizumab in treating patients with small bowel adenocarcinoma	*Futile*: ORR ≤0.2 *Promising*: ORR ≥0.4.
Example 2: **nested**	CR PR PD SD	Evaluate the efficacy of nivolumab in patients with Hodgkin's lymphoma	*Promising*: CR + PR ≥ 0.3 or CR > 0.15,
Example 3: **coprimary**	ORR, EFS rate at 6 months (EFS6)	Evaluate the efficacy of trebananib administered at 15 mg/kg IV per week in patients with persistent or recurrent carcinoma of the endometrium (52)	*Futile*: ORR ≤0.1 and EFS6 ≤0.2 *Promising*: ORR ≥0.3 and EFS6 >0.35
Example 4: **joint**	ORR and toxicity rate	Evaluate the safety and efficacy of lenalidomide in combination with rituximab in patients with recurrent indolent nonfollicular lymphoma (53)	*Promising*: ORR ≥0.45 and toxicity rate ≤0.3

CR, complete remission; EFS, event-free survival; IV, intravenous; ORR, objective response rate; PD, progressive disease; PR, partial remission; RECIST, Response Evaluation Criteria in Solid Tumors; SD, stable disease.

Source: Zhou H, Lee JJ, Yuan Y. BOP2: Bayesian optimal design for phase II clinical trials with simple and complex endpoints. *Stat Med.* 2017;36(21):3302–3314. doi:10.1002/sim.7338

Table 21.5 provides the category mapping for the four examples. Under the Bayesian paradigm, we assign θ a Dirichlet prior distribution:

$$(\theta_1, \ldots, \theta_k) \sim \text{Dirichlet}\ (a_1, \ldots, a_K)$$

where $a_1, \ldots, a_K$ are hyperparameters. In general, we can set $\sum_{k=1}^{K} a_k = 1$ such that the prior information is vague and equivalent to a prior sample size of 1. Suppose that at an interim time, a total of n patients have been enrolled in the trial and their endpoints have been fully evaluated. Let $D_n = (x_1, \ldots, x_n)$ denote the interim data, and x_k denote the number of patients with $Y = k$. The posterior distribution of θ arises as

$$(\theta_1, \ldots, \theta_k) \mid D_n \sim \text{Dirichlet}\ (a_1 + x_1, \ldots, a_K + x_K)$$

BOP2 TRIAL DESIGN

The BOP2 design consists of R interim looks, which occur when the number of enrolled patients reaches $n_1, \ldots n_R$, and a final look when all N patients are enrolled. At each of the looks, the go/no-go decision is made based on the posterior probabilities of one or more linear combinations of the model parameters θ in the form of

$$Pr(b\,\theta \leq \phi \mid D_n) > C(n) \tag{6}$$

where b is a design vector with elements of 0 and 1; ϕ is a prespecified limit; and $C(n)$ is a probability cutoff, which is a function of interim sample size n. Specifically, the posterior probability based stopping rules for the four trial examples are as follows:

TABLE 21.5 DESIGN PARAMETER FOR EACH EXAMPLE, WHERE $\theta_K = PR(Y = K)$, $K = 1,2$ IN EXAMPLE 1 AND $K = 1, \ldots, 4$ FOR EXAMPLES 2–4

	Outcomes	Probability (θ)	Design parameter (b)
Example 1	Y = {1,2} with 1 = OR and 2 = no OR	(θ_1,θ_2)	b = {1,0}
Example 2	Y = {1,2,3,4} with 1 = CR, 2 = PR, 3 = SD, 4 = PD	$(\theta_1,\theta_2,\theta_3,\theta_4)$	b = {1,0,0,0} and b = {1,1,0,0}
Example 3	Y = {1,2,3,4} with 1 = (OR, EFS6), 2 = (OR, no EFS6), 3 = (no OR, EFS6), 4 = (no OR, no EFS6)	$(\theta_1,\theta_2,\theta_3,\theta_4)$	b = {1,1,0,0} and b = {1,0,1,0}
Example 4	Y = {1,2,3,4} with 1 = (toxicity, OR), 2 = (no toxicity, OR), 3 = (toxicity, no OR), 4 = (no toxicity, no OR)	$(\theta_1,\theta_2,\theta_3,\theta_4)$	b = {1,1,0,0} or b = {1,0,1,0}

CR, complete remission; EFS6, event-free survival at 6 months; OR, objective response; PR, partial remission; SD, stable disease.

- *Example 1:* $Pr(\theta_1 \le 0.2 \mid D_n) > C(n)$
- *Example 2:* $Pr(\theta_1 \le 0.15 \mid D_n) > C(n)$ and $Pr(\theta_1 + \theta_2 \le 0.3) > C(n)$
- *Example 3:* $Pr(\theta_1 + \theta_2 \le 0.1 \mid D_n) > C(n)$ and $Pr(\theta_1 + \theta_3 \le 0.2) > C(n)$
- *Example 4:* $Pr(\theta_1 + \theta_2 \le 0.45 \mid D_n) > C(n)$ or $Pr(\theta_1 + \theta_3 \le 0.3 \mid D_n) > C(n)$

We summarize the outcomes Y, corresponding probabilities θ, and design vector b in Table 21.5.

The BOP design considers the following adaptive cutoff function:

$$C(n) = 1 - \lambda\left(\frac{n}{N}\right)^{\gamma}$$

where λ determines the cutoff at the end of the trial, and γ controls how fast the cutoff changes with the fraction of interim information. The stopping cutoff $C(n)$ is adaptive and depends on the interim sample size n, such that the stopping criteria are lenient at the beginning of the trial and become increasingly stricter when the trial proceeds. It reflects the practical consideration that at the beginning of the trial, clinicians prefer a lenient efficacy requirement to avoid incorrectly stopping the trial too early (caused by spare data) so that more data can be collected to learn more on the characteristics of the agent; whereas toward the end of the trial, as more data accumulate, a stringent requirement is preferred so that the futile treatment can be stopped timely. Given a prespecified type I error rate and the maximum sample size N, the BOP design chooses the values of design parameters (λ,γ) to maximize the power. See Zhou et al. (54) for the technical details of this optimization.

Similar to Simon's two-stage design, one important advantage of the BOP2 design is that its stopping boundary can be enumerated and included in the trial protocol prior to the onset of the trial. When conducting the trial, clinicians simply count the number of relevant events and make the go/no-go decision based on whether that count exceeds the boundary. Table 21.6 presents the corresponding stopping boundaries for each trial example, given the null and alternative hypotheses shown in Table 21.7. The Shiny application is freely available at www.trialdesign.org to obtain the stopping boundaries.

TABLE 21.6 STOPPING BOUNDARIES FOR EACH EXAMPLE IN TABLE 21.7 GIVEN TYPE I ERROR RATE AT 0.1

			Number of patients treated						
Trial	Stop the trial if		10	15	20	25	30	35	40
Example 1		# of OR ≤	1	2	4	5	7	9	12
Example 2		# of CR ≤	0	1	3	4	5	7	10
	and	# of CR/PR ≤	2	3	6	8	10	13	17
Example 3		# of OR ≤	1	2	2	3	4	6	7
	and	# of EFS6 ≤	2	3	5	6	8	10	12
Example 4		# of OR ≤	3	5	8	11	14	16	19
	or	# of Toxicity ≥	5	6	7	8	9	10	11

CR, complete remission; OR, objective response; EFS6, event-free survival at 6 months; PR, partial remission.

Compared to most of the existing Bayesian phase II designs, such as Thall et al. (55) and Thall and Sung (56), the advantages of the BOP2 design include (a) offering a more flexible framework to monitor multiple events simultaneously, including nested or coprimary endpoints; (b) explicitly controlling the type I error rate, thereby bridging the gap between Bayesian designs and frequentist designs and also rendering the proposed Bayesian design more accessible to a wide range of

TABLE 21.7 NULL HYPOTHESIS AND ALTERNATIVE HYPOTHESIS FOR THE FOUR EXAMPLES

	Null hypothesis H_0 and alternative hypothesis H_1
Example 1	H_0: $Pr(OR) = Pr(\theta_1) = 0.2$
	H_1: $Pr(OR) = Pr(\theta_1) = 0.4$
Example 2	H_0: $Pr(CR) = Pr(\theta_1) = 0.15$, $Pr(CR \text{ or } PR) = Pr(\theta_1 + \theta_2) = 0.30$
	H_1: $Pr(CR) = Pr(\theta_1) = 0.25$, $Pr(CR \text{ or } PR) = Pr(\theta_1 + \theta_2) = 0.35$
Example 3	H_0: $Pr(OR) = Pr(\theta_1 + \theta_2) = 0.1$, $Pr(EFS6) = Pr(\theta_1 + \theta_3) = 0.20$
	H_1: $Pr(OR) = Pr(\theta_1 + \theta_2) = 0.3$, $Pr(EFS6) = Pr(\theta_1 + \theta_3) = 0.35$
Example 4	H_0: $Pr(OR) = Pr(\theta_1 + \theta_2) = 0.45$, $Pr(Toxicity) = Pr(\theta_1 + \theta_3) = 0.3$
	H_1: $Pr(OR) = Pr(\theta_1 + \theta_2) = 0.60$, $Pr(Toxicity) = Pr(\theta_1 + \theta_3) = 0.2$

CR, complete remission; OR, objective response; EFS6, event-free survival at 6 months; PR, partial remission.

users and regulatory agencies; and (c) maximizing the power of the design by choosing appropriate cutoffs for the stopping rule.

The BOP2 design is flexible in terms of the number of interim looks to be conducted during the trial. The choice of the number of interim looks hinges on logistical considerations. For example, if the endpoints are quickly ascertainable and frequent updating of the interim data is feasible, full sequential or frequent interim monitoring may be used. However, if the endpoints take a long time to be evaluated, we may limit the number of interim looks to avoid frequently suspending the accrual of patients. When desirable, the method of Cai et al. (43) can be adopted to eliminate the requirement of suspending the accrual.

GLOSSARY

maximum tolerated dose (MTD): the dose with the dose-limiting toxicity (DLT) probability closest to the target DLT rate.

dose-limiting toxicity (DLT): side effects of a treatment that are serious enough to prevent an increase in the dose of the drug.

algorithm-based designs: trial designs that use a set of simple, prespecified rules to determine dose escalation and de-escalation, without assuming any model on the dose–toxicity curve.

3 + 3 design: the most widely used algorithm-based trial design.

operating characteristics: the key aspects of a chosen trial design.

model-based designs: trial designs that use a parametric dosetoxicity model to guide the dose escalation and de-escalation process.

continual reassessment method (CRM): a typical model-based design that assumes a parametric model for the dose–toxicity curve.

skeleton: in a CRM, the set of prior estimates of the dose-limiting toxicity rates.

indifference interval: an interval of DLT rates associated with the neighboring doses, such that these neighboring doses may be selected instead of the true MTD.

Bayesian Model-Averaging CRM (BMA-CRM): an approach that improves the robustness of the CRM to the choice of skeleton.

model-assisted design: trial design that utilizes a statistical model to derive the design but also includes a rule of dose escalation and de-escalation that is pretabulated before the onset of the trial.

modified toxicity probability interval (mTPI) design: a model-assisted trial design that starts by defining three dosing intervals.

BOIN design: Bayesian optimal interval design, which is a model-assisted trial design.

Keyboard design: a model-assisted trial design.

escalation and de-escalation boundaries: lower and upper dose limiting toxicity (DLT) rates used to guide dose escalation and de-escalation.

molecularly targeted agents (MTAs): substances developed to modulate specific aberrant pathways in cancer cells while sparing normal tissue.

immunotherapy/immuno-oncology agents (IOAs): substances designed to stimulate a patient's antitumor immune response.

waterfall design: a model for determining MTD contours for more than one drug.

REFERENCES

1. Jaki T, Clive S, Weir CJ. Principles of dose finding studies in cancer: a comparison of trial designs. *Cancer Chemother Pharmacol.* 2013;71(5):1107–1114. doi:10.1007/s00280-012-2059-8
2. Yuan Y, Yin G. Bayesian hybrid design in phase I oncology clinical trials. *Stat Med.* 2011;30(17):2098–2108. doi:10.1002/sim.4164
3. Yan F, Mandrekar SJ, Yuan Y. Keyboard: a novel Bayesian toxicity probability interval design for phase I clinical trials. *Clin Cancer Res.* 2017;23(15):3994–4003. doi:10.1158/1078-0432.CCR-17-0220
4. Lee S, Cheung Y. Model calibration in the continual reassessment method. *Clin Trials.* 2009;6(3):227–238. doi:10.1177/1740774509105076
5. Yin G, Yuan Y. Bayesian model averaging continual reassessment method in phase I clinical trials. *J Am Stat Assoc.* 2009;104(487):954–968. doi:10.1198/jasa.2009.ap08425
6. Zhou H, Murray T, Pan H, Yuan Y. Comparative review of toxicity probability interval designs for phase I clinical trials. *Stat Med.* 2018;37(14):2208–2222. doi:10.1002/sim.7674
7. Ji Y, Liu P, Li Y, Nebiyou Bekele B. A modified toxicity probability interval method for dose-finding trials. *Clin Trials.* 2009;7(6):653–663. doi:10.1177/1740774510382799
8. Liu S, Yuan Y. Bayesian optimal interval designs for phase I clinical trials. *J R Stat Soc Ser A Stat Soc.* 2015;64(3):507–523. doi:10.1111/rssc.12089
9. Yuan Y, Hess K, Hilsenbeck S, Gilbert M. Bayesian optimal interval design: a simple and well-performing design for phase I oncology trials. *Clin Cancer Res.* 2016;22:4291–4301. doi:10.1158/1078-0432.ccr-16-0592
10. Vincze I, Barlow R, Bartholomew D, et al. Statistical inference under order restrictions: the theory and application of isotonic regression. *Int Stat Rev.* 1973;41(3):395. doi:10.2307/1402630
11. Guo B, Yuan Y. Bayesian phase I/II biomarker-based dose finding for precision medicine with molecularly targeted agents. *J Am Stat Assoc.* 2017;112(518):508–520. doi:10.1080/01621459.2016.1228534
12. Berger JO. *Statistical Decision Theory and Bayesian Analysis.* Berlin, Germany: Springer Science Business Media; 2013.
13. Simon R, Freidlin B, Rubinstein L, et al. Accelerated titration designs for phase I clinical trials in oncology. *J Natl Cancer Inst.* 1997;89(15):1138–1147. doi:10.1093/jnci/89.15.1138
14. Clertant M, O'Quigley J. Semiparametric dose finding methods. *J R Stat Soc Series B Stat Methodol.* 2017;79(5):1487–1508. doi:10.1111/rssb.12229
15. Zhou H, Yuan Y, Nie L. Accuracy, safety and reliability of novel phase I trial designs. *Clin Cancer Res.* 2018; 24(18):4357–4364. doi:10.1158/1078-0432.CCR-18-0168
16. Lin R, Yin G. Bayesian optimal interval design for dose finding in drug-combination trials. *Stat Methods Med Res.* 2015;26:2155–2167. doi: 10.1177/0962280215594494
17. Zhang L, Yuan Y. A practical Bayesian design to identify the maximum tolerated dose contour for drug combination trials. *Stat Med.* 2016;35(27):4924–4936. doi:10.1002/sim.7095
18. Yuan Y, Lin R, Nie L, et al. Time-to-event Bayesian optimal interval design to accelerate phase I trials. *Clin Cancer Res.* 2018. doi:10.1158/1078-0432.CCR-18-0246. [Epub ahead of print]
19. Mu R, Yuan Y, Xu J, et al. gBOIN: a unified model-assisted phase I trial design accounting for toxicity grades, binary or continuous endpoint. *J R Stat Soc Ser C.* 2018. https://rss.onlinelibrary.wiley.com/doi/abs/10.1111/rssc.12263
20. The University of Texas MD Anderson Cancer Center. Bayesian Optimal Interval (BOIN) design desktop program. https://biostatistics.mdanderson.org/softwaredownload/SingleSoftware.aspx?Software_Id=99. Updated August 17, 2018.
21. Korn E. Nontoxicity endpoints in phase I trial designs for targeted, non-cytotoxic agents. *J Natl Cancer Inst.* 2004;96:977–978. doi:10.1093/jnci/djh208
22. Postel-Vinay S, Arkenau HT, Olmos D, et al. Clinical benefit in phase-I trials of novel molecularly targeted agents: does dose matter? *Br J Cancer.* 2009;100(9):1373–1378. doi:10.1038/sj.bjc.6605030
23. Robert C, Ribas A, Wolchok JD, et al. Anti-programmed-death-receptor-1 treatment with pembrolizumab in ipilimumab-refractory advanced melanoma: a randomised dose-comparison cohort of a phase 1 trial. *Lancet.* 2014;384(9948):1109–1117. doi:10.1016/S0140-6736(14)60958-2
24. Food and Drug Administration. Guidance for industry: clinical considerations for therapeutic cancer vaccines. https://www.fda.gov/downloads/biologicsbloodvaccines/guidancecomplianceregulatoryinformation/guidances/vaccines/ucm278673.pdf. 2011.
25. Yuan Y, Nguyen HQ, Thall PF. *Bayesian Designs for Phase I/II Clinical Trials.* Boca Raton, FL: CRC Press; 2016.
26. Hunsberger S, Rubinstein LV, Dancey J, Korn EL. Dose escalation trial designs based on a molecularly targeted endpoint. *Stat Med.* 2005;24(14):2171–2181. doi:10.1002/sim.2102
27. Riviere MK, Yuan Y, Jourdan JH, et al. Phase I/II dose-finding design for molecularly targeted agent: plateau determination using adaptive randomization. *Stat Methods Med Res.* 2016;27(2):466–4791. doi:10.1177/0962280216631763
28. Zang Y, Lee JJ, Yuan Y. Adaptive designs for identifying optimal biological dose for molecularly targeted agents. *Clin Trials.* 2014;11(3):319–327. doi:10.1111/j.0006-341x.2004.00215.x
29. Liu S, Guo B, Yuan Y. A Bayesian phase i/ii design for immunotherapy trial. *J Am Stat Assoc.* 2017:1–12. doi:10.1080/01621459.2017.1383260
30. Guo W, Wang S, Yang S, et al. A Bayesian interval dose-finding design addressing Ockham's razor: mtpi-2. *Contemp Clin Trials.* 2017;58:2333. doi:10.1016/j.cct.2017.04.006
31. Barlow RE, Bartholomew DJ, Bremner JM, Brunk HD. *Statistical Inference Under Order Restrictions.* Hoboken, NJ: John Wiley & Sons; 1972.
32. Robertson T, Wright FT, Dykstra RL. *Order Restricted Statistical Inference.* Hoboken, NJ: John Wiley & Sons; 1988.

33. Turner T, Wollan P. Locating a maximum using isotonic regression. *Comput Stat Data Anal.* 25(3):305–320. doi:10.1016/s0167-9473(97)00009-1
34. Conaway M, Dunbar S, Peddada SD. Designs for single- or multiple-agent phase I trials. *Biometrics.* 2004;60(3):661–669. doi:10.1111/j.0006-341x.2004.00215.x
35. Yin G, Yuan, Y. A latent contingency table approach to dose finding for combinations of two agents. *Biometrics.* 2009;65(3):866–875. doi:10.1111/j.1541-0420.2008.01119.x
36. Yin G, Yuan Y. Bayesian dose finding in oncology for drug combinations by copula regression. *J R Stat Soc Series C.* 2009;58(2):211–224. doi:10.1111/j.1467-9876.2009.00649.x
37. Braun T, Wang S. A hierarchical Bayesian design for phase I trials of novel combinations of cancer therapeutic agents. *Biometrics.* 2010;66(3):805–812. doi:10.1111/j.1541-0420.2009.01363.x
38. Wages N, Conaway M, O'Quigley J. Continual reassessment method for partial ordering. *Biometrics.* 2011;67(4):1555–1563. doi:10.1111/j.1541-0420.2011.01560.x
39. O'Quigley J, Pepe M, Fisher L. Continual reassessment method: a practical design for phase I clinical trials in cancer. *Biometrics.* 1990;46(1):33–48. doi:10.1111/j.1541-0420.2011.01560.
40. Braun T, Jia N. (2013). A generalized continual reassessment method for two-agent phase I trials. *Stat Biopharm Res.* 2013;5:105–115. doi:10.1080/19466315.2013.767213
41. Riviere M, Yuan Y, Dubois F, Zohar S. (2014). A Bayesian dose-finding design for drug combination clinical trials based on the logistic model. *Pharm Stat.* 2014;13(4):247–257. doi:10.1002/pst.1621
42. Cai C, Liu S, Yuan Y. A Bayesian design for phase II clinical trials with delayed responses based on multiple imputation. *Stat Med.* 2014;33(23):4017–4028. doi:10.1002/sim.6200
43. Cai C, Yuan Y, Ji Y. A Bayesian phase I/II design for oncology clinical trials of combining biological agents. *J R Stat Soc Series C.* 2014;63: 159–173. doi:10.1111/rssc.12039
44. Riviere M, Yuan Y, Dubois F, Zohar S. A Bayesian dose-finding design for clinical trials combining a cytotoxic agent with a molecularly targeted agent. *J R Stat Soc Series C.* 2015;64:215–229. doi:10.1111/rssc.12072
45. Thall P, Millikan R, Mueller P, Lee S. Dose-finding with two agents in phase I oncology trials. *Biometrics.* 2003;59(3):487–496. doi:10.1111/1541-0420.00058
46. Wang K, Ivanova A. Two-dimensional dose finding in discrete dose space. *Biometrics.* 2005;61(1):217–222. doi:10.1111/j.0006-341X.2005.030540.x
47. Yuan Y, Yin G. Sequential continual reassessment method for two-dimensional dose finding. *Stat Med.* 2008;27(27):5664–5678. doi:10.1002/sim.3372
48. Mander A, Sweeting M. A product of independent beta probabilities dose escalation design for dual-agent phase I trials. *Stat Med.* 2015;34(8):1261–1276. doi:10.1002/sim.6434
49. Gordon B, Richard D, Carolyn P, Tim R. Isotonic regression in two independent variables. *J R Stat Soc Series B Stat Methodol.* 1984;33(3):352–357. doi:10.2307/2347723
50. Simon R. Optimal two-stage designs for phase II clinical trials. *Contemp Clin Trials.* 1989;10(1):1–10. doi:10.1016/0197-2456(89)90015-9
51. Cheson BD, Pfistner B, Juweid ME, et al. Revised response criteria for malignant lymphoma. *J Clin Oncol.* 2007;25(5):579. doi:10.1200/JCO.2006.09.2403
52. Moore KN, Sill MW, Tenney ME, et al. (2015). A phase II trial of trebananib (AMG 386; IND# 111071), a selective angiopoietin 1/2 neutralizing peptibody, in patients with persistent/recurrent carcinoma of the endometrium: an NRG/Gynecologic Oncology Group trial. *Gynecol Oncol.* 2015;138(3):513–518. doi:10.1016/j.ygyno.2015.07.006
53. Sacchi S, Marcheselli R, Bari A, et al. Safety and efficacy of lenalidomide in combination with rituximab in recurrent indolent non-follicular lymphoma: final results of a phase II study conducted by the Fondazione Italiana Linfomi. *Haematologica.* 2016;101(5):e196–e199. doi:10.3324/haematol.2015.139329
54. Zhou H, Lee JJ, Yuan Y. BOP2: Bayesian optimal design for phase II clinical trials with simple and complex endpoints. *Stat Med.* 2017;36(21):3302–3314. doi:10.1002/sim.7338
55. Thall PF, Simon RM, Estey EH. Bayesian sequential monitoring designs for single-arm clinical trials with multiple outcomes. *Stat Med.* 1995;14(4):357–379. doi:10.1002/sim.4780140404
56. Thall PF, Sung HG. Some extensions and applications of a Bayesian strategy for monitoring multiple outcomes in clinical trials. *Stat Med.* 1998;17(14):1563–1580. doi:10.1002/(SICI)1097-0258(19980730)17:14<1563::AID-SIM873>3.0.CO;2-L

APPENDIX

BAYESIAN MODEL AVERAGING CONTINUOUS REASSESSMENT METHOD (BMA-CRM)

Let $(M_1, \ldots, M_K)$ be the models corresponding to the K prespecified skeletons $\{(\pi_{11} \ldots \pi_{1J}), \ldots, (\pi_{K1}, \ldots \pi_{KJ})\}$, where M_k ($k = 1, \ldots, K$) takes a form $p_{kj}(a_k) = \pi_{kj}^{\exp(a_k)}, j = 1, \ldots, J$, obtained using the kth skeleton $(\pi_{k1}, \ldots \pi_{kJ})$. Let $\Pr(M_k)$ be the prior probability that model M_k is the true model, that is, the probability that the kth skeleton $(\pi_{k1}, \ldots \pi_{k,J})$ matches the true dose–toxicity curve. When there is prior information on the importance of each set of the prespecified DLT rates, we can incorporate such information into $Pr(M_k)$. For example, if a certain set of prespecified models is more likely to be true, we can assign it a higher prior probability. Otherwise we can take a noninformative approach of assigning equal weights to the different skeletons with $Pr(M_k) = 1/K$.

At a certain stage of the trial, based on the observed data $D = \{(n_j, y_j) : j = 1, \ldots, J\}$, the likelihood function under model M_k is

$$L(D \mid a_k, M_k) = \prod_{j=1}^{J} \left\{\pi_{kj}^{\exp(a_k)}\right\}^{y_j} \left\{1 - \pi_{kj}^{\exp(a_k)}\right\}^{n_j - y_j}.$$

Applying the Bayes theorem, the posterior model probability for M_k is given by

$$Pr(M_k \mid D) = \frac{L(D \mid M_k) Pr(M_k)}{\sum_{i=1}^{K} L(D \mid M_i) Pr(M_i)},$$

where $L(D \mid M_k)$ is the marginal likelihood of model M_k,

$$L(D \mid M_k) = \int L(D \mid a_k, M_k) f(a_k \mid M_k) da_k,$$

where α_k is the power parameter in the CRM associated with model M_k and $f(\alpha_k \mid M_k)$ is the prior distribution of α_k under model M_k.

The BMA estimate for the DLT rate at each dose level is given by

$$\bar{p}_j = \sum_{k=1}^{K} \hat{p}_{kj} Pr(M_k \mid D), j = 1, \ldots, J, \tag{7}$$

where $\hat{p}_{kj}$ is the posterior mean of the DLT rate of dose level j under model M_k, that is,

$$\hat{p}_{kj} = \int \pi_{kj}^{\exp(a_k)} \frac{L(D \mid a_k) f(a_k)}{\int L(D \mid a_k, M_k) f(a_k \mid M_k) da_k} da_k.$$

By assigning $\hat{p}_{kj}$ a weight of $\Pr(M_k \mid D)$, the BMA method automatically identifies and favors the best fitting model; thus $\bar{p}_j$ is always close to the best estimate. The dose-finding algorithm of the BMA-CRM is the same as that of the CRM described previously, except that the DLT rate estimate $\hat{p}_j$ is replaced by $\bar{p}_j$ given in equation (7). In other words, the decision of dose escalation or de-escalation in the trial is based on $\bar{p}_j$, which is estimated with multiple skeletons, as opposed to $\hat{p}_j$, which is calculated with a single skeleton.

22

Late Phase Clinical Trials

KARLA V. BALLMAN

There are two general types of late phase clinical trials: phase III trials and phase IV trials. A phase III trial usually compares a new treatment with the best currently available treatment, which is generally the current standard of care. The objective of a phase III trial is to change clinical practice if the new treatment is found to be superior to the current standard of care. Often, a drug company will apply for Food and Drug Administration (FDA) approval of a drug on the basis of phase III data that demonstrate their drug is superior to the current standard of care. Phase IV trials are performed after a drug has obtained approval by the FDA. The main reasons for performing a phase IV trial include (a) identification of rare adverse events (AEs), (b) determination of long-term risks and benefits, and (c) evaluation of how well the drug works when it is used in the general population. These trials often require thousands of patients. This chapter focuses on phase III trials.

The goal of a phase III trial is to compare the efficacy of a new treatment regimen to the accepted standard of care, which acts as a control. The new treatment regimen has already been tested in early phase trials and has been demonstrated to have an acceptable safety profile and found to have some antitumor activity. The question now is whether the new treatment is better than the current standard of care. The primary objective for a phase III trial is to compare the overall survival (OS), or disease-free survival (DFS) or progression-free survival (PFS), of patients assigned to the different treatment arms.

Phase III trials use accepted scientific principles of good experimental design, including an explicit statement of primary and secondary objectives, specification of the types of patients appropriate for the trial, details of the treatment arms being compared, specifics for how the randomization will be done, clear definitions of endpoints, statistical considerations (hypotheses tested, sample size and expected trial duration, interim and final analysis plans), and study monitoring. There are different designs that can be used to determine whether an experimental treatment (or experimental treatments) is (are) better than the standard of care (control arm). The most commonly used design is a **two-arm trial**. Two other commonly used designs that are discussed include designs with more than two treatment arms, generally called **multiarm trials**, and **factorial designs**.

Designing a phase III clinical trial is a true team effort. It is important that key individuals work together from the start, especially the primary investigator (or trial chair) and the trial statistician. Depending on the interventions being tested and the trial secondary objectives, it may require that additional individuals with relevant expertise be included in the study design discussions. For example, if the intervention requires the combination of a new drug and radiation therapy, it would be important to have a radiation oncologist as a key study team member, assuming that a medical oncologist is the trial chair. Finally, the design of phase III clinical trial is an iterative process. Frequently there are major modifications made in the study design from what was initially proposed to what is eventually opened for accrual. This iterative process generally yields a well-designed trial.

TWO-ARM TRIAL DESIGNS

PRIMARY OBJECTIVE

Identifying the primary objective requires careful thought about what conclusion is of most interest at the completion of the trial. An objective also has to be specific so that it contains a testable hypothesis. Merely stating that the objective is to compare the experimental treatment to the standard of care is not sufficient. Is the goal to definitively determine which treatment should be used to treat future patients with a particular cancer? Is the goal to determine whether the combination of another treatment to the standard of care improves survival for patients with a specific cancer? Answering the first question would require a two-sided **superiority test** because it is not known which treatment is better, if either. If the combination is found to be significantly (both clinically and statistically) superior, it would become the new standard of care. If the current standard of care is significantly superior to the combination, there would be no change in standard of care. Likewise, if it is found that neither is significantly superior to the other, there would be no change in the standard of care. Studies to answer the second question would likely use a one-sided superiority test because there would be no interest in the unlikely (though possible) scenario that the combination confers significantly worse survival compared to the control arm. The only outcome of interest is whether the combination significantly improves patient outcomes compared to the standard of care alone: if it does, the combination would become the new standard of care. If the combination were not found to be significantly superior, it would not become the new standard of care because it is likely more expensive due to the addition of another drug and likely has more AEs. Clearly, if the combination is significantly worse, the standard of care would not change.

ELIGIBILITY

There is an inherent trade-off between restricting a trial to patients most likely to benefit from the new treatment and the **generalizability** of the results to a broader patient population. For example, many past phase III oncology trials would restrict patient age to adults (those 18 and older) who were younger than 65 years of age. This has caused issues for treating oncologists regarding the use of treatments known to have a substantial AE burden in patients older than 65 years. Because trials did not include these patients, it is not known whether such patients can tolerate a number of cycles sufficient to gain benefit from the treatment or whether the treatment may be detrimental with respect to survival of these already frail patients by hastening their death as a result of their comorbidities. This is a serious issue as, for many cancers, the average age at diagnosis is above 65 years. Generalizability can be comprised if eligibility criteria are too narrow. In contrast, if the eligibility criteria are too broad, the effectiveness of a new treatment may be diluted, because the trial contains a significant proportion of patients who would not be expected to benefit from it.

Determining the correct patient population (e.g., trial eligibility) in the current era of **targeted therapies** has become even more challenging. Targeted treatments take advantage of a specific aberration in a tumor as a means to only kill cancer cells versus cytotoxic treatment that indiscriminately kills all cells. One issue is that a treatment designed for a specific tumor aberration may not effectively target it as expected. This would mean the agent does not have efficacy in a patient population with tumors containing the aberration. Another issue is that a targeted treatment may have off-target effects that render it effective in tumors that do and do not have the target aberration. This illustrates that it may not be well understood which tumor and patient characteristics are more predictive of patient benefit from targeted treatments. Many new trial designs have been proposed for targeted agents with accompanying biomarkers (1,2).

TREATMENT ARMS

Two-arm phase III trials generally compare a new treatment (Arm E) to the current standard of care, which is the control arm (Arm C). To ensure scientific rigor, the selected treatment arms must align with the objectives of the trial; this means that the arms should be as similar as possible other than the aspect of treatment that is under investigation. If the objective is to demonstrate that the new treatment should become the new standard of care, then Arm C should be the current standard of care and not a variation of it. Obviously, Arm C should not be another experimental treatment that is not the standard of care for this objective. If Arm C is not the current standard of care, at the end of the trial there will be no evidence that Arm E is better than the current standard of care, even if it is found to be superior to some variant of it or found to be superior to another experimental treatment. If the objective is to demonstrate that the addition of a new treatment to the current standard of care is better than the current standard of care, then the current standard of care has to be exactly the same in both arms. If the current standard of care is modified in the arm with the combination (perhaps to make it more tolerable when combined with the new treatment), at the end of the trial it will not be clear whether the addition of the new treatment or the modification of the current standard of care is responsible for observed differences between the treatment arms.

RANDOMIZATION

Randomization is used in phase III trials to ensure that the two comparator arms are as balanced as possible in baseline patient and tumor characteristics, with the only systematic difference between the arms being the protocol treatments. If the trial sample size is fixed at N patients, the most information obtained (or the greatest power for a given difference of interest) is from a **1:1 randomization**, which assigns $N/2$ patients to each arm. In this scenario, a patient has an equal chance of being assigned to either arm.

Sometimes a **2:1 randomization** scheme is used to motivate patients to enroll in the trial. In this case, the patient has a 2/3 probability of being assigned to the experimental arm compared to a 1/3 probability of being assigned to the control arm. Occasionally, other randomization balances have been used as well (3). An unbalanced randomization can be attractive to patients who perceive the experimental arm to be more desirable (e.g., will have more survival benefit, has fewer AEs) than the control arm. However, if all other trial aspects are kept constant (e.g., power, accrual rate, minimal detectable difference, and significance), a trial with an unbalanced randomization requires more patients than a trial with a 1:1 randomization. The increase in sample size must be weighed against the (theoretical) expected increase in patient enrollment rates. Another type of randomization gaining in popularity is adaptive randomization (see Chapter 25). There should be a strong justification for using a randomization scheme that is not 1:1, due to the increased resources required for the other randomization schemes.

Randomization does not guarantee that all baseline variables will be balanced between the treatment arms, unless the sample size is quite large. There is the chance, though small, that an imbalance in an important patient characteristic happens by chance in small or modestly sized trials. The use of **stratification factors** protects against imbalances of important prognostic variables.

For example, suppose it is most important that sex, out of all other baseline variables, be balanced between the treatment arms. Sex would be a stratification variable, which means that there is a separate randomization scheme for males and a separate randomization scheme for females, in contrast to a single randomization scheme across all patients enrolled. If 80% of the patients are female and 20% are male, there will be an essentially equal proportion of females (males) randomized to each arm, ensuring that proportion of females (males) in each arm is the same, namely 80% females in each arm. If sex is not used as a stratification variable there is a greater chance, although small, that one arm could have 70% females and the other arm have 90% females.

Variables to be considered for stratification are those known to be strongly prognostic for or strongly associated with patient outcome. If a small trial is to enroll patients with stage II or stage III lung cancer with DFS as the primary endpoint, stage might be a reasonable choice for a stratification variable because of its established strong association with DFS. It is important for the study team to discuss the use of and then number of stratification variables for a trial. After agreeing to the use of a number of stratification factors, the team then needs to select which are the important ones to be included. For a small to moderately sized trial, it is best to limit the number of stratification factors to 2 or 3. Having too many stratification factors increases the logistical burden and complicates the analysis of trial results. Many times, members of the study team advocate for an unreasonable number of stratification factors. It should be remembered that randomization balances the arms across important variables the majority of the time. For a large trial, stratification variables are likely not necessary.

Randomization is not preserved if there are a sizable number of patient cancellations. A *canceled patient* is a person who withdraws from the trial after he or she was randomized but before he or she receives his or her assigned treatment. A common scenario is one in which the patient strongly prefers the experimental treatment and is informed that he or she was randomized to the control arm. Unhappy about this, the patient discovers it is possible to be treated with the experimental treatment outside of a clinical trial and so chooses to withdraw from the trial in order to be treated with the experimental treatment.

To avoid systematic biases due to uneven patient cancellations on the two arms, good clinical trial practice mandates that the analysis be done according to the **intention-to-treat principle** (see Chapter 27). This means that a patient randomized to the control arm who cancels and receives the experimental treatment outside of the trial is followed for the primary endpoint and remains as part of the experimental arm for the analysis. If there is a considerable proportion of canceled patients, this will dilute the true treatment effect, essentially reducing the power of the study. It is important to minimize the number of patients who cancel prior to treatment initiation. One way to achieve this is to blind patients with respect to the treatment to which they were randomized. Cancellation rates should be closely monitored, especially at the start of a trial, so that the study team can intervene early to reduce an unacceptably high cancellation rate.

ENDPOINTS

A common phase III trial objective is to define the standard of care for future patients. The selected endpoint for this purpose should reflect patient benefit. endpoints that reflect patient benefit include OS, DFS, PFS, and quality of life (QOL). Recently, there are an increasing number of trials that have QOL or patient-reported outcomes (PROs) as their primary endpoint (see Chapter 23). Additional discussion of endpoints for time-to-event analysis appears in Chapter 16.

OVERALL SURVIVAL

Overall survival is defined as the time from study enrollment to time of death due to any cause. This a straightforward and objective cancer endpoint. Nonetheless, there are some issues with using OS as a primary endpoint. Bias can result if a substantial number of patients are lost to follow-up and the proportion lost to follow-up differs between the arms. Even in cases where the proportion lost to follow-up is balanced between the arms, more subtle biases could arise if sicker patients who are more likely to die are also more likely to be lost to follow-up. Then, the worse performing arm would be more likely to lose sicker patients to follow-up. It could also be the case that patients who are feeling better due to treatment may decide they do not need to participate in the trial any longer, which may be more likely to happen on the better performing arm.

If most patients are still alive at the time of analysis, estimates of survival differences may be unstable or undefined due to the small number of events, especially in phase II trials. Another concern is that if patients die of a cause other than the cancer of interest, the interpretation of survival can be challenging, especially with regard to the effect of the treatment on the cancer under study. In particular, if arms are not balanced with respect to factors associated with causes of death other than cancer (such as age and comorbidity status), biased estimates of the treatment effect can result (4). Large proportions of deaths from noncancer causes also dilute the power of trials of cancer therapies (5,6).

Using cancer-specific survival as a primary endpoint, however, can also be problematic. Cancer-specific survival is defined the same as OS except that patients are censored at the time of death if the death was not due to the cancer of interest (e.g., death due to a car accident). One problem with this approach is that a cause-specific endpoint does not account for all of a cancer treatment's effects on survival. For example, early deaths directly due to AEs or late deaths due to secondary malignancies arising as a consequence of treatment for the first cancer would not be counted as cause-specific cancer deaths. It could be argued that if the patients had not developed the cancer, they would not have developed the second cancer from which they died and thus would not have died from the cancer treatment.

More importantly, the unreliability in ascribing a cause of death becomes methodologically problematic. It may be difficult to determine definitively whether the cause of death is or is not related to the cancer. For example, it may be impossible to decide whether a death from a pulmonary embolism is cancer related, given that cancer increases the risk of thrombus formation. Certain downstream AEs, such as aspiration pneumonia, may also be indirectly associated with sequelae of treatment, making it challenging to decide whether a fatal outcome is cancer related. Finally, it would be difficult to know precisely how to attribute a death that occurred by accident while the patient is at the cancer treatment facility—although it is not quite fair to call such an event cancer related, the patient never would have been there were it not for the treatment.

Finally, interpreting effects of a new treatment on a survival endpoint may be confounded by treatments the patient receives after cancer recurrence or cancer progression. Some trials allow patients on the control arm to cross over to the experimental arm when they experience a treatment failure (e.g., cancer recurrence/progression, unacceptable AEs), and vice versa. Even if the new treatment is truly effective, there may be no difference in survival in this case if the timing of the treatment delivery is not relevant to its effectiveness. Specifically, patients assigned to the experimental arm could realize benefit from the effective treatment and those who fail on the control arm treatment also realize subsequent benefit from the experimental treatment. Such a scenario might be reflected by an improvement in DFS (or PFS) for the experimental arm compared to the control arm but no difference in OS between the arms.

DFS AND PFS

DFS and PFS are common primary endpoints used in adjuvant (metastatic) cancer trials. These endpoints are similarly defined as the time from study enrollment to the first recurrence (or progression) of the cancer, or death due to any cause. An advantage of DFS and PFS as primary endpoints is that in many settings they serve as effective **surrogate endpoints** for OS: that is, they are highly correlated with OS, yet have much higher event rates, leading to faster and less expensive evaluations of the effectiveness of new treatments (7). Often a cancer treatment that improves OS will have substantial effects on DFS and PFS. However, just because these endpoints are correlated with OS does not guarantee that they are always a reliable substitute. For example, a treatment may be effective at temporarily delaying the progression of a cancer, as evaluated by scans or blood tests, without ultimately affecting patient mortality. Hence, even if a new treatment improves DFS or PFS, it may not be clearly superior to the standard of care if an effect on OS cannot be proven.

Another difficulty with these endpoints is that the time of cancer recurrence (progression) is not known exactly. The cancer recurrence (or progression) is only known to have occurred sometime between two successive cancer assessments. As a result, the estimate of DFS (PFS) depends on the **schedule of assessments**. For unbiased comparisons, it is required that the cancer assessment schedules be identical for the two treatment arms. Another potential bias in DFS (PFS) measurement occurs when the disease is no longer assessed after the patient stops protocol treatment, due to toxicity or patient refusal to continue. Censoring DFS (PFS) at the time the patient discontinues treatment introduces bias when the reasons for early treatment discontinuation are related to disease outcome: that is, a patient may stop early because he or she is not perceiving benefit (which happens more often when a patient knows he or she is assigned to the control arm), or a patient may stop early because he or she is feeling well and wants a break from treatment. To minimize biases in DFS, it is recommended that both the patient and physician be blinded, that is, that the trial should be double-blinded (8). Similar to the previous discussion for OS, the use of DFS, PFS, or any event-free survival endpoint that includes death from any cause as an event may be adversely affected by high background rates of competing mortality; as discussed in Chapter 16, special considerations are needed in such situations.

OTHER CONSIDERATIONS

Sometimes the choice of a trial endpoint is made on the basis of available resources. For example, women with early-stage breast cancer have a good prognosis and tend to live for a long time on average, with median survival times in excess of 20 years. In this population, a trial with OS as an endpoint would require extremely large sample sizes and/or would be of very long duration. Given this, a DFS endpoint is often preferred because the median time to DFS is considerably shorter than median OS. Another factor that favors DFS versus OS in this population is the existence of a number of effective second- and third-line treatments. This could lead to no difference in OS, even for an effective treatment, because patients assigned to the effective treatment have good outcomes and those assigned to the less effective treatment can be treated with effective second- and third-line treatments. This would be another situation in which there would be a difference in DFS but not OS. As with other components of a clinical trial, the selection of a primary endpoint should be done collaboratively among the key study team members. Input from the FDA should be sought (early) if there is a possibility that the trial data will be used for FDA label approval.

STATISTICAL CONSIDERATIONS

STUDY DESIGN

A major question of interest in study design is how many patients are required for the clinical trial. The trial sample size is a major driver of the resources needed for the trial; the greater the sample size, the more the trial will cost and the longer it will take. Sample size is influenced by the desired **type I error** (α) and **type II error** (β), the event rate for the control arm, the minimum detectable difference of interest, and the anticipated accrual rate. A clinical trial is based on a statistical hypothesis testing framework. The **null hypothesis** for a superiority trial is that there is no difference in patient benefit (e.g., OS) between the two treatment arms. The alternative hypothesis is that there is a difference in OS between the two arms (two-sided test), or that the experimental arm has better outcomes than the control arm (one-sided).

The specific desired error rates are set a priori by the study team, usually in alignment with standard practices and conventions. The level of **significance** (type I error) is the probability of rejecting the null hypothesis when it is true. Specifically, it is the probability of concluding one treatment is better than the other when in reality there is no difference. **Power**, in contrast, is defined as 1 – β, with β defined as the probability of failing to reject the null hypothesis when in fact one treatment is superior to the other. Conversely, power is the probability of correctly rejecting the null hypothesis when there truly is a difference between the two treatment arms.

To determine a trial's power, a specific minimum difference must be specified. This is usually the minimum difference that is felt to be clinically meaningful. Often for time-to-event data, this difference is stated either as a **hazard ratio (HR)**, or as a difference in the survival probability at a specific time point, or as a difference in median survival. Typically, the time-to-event data are assumed to follow an exponential distribution, such that it is possible to determine the other two quantities when given one of them. Specifically, if a desired difference between survival rates at time point t is given, then the HR and the difference in median survival times can be calculated. For example, suppose that the control arm has a 5-year OS of 30% and the investigators want to determine if the treatment improves the rate to 40%. This corresponds to a difference in median survival time of 2.9 years for the control versus 3.8 years for the experimental arm. The corresponding minimal detectable HR is 0.76.

In addition to being clinically meaningful, it is crucial that the minimum difference also be realistically achievable and, ideally, supported by prior evidence, in order to avoid wasting resources on underpowered studies. For example, by specifying a minimum clinically important difference, it is technically possible to render a sample size with a desired level of power for a hypothetical randomized trial that compares precisely the same treatment in each arm. Although a sample size calculation will yield an answer that is finite, clearly the true power of such a study is nil and the sample size is infinite (no sample will ever be sufficiently large to detect a difference that does not exist). Overzealous tinkering with effect sizes can lead to a problem called **optimism bias**, or the tendency to exaggerate the hypothesized effects of novel treatments in order to suppress sample sizes (9).

One approach to determine the trial sample size is to set the level of significance, often 0.025 or 0.05, and then to find the minimum sample size to achieve power of at least some specified value, often 80% or 90%, at some specified minimum detectable difference of interest. The minimum detectable difference of interest is the smallest difference that would be of clinical interest; that is, the difference that would convince care providers to adopt a new standard of care, provided it is hypothetically achievable. For a time-to-event endpoint such as OS, DFS, or PFS, power is a function of the number of events: deaths, disease events, or progression events, respectively. The relationship between the number of events and the trial sample size is governed by the event rates of the treatment arms and the anticipated accrual time.

To observe the requisite number of events for the final analysis, patients enrolled on the trial have to be followed over time until the events are observed. At one extreme, if the required number of events is D, the trial could enroll exactly D patients and follow them until they each experience an event; for a survival endpoint, all patients would be followed to death before the final analysis. This would require the least number of patients but the maximum duration of the study. At the other extreme, patients could continue to be enrolled in the trial until D events have been observed. This would ensure the shortest duration of the trial but would require the maximum number of patients to be enrolled. Both designs yield the same power, the same level of significance, and the minimum detectable difference. Trials are rarely, if ever, designed for either of the two extremes; rather, some intermediate approach is used. Luckily, there are a number of available software packages that facilitate exploration of the intermediate approaches.

EXAMPLE SAMPLE SIZE DETERMINATION

Suppose we want to design a trial that has a two-sided level of significance of 0.05 and power of 90%. The desire is to be able to detect a difference in 5-year OS of 30% in the control arm (obtained from historical data in published studies) and 40% in the experimental arm. This would require a sample size of 960 patients (480 in each arm) and the final analysis could be done after 564 total deaths across both arms have been observed. Assuming an accrual rate of 20 patients per month, the expected accrual time is 4 years and the total study duration (time at which the 960th death would be observed) is 6.3 years. The estimates for the study accrual duration and length of the study are just estimates or expected times based on past experience accruing similar patient

TABLE 22.1 SUMMARY OF THE DIRECTION OF CHANGE IN THE SAMPLE SIZE AS A FUNCTION OF THE DIRECTION OF CHANGE IN THE INDICATED CLINICAL TRIAL PARAMETER

Change in...	Change in sample size...
level of significance increases decreases	 decreases increases
power increases decreases	 increases decreases
minimum detectable difference increases decreases	 decreases increases

populations onto trials. Even if the assumptions are exactly correct, the actual time at which the required number of events will occur during any clinical trial might be considerably different from the expected time.

The clinical trial parameters, level of significance, power, and minimum detectable difference all influence the sample size. Table 22.1 summarizes the direction of change in sample size as a function of the direction of change in each clinical trial parameter. These relationships can also be graphed. For example, Figure 22.1A has a graph of how the power of the trial changes for different sample sizes, keeping all other aspects of the design the same. If the investigator wanted to enroll only 400 patients, the trial would have 60% power. If the investigator wanted to change the power from 90% to 80%, the sample size would only be 664 patients compared to 960 patients for 90% power. Relationships also exist among the other trial parameters.

There is a relationship between power and the minimal detectable difference between the treatment arms. Figure 22.1B illustrates how the minimum detectable difference, as measured by HR, is related to power keeping all the other trial design values the same. The smaller the detectable differences, in magnitude, the lower the power. If the minimum detectable difference is increased from 0.76 to 0.80, the power of the study would decrease from 90% to approximately 78%. A final example shows how the accrual is related to the study duration with all other aspects of the clinical trial kept the same. In the original design, the accrual rate was 20 patients per month, which meant the study would accrue the 960 patients in 48 months, or 4 years, and the total study duration would be 6.3 years (approximately 75.6 months). If the accrual time was reduced to 36 months (3 years), the sample size would reduce to 720 patients. This would increase the total study duration from 6.3 years to 9.0 years (or approximately 109 months). This illustrates the trade-off between the accrual period and total study duration, assuming the accrual rate is held constant (see Figure 22.1C).

Determining the sample size for a trial is an iterative process, which is facilitated by software. Rarely is a single sample size calculation performed for a trial. When designing a study, it is recommended that matrix of sample sizes for combinations of different values of the design parameters be generated. Again, it is important to ensure that each parameter is realistic and feasible. Often, the sample size that corresponds to the desired values for each trial parameter may not be feasible due to limited resources (specifically, the sample size may exceed the available resources). Generating a matrix of sample sizes for different values of the design parameters allows the study team to weigh the trade-offs among the trial characteristics when making a decision regarding the trial sample size.

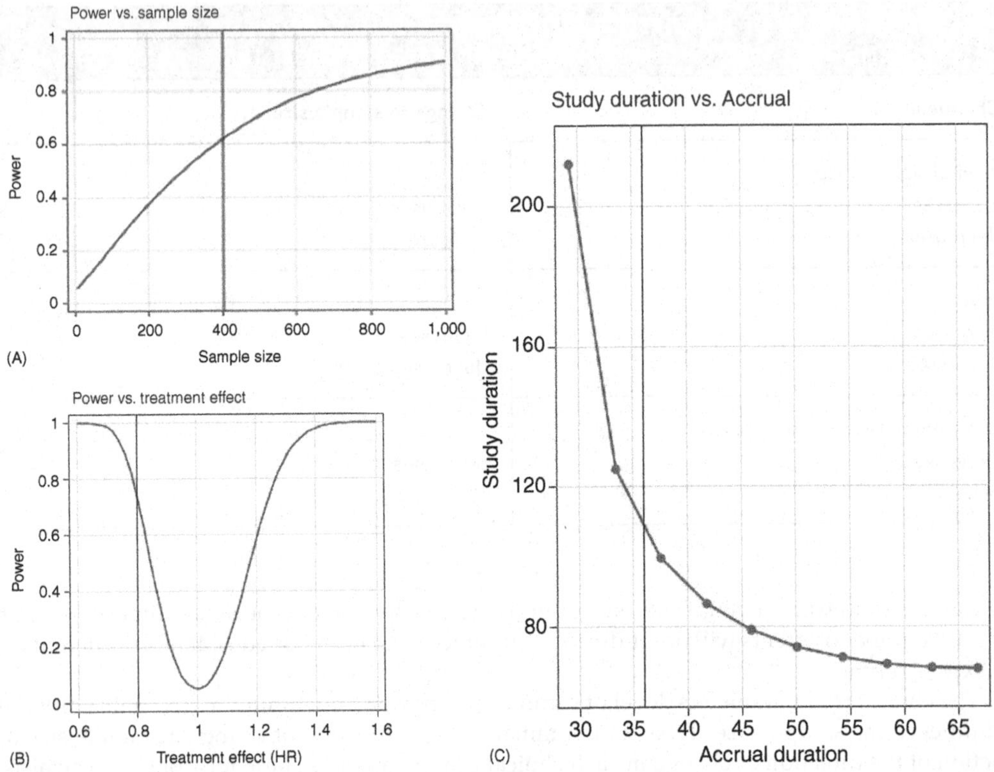

FIGURE 22.1 (A) A plot of power for the example clinical trial design as a function of sample size. (B) A plot of power for the example clinical trial design as a function of minimum detectable difference. (C) A plot of study duration versus accrual duration for the example clinical trial design.

HR, hazard ratio.

ANALYSIS PLANS

The trial analysis plans are specified in the study protocol and finalized prior to the trial being launched. Sometimes, a study team may generate a **statistical analysis plan** that provides more details than might be in the protocol. The analysis plan provides definitions of which patients will be included in the analyses and specific statistical methods that will be used for the primary and secondary analyses. There is often a different set of patients for the efficacy analyses and for the safety and tolerability analyses. In a late phase trial, the scientifically rigorous analysis for a superiority trial is an intent-to-treat analysis, which requires that all randomized patients be included in the analysis even if they were deemed to be ineligible postrandomization or if they canceled prior to receiving any protocol treatment. These patients are analyzed according to the treatment arm to which they were randomized, regardless of whether they received that treatment or not.

An intent-to-treat analysis minimizes potential biases that arise when patients are removed from their assigned arms. The efficacy objective is meant to determine if the experimental treatment should become the new standard of treatment. An intent-to-treat analysis is considered to be conservative because occasionally patients may receive the treatment on an arm other than the one to which they were randomized, and the reason for the change could be related to the primary endpoint. Although this can bias the results toward the null hypothesis, raising the bar for the level of evidence required, in exchange an intent-to-treat analysis provides a stringent evaluation of whether that the experimental treatment is truly superior to the control arm, factoring in patients' behaviors.

In contrast, safety and tolerability analyses typically only include patients who received at least one dose of the treatment (assuming that the primary endpoint is not a safety endpoint). Patients are assigned to groups on the basis of the treatment they received, even if it differed from the treatment to which they were randomized, for the analysis. Patients who did not receive at least one dose of any protocol treatment are omitted from this analysis. Analyzing patients according to the treatment they received allows an evaluation of the potential side effects of the treatment. Generally, there is no formal statistical testing to compare the AE rates between the two arms. Rather, the goal is to describe the AEs observed and to estimate the rates for the individual treatment arms.

The statistical analyses should be aligned with the study design and the type of data. If the trial endpoint is time-to-event data with censored data, the analysis method must properly account for censored values. If the design includes stratification factors, the analysis plan must properly account for this; specifically, a **stratified log-rank test** should be done, for time-to-event endpoints (OS, DFS, PFS) and/or a stratified Cox regression analysis. To ensure scientific rigor, all analyses that are intended to be conducted, primary and secondary, should be prespecified in the protocol. If the study team intends to perform subgroup analyses, these analyses should be detailed in the statistical plan prior to starting the analysis. The level of detail in the statistical analysis plan should be such that the analyses can be conducted by a different group at the end of the trial if they are provided the plan.

STUDY MONITORING

There are two types of formal study monitoring. The first is embedded within the trial and provides formal stopping boundaries, or rules for continuing or discontinuing the trial. This is called **interim monitoring**, and includes interim analyses for either efficacy or futility (or both). The second form of monitoring is conducted by an independent **data safety monitoring board (DSMB)**. This group reviews the study data to date and makes recommendations as to whether the protocol needs to be modified and whether a trial should stop or proceed as planned.

INTERIM MONITORING

The monitoring of trial data for efficacy and AEs is an important component of human subjects' protection. Monitoring a clinical trial ensures the protection of human subjects while allowing sufficient information to be collected so that study objectives can be evaluated. Trials may be stopped as soon as there is compelling evidence of efficacy, lack of benefit, patient harm, or unacceptable AEs. An interim monitoring plan consists of prespecified stopping rules that describe when data will be analyzed and the results that would cause the trial to be stopped early. Rules that describe conditions under which the trial would stop early due to evidence of superiority or harm of the experimental arm are referred to as efficacy **stopping rules**. Criteria for early closure due to lack of evidence for there being benefit or harm are referred to as futility stopping rules. Rules for when a trial should close early because an unacceptable AE rate has been observed are referred to as AE (or toxicity) stopping rules.

Interim analyses for efficacy are motivated by an ethical imperative that a study be stopped if there is exceptionally strong evidence of the superiority of one treatment, especially for cancers in which there are limited treatment options. Stopping early for efficacy allows patients access to an effective treatment as soon as possible. One approach is to continuously evaluate the treatment arms to determine if one is superior. However, frequent analysis of the data for evidence of superiority will inflate the type I error, invalidating the initially specified level of significance.

This inflation occurs because each successive look at the data raises the chance of rejecting the null hypothesis (similar to the multiple hypothesis testing problem; see Chapter 11).

The statistical solution to the interim analysis is to use designs that allow for early stopping for superiority of one arm but still maintain the specified trial level of significance. This is accomplished by limiting the number of times the data are analyzed and the use of conservative stopping boundaries. Rather than evaluating the data on a continuous basis and stopping when the p value is below .05 (if this is the trial level of significance), well-designed interim analyses stop only when the p values are substantially below .05 at only a few prespecified times (10). Most trials usually have between one and three interim analyses. There are different approaches for determining the p-value boundaries that would stop a trial for efficacy.

One approach is to use small, and approximately equal, probabilities of stopping at each interim time (11,12). Another approach for interim testing is to use a spending function (13,14). These approaches start with the overall desired level of significance and allocate (spend) a part of this at each analysis. The final analysis will yield a level of significance equal to the trial level of significance minus what has already been spent. For example, in the **O'Brien–Fleming approach**, the times of analysis are specified up front. The **Lan–DeMets approach** provides a way to determine what interim testing levels should be without prespecifying the times of the tests. Essentially, the level is equal to the area under the curve between two points of a specified function for which the total area under the curve is the overall level of significance (e.g., 0.05).

Trials can also be stopped for futility. One such approach is based on **conditional power** or **stochastic curtailment** (15,16). This approach allows early stopping when, given the current results, the probability of a significant result becomes so small that it is clear a trial is not going to result in a significant difference. Another approach for futility monitoring was proposed by Wieand et al. (17). They propose using one interim look at the data and recommending the trial be stopped if there is no indication of improved outcome for the experimental treatment. Using this approach, the data are analyzed when half the required events have been observed. At this time, if the HR exceeds one (for comparing the experimental treatment to the control treatment), the recommendation would be to terminate the trial due to futility. The conclusion would be that there is no evidence for the superiority of the experimental treatment. Note that this rule is only useful for trials for which the planned accrual period is longer than the median survival time for the control treatment. An approach investigated by Zhang et al. (18) extended the aforementioned method to more than one futility analysis. Their results showed that the linear inefficacy boundary provided the best results among all futility rules considered using data from 52 cancer trials. Statistical software is available for incorporating interim analyses into the study design, with most packages offering a choice of methodology for generating the stopping boundaries.

Increasingly, studies include a stopping rule for unacceptable AE rates. Often the DSMB may request that such rules be part of the trial monitoring plan. AE stopping rules can be based on expert opinion or could be statistically grounded based on the known background rate (19). Often rules that are not based on formal statistical methods specify a boundary for the AE rate that if crossed, would alert the study team to a potential problem. The boundary rate is typically expressed in terms of a global AE rate of a certain grade (i.e., grade 4 or higher, including deaths) or could be based on a specific AE. Unlike formal interim analyses of the primary endpoint, AE stopping rules assume that the study team will analyze the AEs frequently (e.g., monthly), with the frequency driven by the accrual rate or the anticipated potential of a safety or tolerability issue. Analysis of AEs will not inflate the type I error for the primary endpoint because the AE and the primary endpoint are mostly independent. If the AE stopping boundary is crossed, the study team will suspend accrual, notify the DSMB, notify the study sponsor, notify the institutional review board (IRB), and perform a thorough review of the AE data. In consultation with the DSMB and potentially other key groups (e.g., study sponsor, IRB), a decision will be made with respect to the trial disposition. Possible decisions include (a) termination of the study due to unacceptable toxicity, (b) modification of the protocol to reduce the toxicity (e.g., modification of the treatment doses, stricter eligibility criteria), or (c) continue the protocol as written.

DATA SAFETY MONITORING BOARDS

Another common name for a data safety monitoring board is a **data monitoring committee (DMC)**. Safety monitoring is the most critical function of a DSMB. Deciding whether there is sufficient evidence of unacceptable toxicity to terminate or modify the trial can be difficult if not done carefully. The stated AE stopping rules provide guidance, but the DSMB is also charged with careful review of all aspects of the trial and is free to make recommendations even if the formal AE stopping boundary is not crossed. It is generally agreed that the primary responsibility of the DSMB is participant safety and study integrity. Additional oversight responsibilities assumed by a DSMB depend somewhat on the resources and infrastructure supporting the trial study team. Other potential responsibilities of a DSMB may include the approval of the study design, study site performance review, accrual monitoring, and quality and timeliness of data assessment. The responsibilities of the DSMB should be explicitly described in the DSMB charter. Different DSMBs might arrive at different answers to the same monitoring questions because individuals who comprise a DSMB have different perspectives. As such, it is important to balance opinions by including a variety of knowledgeable people, those with complementary knowledge and perspectives, as members of the committee. Much has been written on monitoring committees for oncology trials (20,21).

REAL-WORLD EXAMPLE

Patients with acute myeloid leukemia (AML) and fms-related tyrosine kinase 3 gene (*FLT3*) mutations have poor outcomes. *FLT3* mutations are present in 30% of adults with newly diagnosed AML. Midostaurin is a multitargeted kinase inhibitor for which preclinical studies demonstrated synergy with chemotherapy. In addition, early phase studies yielded encouraging efficacy results of midostaurin plus chemotherapy in patients with AML and an *FLT3* mutation, also demonstrating that the combination was safe and tolerable. This provided the rationale for conducting a multi-institutional, multinational, randomized, double-blind, placebo-controlled trial initiated by the Cancer and Leukemia Group B (CALGB), which is now part of the Alliance for Clinical Trials in Oncology (Alliance). This trial is known as CALGB 10603 or the RATIFY trial (22).

The patient population consisted of adults (18 to 59 years) who had newly diagnosed AML with a *FLT3* mutation. This is an example of an **enrichment design** where there was enough evidence to convince the study team that only patients with the *FLT3* mutation would benefit from the addition of midostaurin. The treatment arms were standard chemotherapy plus midostaurin (experimental arm) and standard chemotherapy plus placebo (control arm). Patients were randomized in a 1:1 fashion and the randomization included one stratification factor: the subtype of *FLT3* mutation (TKD vs. ITD low vs. ITD high). This stratification factor was included because there was evidence that ITD mutations are associated with poor prognosis and the association of TKD mutations on prognosis is uncertain. The study team felt it was important that the treatment arms be balanced according to the subtype of *FLT3* mutations because of the prognostic importance, especially for treatment meant to target *FLT3* mutations.

The primary endpoint was OS. Based on historical data, it was assumed that the median survival in the control group would be 15 months. The minimal detectable HR was set to 0.714, which corresponds to a median survival for the midostaurin arm of 21 months. There was one planned formal interim analysis for efficacy after 50% of the events occurred. The trial power was set at 90% and a 0.025 one-sided level of significance was used. A one-sided level of significance was selected because the comparison was between standard chemotherapy and the standard chemotherapy plus midostaurin. Since chemotherapy was already the standard of care, definitively establishing that it is superior to it plus midostaurin would not change the standard of care (less therapy is always preferred to combination therapy). The anticipated accrual rate was 25 AML patients with an *FLT3* mutation. The output for the sample size calculation (obtained from EAST) is presented in Figure 22.2. The required sample size is 514 patients and the final analysis can occur after 373

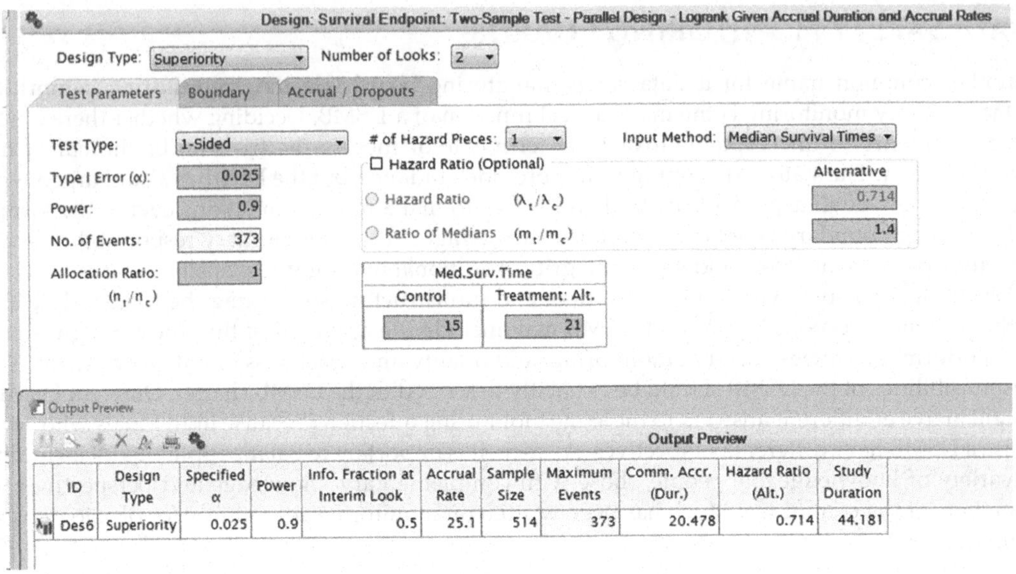

FIGURE 22.2 Example output of EAST® software with input fields and output results.

Source: Reprinted with permission from Cytel, Inc.

deaths have been observed. The minor differences between the numbers presented here and the output in Figure 22.2 are due to rounding errors.

As the study was accruing, it was observed that the proportion of patients who had undergone allogeneic hematopoietic stem cell transplantation was higher than expected (expected 15% and observed 25%). In addition, the proportion of patients who had an *FLT3* mutation of the TKD subtype was also higher than expected (expected was 14% and the observed was 36%). This changed the median expected survival in the control arm; hence, an amendment expanded the target accrual to 714 patients requiring 509 deaths at the time of final analysis. Mid-trial changes like this are not uncommon, underscoring the need to monitor key trial design assumptions while the trial is ongoing. If the assumptions that affect sample size substantially deviate from what is observed, amendments might have to be made so that the study power is preserved. The scientific rigor of a study is maintained if the amendments were without knowledge of the study efficacy data.

A planned interim analysis for efficacy was to occur after 187 (= 373/2, rounded) deaths had been observed. The alpha spending for this analysis was p value = .005 and the remaining alpha (0.02) was to determine whether the experimental arm was superior to the control arm at the final analysis. This controlled the overall trial level of significance at 0.025 (0.005 at the interim analysis plus 0.02 at the final analysis, which equals 0.025).

The primary analysis was conducted using a stratified log-rank test. The p values for the primary analyses were one-sided, in accordance with the study design. The trial had an independent DSMB that reviewed the trial every six months for safety, accrual issues, and data quality and timeliness. The DSMB also reviewed the results of the planned interim analysis results and decided that the trial should continue as planned. Because this was a double-blind trial, the study team was blinded to the arm assignment and results of the interim analyses. Even if a study is not double-blinded, it is a good clinical trial practice to blind the study team to interim analysis results, to prevent subsequent biases in the trial conduct.

At the trial completion, there were 717 patients enrolled. The median OS time in the midostaurin treatment arm was 74.7 months compared to 25.6 months in the control arm (one-sided p value = .009 by stratified log-rank test). As is typical, there were differences between the trial design assumptions and what was subsequently observed. Of interest, the observed median survival was substantially larger for the control group than expected, and was even larger than what was anticipated for the experimental group. A potential explanation for the unexpectedly high OS in the control group may be a higher than expected transplantation rate, which is associated with better patient prognosis. However, the observed HR aligned with what was expected in the amended protocol and was found to be statistically significant.

OTHER TRIAL DESIGNS

A number of phase III clinical trials compare $k > 2$ treatments. If a two-arm trial has N patients with $N/2$ patients in each arm, the addition of another arm increases the sample size by more than $N/2$ patients. The sample size is inflated as a consequence of having to control the global error rates (e.g., the level of significance and power) when more than one comparison is being made in the primary analysis.

TWO OR MORE EXPERIMENTAL ARMS INCLUDING A CONTROL ARM

The most common k-arm design is one with $k - 1$ experimental arms tested alongside a control (standard of care) arm. The complexity of multiarm trials increases dramatically above that of a two-arm trial. In a two-arm trial, there is a single primary comparison of interest. With a four-arm trial, there are six possible pairwise comparisons, 19 ways of pooling and comparing two groups, and 24 ways of ordering the arms with respect to the outcome. This yields up to 50 possible hypothesis tests. In order for the sample size of a multiarm trial to be feasible, a few key comparisons of interest among these 50 hypotheses must be identified. The most common design is to compare each of the experimental arms to the standard of care (control arm) to determine whether any of the new treatments is superior to the control arm.

An example of a three-arm trial is the North Central Cancer Treatment Group (NCCTG) trial, N9831 (23). This was a phase III trial for women with HER2-positive breast cancer undergoing adjuvant treatment. Women were randomized in a 1:1:1 fashion to standard chemotherapy (Arm A), standard chemotherapy followed by trastuzumab treatment (Arm B), or standard chemotherapy with concurrent administration of trastuzumab followed by trastuzumab (Arm C). The primary endpoint for the trial was DFS. Three pairwise comparisons were planned: (a) the comparison of Arms A and B at a 0.01 level of significance, (b) the comparison of Arms A and C at a 0.01 level of significance, and (c) the comparison of Arms B and C at a 0.03 level of significance. The sample size for each treatment arm was 1,000 eligible patients, for a total sample size of 3,000 patients. The trial had 88% power to detect a difference in median DFS of 6 years for the control arm (Arm A) versus 8 years in each of the experimental arms (Arms B and C). There was 83% power to detect an increase in median DFS in the poorer performing arm, neither Arm B nor C was considered a control arm for this comparison, of 7 years to 9 years in the better performing arm. The global level of significance for the trial with the three planned comparisons was 0.05 (0.01 + 0.01 + 0.03). Note that had the trial been designed to compare only two arms, the necessary sample size with a 0.05 level of significance and keeping all other parameters the same would have been less than 2,000 total patients. This is because a 0.05 level of significance could have been used for the one comparison rather than having to be spread across the three planned comparisons.

FACTORIAL DESIGNS

A clinical trial with a factorial design is used when there are several treatments to be tested in combination. The simplest is a **2 x 2 factorial design**: treatment A at two levels and treatment B at two levels. The levels of treatment are typically (a) administered versus not administered, (b) two different doses of schedules of the treatment, or (c) two different modes of the treatment (e.g., surgery versus radiation).

For example, suppose the dose levels are treatment administration versus not. This would yield four different treatment combinations: A administered and B administered, only A administered (B not administered), only B administered (A not administered), and neither treatment administered. Factorial designs are not limited to factors with only two levels. If treatment A has R levels and treatment B has C levels, this would lead to a R × C factorial design. It is rare for a treatment to have more than three levels, however. It could also be the case that there are three factors and if each had two levels, this would be a 2 × 2 × 2 design. Overall, the most common factorial design is a 2 × 2 trial.

A factorial design allows an assessment of each of the treatments separately as well as an evaluation of interaction effects between the treatments. An interaction between the treatments implies that the treatment effect depends on the presence or absence of another treatment. In a 2 × 2 trial with a survival endpoint, if there is no interaction, the effect of treatment A is $HR = hr_A$, regardless of whether treatment B is administered or not. Likewise, the effect for treatment B is $HR = hr_B$, regardless of whether treatment A is given or not. A *positive* interaction implies that there is *synergy* between treatments, that is, the effect of each treatment is increased in the presence of the other. For example, the effect for A is $HR = hr_A$ when B is not administered but the effect for A is $HR = hr_{AB}$ when B is present, and $hr_{AB} > hr_A$. A *negative* interaction is when the effect of each treatment is decreased by the presence of the other treatment or there is *antagonism* between the treatments. For example, the effect for B is $HR = hr_B$ when A is not administered but the effect for B is $HR = hr_{AB}$ when A is administered and $hr_{AB} < hr_B$.

If it is expected that there will be no interaction between the treatments, then a factorial design is efficient in the sense that two trials are completed for the price of one. If n_A and n_B are the required sample sizes for two individual trials comparing treatment A against a control and comparing treatment B against a control, respectively, a single factorial trial would have a sample size equal to the maximum of the two individual trial sample sizes, that is, $n = \max\{n_A, n_B\}$. This factorial trial will achieve at least the same power for each individual treatment comparison as doing the two individual trials for treatments A and B with sample sizes n_A and n_B respectively. Doing the two separate trials would require $n_A + n_B$ total patients, whereas the 2 × 2 trial would only require the $\max\{n_A, n_B\}$.

However, if there is an interaction between the treatments, this may potentially reduce the power of the individual comparisons, making the interpretation of treatment effects more difficult. If the intent of the 2 × 2 trial is to determine whether two treatments are synergistic (a positive interaction), the required sample size to formally test for an interaction is considerably larger than for a 2 × 2 trial meant only to test the main effects of each treatment. The best use for a factorial design is to evaluate treatments that are likely to be used in combination in practice and for which no interaction is expected between the treatments. This allows an evaluation of the joint effects of the treatments. However, if the combination of the two treatments is not likely to be used in practice, factorial designs should not be used, because of the potential loss of power if there is a treatment interaction.

An example of a 2 × 2 factorial design is the CALGB trial, C9741. This was a trial to test adjuvant chemotherapy for women with axillary node positive breast cancer. The two factors assessed were dose density (2-week intervals versus 3-week intervals) and treatment sequence (sequential versus concurrent). It was expected that dose density and schedule would not be synergistic; in other words, no interaction was expected between the two treatment approaches. The treatment sequences were doxorubicin followed by paclitaxel followed by cyclophosphamide (sequential) or doxorubicin and cyclophosphamide concurrently followed by paclitaxel (concurrent). The primary endpoint for the trial was DFS. The study was powered for the two main comparisons: (a) 2-week intervals for doses versus 3-week intervals and (b) concurrent administration of doxorubicin and cyclophosphamide versus sequential administration. The target sample size was 1,584 total patients (396 in each of the four treatment groups) to detect a 33% difference in hazard at a 0.05 level of significance. The analysis groups for the dose density questions were patients treated every 2 weeks, regardless of treatment sequence and compared patients treated every 3 weeks, regardless of treatment sequence. Similarly, the analysis for the sequence question compared the sequential schedule, by pooling patients treated on 2-week or 3-week intervals who were receiving sequential treatment, to the concurrent schedule, by pooling patients treated on 2-week or 3-week intervals who were receiving concurrent treatment. The objective of this trial was to determine a dose density and treatment sequence combination that was the best for treating future patients, so a factorial design was appropriate.

SOFTWARE FOR CLINICAL TRIAL DESIGN

There are a number of commercial and free software packages for the design of phase III trials. Individuals at many institutions have access to at least one clinical trial design package. It is important to understand the input and output parameters of the software, which can be done by reading the manuals or going through the tutorials, if available. Different software packages may do specific things better than others. It is a good idea to compare the capabilities of available packages and choose one that best fits the needs for designing the specific clinical trial. In addition, before committing to a particular trial design, including sample size, it is important that input be provided by all the key study team members. All well-designed phase III trials have an identified trial statistician. This is the individual who will generate the sample size estimations, using software that is available. As discussed earlier, it is good to consider different design scenarios so that the trade-offs among the different study parameters (e.g., between power and minimum detectable difference, between sample size and minimum detectable difference, between accrual rate and study duration) can be better understood and an informed decision can be made.

EAST is a widely used commercial software package for trial design. The types of endpoints it can handle are normal, binomial, and survival. It can include interim analyses (efficacy and/or futility) and can be used to design superiority, noninferiority, and equivalence trials. The spending functions include Pocock (12), O'Brien–Fleming (13), and Wang–Tsiatis (24). The output provides stopping boundaries, power, required number of events, and sample size. It also allows users to plot the relationship between key study parameters to better understand trade-offs (as done in Figure 22.1). Overall, this software facilitates the exploration and comparison of the impact on sample size for different trial assumptions, which provides insights for the trade-offs among the study parameters.

An example of a free package is **gsDesign** (25), which is an R package among many listed on the CRAN Task View: Clinical Trial Design, Monitoring, and Analysis (cran.r-project.org/web/views/ClinicalTrials.html). It allows designs with interim analyses, and common spending functions that are included are Pocock (12), O'Brien–Fleming (13), and Hwang–Shih–DeCani (26). This package is not as easy to use as EAST, making it more difficult to quickly explore different scenarios. However, it does offer flexibility for accommodating nonstandard designs, and it is free. The popular statistical software SAS also has procedures for group sequential design and testing, including PROC SEQDESIGN and SEQTEST (27).

CONCLUSION

The development and implementation of a phase III trial requires a group of individuals with different domains of expertise. Given the amount of resources required for a phase III trial, it is worth the effort and time necessary to produce a well-designed trial. As individuals work on the trial design, it is worthwhile to review the CONsolidated Standards of Reporting Trials (CONSORT) guidelines (28). Randomized trials are the gold standard for evaluating cancer interventions. However, they must be appropriately designed and conducted to ensure unbiased results and scientific rigor. Although the CONSORT guidelines are meant to improve the reporting of clinical trial results, they also provide a useful road map for how to develop a well-designed trial and perform quality analysis. Knowing what is required to generate a high-quality report should inform trial design, conduct, and analysis decisions.

GLOSSARY

two-arm trial: generally compares a new treatment (Arm E) to the current standard of care, which is the control arm (Arm C).

multiarm trial: a clinical trial with more than two arms.

factorial designs: clinical trial designs used when there are several treatments to be tested in combination.

superiority test: investigation to determine which of two treatments is better.

generalizability: applicability.

targeted therapies: treatments that take advantage of a specific aberration in a tumor as a means to kill only cancer cells, versus cytotoxic treatment that indiscriminately kills all cells.

1:1 randomization: two-arm (phase III) trial scheme that assigns N/2 patients to each arm.

2:1 randomization: two-arm (phase III) trial scheme that assigns 2/3 of patients to the experimental arm and 1/3 of patients to the control arm.

stratification factors: experimental design parameter that protects against imbalances of important prognostic variables.

intention-to-treat principle: the principle that outcomes should be compared according to the study group to which subjects were assigned, rather than how they were ultimately treated.

surrogate endpoints: endpoints that are highly correlated with a different endpoint, yet have much higher event rates, leading to faster and less expensive evaluations of the effectiveness of new treatments.

schedule of assessments: element of a phase III trial design specifying when interim assessment(s) of data are to be made.

type I error (α): the probability of rejecting the null hypothesis even though it is false.

type II error (β): the probability of failing to reject the null hypothesis even though it is true.

null hypothesis: The hypothesis that there is no significant difference between specified populations, with any observed difference being due to sampling or experimental error.

statistical significance: a predetermined level of type I error that will be accepted in order to reject the null hypothesis.

power: the probability of correctly rejecting the null hypothesis when there truly is a difference between two treatment arms.

hazard ratio: the ratio of hazard functions between two groups, such as between a treatment and control (i.e., treatment effect) or change in hazard from baseline per unit change of a covariate.

optimism bias: the tendency to exaggerate the hypothesized effects of novel treatments in order to suppress sample sizes.

statistical analysis plan: provides definitions of which patients will be included in the analyses and specific statistical methods that will be used for the primary and secondary analyses of a clinical trial.

stratified log-rank test: a statistical analysis done to properly account for stratification factors in phase III clinical trial designs.

interim monitoring: type of formal study monitoring that is embedded within the trial and provides formal stopping boundaries, or rules for continuing or discontinuing the trial; includes interim analyses for either efficacy or futility (or both).

data safety monitoring board (DSMB) (data monitoring committee [DMC]): independent group that reviews the data in a clinical trial to date and makes recommendations as to whether the protocol should be modified and whether a trial should stop or proceed as planned. A DSMB's primary responsibility is participant safety and study integrity.

stopping rules: describe conditions under which a trial would stop early (e.g., due to evidence of superiority or harm of the experimental arm; lack of evidence for a benefit or harm; unacceptable adverse effect rate).

O'Brien–Fleming approach: plan for interim testing in which the times of analysis are specified up front.

LanDeMets approach: plan for interim testing that provides a way to determine what interim testing levels should be without prespecifying the times of the tests.

conditional power (stochastic curtailment): approach to stopping a trial for futility when, given the current results, the probability of a significant result becomes so small that it is clear a trial is not going to result in a significant difference.

data monitoring committee (DMC): see *data safety monitoring board.*

enrichment design: a study design in which subjects are selected for participation on the basis of a factor that will increase the desired event rate, usually to increase power or shorten the length of a trial.

2 × 2 factorial design: a clinical trial with a factorial design used when there are several treatments to be tested in combination.

EAST: a widely used commercial software package for trial design.

gsDesign: a free R software package that allows designs with interim analyses.

REFERENCES

1. Shih WJ, Lin Y. On study designs and hypotheses for clinical trials with predictive biomarkers. *Contemp Clin Trials.* 2017;62:140–145. doi:10.1016/j.cct.2017.08.014
2. Renfro LA, Mallick H, An MW, et al. Clinical trial designs incorporating predictive biomarkers. *Cancer Treat Rev.* 2016;43:74–82. doi:10.1016/j.ctrv.2015.12.008
3. Dumville JC, Hahn S, Miles JNV, Torgerson DJ. The use of unequal randomisation ratios in clinical trials: a review. *Cont Clin Trials.* 2006;27:1–12. doi:10.1016/j.cct.2005.08.003
4. Zakeri K, Rose BS, Gulaya S, et al. Competing event risk stratification may improve the design and efficiency of clinical trials: secondary analysis of SWOG 8794. *Contemp Clin Trials.* 2013;34(1):74–79. doi:10.1016/j.cct.2012.09.008
5. Mell LK, Jeong JH. Pitfalls of using composite primary endpoints in the presence of competing risks. *J Clin Oncol.* 2010;28(28):4297–4299. doi:10.1200/JCO.2010.30.2802
6. Gómez G, Lagakos SW. Statistical considerations when using a composite endpoint for comparing treatment groups. *Stat Med.* 2013;32(5):719–738. doi:10.1002/sim.5547
7. Baker SG, Kramer BS. Surrogate endpoint analysis: an exercise in extrapolation. *J Natl Cancer Inst.* 2013;105(5):316–320. doi:10.1093/jnci/djs527
8. Dodd LE, Korn EL, Friedlin B, et al. Blinded independent central review of progression-free survival in phase III oncology trials: important design element or unnecessary expense? *J Clin Oncol.* 2008;26:3791–3795. doi:10.1200/JCO.2008.16.1711
9. Djulbegovic B, Kumar A, Magazin A, et al. Optimism bias leads to inconclusive results—an empirical study. *J Clin Epidemiol.* 2011;64(6):583–593. doi:10.1016/j.jclinepi.2010.09.007
10. Haybittle JL. Repeated assessment of results in clinical trials of cancer treatment. *Brit J Radiology.* 1971;44:793–797. doi:10.1259/0007-1285-44-526-793

11. Crowley J, Green S, Liu PY, Wolf M. Data monitoring committees and early stopping guidelines: the Southwest Oncology Group experience. *Stat Med*. 1994;13(13–14):1391–1399. doi:10.1002/sim.4780131314
12. Pocock SJ. Interim analyses for randomized clinical trials: the group sequential approach. *Biometrics*. 1982;38:153–162. doi:10.2307/2530298
13. O'Brien PC, Fleming TR. A multiple testing procedure for clinical trials. *Biometrics*. 1979;35(3):549–556. doi:10.2307/2530245
14. Lan KKG, DeMets DL. Discrete sequential boundaries for clinical trials. *Biometrika*. 1983;70:659–663. doi:10.2307/2336502
15. Anderson PK. Conditional power calculations as an aid in the decision whether to continue a clinical trial. *Control Clin Trials*. 1987;8:67–74. do:i10.1016/0197-2456(87)90027-4
16. Spiegelhalter DJ, Freedman LS, Blackburn PR. Monitoring clinical trials: conditional or predictive power? *Control Clin Trials*. 1986;7:8–17. doi:10.1016/0197-2456(86)90003-6
17. Wieand S, Schroeder G, O'Fallon JR. Stopping when the experimental regimen does not appear to help. *Stat Med*. 1994;13(13-14):1453–1458. doi:10.1002/sim.4780131321
18. Zhang Q, Freidlin B, Korn E, et al. Comparison of futility monitoring guidelines using completed phase III oncology trials. *Clin Trials*. 2017;14(1):48–58. doi:10.1177/1740774516666502
19. Zhu L, Yao B, Xia HA, Jiang Q. Statistical monitoring of safety in clinical trials. *Stat Biopharm Res*. 2016;8:88–105. doi:10.1080/19466315.2015.1117017
20. Ellenberg SS, Fleming TR, DeMets DL. *Data Monitoring Committees in Clinical Trials: A Practical Perspective*. Chichester, UK: John Wiley & Sons; 2007.
21. DeMets D, Furberg CD, Friedman LM, eds. *Data Monitoring in Clinical Trials: A Case Studies Approach*. New York, NY: Springer-Verlag; 2006.
22. Stone RM, Mandrekar SJ, Sanford BL, et al. Midostaurin plus chemotherapy for acute myeloid leukemia with a FLT3 mutation. *N Engl J Med*. 2017;377(5):454–464. doi:10.1056/NEJMoa1614359
23. Romond EH, Perez EA, Bryant J, et al. Trastuzumab plus adjuvant chemotherapy for operable HER2-positive breast cancer. *N Engl J Med*. 2005;353(16): 1673–1684. doi:10.1056/NEJMoa052122
24. Wang SK, Tsiatis AA. Approximately optimal one-parameter boundaries for group sequential trials. *Biometrics*. 1987;43(1):193–199. doi:10.2307/2531959
25. Anderson K. gsDesign: Group Sequential Design [computer software]. https://cran.r-project.org/web/packages/gsDesign/index.html. 2016.
26. Hwang IK, Shih WJ, DeCani JS. Group sequential designs using a family of type I error probability spending functions. *Statistics in Medicine*. 1990;9:1439–1445. doi:10.1002/sim.4780091207
27. SAS Institute Inc. *SAS/STAT® 14.1 User's Guide*. Cary, NC: Author; 2015.
28. Schulz KF, Altman DG, Moher D, for the CONSORT Group. CONSORT 2010 statement: updated guidelines for reporting parallel group randomised trials. *Trials*. 2010;11:32. doi:10.1186/1745-6215-11-32

23

Quality of Life and Patient-Reported Outcome Analysis

MINH TAM TRUONG ■ MICHAEL A. DYER

The World Health Organization (WHO) defines **health** as "a state of complete physical, mental and social well-being, and not merely the absence of disease and infirmity" (1) and **quality of life (QOL)** as "individuals' perception of their position in life in the context of culture and value systems in which they live, and in relation to their goals, expectations, standards, and concerns" (1). In the context of an individual's health, **health-related quality of life (HR-QOL)** refers to a complex multidimensional concept, which describes the patient's perception of the effects of disease and treatment, and its impact on the individual's physical functioning, psychological and social well-being, personal beliefs, level of independence, and relationship to the environment (2). The focus of this chapter is HR-QOL; for ease, the term QOL, unless otherwise stated, refers specifically to HR-QOL.

Wilson and Cleary developed a conceptual model to understand the relationship among different health outcomes: biological and physiologic factors, symptoms, functioning, general health perceptions, and overall quality of life (3). Figure 23.1 illustrates this model: on the left are biological and physiological factors of health and disease, which affect symptoms. Symptoms then affect functional status, and functional status measures the ability of the individual to perform particular tasks. Four domains of functioning include physical, role, social, and psychological function. Functional status has an impact on general health perceptions, which can be modified by cognitive, emotional, socioeconomic, cultural, and demographic factors. Characteristics of the individual and of the environment may have a positive or negative impact on symptoms, functional status, and general health perceptions. These outcomes combined with biological and physiological variables affect overall HR-QOL, shown on the far right of the model. As one moves from left to right, there is increasing interaction between the individual and his or her environment, such that the concepts at each level are increasingly integrated and difficult to define and measure, with multiple inputs that cannot be controlled by clinicians or the healthcare system (3). QOL is inherently subjective and ideally should be evaluated by directly asking the patient. However, the goal of HR-QOL measurement is to be able to quantify how disease or treatment affects an individual's life in a reproducible way (2). The challenge is that a patient's perception of his or her QOL may also change over time. Patients with chronic symptoms may learn to adapt to problems, leading

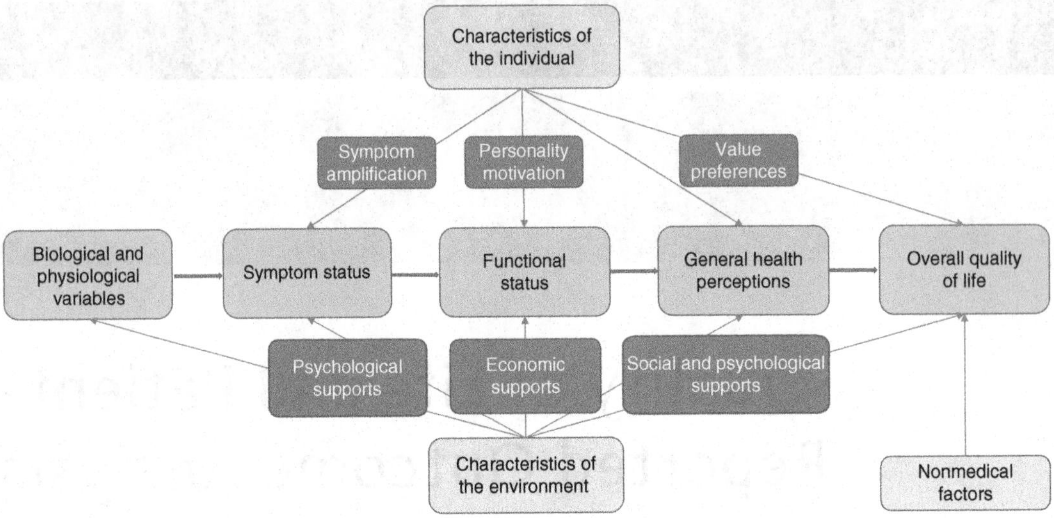

FIGURE 23.1 Wilson and Cleary model of patient outcomes.

Source: Wilson IB, Cleary PD. Linking clinical variables with health-related quality of life: a conceptual model of patient outcomes. *JAMA.* 1995;273(1):59–65. doi:10.1001/jama.273.1.59

to reporting of better QOL over time; conversely, continuing symptoms may increase patient distress, leading to reporting of worse QOL over time. Subjective changes in patients' perceptions are referred to as **response shift bias** (4,5). Patients may also ignore or under-report symptoms or problems they believe are unrelated to their illness, which may result in selective reporting, thereby introducing bias and interfering with the interpretation of QOL data (6).

Patient-reported outcomes (PROs) measure any clinical outcome reported directly by the patient. In the context of QOL, PROs can measure the patient's direct self-report of the effects of disease and treatment on his or her health and well-being, without the interference of another person's opinion or bias. PROs may be obtained through an interview, provided that the interviewer directly records the patient's response without introducing the interviewer's own bias. PROs can measure absolute severity of a symptom or as a change in score from a previous measure. PROs may also measure endpoints beyond QOL alone, including clinical care metrics, quality and performance metrics, patient adherence to medications, and patient satisfaction, and they can be used in public reporting (7). In general, PROs are considered the gold-standard method for evaluating QOL.

Proxy-reported outcome instruments, in contrast, are instruments that elicit reports from caregivers or clinicians and are not directly from the patient's perspective (8). Proxy reports from caregivers, though indirect and thus more susceptible to a certain bias, can provide some measurement of certain domains of a patient's QOL (9). However, for the purpose of this chapter, we focus on PROs as a tool for measuring patient-reported symptoms and QOL outcomes in clinical research and clinical trials.

Many QOL and PRO instruments have been developed and validated over the past few decades. These instruments measure a patient's report of his or her health through signs, symptoms, function, or complex multidimensional concepts. **Symptom burden** measures the symptom severity and the patient's perception of the impact of the symptoms reported (10). Patient-reported symptom burden can be a subset of QOL (assuming that it also measures some aspect of subjective functional status and/or health perception), which may be incorporated into clinical trials to evaluate new treatments without measuring other QOL domains. **Toxicity** is defined as signs or symptoms related to treatment and is a subset of morbidity, which may be related to treatment or disease effect and is traditionally a clinician-rated measure (11). Toxicity and **adverse events (AEs)** in clinical trials have historically been graded by clinicians and are often used to determine safety or feasibility of a new treatment. However, not all clinician-graded measures accurately represent how these side effects affect the patient. This has raised interest in developing and using patient-reported toxicity scales on clinical trials (12).

Cancer therapy is often complex, requiring a multidisciplinary approach tailored to disease site, stage, and the context of a patient's comorbidities. After accurate diagnosis and staging, the goal of care is to select the most appropriate therapies, which may be drawn from a broad range of options, including surgery, radiotherapy, chemotherapy, or a combination of these, to achieve the best possible outcomes. Such outcomes may include locoregional control, disease-free survival, overall survival, and/or amelioration or prevention of bothersome symptoms. Patient factors, decision preferences of both the patient and caregivers, and potential toxicities and how these toxicities may affect a patient's QOL, both during therapy and long term, are important considerations in choosing the most appropriate treatment strategy (13,14).

When comparing two distinct treatment strategies with a similar probability of disease control, but with different effects on function and QOL, understanding potential impacts on QOL between different therapeutic options is important in deciding the best therapy for a patient or group of patients. Similarly, when cancer therapies are associated with improvements in disease control or survival, it may not be clear whether incremental survival improvement translates to an improvement in QOL. In these situations, research using QOL assessment can be informative for clinical decision making and in subsequent clinical trials.

In this chapter, we discuss the development of QOL and PRO instruments, the instruments commonly used in clinical trials, utilities as a special type of QOL measurement, how to design studies incorporating QOL measurement, analysis and reporting of PROs on clinical trials, and the importance of QOL/PROs and implications for clinical care and decision making.

DEVELOPMENT OF QOL AND PRO INSTRUMENTS

There are generally two types of QOL measurements: health status and patient preference. Health-status measures are based on psychometrics, whereas patient preference measures are based on econometrics (15). Health-status instruments are traditional patient-reported questionnaires that assess QOL or symptom burden. Patient preference measurements usually aim to incorporate QOL into economic analyses, where the derivation of metrics such as **quality-adjusted life years (QALYs)** can help evaluate the trade-offs between quantity of life and quality of life (or evaluate costs of care, or cost-effectiveness analysis) (16).

Measuring QOL requires the development and validation of questionnaires used for assessing QOL in the population of interest. PRO instrument development should consider the patient population being tested, the acceptability of the questionnaire to the patient, practical considerations of administration, and the ability to interpret the scores. Instrument validation using statistical and psychometric techniques is performed so that the instrument performs in the expected manner (17).

The development of a PRO instrument requires testing for appropriateness, reliability, validity, ability to detect change, interpretability, and patient burden. *Appropriateness* refers to developing a conceptual framework to support the measurement of the concept of interest through patient interviews of the target population, focus groups, and qualitative cognitive interviewing. The developers may need to hypothesize the conceptual framework to support the measurement of interest by drafting domains and items to be measured using literature reviews or expert opinion. The conceptual framework is adjusted during drafting of the instrument through patient input, new item generation, and patient cognitive interviews. The instrument is also then assessed for clarity or relevance to the target population, response range and distribution, variability in the ability of the item to detect important differences among patients, reproducibility, interitem correlation, ability to detect change, item discrimination, redundancy, and recall period (18).

Reliability refers to the degree to which an instrument is reproducible, stable, and free from measurement error. **Internal consistency reliability** is the degree to which the items in a multi-item instrument are inter-related. **Test–retest reliability** is the ability of the instrument to be reproducible and provide consistency of scores over time in a stable population. In clinical trials, changes are measured over time, and the PRO instrument selection depends on the instrument's reliability in terms of obtaining consistent reproducible results that reflect the true effect of treatment.

Validity is the degree to which an instrument measures the concept it is aiming to measure. **Content validity** is the extent to which the instrument contains the most relevant and important aspects of a dimension of interest. **Construct validity** is the extent to which an instrument measures the concept that it is designed to measure in relation to other measures. **Criterion validity** refers to the degree to which scores of an instrument relate to a "gold standard" (17). The U.S. Food and Drug Administration (FDA) defines the "ability to detect change" as evidence that a PRO can identify differences in scores over time and in individuals or groups that have changed with respect to their measurement concept (19). The **European Organisation for Research and Treatment of Cancer (EORTC)** group defines the term *responsiveness* as a combination of **reliability** (identical scores in stable subjects over time) and **sensitivity** (the ability to demonstrate changes when a patient's health state improves or deteriorates over time, or to detect treatment effects) (20). Lindeboom et al. state that responsiveness is not a separate psychometric property of health states and is part of reliability. Sensitivity is also referred to as **longitudinal validity** (21,22).

When interpreting QOL scores in clinical research, defining what constitutes a clinically important difference in QOL is vital, as it helps determine the study design, the requirement for sample size, and the ultimate success or failure of the treatment intervention of interest. The **minimum important difference (MID)** is defined as the smallest difference in score in the domain of interest that patients perceive as important, either beneficial or harmful, and which would lead the clinician to consider a change in the patient's management (23–25). The MID is an important method for interpreting the results of QOL studies.

Commonly used methods to estimate the MID include **anchor-based** methods and **distribution-based** methods, the latter using standard error of measurement or effect size (usually between 0.2 and 0.5) (24). Anchor-based methods require an independent standard or anchor. These can include patient change anchors, using retrospective ratings of change in global transition items, symptoms; or external clinical anchors, using commonly utilized clinical scales or classifications, such as performance status. In anchor-based methods, the smallest change in score considered important to the patient (i.e., MID) is defined, and then estimates of the proportion of patients who have achieved that MID are calculated. With distribution methods, an effect is expressed using statistical methods, such as between-person standard deviation units, or within-person standard deviation units, or standard error of measurement or effect size (23).

Using multiple strategies to determine the MID can enhance the interpretability of the instrument. For example, Ringash et al., using a laryngeal cancer cohort, calculated the MIDs using an interpatient method, through comparisons between individuals at a single time point, and compared arithmetic differences in QOL with subjective comparison ratings. MIDs (expressed as a percentage of the total instrument range in the positive and negative directions) for the **Functional Assessment of Cancer Therapy (FACT)**-Head and Neck (FACT-H&N) cancer instrument were 4.3% and 8.6%, respectively. For the FACT-General (FACT-G) scale, these were 4% and 7.7%, respectively. For the **time trade-off (TTO) utility measure**, these were 5% and 6%, respectively. For the Daily Active Time Exchange utility measure, these were 5.5% and 14%, respectively. In summary, they found that the MIDs expressed as a percentage of the total score were estimated to be approximately 5% for a positive change and approximately 10% for a negative change, such that patients were more sensitive to positive changes compared to negative change in QOL (26).

Similarly, Cella et al. found that clinically meaningful group score changes in global QOL are often small for QOL improvements from baseline, whereas worsening global QOL is often associated with much larger negative score changes (27). Often, **clinically important differences** (or minimum clinically important differences) are used interchangeably with MID. Schünemann et al. claims that MID should be used rather than these other terms, because "clinically important difference" does not define to whom the difference is important, and the patients' perspective should provide the basis for the MID (25).

In a study of 812 non-small cell lung cancer (NSCLC) patients where QOL was evaluated using the **EORTC Quality-of-Life Core Questionnaire (EORTC QLQ-C30)**, the MIDs varied depending on which clinical anchor was used (WHO performance status or weight change). MIDs for improvement were greater and approximated more closely to the standard error of the mean (SEM), compared to MIDs for deterioration, which approximated more closely to 0.2 standard deviation estimates (28). Given this, when comparing different treatments, if survival or disease control endpoints are thought to be equivalent, then appropriately powered QOL or PRO designed endpoints, using appropriate estimates of the MID between treatment groups, can be used to determine between-group differences.

Different types of response options used to gather and record PROs include the **visual analogue scale (VAS)**, anchored or categorized VAS, **Likert scale,** rating scale, recording of events as they occur, pictorial scale, and checklists. A VAS is a line of fixed length with words that anchor the scale at each end. Patients are instructed to indicate the place on the line corresponding to their perceived state. The position marked is measured as the score. An anchored VAS has one or more intermediate marks positioned along the line to assist patients in identifying locations between each end of the scale. A Likert scale is a set of discrete terms or statements from which patients are asked to choose the response that best describes their state or experience. A rating scale is a set of numbered categories, from which patients are asked to pick the number that best describes their state/experience. The ends of the rating scales are anchored with words, but the categories are numbered. Recording events as they occur is done with an event log or patient diary. A checklist format is a set of limited-option answers such as yes/no/don't know (19).

QOL instruments depend on the language spoken by the patient and the cultural context of the patient's environment. Many QOL instruments have been translated and validated in different patient populations to determine if the instrument is linguistically and culturally relevant to the population studied. In cross-cultural adaptation of QOL instruments, multiple steps are required, including specific requirements with regard to translation of the QOL instrument, and then its adaptation, including both combining the literal translation of the words and an adaptation with regard to idiom, cultural context, and lifestyle (29). Proposed guidelines exist in terms of execution of forward translations and back translations by qualified linguistic experts, preferably producing several translations to improve accuracy. A multidisciplinary committee review of these translations is then performed to evaluate and compare source and final versions and systematically resolve any discrepancies, while modifying the format as appropriate. Verification of cross-cultural equivalence of the source and final versions is performed, followed by pretesting for equivalence with bilingual or monolingual individuals, and evaluating the weighting of scores and modifications, if necessary, to ensure that the instrument is culturally appropriate.

COMMON QOL AND PRO INSTRUMENTS IN CANCER CLINICAL TRIALS

Several common validated instruments appear in cancer clinical trials, which usually have both a general component focusing on QOL that is pertinent to a wide range of populations and health states, and a cancer disease-specific component focusing on particular disease and treatment-related effects.

The most commonly used validated QOL and PRO instruments used in cancer research include: the EORTC core questionnaire (EORTC QLQ-C30 version 3.0) (30); the FACT-G Questionnaire (31,32); the **MD Anderson Symptom Inventory (MDASI)** (33); and the five-item health utility instrument, the **EuroQol (EQ-5D)** (34,35). The EORTC QLQ-C30, FACT-G, and MDASI have accompanying disease-specific modules. When selecting an instrument in a clinical trial, consideration of the patient population, disease and treatment type, instrument validity for the population being tested, and the individual questions in the instrument are important factors in ensuring that the instrument of interest appropriately addresses the QOL domain or patient-reported symptom pertinent to the study. There are many disease-specific PRO instruments that address unique symptoms, function, and QOL issues facing patients with specific cancers, but their descriptions are beyond the scope of this chapter. The most commonly used PRO instruments in cancer research are summarized in Table 23.1.

TABLE 23.1 FREQUENTLY USED QOL AND PRO INSTRUMENTS IN CANCER RESEARCH

Instrument	General QOL Items	Indication	Time to Complete (Minutes)
EORTC QLQ-C30 (36)	30	QOL from surgery, radiation, and chemotherapy	15–20
FACT-G (31)	27	QOL from surgery, radiation, and chemotherapy	5–10
MDASI (33)	19	Symptom burden from surgery, radiation, and chemotherapy	5–10
PRO-CTCAE (12,37)	78	Patient-reported symptoms	15 depending on item selection
PROMIS (38)	4–10 for item short forms, 95 full item bank (e.g., fatigue)	Patient-reported symptoms/QOL	5–15 depending on instrument selection
EQ-5D (34)	5 + VAS	Health utilities; quality-adjusted survival	1–5

EORTC QLQ-C30, European Organisation for Research and Treatment of Cancer Quality-of-Life Core Questionnaire (EORTC QLQ-C30 version 3.0); EQ-5D, 5-item heath utility instrument of the EuroQol Group; FACT-G, Functional Assessment of Cancer Therapy-General; MDASI, MD Anderson Symptom Inventory; PRO, patient-reported outcome; PRO-CTCAE, Patient-Reported Outcomes version of the Common Terminology Criteria for Adverse Events; PROMIS, Patient-Reported Outcomes Measurement Information System; QOL, quality of life; VAS, visual analogue scale.

The EORTC is an independent, nonprofit cancer research organization, which has extensively developed and validated several QOL instruments that have been widely used in cancer research over the past few decades (39). The EORTC QLQ-C30 consists of a 30-item self-reporting questionnaire developed to assess overall QOL of patients with cancer, with 23 multiple disease-site–specific and patient-specific modules (40). As of 2018, Version 3 is the most recent.

The QLQ-C30 is grouped into five functional subscales with 16 questions (role, physical, cognitive, emotional, and social functioning), four multi-item symptom scales in six questions (fatigue, pain, nausea/vomiting, and appetite), six individual questions concerning common symptoms in cancer patients (constipation, diarrhea, sleep, dyspnea, financial), and two questions assessing overall QOL. This copyrighted instrument has been translated into and validated in more than 100 languages and has been used in more than 3,000 studies worldwide. There are multiple disease-site–specific modules as well.

For example, in head and neck cancer, the H&N35 module is specific for multimodality head and neck cancer therapy and contains an additional 35 questions. In the EORTC QLQ-C30, both of the scales as well as the single-item measures range in score from 0 to 100. A high score for a **functional scale** represents a higher level of functioning (health), while a high score on a **symptom scale** represents a high level of symptomatology (problems). Fifteen outcome profiles can be generated by the EORTC QLQ-C30. A summary score for the questionnaire was recently developed and is calculated from the mean of 13 of the 15 QLQ-C30 scales (41). The summary score combines physical, role, social, emotional, cognitive functioning, fatigue, pain, nausea/vomiting, dyspnea, sleep disturbances, appetite loss, constipation, and diarrhea items/scales. The global QOL scale and financial impact scale are not included. The time for administration is about 7 to 10 minutes for each instrument. Permission to use the EORTC scales may be obtained at http://groups.eortc.be/qol/eortc-qlq-c30 (36).

The Functional Assessment of Chronic Illness Therapy (FACIT.org) organization developed the FACT-G, first validated in 1993 (31). The self-administered 27-item FACT-G assesses patient function in four domains: physical, social/family, emotional, and functional well-being. There are disease-site–specific symptom items for multiple cancer disease sites. Each item is rated on a 0 to 4 Likert-type scale, and then combined to produce subscale scores for each domain, as well as a global QOL score. Higher scores represent better QOL. This copyrighted instrument has been translated into and validated in more than 50 languages. As of 2018, Version 4 is the most current version.

The FACT-G instrument takes about 5 to 10 minutes to complete. FACIT.org investigators have also developed focused disease-site questionnaires, cancer-specific symptom indexes, and treatment- and symptom-specific measures. In clinical trials, social and emotional well-being subscales of the FACT-G do not change significantly over time. Therefore, when evaluating a new treatment on clinical trial the investigator may opt to use the **FACT-Trial Outcome Index (TOI)** as the QOL endpoint, which can be computed for any disease-, treatment-, or condition-specific scale. It is the sum of the physical, functional, and additional concerns subscales.

The FACT-TOI is an efficient summary index of physical and functional PROs. An example of its use is in Radiation Therapy Oncology Group (RTOG) 0617, a randomized controlled trial (RCT) comparing dose-escalated versus standard chemoradiation in unresectable stage III NSCLC. Contrary to expectations, RTOG 0617 found a lower survival in the high-dose radiation therapy arm (74 Gy) compared to the standard-dose arm (60 Gy). The primary QOL hypothesis predicted a clinically meaningful decline in QOL using FACT-TOI of 5 points or more in the high-dose radiation arm at 3 months. The study did find that significantly more patients had a clinically meaningful decline in FACT-TOI scores of 45% versus 30% ($p = .02$) in the 74 Gy versus 60 Gy arm respectively, even though there were few differences in clinician-reported toxicity (42). Permission to use the FACT questionnaires may be obtained at www.facit.org/FACITOrg/Questionnaires (43).

The FACT-G and EORTC-QLQ are the two most commonly used validated QOL instruments in oncology clinical trials. In a meta-review of RCTs reporting QOL using PROs between 2000 and 2012, the EORTC-QLQ and FACT-G accounted for 55% of instruments used (44). Attempts at equating the EORTC and FACT instruments have been made. In a study of 737 cancer patients, a scheme for converting between instruments was devised for physical, emotional, and functional/role domains. Although earlier reports suggested that the instruments have significant overlap, they were found to have poor correlation in the social domain, but good agreement in the physical domain in a sample of breast cancer and Hodgkin lymphoma patients; the overall agreement between the two instruments was only moderate (44).

The FACT-G and EORTC-QLQ are two excellent QOL tools, but instruments that focus on symptom burden have also been developed, such as the MDASI. This is a self-administered multisymptom PRO measure for clinical and research use, which includes 13 core items (pain, fatigue, nausea, disturbed sleep, distress, shortness of breath, lack of appetite, drowsiness, dry mouth, sadness, vomiting, difficulty remembering, and numbness or tingling). These symptoms have the highest frequency and/or severity in patients with various cancers and treatment types. There are also six interference items (general activity, mood, walking ability, normal work, relations with other people, and enjoyment of life). This inventory uses a 0 to 10 numerical rating scale (NRS) to assess the severity of symptoms and interference. The MDASI assesses the severity of symptoms at their worst in the past 24 hours, with 0 being "not present" and 10 being "as bad as you can imagine."

There are various disease-site–specific modules assessing symptom burden unique to each disease site. The MDASI copyrights are held by the University of Texas MD Anderson Cancer Center and administered by the MDASI's developer, Charles S. Cleeland, PhD. Each instrument takes 5 to 10 minutes to complete. The MDASI instrument may be used in clinical trials to evaluate symptom burden or to test therapeutic interventions aimed at amelioration of symptoms. For example, in head and neck cancer, it has been demonstrated that the MDASI head and neck module is able to detect moderate to severe symptoms associated with mucositis better than the FACT-H&N instrument (10,45). Permission to use the MDASI questionnaires may be obtained at www3.mdanderson.org/depts/symptomresearch.

PATIENT- VERSUS CLINICIAN-REPORTED ADVERSE EVENTS

The National Cancer Institute **Common Terminology Criteria for Adverse Events** (NCI-CTCAE) reporting system is routinely used by physicians and on clinical trials to measure toxicity or adverse medical events. Other toxicity scoring systems include the **National Cancer Institute of Canada-Common Toxicity Criteria** (NCIC-CTC), **RTOG Grading System**, and the **Late Effects Normal Tissue/Subjective, Objective, Management, and Analytic** (LENT/SOMA) system (46). More recently, efforts have focused on eliciting toxicity reports directly from patients, as studies suggest that patient-reported toxicity provides additional and complementary information compared to physician-only toxicity reports.

For example, in a retrospective pooled analysis of 2,279 cancer patients from 14 EORTC RCTs, six cancer symptoms (pain, fatigue, vomiting, nausea, diarrhea, and constipation) were analyzed to evaluate the extent of agreement between clinician and patient symptom scoring, using, respectively, the NCI-CTCAE, and items extracted from the EORTC QLQ-C30 (47). Patient-reported fatigue differed from clinician-reported scores. Both clinician- and patient-reported symptoms were independently and positively predictive of survival. This study found that using clinician and patient scores together for fatigue, nausea, vomiting, and constipation was more predictive of survival than clinician scores alone (47). Similarly, in a cross-sectional study of 1,933 cancer patients, patient-reported symptoms using the EORTC QLQ-C30 were compared to provider-reported four-point categorical scales. This study found that providers underestimated symptoms in 10% of patients, and overestimated in 1% of patients. Patients with low Karnofsky performance status or high Mini-Mental State score, or patients who were hospitalized, recently diagnosed, or undergoing opioid titration, were at increased risk of symptom underestimation by providers (48).

Given this discrepancy between physician and patient reporting of toxicity, and the ability of patient-reported toxicities to improve prognostic models compared to models only incorporating clinician-scored toxicities, patient-reported toxicity scoring systems are in development. The NCI-CTCAE library consists of 790 discrete AEs using a five-point scale encompassing three general categories: laboratory events, observable/measurable events, and symptomatic events. Approximately 10% of AEs in the CTCAE library are symptomatic AEs.

The NCI sponsored an initiative to develop the Patient-Reported Outcomes version of the Common Terminology Criteria for Adverse Events (PRO-CTCAE). The purpose was to develop a patient-centered approach to AE reporting, creating a more representative account of patients' treatment experience. An additional goal was to incorporate patient-reported AEs into clinical trials to assess AEs and tolerability of treatment regimens from the patient's perspective. There are currently 78 items identified as appropriate for patient self-reporting using PRO-CTCAE. For each item, a plain-language term in English has one to three items, which characterize frequency, severity, and/or interference with activity. There are a total of 124 PRO-CTCAE items (12). Information on PRO-CTCAE may be found at healthcaredelivery.cancer.gov/pro-ctcae/instrument.html.

The PRO-CTCAE instrument has been validated and tested in 975 patients with cancer undergoing chemotherapy and/or radiotherapy (37). The incorporation of the PRO-CTCAE in a number of multicenter national trials is ongoing, and results of initial feasibility testing appear promising (49). In a head and neck cancer study evaluating chemoradiotherapy, a comparison of the NCI-CTCAE with the PRO-CTCAE found a high concordance between patient-reported and practitioner-reported symptom severity at baseline, when symptoms were absent, but as toxicity increased during therapy, it was noted that clinician-reported toxicity was significantly lower than patient-reported toxicity. This was true even for more objectively clinician-graded symptoms, such as radiation dermatitis (which is almost entirely based on physical exam in the NCI-CTCAE grading system; in the PRO-CTCAE, it is, as all measures are, inherently subjective). There was less concordance with measures that are subjective in both NCI-CTCAE and PRO-CTCAE systems, such as fatigue (50).

Finally, the **Patient-Reported Outcomes Measurement Information System (PROMIS)** Network was a program started in 2004 within the National Institutes of Health Common Fund to develop item banks for measuring major self-reported health domains affected by chronic illness. This was then extended by the NCI to develop PROs relevant for cancer patients and survivors. PROMIS measures physical, mental, and social domains. The symptoms relevant to cancer patients include fatigue, pain, physical functioning, and emotional distress (anxiety and depression). PROMIS includes multiple types of instruments, including short forms (with a fixed set of 4 to 10 items for a single domain), computer adaptive tests (which are dynamically selected for administration from the item bank based on the previous respondent's answers), and profiles (which are a fixed collection of short forms from multiple domains). More information on PROMIS can be found at www.healthmeasures.net/explore-measurement-systems/promis/intro-to-promis (38).

UTILITIES IN CLINICAL TRIALS

A special subtype of QOL measurement is **patient preference**, or **utility, measurement.** *Patient preference* is a broad term, and can mean preference for one given treatment over another, particularly when the outcomes associated with the treatments are known in advance. Patients (and people in general, including people in good health) can also have preferences for one health state over another. The preferences for/against these health states are a way to identify the QOL associated with the health states. When patient preferences are assessed in conditions of uncertainty, they are termed *utilities*, although, in practice, preferences for different health states are often called utilities even when they are not assessed in conditions of uncertainty (51).

The utility for a given health state is measured on a scale from 0 to 1, where 0 represents death, and 1 represents life in perfect health. One of the benefits of preference/utility-based QOL measurement compared to other types of QOL measurement is that utilities can place the QOL of any person and/or health state on this universal scale with death on one end (0) and perfect health on the other (1). Another benefit of utilities is that they can be used to evaluate trade-offs between QOL and survival, for example, by allowing calculation of QALYs, discussed further in what follows (15).

Methods to measure patient preference ratings include the VAS, **TTO discrete choice experiments**, the **standard gamble method**, and certain multiattribute health-status questionnaires, such as the EQ-5D (51–56). Some of these methods are discussed in Chapter 19. The simplest method of utility measurement is the VAS, where the patient is asked to rate his or her QOL on a linear scale anchored from "best" to "worst" possible QOL. TTO is a method for eliciting patient preferences and compares QOL to length of survival. It involves asking respondents whether they would choose a certain amount of time in perfect health versus a longer amount of time in a compromised health state of interest. The discrete choice experiments method is another way to measure utilities; in this method, respondents are presented with a number of hypothetical decision situations ("choice sets") consisting of two or more health profiles, and the respondent selects which health profile is preferable (57).

The standard gamble is the method of utility measurement that involves decisions in the face of uncertainty, and is the method most grounded in econometric utility theory (6,56). It assesses the utility of a health state by asking the respondent (who may be a patient affected by the health state, or, alternatively, a healthy subject) the risk of death he or she would accept to improve or avoid it. Respondents are asked to choose between life in a compromised health state, and a gamble between perfect health and death (51,52,56,58). The odds of perfect health versus death associated with the gamble are changed iteratively until the researcher is able to find the odds of the gamble at which the person becomes indifferent between the gamble and the compromised health state of interest. At this point of indifference between the gamble and the compromised health state, the utility value of the compromised health state is defined by the probability of perfect health associated with the gamble (56).

Generally, standard gamble and TTO techniques are difficult to implement in clinical trials. In clinical trials, it is more common to elicit utilities using a multiattribute health-status questionnaire. Additionally, Noel et al. compared different utility measures in patients with head and neck cancer and found that health-status questionnaire utility measures may better reflect true health status than standard gamble or TTO methods (59).

The most commonly used instrument is the EQ-5D, a multiattribute instrument that has five dimensions, and (in its original EQ-5D-3L form) 243 health states (35,60–62). The EQ-5D is a trademark of the EuroQol Group. It was originally designed to complement other instruments, but is now increasingly used as a stand-alone measure to assess a patient's current health status, and to indirectly measure the utility of this health state (Table 23.1). The EQ-5D is a two-part patient self-administrated questionnaire that takes approximately 1 to 5 minutes to complete. The first part consists of five items covering five dimensions including mobility, self-care, usual activities, pain/discomfort, and anxiety/depression. The EQ-5D-3L version grades each dimension on three levels: 1—no problems, 2—moderate problems, and 3—extreme problems. The EQ-5D-5L version grades each dimension on five levels: 1—no problems, 2—slight problems, 3—moderate problems, 4—severe problems, and 5—unable to/extreme problems. The second part is a VAS valuing current health state, measured on a 20-cm 10-point interval scale (Figure 23.2).

For version EQ-5D-3L, there are 243 distinct health states (i.e., 3 to the 5th power) defined by the unique combinations of answers to the five items in the first part of the questionnaire. Based on the administration of the EQ-5D-3L to members of the general population, and based on utility measurement of different health states using the TTO method in these respondents, researchers have mapped the health states that are defined by answers to the ED-5D-3L to utility values. Therefore, any patient completing the questionnaire can have a utility value assigned to his or her current health state, albeit indirectly (35,60–63). The EQ-5D is available in more than 125 languages, and can be accessed at www.euroqol.org (34). There is some evidence that the EQ-5D-5L may have greater discriminative ability and less ceiling effect than the EQ-5D-3L in patients with cancer (64), and valuation data for derivation of a utility score for the 5L version are available in some, but not all, populations (35). Data from a U.S. study that provided valuation (i.e., patient preference data to convert the EQ-5D-3L health states to utilities) can be found at archive.ahrq.gov/professionals/clinicians-providers/resources/rice/EQ5Dproj.html (62).

The EQ-5D is not specific to patients with cancer and may have issues with ceiling effects and content validity, particularly around health states that are especially relevant to patients with cancer, such as fatigue (58,65). The **EORTC-8D** and EORTC **Quality of Life Utility Measure-Core 10 dimensions** (**QLU-C10D**) are two separate multiattribute health-status measures specific to cancer patients, both derived from the EORTC QLQ-C30 questionnaire. The EORTC-8D assigns utilities to the health state of each particular respondent at a given point in time based on his or her responses to particular items in the EORTC QLQ-C30 (66,67).

EORTC-8D covers eight dimensions: physical, role, emotional, social functioning, pain, fatigue/sleep disturbance, nausea, and constipation/diarrhea. Each dimension has 4 to 5 levels of severity. It is derived from 10 QLQ-30 items and provides utility values based on the 81,920 health states defined by answers to these items and on TTO data from a population in the United Kingdom (66). The QLU-C10D metric is a health state classification system, based on a subset of responses to the EORTC QLQ-C30 (12 items representing 10 dimensions): physical functioning (mobility), role functioning, social functioning, emotional functioning, pain, fatigue, sleep, appetite, nausea, and bowel problems (67). Norman et al. completed a feasibility study to show that a discrete choice experiment can be used to value health states within the QLU-C10D, and collection of full valuation data is ongoing (57). The EORTC-8D may have less of a problem with ceiling effects compared to the EQ-5D in patients with cancer, and the QLU-C10D, having been developed using data from multiple cancer types (as opposed to the EORTC-8D, which was developed using data from multiple myeloma patients), may eventually prove even more useful in cancer patients than the EORTC-8D (68).

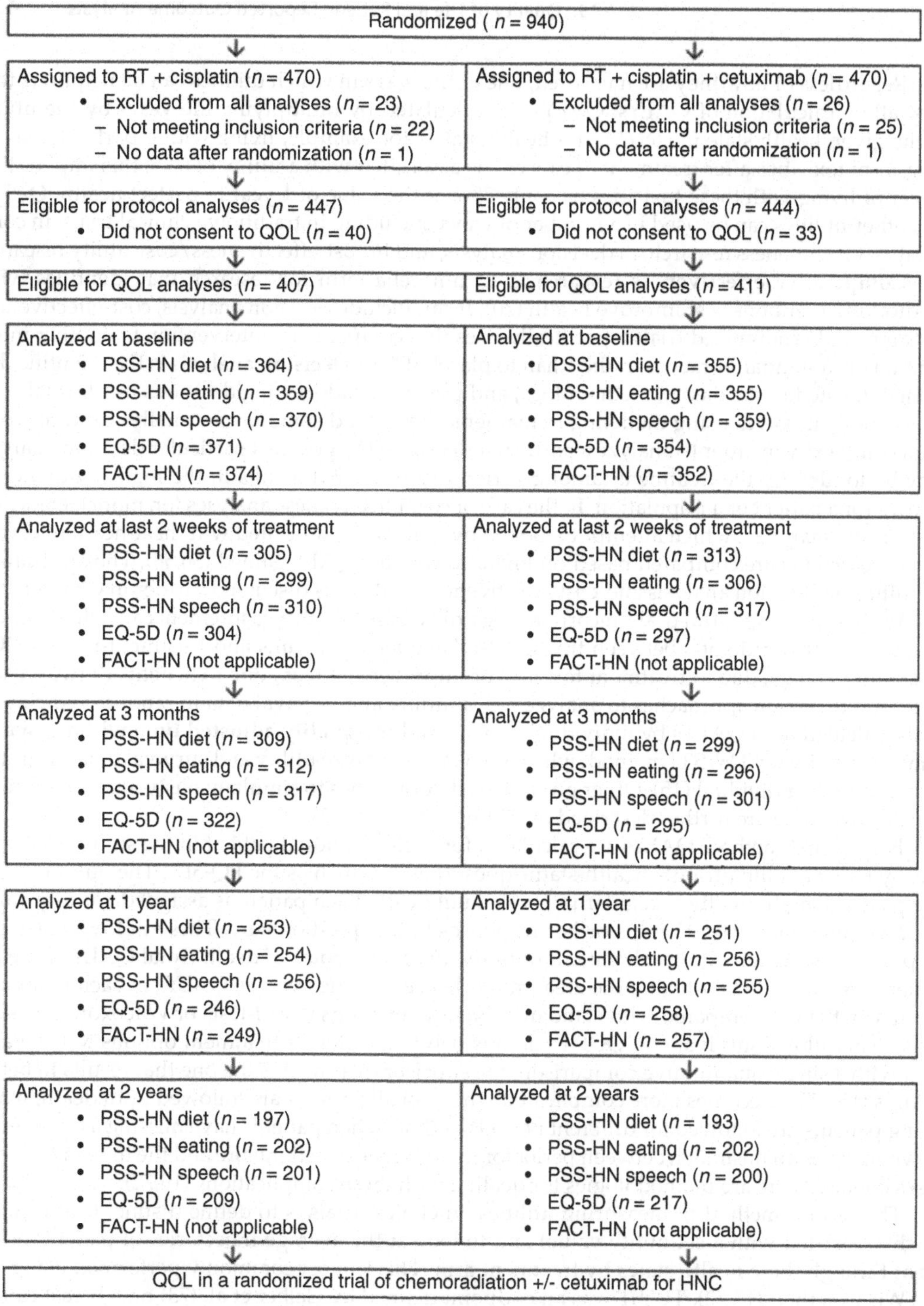

FIGURE 23.2 Example of a CONSORT diagram of a randomized study comparing chemoradiation with and without cetuximab for head and neck cancer, RTOG 0522.

CONSORT, Consolidated Standards of Reporting Trials; EQ-5D, 5-item heath utility instrument of the EuroQol Group; FACT-HN, Functional Assessment of Cancer Therapy-Head and Neck; PS, performance status; PSS-HN, Performance Status Scale for Head and Neck Cancer Patients; QOL, quality of life; RT, radiation therapy.

Source: Truong MT, Zhang Q, Rosenthal DI, et al. Quality of life and performance status from a substudy conducted within a prospective phase 3 randomized trial of concurrent accelerated radiation plus cisplatin with or without cetuximab for locally advanced head and neck carcinoma: NRG Oncology Radiation Therapy Oncology Group 0522. *Int J Radiat Oncol Biol Phys.* 2017;97(4):687–699. doi:10.1016/j.ijrobp.2016.08.003

Regardless of how they are measured, one of the ways in which utilities can be helpful is that they allow calculation of QALYs. QALYs are calculated by multiplying life years by the utility of the given health state (56,58,69). If a health state—for example, living with a particular set of long-term toxicities after treatment of cancer—is associated with a utility of 0.75, this implies that 1 year of living with these toxicities has only 75% of the value of 1 year in perfect health. QALYs and other utilities can be used in a number of ways, including in traditional clinical trials, in comparative effectiveness research, in decision analysis, and in cost-effectiveness/cost-utility research.

Comparative effectiveness research is an umbrella term for research that identifies what medical interventions best improve health (70). It can include decision analysis, cost-effectiveness research, and randomized trials (specifically ones that compare one intervention to another intervention or to standard practice, rather than to placebo) (71). **Decision analysis** is the scientific discipline devoted to the theory, methodology, and practice of addressing decisions in a formal way. This usually involves using modeling to mathematically (and sometimes visually) capture structural complexity in order to analyze a particular decision. The goal of a particular decision analysis may be to identify the treatment (among various options) that results in the highest number of QALYs for a patient or a population. In the case of cost-effectiveness analyses (or, more technically, cost-utility analyses), which attempt to look at overall value associated with healthcare interventions, treatments are compared based on financial cost per QALY gained (56,58). The application of utilities in decision analysis and cost-effectiveness analysis is discussed further in Chapter 19.

With respect to clinical trials, incorporating utility-based QOL measurement can help researchers evaluate the trade-offs between treatment-related survival gains and treatment-related QOL deterioration (e.g., due to treatment toxicity) or improvement (e.g., due to benefits of treatment). There are two main approaches to analyze repeat utility and survival data in randomized clinical trials: calculation of QALYs by individual patient; and the **quality adjusted time without symptoms or toxicity** (**Q-TWiST**) method, which is a way to analyze utility and survival data by group, rather than by individual (15). Other group-based approaches to simultaneously analyzing utility and survival data are further described by Billingham et al. (72).

For the first method, QALYs are calculated for each individual patient in the study, for example, by using a multiattribute health-status questionnaire (such as the EQ-5D). The questionnaire is repeated longitudinally at regular intervals until death. Each patient is assigned a utility value at every time point based on his or her responses to the questionnaire. These utility values can be plotted against time for each patient until the final time point of death. Total QALYs for each patient are calculated by taking the area under this curve. The average QALYs in each treatment group can then be compared with standard statistical methods (e.g., *t*-tests or Wilcoxon rank sum tests). This allows survival and QOL trade-offs between different treatment options to be evaluated with a single quantitative comparison; the superior treatment is the one that results in better QALYs (15). This becomes more complicated when not all patients are followed until death; when living patients are followed for different periods of time; when patients have missing assessments; or when there is a mismatch between period of recall for the questionnaire and the time in between assessments. There are methodologies for dealing with these complications (15,72).

The second method of measuring utilities on clinical trials is to define distinct health states (each associated with a set utility value) and to look at the average trajectories of patient movement through these health states by treatment arm. This is most commonly performed using the Q-TWiST method (15,72). TWiST was an endpoint defined by Gelber et al. (73) on a breast cancer study to represent the duration of time spent without symptoms and toxicity. For patients with toxicity or symptoms, TWiST is calculated by subtracting from overall survival the periods of time during which the patient experienced toxic effects from treatment or from the disease itself. Q-TWiST uses utility scores to adjust the relative value of years survived when health is impaired. It can be useful in clinical trials because it can be applied to censored survival data (6).

To calculate the Q-TWiST, distinct health states are defined for each group of patients. For example, in the method described by Goldhirsch et al. (74), overall survival time was divided into the following different health states: TWiST (i.e., time without symptoms/toxicity); TOX (i.e., time with toxicity); and REL (i.e., time after systemic relapse). TOX and REL were weighted by utility coefficients (u_{tox}, u_{rel}) between 0 and 1 to represent the QOL value of these health states in relation to TWiST. The results were added to give a period of quality-adjusted survival (Q-TWiST) as follows:

$$\text{Q-TWiST} = (u_{tox} * \text{TOX}) + (\text{TWiST}) + (u_{rel} * \text{REL})$$

In clinical trials, for each treatment arm, an estimate is made of the average time the group spends in each health state. Every defined health state is associated with a utility value (which can be based on utilities collected during the clinical trial). The total Q-TWiST value for each treatment arm is calculated by multiplying the time in each health state by the utility of the health state, and then adding these products together. Q-TWiST scores can then be compared between treatment arms (69,72,74–79).

Regarding the incorporation of utility or preference measures into clinical trials, the FDA states that preference weights that were developed "for use in resource allocations (e.g., as in cost-effectiveness analysis that may use predetermined community weights)" should not be used to weight items in a PRO measure to create a composite/summary score "unless the preference weights' relationship to the intended clinical trial population is known and found adequate and appropriate (19)." Utilities, QALYs, or costs per QALY gained are not generally used in the United States to determine whether new therapies should be approved or adopted. In contrast, many other countries, including the United Kingdom, rely on costs, QALYs, and patient preferences/utilities to guide healthcare policy and practice (57).

Whether or not a researcher (or his or her government) is interested in healthcare costs, utilities and QALYs can be a useful tool in clinical trials, particularly if a researcher is interested in an integrated and quantitative comparison of efficacy and toxicity trade-offs between the different treatments he or she is studying. If a researcher is interested in incorporating QALYs, decision analysis, and/or cost-utility analysis into a clinical trial, we recommend using the EQ-5D instrument (specifically the EQ-5D-5L if there are valuation data from the research population's country; otherwise, the EQ-5D-3L can be used) (35). If the researcher is planning to use the EORTC-QLQ-C30 as a PRO measure, he or she can alternatively, or additionally, consider using the EORTC-8D and QLU-C10D to derive utilities, once valuation data become available for the research population of interest. We recommended that researchers interested in incorporating utility measurement and analysis into clinical trials elicit the input of collaborators with particular expertise in collecting and analyzing utilities from the outset of the study, that is, during protocol design, if the researcher does not possess this expertise.

DESIGNING STUDIES WITH QOL/PRO ENDPOINTS

When designing studies that include QOL evaluation, a clear statement of the QOL research question, hypothesis, and selection of the appropriate QOL tool that will best answer the research question, both qualitatively and quantitatively in the target population, should be created. In addition to information regarding the informed consent process, the following factors should be considered and specified in the protocol:

1. Outline of the study design
2. Patient eligibility
3. Rationale for measuring QOL
4. Statement about the QOL variable(s) considered relevant to the primary or secondary endpoint, in terms of acute or late effects
5. QOL instruments and their domains that will be collected
6. Rationale for choice of instrument
7. Rationale for the timing of assessments
8. Method of data collection
9. Methods to enhance compliance and minimize missing data
10. Statistical considerations, including sample size calculations

Because measuring QOL/PROs is resource intensive, they are often not included in phase I or II trials, due to small patient numbers and the intent (usually) to test feasibility and toxicity. However, there may be a rationale to include QOL in early phase studies if the QOL instrument is being piloted for use, prior to a phase III trial, or if a randomized phase II study is likely to continue as a phase III study, and where QOL is considered an important outcome measure (49). QOL assessment may also be included in phase II studies to help inform (in conjunction with results of the primary survival endpoint) which arm should proceed to a phase III study. This strategy is currently being used in a number of ongoing randomized trials, in which QOL endpoints are administered in conjunction with the primary survival endpoint as a "go-no go" decision to inform which arm will move forward into a phase III study (80,81).

Some investigators consider QOL an essential secondary endpoint on all phase III studies (82), whereas others recommend that QOL be used as the primary endpoint when no specific differences in survival or disease-free survival exist, but treatment arms have differing toxicity profiles that could lead to differences in QOL. QOL may also be used to help conduct cost-effectiveness—or, more accurately, cost-utility—analyses.

The FDA released a guidance statement in 2009 on the use of PRO measures for conducting industry-sponsored clinical trials for medical product development to support labeling claims (statement of treatment benefit) (19). Using the FDA definition, a PRO instrument captures patient-reported data to measure treatment benefit (or risk) in medical product clinical trials. PRO data may be used to make conclusions about the treatment effect at the time of medical product approval. The FDA defines the concepts "symptom," "group of symptoms," and "effects on function" in order to measure the severity of a health condition. Concepts can include patient-reported symptoms, quality of life, patient experience, convenience, patient adherence, patient-reported side effects, activities of daily living, and health status. When PROs are used in clinical trials to support labeling claims, the PRO concept measurement should be stated as a specific objective or hypothesis of the study. Other requirements by the FDA include specific instructions on clinical investigator training, instructions for patients on how to complete PRO measures, methods of data filing and storage, and transmission method from the clinical trial site.

When choosing a QOL instrument, researchers should consider a number of specific factors: instrument validation, applicability to the population being studied, methods to obtain permission to use the instrument, scoring and interpretation, number of patients required to power the study, how burdensome the instrument will be for patients (i.e., the adverse physical, emotional, and cognitive strain on patients), whether the instrument is validated in the language(s) and culture(s) of interest, and whether the instrument will capture the potential expected treatment side effects (6). Efforts must be made to ensure that the questionnaire selected is acceptable to patients in terms of method of collection (including the choice of paper or electronic formats), time for completion of the instrument, format and layout appearance, legibility, and literacy level of the target population. These factors should be considered in clinical trial design to maximize the compliance of QOL collection. Researchers should also consider the administrative and resource burden of PRO collection (i.e., the cost and training of staff and the infrastructure costs required to collect and analyze the data).

The timing of PRO assessment usually includes a baseline assessment prior to or immediately after randomization, and assessments at subsequent time points, to assess longitudinal changes caused by the treatment and disease. QOL at baseline has also been demonstrated to be a prognostic factor for outcomes such as survival (83). In selecting the timing of QOL assessments during treatment, researchers should consider methods to maximize compliance and select time points that coincide with other aspects of clinical care (as dictated by the treatment regimen). The optimal schedule of assessments should minimize patient and investigator burden of completing the questionnaires, while capturing the most likely period in which treatment toxicity is expected to occur. A simple method is to schedule PRO collection at similar or identical schedules between arms. **Time-based QOL evaluations** are when the measurements are dictated at regular intervals relative to the baseline or randomization date, whereas **event-based evaluations** may be timed to a specific treatment and may be different between treatment arms, according to the timing of treatment delivery in each trial arm (20).

ANALYSIS OF QOL AND PRO DATA

In a clinical trial designed to evaluate QOL, it is essential to outline a detailed statistical plan. This includes a significance test to assess the weight of evidence and the possibility that observed differences are due to chance. To estimate the sample size, the significance threshold (α), power ($1 - \beta$), and anticipated effect size (Δ) must be specified (84). Tests are usually two-sided, with minimum significance threshold and a power set at 5% and 80%, respectively. The effect size (e.g., MID) is usually best determined based on prior published data or pilot studies. However, in QOL studies, there may be no prior experience to determine appropriate effect size. In the absence of prior data, relative differences are typically employed, with a small effect corresponding to $\Delta = 0.2$, a moderate effect to $\Delta = 0.5$, and a large effect to $\Delta = 0.8$.

QOL variables should be ranked in order of importance, with one primary QOL endpoint specified (6). If there are additional endpoints, multiple hypotheses may be tested, using separate sample size calculations for each endpoint, with appropriate corrections to avoid inflation of error rates (see Chapter 11) (6). One method to analyze serial/longitudinal QOL measurements from baseline to the end of treatment is to calculate a summary score of each individual patient using the area under the curve (AUC) (85). The average of the AUCs for each patient can be calculated by treatment group, and then the group means can be compared using an appropriate statistical test.

The statistical plan must also address how missing data will be handled. **Missing data** is defined as values that are not available and that would be meaningful for analysis if they were observed. This is in contrast to **compliance,** which is defined as the number of completed questionnaires received as a proportion of the number expected, given the study design and number of patients who are alive and enrolled in the study. This latter metric, for example, acknowledges that questionnaires are not expected from patients who have died (86–89).

In QOL research, missing data may include **item nonresponse** (i.e., missing data in a questionnaire where a response has not been provided for a question), and **unit nonresponse** (i.e., the whole questionnaire is missing for a patient). For unit nonresponse, there may be an intermittent missing form, dropout from the study, or late entry into the study (88). Missing data is a problem in PRO and QOL data because it can potentially introduce bias into the study, compromising the ability to compare effects between study groups and increasing the risk of false findings (86). Gathering information on the reasons for missing data is important to minimize additional dropouts and to establish backup plans to ensure continued PRO collection, even if patients have discontinued treatment.

Potentially avoidable sources of missing data may be broadly categorized into methodological factors; logistic and administrative factors; and patient-related factors (89,90). Identifying the types of missingness involves collecting data on why the QOL information was not collected, and then, based on this information, assigning one of the aforementioned categories to each instance of missing data. Another approach is to model the missing data mechanism and perform hypothesis testing to determine the missing data processes.

Rubin defines three mechanisms of missing data: **missing completely at random (MCAR), missing at random (MAR),** and **missing not at random (MNAR)** (90–94). MCAR means the probability of missing is independent of all past, present, and future assessments. An example might be because of administrative errors. MCAR assumes that the patients with missing data are a random sample of the whole patient cohort. If the study is adequately powered, then MCAR should not alter the results if MCAR is ignored in the analysis. MAR means the probability of missing data depends on observed data, but not current or future assessment scores. An example might be where a particular patient group has fatigue. This group may have both worse QOL scores and higher missing data. Using a statistical method that ignores MAR may introduce bias. MNAR means the probability of missing data depends on current and future unobserved scores. If previous scores observed are constant, but a decline after dropout occurred is not observed due to missingness, the extent of decline is unknown. For example, if a patient is too sick to fill out the questionnaires, the rate of dropout and of missing data increases. Patients with a decreasing QOL score may be more likely to drop out (87). In this scenario, MNAR cannot be ignored, as it introduces bias into the analysis.

MCAR and MAR are considered *potentially* ignorable: that is, if the dropout process is random, then unbiased estimates can be obtained. Determining the type of missingness helps to identify the most appropriate statistical analysis method (87). Several methods can be used to determine missingness mechanism. These include **Little's test** of MCAR, **Listin–Schlittgen test** to determine if dropouts are missing at random, **Ridout's logistic regression method**, and **Fairclough's logistic regression method** (95).

Little's test of MCAR assumes that the means of the observed data should be the same regardless of the pattern of missingness if the data are MCAR. The Listin–Schlittgen test can be used to determine if missing data are MAR. Ridout's method is a test for random dropouts in repeated measurement data. Fairclough's method identifies variables within the dataset that are associated with missingness, using logistic regression models created from the significant candidate variables, using a stepwise procedure. Differences between MCAR and MAR are evaluated by testing the association of missing data with observed QOL scores. If the observed QOL score is significant in the model predicting missingness, then there is evidence of MAR data. This method can be used to determine if data are MNAR versus MCAR or MAR.

When analyzing PRO data, the simplest method is **complete-case analysis**, whereby patients who have incomplete data are excluded. This is feasible if the data are thought to be MCAR, but is not appropriate in instances of MAR or MNAR. Hence, several statistical methods may be used, depending on the mechanism of missing data; they include repeated measures methods, mixed effects models, generalized linear models, generalized estimating equations, and methods that jointly model the measurement and missingness process. Multiple imputation methods may also be used to fill in missing values in the dataset (96). For further reference, Fairclough et al. also define several statistical methods of analysis for longitudinal assessment of QOL in cancer trials (97).

INTEGRATING ELECTRONIC TECHNOLOGY TO OBTAIN QOL ASSESSMENTS

Traditionally, QOL data have been collected in paper format. More recently, electronic, web-based, and mobile platforms have been developed to facilitate the collection of PROs (see www.visiontree.com). Such technology allows patients to fill out questionnaires on computers or mobile devices, which has been demonstrated to improve compliance and reduce missing data in clinical trials (98). In practice, there is also increasing interest in using electronic PROs as part of routine cancer care, and in integrating PROs into existing electronic medical health records in order to obtain real-time patient-reported data, which may enhance clinical history and examination findings. Furthermore, real-time electronic PROs may improve communication between the patient and provider, and allow providers to monitor longitudinal QOL, and potentially implement early intervention to mitigate any patient-reported side effects (99).

REPORTING OF QOL AND PRO DATA

Collection of PROs and QOL on RCT can involve significant administrative costs and time to the patient and clinical investigator. Hence, for the inclusion of PROs in an RCT, careful consideration of the study design, analysis, and reporting is required. Inadequate reporting limits interpretation of PROs and, therefore, their applicability to clinical practice (100,101).

The **Consolidated Standards of Reporting Trials** (**CONSORT**) is a statement first published in 1996 and then revised in 2010, which is composed of a quality checklist of 22 items essential for the conduct and reporting of RCTs (102). The CONSORT diagram (Figure 23.2) should illustrate the flow of study participants through a trial to standardize the primary reporting of RCTs with two-group, parallel designs. The objective of CONSORT is to provide guidance to authors to improve the reporting of their study results and also for reviewers and editors to critically appraise and interpret the results of an RCT (102).

The 2013 CONSORT-PRO extension provided specific recommendations on the reporting of PROs and QOL data from randomized trials, which included five items in addition to the 2010 CONSORT checklist to facilitate the optimal reporting of PROs, as primary or secondary endpoints in RCTs (8). More information on CONSORT-PRO may be found at www.consort-statement.org/extensions?ContentWidgetId=560.

The goal of adherence to the CONSORT-PRO statement is the robust reporting and interpretation of PRO and QOL data, which can then inform patient care. The five CONSORT-PRO items recommended for RCTs that include PROs as primary or secondary endpoints are:

1. The PROs should be identified as a primary or secondary outcome in the abstract.
2. The hypothesis/hypotheses relevant to the PROs should be described, and the specific relevant domains being tested if a multidimensional instrument is being used should be outlined.
3. Evidence that the instrument has validity and reliability should be provided and cited.
4. Statistical methods for dealing with missing data should be explicitly stated.
5. PRO-specific limitations of the study findings and generalizability of the results should be described.

A number of studies evaluated the adherence to CONSORT reporting guidelines: in a study of 794 RCTs, 86% of RCTs reported QOL within the initial RCT report, whereas 14% used supplementary reports separate from the first publication to report QOL. Of the 794 studies, QOL was a primary outcome in 25.4% (101). Of these trials, 81% reported on the instrument validity, but more than a third of trials failed to provide a rationale for the tool chosen, to give information on who administered the instrument, to provide a CONSORT flowchart, and/or to state the hypothesis relating to QOL. More than two-thirds failed to provide sample size and power calculations and/or to provide a methodology to address missing data. These findings suggested the need to improve systematic reporting of QOL data.

A systematic review of QOL reporting in NSCLC RCTs from 2002 to 2010 (53 RCTs) found that in 81% there were no significant differences in overall survival. However, 50% of RCTs without differences in overall survival reported a significant difference in QOL scores. This systematic review found that the quality of QOL reporting had improved with regard to reporting clinically significant differences and statistical methods. The EORTC instrument was used in 57% of the studies. Weaknesses in reporting included lack of hypotheses and rationales for choosing QOL instruments. This study demonstrated the importance of including QOL in randomized trials, especially in those where no overall survival differences were found, although the methodology and hypotheses for including QOL required standardization (103).

In a study of 557 RCTs with PRO evaluation, enrolling 254,677 patients overall, PROs were predominantly used in RCT for breast (n = 123), lung (n = 85), and colorectal cancers (n = 66). PROs were the secondary endpoints in 421 RCTs (76%). Four of six CONSORT-PRO items were evaluated in less than 50% of RCTs. The level of reporting was higher in RCTs when PROs were the primary endpoint, and with the use of supplementary reporting (104).

In a study of 325 randomized clinical trials, Bylicki et al. found poor compliance in reporting PROs according to the CONSORT guidelines. Sixty-two percent (201 of 325) of trials did not report on PROs at all (105). Items on the CONSORT checklist that were not reported included: not prespecifying a PRO hypothesis (26%); missing methodology of data collection (16%); and a lack of description of statistical approaches for managing missing data (37%). An improvement in reporting of PROs was found in dedicated secondary manuscripts, which reported solely on PROs in 29% of RCTs (36 of 124) (105).

Ongoing efforts in standardization of QOL reporting include an initiative led by the EORTC group called **Setting International Standards in Analyzing Patient-Reported Outcomes and Quality of Life Endpoints Data (SISAQOL)** (9). This group acknowledges past efforts to standardize the reporting and inclusion of PROs/QOL in clinical trials from different regulatory bodies such as the FDA, European Medicines Agency, academic societies such as the International Society for Quality of Life Research, and the International Society for Pharmacoeconomics and

Outcomes Research. The SISAQOL group aims to identify relevant guidelines and methodology for outcomes research, perform systematic reviews of the data, and interpret this information to develop an international consensus on standardization of statistical methods, analysis and interpretation of QOL data in cancer clinical trials.

IMPORTANCE OF QOL/PRO DATA

QOL AS A PROGNOSTIC FACTOR

QOL has been demonstrated to be an important prognostic factor for survival across multiple cancer sites; see Figure 23.3 (47,83,106,107). In a meta-analysis of individual QOL data for 11 different cancer types across 30 EORTC RCTs conducted between 1986 and 2004, the QOL parameters of physical functioning and pain and appetite loss, in addition to the sociodemographic and clinical factors of age, sex, and distant metastases, were all predictive for overall survival, whereas WHO performance status was not (83). Consideration of the three QOL parameters, as

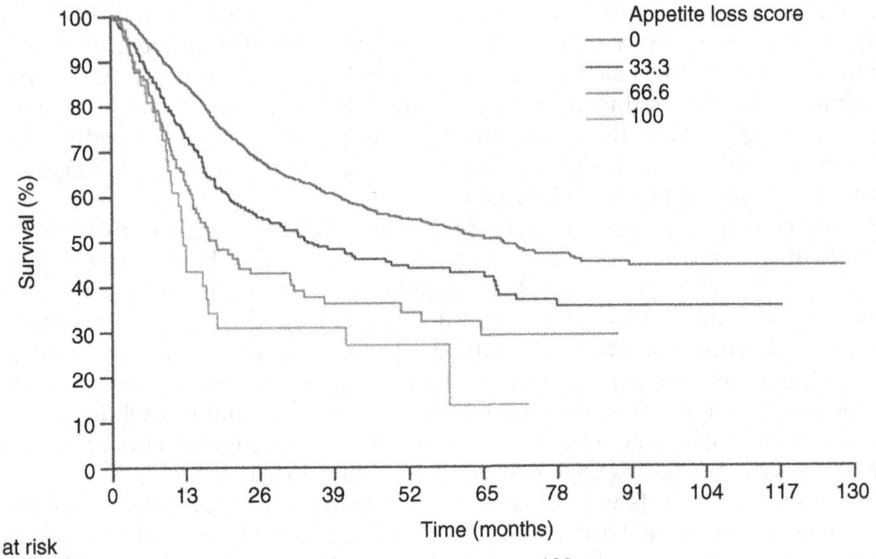

Number at risk

0	1314	984	686	486	310	195	128	46	9	1
33.3	348	205	132	90	60	42	27	12	4	1
66.6	133	65	37	22	17	10	6	0	0	0
100	63	17	9	8	5	1	0	0	0	0

Appetite loss score	Median survival (months; 95% CI)	1-year survival (%; 95% CI)
0	68.86 (58.38–81.12)	86.11 (83.88–87.80)
33.3	35.35 (26.68–59.37)	76.50 (71.38–80.82)
66.6	17.28 (14.39–31.47)	66.19 (56.81–74.00)
100	12.65 (10.64–18.69)	57.94 (42.57–70.63)

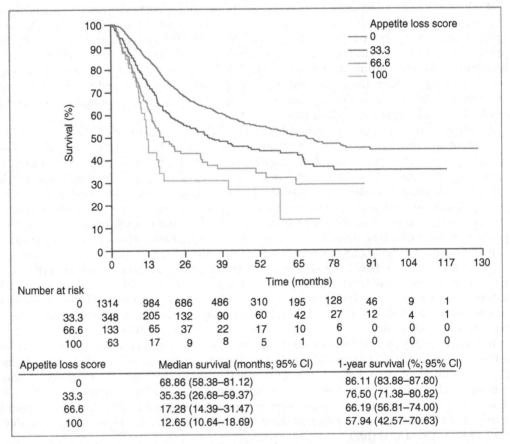

FIGURE 23.3 Overall survival curves stratified by EORTC QLQ-C30 appetite loss score in a study evaluating baseline QOL as a prognostic indicator of survival.

CI, confidence interval; QLQ-C30, Quality-of-Life Core Questionnaire.

Source: Quinten C, Coens C, Mauer M, et al. Baseline quality of life as a prognostic indicator of survival: a meta-analysis of individual patient data from EORTC clinical trials. *Lancet Oncol.* 2009;10(9):865-871. doi:10.1016/S1470-2045(09)70200-12009

well as sociodemographic and clinical data, increased the predictive accuracy for overall survival by 6%, relative to sociodemographic and clinical characteristics alone, in this large dataset of 10,108 patients.

The importance of baseline QOL has also been demonstrated in multiple head and neck cancer randomized trials, where differences in baseline QOL profiles were observed between human papillomavirus (HPV)-positive versus HPV-negative head and neck cancer patients (108–110). HPV-positive patients, who have higher survival compared to HPV-negative patients, had better baseline QOL scores, but greater deterioration in QOL during chemoradiotherapy treatment. These findings suggest that efforts to find less toxic treatment approaches in this population, while maintaining high survival outcomes, are warranted to reduce QOL deterioration, particularly as it relates to treatment-related swallowing pain. Integration of swallowing-related QOL measures are currently being investigated in ongoing head and neck cancer trials to test if therapeutic de-escalation approaches can maintain high survival outcomes but with less swallowing-related QOL deterioration (81,111).

A change in QOL scores also has prognostic significance for survival (106). In a study of 391 advanced NSCLC patients enrolled in the EORTC 08975 study, comparing palliative chemotherapy regimens, QOL was assessed at baseline and after each chemotherapy cycle using the EORTC QLQ-C30 and the lung module QLQ-LC13. For every 10-point increase in baseline pain and dysphagia, there was an associated 11% and 12% increased risk of death, with hazard ratios (HRs) of 1.11 and 1.12, respectively. Every 10-point improvement in physical function (HR = 0.93) and social function (HR = 0.91) at chemotherapy cycle 2 from baseline was associated with 7% and 9% lower risk of death, respectively (106).

QOL INFORMING CLINICAL PRACTICE

Finally, how QOL information from clinical trials is integrated into clinical practice was evaluated in a cross-sectional survey of oncologists from Canada, the United Kingdom, and the Australian clinical trials network (112). This study found that of 396 oncologists (30% response rate), 73% found trial QOL data to be valuable, but only 45% used the data to inform clinical practice and guide decision making, due to the perceived barriers of lack of time, lack of understanding, and lack of generalizability of the results. Most respondents preferred the QOL data to be reported simultaneously in the same journal with the main trial results, and 39% of respondents felt confident in interpreting clinically meaningful change of QOL data. To improve integration of important QOL data into clinical decision making and routine practice, strategies are warranted to enhance dissemination, and to promote the interpretability and clinical relevance of the data combined with other outcomes.

CONCLUSION

In summary, QOL is a complex multidimensional concept with many applications in clinical trials and patient care. Interpretation of QOL and QOL data is challenging due to the inherent subjectivity of measurements, variability across different populations, and complex statistical methodology for handling QOL data. However, several tools have been developed and validated specifically for cancer patients across international patient populations. Incorporating QOL/PROs into clinical trials requires careful planning, which includes thoughtful hypothesis testing, appropriate selection of the PRO instrument(s) to address the study question, and statistical considerations to address meaningful differences in QOL and handling of missing data. International ongoing efforts to standardize reporting of QOL data from clinical trials are in progress.

The hallmark of PROs is that they provide a direct perspective from the patient without interference from the provider. Most QOL data are ideally collected in the form of PROs. Patient preferences and utilities are special QOL measures that allow integrated and quantitative assessment of trade-offs between quality and quantity of life. With evolving electronic platforms, we are likely to see PROs increasingly integrated into electronic heath record systems. This may be a methodology to improve PRO compliance in trials, by means of enhanced ease of data collection and analysis. QOL outcomes can inform both patient care and treatment recommendations, and support labeling claims for new therapies. Moreover, as we enter into an era of evaluating the value of healthcare to the patient and society, PROs and QOL are being used as important measures of value-based health-care delivery. By quantitatively comparing trade-offs between treatment strategies, these measures give critical insight into resource allocation and patient preferences for different health states.

GLOSSARY

health: according to the World Health Organization, "a state of complete physical, mental and social well-being, and not merely the absence of disease and infirmity."

quality of life (QOL): according to the World Health Organization, "individuals' perception of their position in life in the context of culture and value systems in which they live, and in relation to their goals, expectations, standards, and concerns."

health-related quality of life (HR-QOL): a complex multidimensional concept that describes an individual's perception of the effects of disease and treatment, and its impact on his or her physical functioning, psychological and social well-being, personal beliefs, level of independence, and relationship to the environment.

response shift bias: subjective changes in patients' perceptions; also occurs when patients ignore or under-report symptoms or problems they believe are unrelated to their illness (selective reporting).

patient-reported outcome (PRO): any clinical outcome reported directly by the patient.

proxy-reported outcome instruments: instruments that elicit reports from caregivers or clinicians rather than outcomes reported directly by the patient.

symptom burden: measures the symptom severity and the patient's perception of the impact of the symptoms reported.

toxicity: signs or symptoms related to treatment; a subset of morbidity.

adverse events (AEs): detrimental effects or occurrences in clinical trials.

quality-adjusted life years (QALYs): a metric that can help evaluate the trade-offs between quantity of life and quality of life (or evaluate costs of care, or cost-effectiveness analysis).

reliability: the degree to which an instrument is reproducible, stable, and free from measurement error.

internal consistency reliability: the degree to which the items in a multi-item instrument are inter-related.

test–retest reliability: the ability of the instrument to be reproducible and provide consistency of scores over time in a stable population.

validity: the degree to which an instrument measures the concept it is intended to measure.

content validity: the extent to which an instrument contains the most relevant and important aspects of a dimension of interest.

construct validity: the extent to which an instrument measures the concept that it is designed to measure in relation to other measures.

criterion validity: the degree to which scores of an instrument relate to a gold standard.

European Organisation for Research and Treatment of Cancer (EORTC): a multidisciplinary, non-for-profit organization located in Europe dedicated to clinical cancer research to improve treatment, survival, and quality of life for cancer patients.

reliability: the extent to which an instrument yields identical scores in stable subjects over time.

sensitivity (longitudinal validity): in PROs, the ability to demonstrate changes when a patient's health state improves or deteriorates over time, or to detect treatment effects.

longitudinal validity: See *sensitivity*.

minimum important difference (MID): the smallest difference in score in the domain of interest that patients perceive as important, either beneficial or harmful, and which would lead the clinician to consider a change in the patient's management.

anchor-based method: means of estimating minimum important difference that requires an independent standard (*anchor*).

distribution-based method: means of estimating minimum important difference in which an effect is expressed using statistical methods.

Functional Assessment of Cancer Therapy (FACT) instruments: a series of patient-reported outcome measures used to assess QOL in patients with cancer. Individual instruments include the FACT-G (General) and several disease-site specific instruments, such as the FACT-H&N (Head and Neck) and FACT-L (Lung).

Time trade-off (TTO) utility measure: a utility measure derived from TTO discrete choice experiments.

clinically important difference: See *minimum important difference.*

visual analogue scale (VAS): a means of gathering patient-reported outcomes that uses a line of fixed length with words anchoring the scale at each end.

Likert scale: a means of gathering patient-reported outcomes; uses a set of discrete terms or statements from which patients are asked to choose the response that best describes their state or experience.

MD Anderson Symptom Inventory (MDASI): a patient-reported outcome measure used to assess symptom burden from surgery, radiation, and chemotherapy.

EuroQol (EQ-5D): a self-reported multiattribute instrument with five dimensions that can be used to assess a patient's current health status; it can also be used to indirectly measure the utility of the patient's current health state.

functional scale: PRO measure on which a high score represents a higher level of functioning (health).

symptom scale: PRO measure on which a high score represents a high level of symptomatology (problems).

FACT-Trial Outcome Index (TOI): an efficient summary index of physical and functional patient-related outcomes.

Common Terminology Criteria for Adverse Events (NCI-CTCAE): a reporting system routinely used by physicians and in clinical trials to measure toxicity or adverse medical events. There is now also a patient-reported version called the PRO-CTCAE.

National Cancer Institute of Canada-Common Toxicity Criteria (NCIC-CTC): a reporting system used by physicians and in clinical trials to measure toxicity or adverse medical events.

RTOG Grading System: a reporting system used by physicians and in clinical trials to measure toxicity or adverse medical events.

Late Effects Normal Tissue/Subjective, Objective, Management, and Analytic (LENT/SOMA): a reporting system used by physicians and in clinical trials to measure toxicity or adverse medical events.

Patient-Reported Outcomes Measurement Information System (PROMIS): a program started in 2004 within the National Institutes of Health Common Fund to develop item banks for measuring major self-reported health domains affected by chronic illness.

patient preference measurement: a special subtype of quality of life measurement that elicits patient preference for one treatment or health state over another.

utilities: a quantification of patient preference, particularly when preferences are assessed under conditions of uncertainty.

TTO discrete choice experiments: a method for eliciting patient preferences that compares QOL to length of survival.

standard gamble method: a method of utility measurement that involves decisions in the face of uncertainty; the method most grounded in econometric utility theory.

EORTC-8D: a multiattribute health-status measure specific to cancer patients; derived from the EORTC QLQ-C30 questionnaire.

EORTC QLQ-C30: a 30-item, self-reporting questionnaire used to assess overall QOL in patients with cancer.

Quality of Life Utility Measure-Core 10 dimensions (QLU-C10D): a multiattribute health-status measure specific to cancer patients; derived from the EORTC QLQ-C30 questionnaire.

comparative effectiveness research: an umbrella term for research that identifies what medical interventions best improve health.

decision analysis: the scientific discipline devoted to the theory, methodology, and practice of addressing decisions in a formal way; usually involves using modeling to mathematically (and sometimes visually) capture structural complexity in order to analyze a particular decision.

quality adjusted time without symptoms or toxicity (Q-TWiST) method: a way to analyze utility and survival data by group, rather than by individual.

time-based QOL evaluations: evaluations in which the measurements are dictated at regular intervals relative to the baseline or randomization date.

event-based [QOL] evaluations: evaluations that are timed to a specific treatment and may be different between treatment arms, according to the timing of treatment delivery in each trial arm.

missing data: values that are not available and that would be meaningful for analysis if they were observed.

compliance: the number of completed questionnaires received as a proportion of the number expected, given the study design and number of patients who are alive and enrolled in the study.

item nonresponse: situation when data are missing from a questionnaire or dataset, such as where a response has not been provided for a question.

unit nonresponse: situation when an entire questionnaire or dataset is missing.

missing completely at random (MCAR): one of three mechanisms of missing data; indicates that the probability of missing is independent of all past, present, and future assessments and assumes that the patients with missing data are a random sample of the whole patient cohort.

missing at random (MAR): one of three mechanisms of missing data; indicates that the probability of missing data depends on observed data, but not current or future assessment scores.

missing not at random (MNAR): one of three mechanisms of missing data; indicates that the probability of missing data depends on current and future unobserved scores.

Little's test: assumes that the means of the observed data should be the same regardless of the pattern of missingness if the data are missing completely at random (MCAR).

Listin–Schlittgen test: used to determine if dropouts (missing data) are missing at random (MAR).

Ridout's logistic regression method: a test for random dropouts (missing data) in repeated measurement data.

Fairclough's logistic regression method: identifies variables within the dataset that are associated with missingness, using logistic regression models created from the significant candidate variables, using a stepwise procedure.

complete-case analysis: analysis method that excludes patients who have incomplete data.

Consolidated Standards of Reporting Trials (CONSORT): a quality checklist of 22 items essential for the conduct and reporting of RCTs.

Setting International Standards in Analyzing Patient-Reported Outcomes and Quality of Life Endpoints Data (SISAQOL): a group that aims to identify relevant guidelines and methodology for outcomes research, perform systematic reviews of the data, and interpret this information to develop an international consensus on standardization of statistical methods, analysis, and interpretation of QOL data in cancer clinical trials.

REFERENCES

1. Hubanks L, Kuyken W, World Health Organization. *Quality of Life Assessment: An Annotated Bibliography*. Geneva, Switzerland: World Health Organization; 1994.
2. International Society for Quality of Life Research. What is health-related quality of life research? http://www.isoqol.org/about-isoqol/what-is-health-related-quality-of-life-research. 2017.
3. Wilson IB, Cleary PD. Linking clinical variables with health-related quality of life. A conceptual model of patient outcomes. *JAMA*. 1995;273(1):59–65. doi:10.1001/jama.1995.03520250075037
4. Schwartz CE, Sprangers MA. Methodological approaches for assessing response shift in longitudinal health-related quality-of-life research. *Soc Sci Med*. 1999;48(11):1531–1548. doi:10.1016/S0277-9536(99)00047-7
5. Sprangers MA, Schwartz CE. Integrating response shift into health-related quality of life research: a theoretical model. *Soc Sci Med*. 1999;48(11):1507–1515. doi:10.1016/s0277-9536(99)00045-3
6. Fayers PM, Machin D. *Quality of Life: The Assessment, Analysis, and Interpretation of Patient Reported Outcomes*. 2nd ed. Hoboken, NJ: Wiley; 2007.
7. Wu AW, Jensen RE, Salzberg C, Snyder C. Advances in the use of patient reported outcome measures in electronic health records. Baltimore, MD: Center for Health Services and Outcomes Research, Johns Hopkins Bloomberg School of Public Health. http://www.pcori.org/assets/2013/11/PCORI-PRO-Workshop-EHR-Landscape-Review-111913.pdf. 2013.
8. Calvert M, Blazeby J, Altman DG, et al. Reporting of patient-reported outcomes in randomized trials: the CONSORT PRO extension. *JAMA*. 2013;309(8):814–822. doi:10.1001/jama.2013.879

9. Bottomley A, Pe M, Sloan J, et al. Analysing data from patient-reported outcome and quality of life endpoints for cancer clinical trials: a start in setting international standards. *Lancet Oncol.* 2016;17(11):e510–e514. doi:10.1016/s1470-2045(16)30510-1
10. Rosenthal DI, Mendoza TR, Chambers MS, et al. Measuring head and neck cancer symptom burden: the development and validation of the M.D. Anderson symptom inventory, head and neck module. *Head & Neck.* 2007;29(10):923–931. doi:10.1002/hed.20602
11. Ringash J, Bernstein LJ, Cella D, et al. Outcomes toolbox for head and neck cancer research. *Head & Neck.* 2015;37(3):425–439. doi:10.1002/hed.23561
12. Basch E, Reeve BB, Mitchell SA, et al. Development of the National Cancer Institute's patient-reported outcomes version of the common terminology criteria for adverse events (PRO-CTCAE). *J Natl Cancer Inst.* 2014;106(9). doi:10.1093/jnci/dju244
13. Fleissig A, Jenkins V, Catt S, Fallowfield L. Multidisciplinary teams in cancer care: are they effective in the UK? *Lancet Oncol.* 2006;7(11):935–943. doi:10.1016/S1470-2045(06)70940-8
14. Shah BA, Qureshi MM, Jalisi S, et al. Analysis of decision making at a multidisciplinary head and neck tumor board incorporating evidence-based National Cancer Comprehensive Network (NCCN) guidelines. *Pract Radiat Oncol.* 2016;6(4):248–254. doi:10.1016/j.prro.2015.11.006
15. Fairclough DL. *Design and Analysis of Quality of Life Studies in Clinical Trials.* 2nd ed. Boca Raton, FL: Taylor and Francis Group; 2010.
16. Mandelblatt JS, Eisenberg JM. Historical and methodological perspectives on cancer outcomes research. *Oncology.* 1995;9(11 Suppl):23–32.
17. Walters SJ. *Quality of Life Outcomes in Clinical Trials and Health-Care Evaluation.* 1st ed. Hoboken, NJ: John Wiley & Sons; 2009.
18. Tarver, M. Development of validated instruments. https://www.fda.gov/downloads/MedicalDevices/NewsEvents/WorkshopsConferences/UCM391583.pdf. 2014.
19. U.S. Department of Health and Human Services, U.S. Food and Drug Administration. *Guidance for Industry: Patient-Reported Outcome Measures: Use in Medical Product Development to Support Labeling Claims.* http://www.fda.gov/downloads/Drugs/GuidanceComplianceRegulatoryInformation/Guidances/UCM193282.pdf. 2009.
20. European Organisation for Research and Treatment of Cancer. *Guidelines for Assessing Quality of Life in EORTC Clinical Trials.* http://groups.eortc.be/qol/sites/default/files/archives/clinical_trials__guidelines_qol.pdf. 2012.
21. Lindeboom R, Sprangers MA, Zwinderman AH. Responsiveness: a reinvention of the wheel? *Health Qual Life Outcomes.* 2005;3:8. doi:10.1186/1477-7525-3-8
22. Terwee CB, Dekker FW, Wiersinga WM, et al. On assessing responsiveness of health-related quality of life instruments: guidelines for instrument evaluation. *Qual Life Res.* 2003;12(4):349–362. doi:10.1023/A:1023499322593
23. Guyatt GH, Osoba D, Wu AW. Methods to explain the clinical significance of health status measures. *Mayo Clin Proc* 2002;77(4):371–383. doi:10.4065/77.4.371
24. King MT. A point of minimal important difference (MID): a critique of terminology and methods. *Expert Rev Pharmacoecon Outcomes Res.* 2011;11(2):171–184. doi:10.1586/erp.11.9
25. Schunemann HJ, Guyatt GH. Commentary–goodbye M(C)ID! Hello MID, where do you come from? *Health Serv Res.* 2005;40(2):593–597. doi:10.1111/j.1475-6773.2005.00374.x
26. Ringash J, O'Sullivan B, Bezjak A, Redelmeier DA. Interpreting clinically significant changes in patient-reported outcomes. *Cancer.* 2007;110(1):196–202. doi:10.1002/cncr.22799
27. Cella D, Hahn EA, Dineen K. Meaningful change in cancer-specific quality of life scores: differences between improvement and worsening. *Qual Life Res.* 2002;11(3):207–221. doi:10.1023/A:1015276414526
28. Maringwa JT, Quinten C, King M, et al. Minimal important differences for interpreting health-related quality of life scores from the EORTC QLQ-C30 in lung cancer patients participating in randomized controlled trials. *Support Care Cancer.* 2011;19(11):1753–1760. doi:10.1007/s00520-010-1016-5
29. Guillemin F, Bombardier C, Beaton D. Cross-cultural adaptation of health-related quality of life measures: literature review and proposed guidelines. *J Clin Epidemiol.* 1993;46(12):1417–1432. doi:10.1016/0895-4356(93)90142-n
30. Aaronson NK, Ahmedzai S, Bergman B, et al. The European Organization for Research and Treatment of Cancer QLQ-C30: a quality-of-life instrument for use in international clinical trials in oncology. *J Natl Cancer Inst.* 1993;85(5):365–376. doi:10.1093/jnci/85.5.365
31. Cella DF, Tulsky DS, Gray G, et al. The Functional Assessment of Cancer Therapy scale: development and validation of the general measure. *J Clin Oncol.* 1993;11(3):570–579. doi:10.1200/jco.1993.11.3.570
32. D'Antonio LL, Zimmerman GJ, Cella DF, Long SA. Quality of life and functional status measures in patients with head and neck cancer. *Arch Otolaryngol Head Neck Surg.* 1996;122(5):482–487. doi:10.1001/archotol.1996.01890170018005
33. Cleeland CS, Mendoza TR, Wang XS, et al. Assessing symptom distress in cancer patients: the M.D. Anderson Symptom Inventory. *Cancer.* 2000;89(7):1634–1646. doi:10.1002/1097-0142(20001001)89:7<1634::AID-CNCR29>3.0.CO;2-V
34. EuroQol EQ-5D instrument. http://www.euroqol.org. 2017.
35. Devlin NJ, Brooks R. EQ-5D and the EuroQol Group: past, present and future. *Appl Health Econ Health Policy.* 2017;15(2):127–137. doi:10.1007/s40258-017-0310-5
36. EORTC-QLQ questionnaire. http://groups.eortc.be/qol/eortc-qlq-c30. 2017.
37. Dueck AC, Mendoza TR, Mitchell SA, et al. Validity and reliability of the US National Cancer Institute's patient-reported outcomes version of the Common Terminology Criteria for Adverse Events (PRO-CTCAE). *JAMA Oncol.* 2015;1(8):1051–1059. doi:10.1001/jamaoncol.2015.2639
38. HealthMeasures. Intro to PROMIS®. http://www.healthmeasures.net/explore-measurement-systems/promis/intro-to-promis. 2017.
39. European Organisation for Research and Treatment of Cancer. http://www.eortc.org. 2017.

40. Sherman AC, Simonton S, Adams DC, et al. Assessing quality of life in patients with head and neck cancer: cross-validation of the European Organization for Research and Treatment of Cancer (EORTC) Quality of Life Head and Neck module (QLQ-H&N35). *Arch Otolaryngol Head Neck Surg.* 2000;126(4):459–467. doi:10.1001/archotol.126.4.459
41. Giesinger JM, Kieffer JM, Fayers PM, et al. Replication and validation of higher order models demonstrated that a summary score for the EORTC QLQ-C30 is robust. *J Clin Epidemiol.* 2016;69:79–88. doi:10.1016/j.jclinepi.2015.08.007
42. Movsas B, Hu C, Sloan J, et al. Quality of life analysis of a radiation dose-escalation study of patients with non-small-cell lung cancer: a secondary analysis of the Radiation Therapy Oncology Group 0617 randomized clinical trial. *JAMA Oncol.* 2016;2(3):359–367. doi:10.1001/jamaoncol.2015.3969
43. FACIT.org. Functional assessment of cancer therapy questionnaires. http://www.facit.org/FACITOrg/Questionnaires. 2017.
44. Kemmler G, Holzner B, Kopp M, et al. Comparison of two quality-of-life instruments for cancer patients: the Functional Assessment of Cancer Therapy-General and the European Organization for Research and Treatment of Cancer Quality of Life Questionnaire-C30. *J Clin Oncol.* 1999;17(9):2932–2940. doi:10.1200/JCO.1999.17.9.2932
45. Rosenthal DI, Mendoza TR, Chambers MS, et al. The M.D. Anderson Symptom Inventory-Head and Neck Module, a patient-reported outcome instrument, accurately predicts the severity of radiation-induced mucositis. *Int J Radiat Oncol Biol Phys.* 2008;72(5):1355–1361. doi:10.1016/j.ijrobp.2008.02.072
46. Denis F, Garaud P, Bardet E, et al. Late toxicity results of the GORTEC 94-01 randomized trial comparing radiotherapy with concomitant radiochemotherapy for advanced-stage oropharynx carcinoma: comparison of LENT/SOMA, RTOG/EORTC, and NCI-CTC scoring systems. *Int J Radiat Oncol Biol Phys.* 2003;55(1):93–98. doi:10.1016/S0360-3016(02)03819-1
47. Quinten C, Maringwa J, Gotay CC, et al. Patient self-reports of symptoms and clinician ratings as predictors of overall cancer survival. *J Natl Cancer Inst* 2011;103(24):1851–1858. doi:10.1093/jnci/djr485
48. Laugsand EA, Sprangers MA, Bjordal K, et al. Health care providers underestimate symptom intensities of cancer patients: a multicenter European study. *Health Qual Life Outcomes.* 2010;8:104. doi:10.1186/1477-7525-8-104
49. Basch E, Pugh SL, Dueck AC, et al. Feasibility of patient reporting of symptomatic adverse events via the Patient-Reported Outcomes version of the Common Terminology Criteria for Adverse Events (PRO-CTCAE) in a chemoradiotherapy cooperative group multicenter clinical trial. *Int J Radiat Oncol Biol Phys.* 2017;98(2):409–418. doi:10.1016/j.ijrobp.2017.02.002
50. Falchook AD, Green R, Knowles ME, et al. Comparison of patient- and practitioner-reported toxic effects associated with chemoradiotherapy for head and neck cancer. *JAMA Otolaryngol Head Neck Surg.* 2016;142(6):517–523. doi:10.1001/jamaoto.2016.0656
51. Torrance GW. Measurement of health state utilities for economic appraisal. *J Health Econ.* 1986;5(1):1–30. doi:10.1016/0167-6296(86)90020-2
52. Martin AJ, Glasziou PP, Simes RJ, Lumley T. A comparison of standard gamble, time trade-off, and adjusted time trade-off scores. *Int J Technol Assess Health Care.* 2000;16(1):137–147. doi:10.1017/s0266462300161124
53. McNeil BJ, Weichselbaum R, Pauker SG. Speech and survival: tradeoffs between quality and quantity of life in laryngeal cancer. *N Engl J Med.* 1981;305(17):982–987. doi:10.1056/NEJM198110223051704
54. Torrance GW, Feeny D. Utilities and quality-adjusted life years. *Int J Technol Assess Health.* 1989;5(4):559–575. doi:10.1017/S0266462300008461
55. Torrance GW, Thomas WH, Sackett DL. A utility maximization model for evaluation of health care programs. *Health Serv Res.* 1972;7(2):118–133.
56. Hunink MGM, Weinstein MC, Wittenberg E, et al. *Decision Making in Health and Medicine: Integrating Evidence and Values.* Cambridge, UK: Cambridge University Press; 2014.
57. Norman R, Viney R, Aaronson NK, et al. Using a discrete choice experiment to value the QLU-C10D: feasibility and sensitivity to presentation format. *Qual Life Res.* 2016;25(3):637–649. doi:10.1007/s11136-015-1115-3
58. Devlin NJ, Lorgelly PK. QALYs as a measure of value in cancer. *J Cancer Policy.* 2017;11:19–25. doi:10.1016/j.jcpo.2016.09.005
59. Noel CW, Lee DJ, Kong Q, et al. Comparison of health state utility measures in patients with head and neck cancer. *JAMA Otolaryngol Head Neck Surg.* 2015;141(8):696–703. doi:10.1001/jamaoto.2015.1314
60. Brooks R. EuroQol: the current state of play. *Health Policy.* 1996;37(1):53–72. doi:10.1016/0168-8510(96)00822-6
61. Agota, S, Mark O, Nancy D, eds. *EQ-5D Value Sets: Inventory, Comparative Review and User Guide.* New York, NY: Springer; 2007.
62. Herdman M, Gudex C, Lloyd A, et al. Development and preliminary testing of the new five-level version of EQ-5D (EQ-5D-5L). *Qual Life Res.* 2011;20(10):1727–1736. doi:10.1007/s11136-011-9903-x
63. Agency for Healthcare Research and Quality. U.S. Valuation of the EuroQol EQ-5 Health States. archive.ahrq.gov/professionals/clinicians-providers/resources/rice/EQ5Dproj.html. 2012.
64. Pickard AS, De Leon MC, Kohlmann T, et al. Psychometric comparison of the standard EQ-5D to a 5 level version in cancer patients. *Med Care.* 2007;45(3):259–263. doi:10.1097/01.mlr.0000254515.63841.81
65. Rowen D, Young T, Brazier J, Gaugris S. Comparison of generic, condition-specific, and mapped health state utility values for multiple myeloma cancer. *Value Health.* 2012;15(8):1059–1068. doi:10.1016/j.jval.2012.08.2201
66. Rowen D, Brazier J, Young T, et al. Deriving a preference-based measure for cancer using the EORTC QLQ-C30. *Value Health.* 2011;14(5):721–731. doi:10.1016/j.jval.2011.01.004
67. King MT, Costa DS, Aaronson NK, et al. QLU-C10D: a health state classification system for a multi-attribute utility measure based on the EORTC QLQ-C30. *Qual Life Res.* 2016;25(3):625–636. doi:10.1016/j.jval.2011.01.004
68. Lorgelly PK, Doble B, Rowen D, Brazier J. Condition-specific or generic preference-based measures in oncology? A comparison of the EORTC-8D and the EQ-5D-3L. *Qual Life Res.* 2017;26(5):1163–1176. doi:10.1007/s11136-016-1443-y
69. Glasziou PP, Simes RJ, Gelber RD. Quality adjusted survival analysis. *Stat Med.* 1990;9(11):1259–1276. doi:10.1002/sim.4780091106

70. O'Leary TJ, Slutsky JR, Bernard MA. Comparative effectiveness research priorities at federal agencies: the view from the Department of Veterans Affairs, National Institute on Aging, and Agency for Healthcare Research and Quality. *J Am Geriatr Soc.* 2010;58(6):1187–1192. doi:10.1111/j.1532-5415.2010.02939.x
71. Harvard T.H. Chan. "What Is CER?" Comparative Effectiveness Research Initiative, 2012:. what is CER? https://www.hsph.harvard.edu/comparative-effectiveness-research-initiative/definition. 2017.
72. Billingham LJ, Abrams KR. Simultaneous analysis of quality of life and survival data. *Stat Methods Med Res.* 2002;11(1):25–48. doi:10.1191/0962280202sm269ra
73. Gelber RD, Goldhirsch A. A new endpoint for the assessment of adjuvant therapy in postmenopausal women with operable breast cancer. *J Clin Oncol.* 1986;4(12):1772–1779. doi:10.1200/JCO.1986.4.12.1772
74. Goldhirsch A, Gelber RD, Simes RJ, et al. Costs and benefits of adjuvant therapy in breast cancer: a quality-adjusted survival analysis. *J Clin Oncol.* 1989;7(1):36–44. doi:10.1200/JCO.1989.7.1.36
75. Till JE, de Haes JC. Quality-adjusted survival analysis. *J Clin Oncol.* 1991;9(3):525–526. doi:10.1200/JCO.1991.9.3.525
76. Fairclough DL, Fetting JH, Cella D, et al. Quality of life and quality adjusted survival for breast cancer patients receiving adjuvant therapy. *Qual Life Res.* 1999;8(8):723–731. doi:10.1023/A:1008806828316
77. Porcher R, Levy V, Fermand JP, et al. Evaluating high dose therapy in multiple myeloma: use of quality-adjusted survival analysis. *Qual Life Res.* 2002;11(2):91–99. doi:10.1023/a:1015096313594
78. Marino P, Sfumato P, Joly F, et al. Q-TWiST analysis of patients with metastatic castrate naive prostate cancer treated by androgen deprivation therapy with or without docetaxel in the randomised phase III GETUG-AFU 15 trial. *Eur J Cancer.* 2017;84:27–33. doi:10.1016/j.ejca.2017.07.008
79. Marcus R, Aultman R, Jost F. A quality-adjusted survival analysis (Q-TWiST) of rituximab plus CVP vs CVP alone in first-line treatment of advanced follicular non-Hodgkin's lymphoma. *Br J Cancer.* 2010;102(1):19–22. doi:10.1038/sj.bjc.6605443
80. Radiation Therapy Oncology Group. RTOG 1216 Protocol Information. RTOG Clinical Trials Study Number 1216. https://www.rtog.org/ClinicalTrials/ProtocolTable/StudyDetails.aspx?study=1216. 2017.
81. Yom SS. NRG-HN002: A randomized phase II trial for patients with p16 positive, non-smoking associated, locoregionally advanced oropharyngeal cancer. https://www.nrgoncology.org/Clinical-Trials/Protocol-Table. 2017.
82. Osoba D. The Quality of Life Committee of the Clinical Trials Group of the National Cancer Institute of Canada: organization and functions. *Qual Life Res.* 1992;1(3):211–218. doi:10.1007/bf00635620
83. Quinten C, Coens C, Mauer M, et al. Baseline quality of life as a prognostic indicator of survival: a meta-analysis of individual patient data from EORTC clinical trials. *Lancet Oncol.* 2009;10(9):865–871. doi:10.1016/S1470-2045(09)70200-1
84. Julious SA, Campbell MJ, Walker SJ, et al. Sample sizes for cancer trials where health related quality of life is the primary outcome. *Br J Cancer.* 2000;83(7):959–963. doi:10.1054/bjoc.2000.1383
85. Matthews JN, Altman DG, Campbell MJ, Royston P. Analysis of serial measurements in medical research. *BMJ.* 1990;300(6719):230–235. doi:10.1136/bmj.300.6719.230
86. Mercieca-Bebber R, Palmer MJ, Brundage M, et al. Design, implementation and reporting strategies to reduce the instance and impact of missing patient-reported outcome (PRO) data: a systematic review. *BMJ Open.* 2016;6(6):e010938. doi:10.1136/bmjopen-2015-010938
87. Curran D, Bacchi M, Schmitz SF, et al. Identifying the types of missingness in quality of life data from clinical trials. *Stat Med.* 1998;17(5–7):739–756. doi:10.1002/(sici)1097-0258(19980315/15)17:5/7<739::aid-sim818>3.0.co;2-m
88. Curran D, Molenberghs G, Fayers PM, Machin D. Incomplete quality of life data in randomized trials: missing forms. *Stat Med.* 1998;17(5–7):697–709. doi:10.1002/(sici)1097-0258(19980315/15)17:5/7<697::aid-sim815>3.0.co;2-y
89. Kurland BF, Egleston BL. For health-related quality of life and other longitudinal data, analysis should distinguish between truncation by death and data missing because of nonresponse. *J Clin Oncol.* 2016;34(36):4449. doi:10.1200/JCO.2016.69.1220
90. Bernhard J, Cella DF, Coates AS, et al. Missing quality of life data in cancer clinical trials: serious problems and challenges. *Stat Med.* 1998;17(5–7):517–532. doi:10.1002/(sici)1097-0258(19980315/15)17:5/7<517::aid-sim799>3.0.co;2-s
91. Troxel AB, Fairclough DL, Curran D, Hahn EA. Statistical analysis of quality of life with missing data in cancer clinical trials. *Stat Med.* 1998;17(5–7):653–666. doi:10.1002/(sici)1097-0258(19980315/15)17:5/7<653::aid-sim812>3.0.co;2-m
92. Fairclough DL, Peterson HF, Chang V. Why are missing quality of life data a problem in clinical trials of cancer therapy? *Stat Med.* 1998;17(5–7):667–677. doi:10.1002/(sici)1097-0258(19980315/15)17:5/7<667::aid-sim813>3.3.co;2-y
93. Hahn EA, Webster KA, Cella D, Fairclough DL. Missing data in quality of life research in Eastern Cooperative Oncology Group (ECOG) clinical trials: problems and solutions. *Stat Med.* 1998;17(5–7):547–559. doi:10.1002/(sici)1097-0258(19980315/15)17:5/7<547::aid-sim802>3.3.co;2-6
94. Rubin DB. Inference and missing data. *Biometrika.* 1976;63(3):581–592. doi:10.1093/biomet/63.3.581
95. Fielding S, Fayers PM, Ramsay CR. Investigating the missing data mechanism in quality of life outcomes: a comparison of approaches. *Health Qual Life Outcomes.* 2009;7:57. doi:10.1186/1477-7525-7-57
96. Little RJ, Raghunathan T. On summary measures analysis of the linear mixed effects model for repeated measures when data are not missing completely at random. *Stat Med.* 1999;18(17–18):2465–2478. doi:10.1002/(sici)1097-0258(19990915/30)18:17/18<2465::aid-sim269>3.0.co;2-2
97. Fairclough DL, Peterson HF, Cella D, Bonomi P. Comparison of several model-based methods for analysing incomplete quality of life data in cancer clinical trials. *Stat Med.* 1998;17(5–7):781–796. doi:10.1002/(sici)1097-0258(19980315/15)17:5/7<781::aid-sim821>3.3.co;2-f
98. Movsas B, Hunt D, Watkins-Bruner D, et al. Can electronic web-based technology improve quality of life data collection? Analysis of Radiation Therapy Oncology Group 0828. *Pract Radiat Oncol.* 2014;4(3):187–191. doi:10.1016/j.prro.2013.07.014
99. Niska JR, Halyard MY, Tan AD, et al. Electronic patient-reported outcomes and toxicities during radiotherapy for head-and-neck cancer. *Qual Life Res.* 2017;26(7):1721–1731. doi:10.1007/s11136-017-1528-2

100. Staquet M, Berzon R, Osoba D, Machin D. Guidelines for reporting results of quality of life assessments in clinical trials. *Qual Life Res.* 1996;5(5):496–502. doi:10.1007/bf00540022
101. Brundage M, Bass B, Davidson J, et al. Patterns of reporting health-related quality of life outcomes in randomized clinical trials: implications for clinicians and quality of life researchers. *Qual Life Res.* 2011;20(5):653–664. doi:10.1007/s11136-010-9793-3
102. Moher D, Hopewell S, Schulz KF, et al. CONSORT 2010 explanation and elaboration: updated guidelines for reporting parallel group randomised trials. *BMJ.* 2010;340:c869. doi:10.1136/bmj.c869
103. Claassens L, van Meerbeeck J, Coens C, et al. Health-related quality of life in non-small-cell lung cancer: an update of a systematic review on methodologic issues in randomized controlled trials. *J Clin Oncol.* 2011;29(15):2104–2120. doi:10.1200/JCO.2010.32.3683
104. Efficace F, Fayers P, Pusic A, et al. Quality of patient-reported outcome reporting across cancer randomized controlled trials according to the CONSORT patient-reported outcome extension: a pooled analysis of 557 trials. *Cancer.* 2015;121(18):3335–3342. doi:10.1002/cncr.29489
105. Bylicki O, Gan HK, Joly F, et al. Poor patient-reported outcomes reporting according to CONSORT guidelines in randomized clinical trials evaluating systemic cancer therapy. *Ann Oncol.* 2015;26(1):231–237. doi:10.1093/annonc/mdu489
106. Ediebah DE, Coens C, Zikos E, et al. Does change in health-related quality of life score predict survival? Analysis of EORTC 08975 lung cancer trial. *Br J Cancer.* 2014;110(10):2427–2433. doi:10.1038/bjc.2014.208
107. Quinten C, Martinelli F, Coens C, et al. A global analysis of multitrial data investigating quality of life and symptoms as prognostic factors for survival in different tumor sites. *Cancer.* 2014;120(2):302–311. doi:10.1002/cncr.28382
108. Truong MT, Zhang Q, Rosenthal DI, et al. Quality of life and performance status from a substudy conducted within a prospective phase 3 randomized trial of concurrent accelerated radiation plus cisplatin with or without cetuximab for locally advanced head and neck carcinoma: NRG Oncology Radiation Therapy Oncology Group 0522. *Int J Radiat Oncol Biol Phys.* 2017;97(4):687–699. doi:10.1016/j.ijrobp.2016.08.003
109. Xiao C, Zhang Q, Nguyen-Tan PF, et al. Quality of life and performance status from a substudy conducted within a prospective phase 3 randomized trial of concurrent standard radiation versus accelerated radiation plus cisplatin for locally advanced head and neck carcinoma: NRG Oncology RTOG 0129. *Int J Radiat Oncol Biol Phys.* 2017;97(4):667–677. doi:10.1016/j.ijrobp.2016.07.020
110. Ringash J, Fisher R, Peters L, et al. Effect of p16 status on the quality-of-life experience during chemoradiation for locally advanced oropharyngeal cancer: a substudy of randomized trial Trans-Tasman Radiation Oncology Group (TROG) 02.02 (HeadSTART). *Int J Radiat Oncol Biol Phys.* 2017;97(4):678–686. doi:10.1016/j.ijrobp.2016.03.017
111. Ferris R. Eastern Cooperative Oncology Group (ECOG) 3311: Transoral surgery followed by low-dose or standard-dose radiation therapy with or without chemotherapy in treating patients with HPV positive stage III-IVA oropharyngeal cancer. https://clinicaltrials.gov/ct2/show/NCT01898494. 2017.
112. Rouette J, Blazeby J, King M, et al. Integrating health-related quality of life findings from randomized clinical trials into practice: an international study of oncologists' perspectives. *Qual Life Res.* 2015;24(6):1317–1325. doi:10.1007/s11136-014-0871-9

24

Trials in Cancer Screening, Prevention, and Public Health

RISHI DEKA ■ LOREN K. MELL

SCREENING AND PUBLIC HEALTH

One of the major goals of public health is to protect and promote health. There are four types of prevention activities aimed to protect health: **primordial**, **primary**, **secondary**, and **tertiary**. Primordial prevention prevents future hazards to health; for example, reducing workplace hazards like asbestos exposure reduces the incidence of mesothelioma. Primary prevention exerts its effects through cellular-level change; for example, vaccination for human papillomavirus (HPV) can prevent genitourinary and oropharyngeal cancers caused by the virus. Secondary prevention reduces the impact of cellular-level change; for example, surgical removal of premalignant skin conditions like melanoma in situ could prevent the later development of malignant melanoma. Finally, tertiary prevention aims to reduce the severity of disease after it has been diagnosed; for example, delivery of bisphosphonates can retard pathologic bone resorption, making bisphosphonates useful in the management of patients with osseous metastases (1).

The role of screening in prevention is to diagnose individuals at an earlier stage of disease than if they waited for symptoms to arise (Figure 24.1). Earlier diagnosis in principle should allow for more effective treatments than if treatment were initiated at clinical presentation. Primary prevention involves screening for risk factors, variables associated with an increased risk of a disease (e.g., Pap smear to detect premalignant cervical changes), whereas secondary prevention involves screening for disease itself. Examples of screening tests include questionnaires (e.g., depression and mental health inventories), physical examinations (e.g., self-breast exam), laboratory and blood tests (e.g., prostate-specific antigen [PSA]), or imaging (e.g., high-resolution chest CT for lung cancer).

Screening has both benefits and risks. In order to justify screening, the disease must be a significant public health problem in terms of frequency and severity. In addition, the **natural history** of a disease—the course of a disease from its inception to its resolution—should present a suitable time frame for screening. Furthermore, treatment should be more effective in the presymptomatic stage than in the symptomatic stage. Finally, a good screening test should be inexpensive, safe, acceptable to the public, and accurately discriminate between diseased and

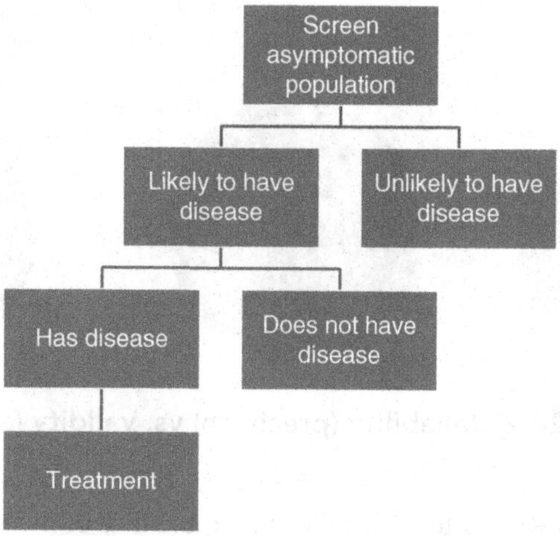

FIGURE 24.1 Screening process.

nondiseased individuals. Many examples of effective screening and public health interventions are discussed in this chapter. Risks and downsides of screening, however, may include a labeling effect on individuals accurately identified with disease, delayed intervention and a false sense of security for individuals who have the disease but who are not positively identified, costs for those who are accurately identified as not having the disease, and anxiety associated with confirmatory tests for individuals who do not have the disease but who are positively identified. In addition, several biases (discussed in the following section) can result from screening that can lead to inflated evaluations of the benefit of screening on overall public health. Nonetheless, the impact of screening tests for some of the most prevalent and virulent cancers has greatly reduced the global morbidity and mortality from cancer over the past century.

SENSITIVITY AND SPECIFICITY OF SCREENING TESTS

An effective screening test first must discern individuals with and without disease. This is measured through **reliability** and **validity** (Figure 24.2). Reliability, or precision, concerns the ability of a screening test to give consistent results in repeated applications. Validity, or accuracy, concerns the ability of a test to measure what it purports to measure. The validity of a screening test encompasses several properties, including its **sensitivity, specificity, positive predictive value** (**PPV**), and **negative predictive value** (**NPV**); see Table 24.1. Sensitivity refers to the percentage of those with disease who will have a positive test result, that is

$$\text{Sensitivity} = \frac{\text{True positives}}{\text{All diseased}} = \frac{A}{(A+C)}.$$

In contrast, specificity refers to the percentage of those without disease who will have a negative test result:

$$\text{Specificity} = \frac{\text{True negatives}}{\text{All nondiseased}} = \frac{D}{(B+D)}.$$

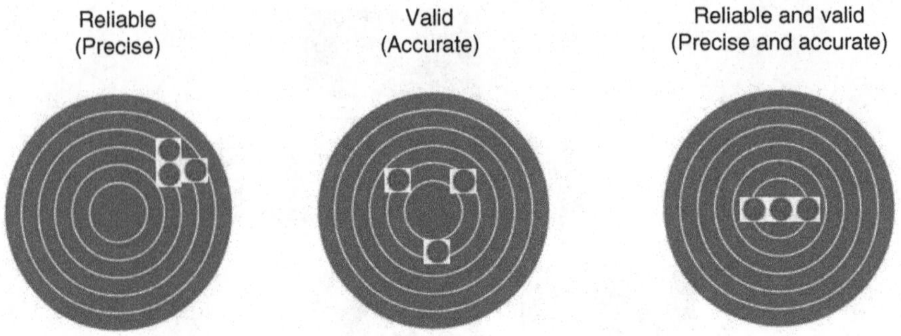

FIGURE 24.2 Reliability (precision) vs. validity (accuracy).

The **false positive rate (FPR)** of a test refers to the probability of incorrectly identifying a tested individual as having the disease:

$$\text{FPR} = \frac{\text{False positives}}{\text{All negatives}} = \frac{B}{(B+D)}.$$

Similarly, the **false negative rate (FNR)** of a test refers to the probability of incorrectly identifying a tested individual as not having the disease:

$$\text{FNR} = \frac{\text{False negatives}}{\text{All positives}} = \frac{C}{(A+C)}.$$

The relationships between the sensitivity and FNR and the specificity and FPR are the following:

$$\text{Sensitivity} + \text{FNR} = 100\%$$

$$\text{Specificity} + \text{FPR} = 100\%.$$

The **PPV** is defined as the percentage of individuals with a positive screening test who truly have the disease:

$$\text{PPV} = \frac{\text{True positives}}{\text{All positives}} = \frac{A}{(A+B)}.$$

The **NPV** is defined as the percentage of individuals with a negative screening test who are truly disease free:

$$\text{NPV} = \frac{\text{True negatives}}{\text{All negatives}} = \frac{D}{(C+D)}.$$

TABLE 24.1 TEST CHARACTERISTICS: SENSITIVITY AND SPECIFICITY

	Disease Present (Gold Standard Positive)	Disease Absent (Gold Standard Negative)
Screening test positive	A True positives	B False positives
Screening test negative	C False negatives	D True negatives

TABLE 24.2 EXAMPLE CA-125 TEST FOR OVARIAN CANCER		
	Ovarian Cancer Present (By Biopsy)	Ovarian Cancer Absent (By Biopsy)
CA-125 positive	60	11
CA-125 negative	26	200

For example, let us compare a blood screening test (CA-125) versus biopsy for ovarian cancer. Consider the counts given in Table 24.2. The sensitivity of the CA-125 test = 60/(60 + 26) = 60/86 = 69.7%. Thus, approximately 70% of those with ovarian cancer will have a positive CA-125 test. The specificity = 200/(200 + 11) = 200/211 = 94.7%. Thus, approximately 95% of those without ovarian cancer will have a negative CA-125 test. The PPV = 60/(60 + 11) = 60/71 = 84.5%, so approximately 85% of those with a positive CA-125 test have ovarian cancer. The NPV = 200/(200 + 26) = 200/226 = 88.5%, so approximately 89% of those with a negative CA-125 test do not have ovarian cancer.

The **likelihood ratio** (**LR**) is a critical property of a screening test that incorporates both its sensitivity and specificity. It provides a direct estimate of how much a test result will change the odds of having disease. The **positive LR** (**LR**$^+$) indicates the extent to which the odds of having the disease increase when a test is positive:

$$LR^{+} = \frac{\text{Sensitivity}}{1-\text{specificity}} = \frac{\text{Sensitivity}}{\text{FPR}} = \frac{A/(A+C)}{B/(B+D)}.$$

A **negative LR** (**LR**$^-$) indicates the extent to which the odds of having the disease decrease when a test is negative:

$$LR^{-} = \frac{1-\text{sensitivity}}{\text{Specificity}} = \frac{\text{FNR}}{\text{Specificity}} = \frac{C/(A+C)}{D/(B+D)}.$$

These relationships can be plotted with receiver operating characteristic (ROC) curves, as discussed in Chapters 8, 11, and 25.

Recall that ***odds*** is defined as the ratio of a probability (p) to its complement (Chapters 11 and 13). If p represents the probability of disease being present, the odds of the disease being present given by

$$\text{Odds} = \frac{p}{1-p} = \frac{A+C}{B+D}$$

and

$$p = \frac{\text{Odds}}{1+\text{odds}} = \frac{(A+C)/(B+D)}{(A+B+C+D)/(B+D)} = \frac{(A+C)}{(A+B+C+D)}.$$

Then it follows that

$$\text{Odds} * LR^{+} = \frac{A+C}{B+D} * \frac{\frac{A}{A+C}}{\frac{B}{(B+D)}} = \frac{A}{B}$$

and

$$\text{Odds} * LR^- = \frac{A+C}{B+D} * \frac{\frac{C}{A+C}}{\frac{D}{(B+D)}} = \frac{C}{D}.$$

Note also that the **odds ratio (OR)** is defined as

$$OR = \frac{LR^+}{LR^-} = \frac{AD}{BC}.$$

A screening test with a high LR^+ will substantially increase the odds of actually having the disease whenever it is positive. However, note that the overall odds of having the disease also depend on the **pretest probability** of having the disease, which relates to its background prevalence. Thus, an individual with a low pretest probability (i.e., if the disease is rare, or the clinical suspicion of having the disease is low) may still have overall low odds of having the disease, even in the face of a positive result from a highly effective screening test. Similarly, a screening test with a high LR^- substantially reduces the odds of actually having the disease whenever it is negative, but the overall odds of having the disease for an individual with a high pretest probability may remain high even with a negative test result.

In the ovarian cancer example, the sensitivity was 0.697 and the specificity was 0.947. Then, $LR^+ = 0.697/(1 - 0.947) = 0.697/0.053 = 13.1$, and $LR^- = (1 - 0.697)/0.947 = 0.303/0.947 = 0.32$. Thus, a positive CA-125 test raises the odds of having ovarian cancer by a factor of 13.1, while a negative test lowers the odds of having ovarian cancer by a factor of 0.32. The reciprocal of LR^+ (13.1) is 0.076, while the reciprocal of LR^- (0.32) is only 3.1, indicating that a positive test is much more powerful at indicating the presence of ovarian cancer than a negative test is in indicating its absence.

Note that the **Bayes theorem** states that the **conditional probability** of an event (*E*) in the present of a condition (*C*) is expressed by the relationship:

$$P(E \mid C) * P(C) = P(C \mid E) * P(E).$$

In regard to screening tests, this can be applied to the sensitivity, specificity, PPV, and NPV in the following way. Consider an "event" as a test result and the "condition" as the presence or absence of the disease. Then

$$P(E^+ \mid C^+) = \text{Sensitivity}$$

$$P(C^+ \mid E^+) = \text{PPV}$$

$$P(C^+) = \frac{A+C}{A+B+C+D} = \frac{O_D}{1+O_D},$$

where E^+ indicates a positive test, C^+ indicates the presence of disease, and is the odds of the disease being present. Thus the overall probability of a positive test depends on its sensitivity, PPV, and the odds of having the disease:

$$P(E^+) = \frac{\text{Sensitivity}}{\text{PPV}} * \frac{O_D}{1+O_D}.$$

Analogously, the probability of a test being negative depends on its specificity, NPV, and the odds of having the disease:

$$P(E^-) = \frac{\text{Specificity}}{\text{NPV}} * \frac{1}{1+O_D},$$

where E^- indicates a negative test, C^- indicates the absence of disease, and is the odds of the disease being present.

BIAS IN SCREENING TESTS

The evaluation of a screening program must consider the potential effects of bias related to the selected outcome measures. **Lead time** is defined as the amount of time gained by earlier detection of a cancer by screening compared to later detection after the appearance of symptoms. **Lead time bias** (Figure 24.3) occurs when screening detects disease, but does not ultimately change its course (i.e., natural history). Lead time bias makes it appear that there was an increase in life expectancy after screening, even though this is not true—the disease was simply caught earlier.

Length time is defined as the period of time a patient who has the disease will be asymptomatic. **Length time bias** (Figure 24.4) occurs when screening preferentially picks up disease that is progressing more slowly (i.e., is more indolent). Individuals with indolent disease are more likely to have screen-detected cancers compared to individuals with more aggressive tumors. Length time bias occurs when it is concluded that individuals with screen-detected diseases have better survival rates, because patients with slowly progressing disease usually have better prognoses. The improved survival rates are not related to screening itself, but rather the indolent nature of the screen-detected illness.

Overdiagnosis bias (Figure 24.5) is caused by improvements in imaging/disease detection. It occurs when screening identifies an illness that would not have shown clinical symptoms. Overdiagnosis can inflate survival rates without any actual benefits of screening. A phenomenon related to overdiagnosis is known as the **Will Rogers effect** (2). Will Rogers (1879–1935) was a humorist, at the turn of the 20th century, who hailed from Oklahoma. He was famous for saying "I never met a man I didn't like." Perhaps he harbored a certain contempt for Californians, however, for he is also credited for saying that "when the Okies left Oklahoma and moved to California, they raised the average intelligence level in both states."

As this relates to screening and imaging tests, the Will Rogers effect indicates that when individuals are reclassified between categories (such as when a staging system changes), it is easy to falsely attribute differences in outcomes to improvements in therapy over time. Specifically, when patients are upstaged due to the acquisition of new information (such as an elevated blood test, or an imaging study showing distant metastases), the observed outcomes (e.g., survival) will appear to improve in both categories. This is because the individuals with the worst prognosis in the lower stage category (because of occult high-risk disease) have now been shifted into the

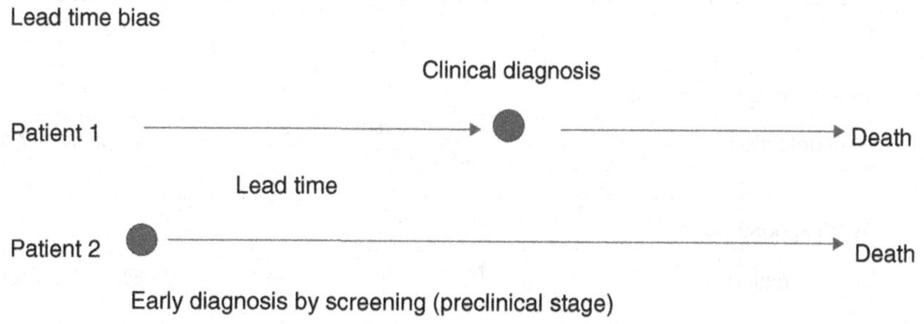

FIGURE 24.3 Lead time bias.

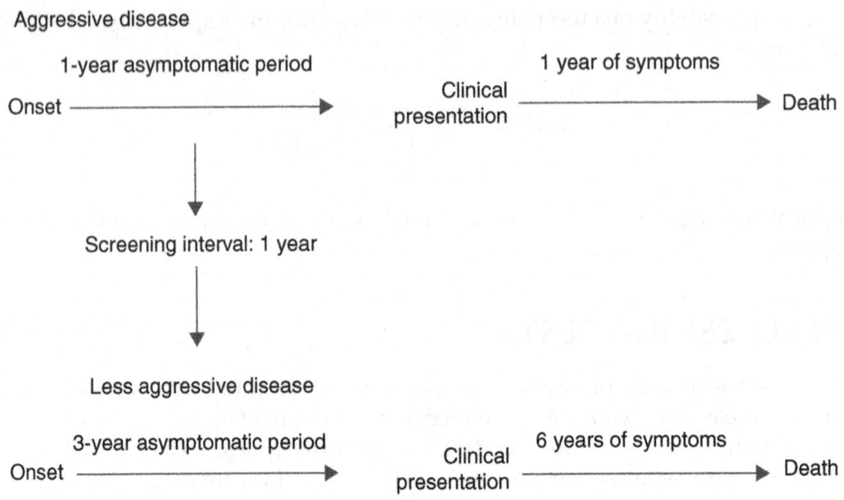

FIGURE 24.4 Length time bias.

higher risk category (where they comparatively fare better, due to their lower disease burden). The survival rates for both groups appear better, when all that has happened in reality is a change in the classification system. The tendency for new technologies to upstage patients over time is also known as **stage migration** (Figure 24.6).

Volunteer bias is a form of bias that occurs in observational studies of screening efficacy. The decision to be screened could be influenced by an individual's health awareness and related to his or her underlying morbidity. If healthy people are more likely to volunteer, then the benefits of a screening test will be overestimated; in contrast, if sicker people are more likely to volunteer, then the benefits of a screening test will be underestimated. Regardless, sampling characteristics can confound the interpretation of the benefits (or lack thereof) of a screening test in the population.

Several outcome measures may be used to evaluate the benefit of a screening program. Simply comparing the survival time for screen-detected cases to unscreened cases, however, may be complicated by lead time, length, or volunteer biases that inflate the perceived benefits of screening. The overall mortality rate (e.g., deaths per capita per year) is a more robust way to assess population trends, because this measure is not subject to these forms of bias; however, if the disease in question only accounts for a small proportion of deaths (such as prostate cancer), death from any cause may be an inadequate yardstick by which to measure the value of a cancer-specific intervention. Thus, disease-specific mortality is often considered the best outcome measure for evaluating the effectiveness of a screening test.

The role of screening in public health is to identify disease before it becomes symptomatic. Serious and prevalent diseases with severe consequences, notably prostate, breast, lung, cervical, and colorectal cancer, are commonly considered for screening. Many notable clinical trials

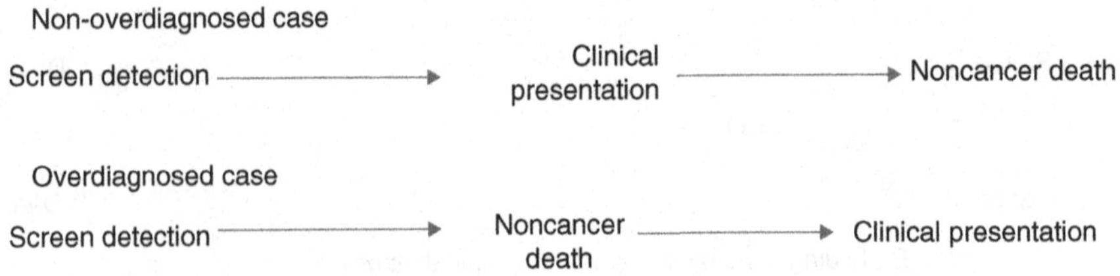

FIGURE 24.5 Overdiagnosis bias.

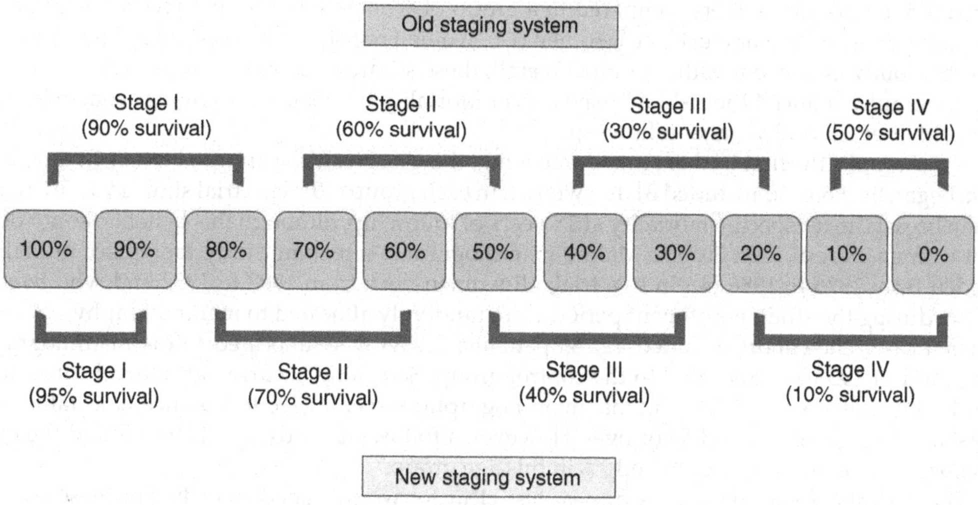

FIGURE 24.6 Stage migration. Survival differences according to stage differ depending on the classification system used, even though the survival for the group overall is unchanged.

in cancer screening and prevention are discussed in the following. Because of the significant potential for the aforementioned biases affecting clinical trials, randomized trials are considered essential for determining the benefit of screening/prevention programs and interventions on the public writ large. Because most study participants in such trials do not have the disease in question, these studies typically involve very large samples of individuals studied for long periods of time. Consequently, these studies tend to be quite expensive and are often undertaken by government agencies and large public health organizations with sufficient resources to carry out careful studies.

Identifying certain at-risk populations can help increase the specificity of the target population through **enrichment**, leading to more efficient and cost-effective trials with a higher likelihood of impact. In order to ensure generalizability of results, however, it is important to ensure access to wide, diverse, and unselected segments of the target population, which often involves taking active steps to engage the public through advertisements and campaigns to bolster participation. Moreover, attention to careful follow-up of participants is necessary to ensure adequate collection of long-term endpoints and that the propensity for follow-up is not biased by the intervention. Often, blinding study participants to the intervention assignment is infeasible or impractical, which can additionally expose the results to erroneous interpretation. Finally, **crossover contamination** is a principal concern in evaluating results of randomized trials, because often patients in the control arm may feel uncomfortable forgoing or accepting reduced cancer screening or prevention efforts, on the presupposition that such efforts are beneficial. This effect can lead to bias toward the null hypothesis of no benefit. Thus, careful attention to design details, including minimizing contamination, is essential when designing screening trials.

SCREENING TRIALS

BREAST CANCER SCREENING

Several randomized controlled trials have investigated the efficacy of mammography on breast cancer mortality (3–10). These studies have taken place in Europe, Canada, and the United States and have followed nearly 500,000 women for up to 18 years, in which a group of women who received mammography were compared to a group of women who did not receive mammography. Individual women or clusters of women (i.e., women registered in a certain medical practice) were randomly assigned to either group. Overall, these studies indicated that the use of screening mammography reduced the risk of breast cancer mortality by about 30% among women 50 to 69 years old after 10 to 12 years of follow-up.

For example, the first trial of annual screening, the U.S. Health Insurance Plan of Greater New York, began in 1963 and included 31,100 women in each group (10). This trial showed a 25% reduction in breast cancer specific mortality at 18 years of follow-up, although this benefit did not occur until women were at least 50. The Malmo mammographic screening study took place in Malmo, Sweden from 1976 to 1986 (4). In this trial, all women born from 1908 to 1932 and who lived in Malmo during the study enrollment period were randomly allocated to mammography screening or usual care. The cohort included 42,283 patients; 21,088 were allocated to the mammography group and 21,195 were allocated to the control group. Screening occurred at intervals of 18 to 24 months. Overall, the authors found that mammographic screening led to a reduced mortality from breast cancer in women aged 55 or over. However, a follow-up study to this trial found the overdiagnosis rate of breast cancer to be 10% in this age group.

The benefits of mammography appear less clear for women aged 40 to 49. For these women, randomized controlled trials have found no significant decrease in mortality after 5 to 7 years of follow-up and only a marginal benefit after 10 to 12 years. Furthermore, the risk of a false positive in this age group was 56.2% after 10 years. This is a significant drawback of screening because false positive mammography results carry a significant burden due to more outpatient visits, mammograms, biopsies, and emotional stress.

The 2015 U.S. Preventive Services Task Force (USPSTF) systematic review concluded that mammographic screening benefits women over 50 and that biennial screening was recommended for women aged 50 to 74 (11). Screening was not routinely recommended for women in their 40s. For these women, the USPSTF suggested a personalized approach taking into consideration individual patient risk and personal preference. In contrast, the 2017 Guidelines from the American College of Radiology and the Society of Breast Cancer Imaging recommended annual screening starting at age 40. The Women Informed to Screen Depending on Measures of risk (WISDOM) study was initiated in 2015 to address these conflicting guidelines. The goal of the trial is to enroll 100,000 women aged 40 or older across five University of California medical centers to determine whether risk-based screening is noninferior to annual mammographic screening for late-stage breast cancers.

PROSTATE CANCER SCREENING

PSA screening for prostate cancer remains controversial due to risks from overdiagnosis and overtreatment. Most men without prostate cancer have PSA levels under 4 nanograms per milliliter (ng/mL) of blood (12). The Cluster Randomized Trial of PSA Testing for Prostate Cancer (CAP) included 419,582 men aged 50 to 69 years and took place across 573 primary care practices in the United Kingdom (13). Randomization and recruitment occurred between 2001 and 2009 and follow-up ended in 2016. The objective of CAP was to evaluate the effect of a single PSA test on prostate cancer specific mortality. There were 189,386 men enrolled in the PSA test group and 219,439 enrolled in the unscreened group. After 10 years, 549 patients died of prostate cancer in the PSA group versus 647 in the unscreened group; the rate ratio of 0.96 (95% confidence interval [CI]: 0.85–1.08, $p = .50$) was not statistically significant. Furthermore, the number diagnosed with prostate cancer was significantly higher in the PSA screened group (relative risk [RR]: 1.19, 95% CI: 1.14–1.25, $p < .0001$). Thus, among men randomized to a single PSA screening intervention versus standard practice without screening, there was no significant difference in prostate cancer mortality. However, detection of low-risk prostate cancer cases significantly increased in those who were screened.

The European Randomized Study of Screening for Prostate Cancer (ERSPC) was initiated in the early 1990s and is the largest trial of PSA screening (14). ERSPC included 162,243 European men in seven countries aged 55 to 69 years who were randomly assigned to PSA screening or usual care. Those in the screening group were tested an average of once every 4 years. During a median follow-up of 9 years, PSA-based screening reduced the rate of death from prostate cancer by 20%. However, PSA-based screening was also associated with a high risk of overdiagnosis. A similar randomized controlled trial was initiated in the United States but yielded different results (15).

The Prostate, Lung, Colorectal, and Ovarian (PLCO) Screening Trial examined the efficacy of screening with PSA testing and digital rectal examination on prostate cancer specific mortality (15). From 1993 to 2001, 76,693 men across 10 U.S. study centers were randomly assigned to annual screening or usual care. The screening group included annual PSA testing for 6 years and digital rectal examination for 4 years. All incident prostate cancers or deaths from prostate cancer through 7 and 13 years of follow-up were obtained. At 7 and 13 years, the rate of death from prostate cancer was very low and did not significantly differ between the screened and unscreened groups. However, this trial was plagued by many biases. For example, many men in the control group were screened, which reduced differences in the two groups and biased study results. A 2017 statistical modeling reanalysis of the PLCO revealed that PSA screening in fact produced a 27% to 32% reduction in prostate cancer specific mortality. In 2018, the USPSTF dropped its total opposition to PSA screening and recommended shared decision making for patients aged 55 to 69 (16).

CERVICAL CANCER SCREENING

In the late 2000s, the Addressing the Need for Advanced HPV Diagnostics (ATHENA) trial evaluated the performance of an HPV test as a primary screening for cervical cancer (17). A total of 42,209 women greater than or equal to 25 years old across multiple sites in the United States were enrolled and had cytology-based Pap smear and high-risk HPV testing. The purpose of screening with Pap smear is to detect abnormal cells that may develop into cancer if left untreated. HPV actually comprises a family of more than 200 viruses, with many strains that can cause cervical cancer and premalignant conditions, such as cervical intraepithelial neoplasia (CIN). HPV-positive women and those with abnormal cytology (atypical squamous cells of undetermined significance) were referred to colposcopy. Women who did not reach the study endpoint of moderate (CIN2+) or severe (CIN3+) cervical dysplasia were not enrolled in the 3-year follow-up phase. HPV screening in women over 25 was found to be as effective as a hybrid screening strategy that uses cytology if 25 to 29 years and cotesting if greater than 30 years. Although HPV testing detected significantly more cases of CIN3+ in women over 25 than either cytology or hybrid strategy, it required significantly more colposcopies. However, the number of colposcopies required to detect a single CIN3+ is the same as for the hybrid strategy. Furthermore, HPV primary screening requires fewer screening tests.

The 2018 USPSTF recommends screening for cervical cancer in women aged 21 to 65 years with Pap smear every 3 years (18). For women aged 30 to 65 years, those who want to lengthen the screening interval are recommended to do so with a combination of cytology and HPV testing every 5 years. For women younger than 30, the USPSTF recommends against screening for cervical cancer with HPV testing, alone or in combination with cytology. For women younger than 21, the USPSTF recommends against screening for cervical cancer.

LUNG CANCER SCREENING

The National Lung Screening Trial (NLST) compared two different ways of detecting lung cancer: low-dose helical CT and standard chest x-ray (19). The NLST enrolled 53,454 current or former heavy smokers aged 55 to 74 from 2002 to 2004. Participants were required to have a smoking history of at least 30 pack-years and were either current or former smokers without signs, symptoms, or history of lung cancer. Participants were randomly assigned to receive three annual screens with either low-dose helical CT or standard chest x-ray. Helical CT uses x-rays to obtain a multiple image scan of the entire chest, whereas a standard chest x-ray produces a single image of the whole chest. The study results revealed that patients who received low-dose helical CT scans had a 15% to 20% lower risk of dying from lung cancer compared to patients who received standard chest x-rays. This is equivalent to approximately three fewer deaths per 1,000 people in the CT group compared to the chest x-ray group over the 7-year follow-up period. Adenocarcinomas and squamous cell carcinomas were detected more frequently at the earliest stage by low-dose helical CT compared to chest x-ray. Small cell lung cancers were infrequently detected at early stages by either low-dose helical CT or chest x-ray. The USPSTF recommends annual screening for lung cancer with low-dose CT in adults aged 55 to 80 years who have a 30 pack-year smoking history and currently smoke or have quit within the past 15 years (20).

COLORECTAL CANCER SCREENING

A total of nine trials have compared screening with flexible sigmoidoscopy or fecal occult blood test (FOBT) to no screening for colorectal cancer (21–29). A flexible sigmoidoscopy evaluates the lower part of the colon through a thin, flexible tube that is inserted into the rectum. A fecal occult blood test is a lab test that is used to check stool samples for hidden (occult) blood that indicates the presence of polyps. The nine trials have comprised 338,467 individuals randomized to screening and 405,919 individuals to control groups. Five trials compared flexible sigmoidoscopy to no screening and four compared repetitive FOBT (annually and biannually) to no screening. When compared to no screening, colorectal cancer mortality was 28% lower with flexible sigmoidoscopy and 14% lower with FOBT. Although there are currently no randomized trials on colonoscopy screening, evidence from case–control and observational cohort studies indicates that colonoscopy reduces colorectal cancer mortality anywhere from 0% to 70%. Overall, the USPSTF recommends screening for colorectal cancer using FOBT testing annually, flexible sigmoidoscopy every 5 years, or colonoscopy every 10 years in adults beginning at age 50 years and continuing until 75 (30).

PREVENTION TRIALS

BREAST CANCER PREVENTION

The Women's Healthy Eating and Living (WHEL) randomized trial investigated the influence of a diet very high in vegetables, fruit, and fiber and low in fat on prognosis following treatment of breast cancer (31). Women were enrolled between 1995 and 2000 and followed up through June 1, 2006. A total of 3,088 women treated for early-stage breast cancer and who were 18 to 70 years old at diagnosis were included in the trial. The intervention group was randomly assigned to a counseling program supplemented with cooking classes and newsletters that promoted daily targets of 5 vegetable servings plus 16 ounces of vegetable juice; 3 fruit servings; 30 grams of fiber; and 15% to 20% energy intake from fat. The control group was provided with print materials on "5-A-Day" dietary guidelines. During an approximately 7-year mean follow-up period, adoption of a diet very high in vegetables, fruit, and fiber and low in fat did not reduce additional breast cancer events or breast cancer specific mortality.

In contrast, numerous studies have shown a protective effect with the medication tamoxifen (32–34). For women with early-stage breast cancer, treatment with tamoxifen significantly reduces breast cancer mortality the first 15 years after diagnosis. In the Adjuvant Tamoxifen: Longer Against Shorter (ATLAS) trial, 12,894 women with early-stage breast cancer who had completed 5 years of treatment with tamoxifen were randomly assigned to continue tamoxifen to 10 years or to stop at 5 years (34). ATLAS recruited women from 36 countries during 1996–2005. Overall, for women with early-stage breast cancer, continuing tamoxifen to 10 years instead of 5 years produced a further reduction in recurrence and mortality, particularly after 10 years. This suggests that 10 years of tamoxifen treatment can approximately halve breast cancer mortality the second decade after cancer diagnosis.

Similarly, the National Surgical Adjuvant Breast and Bowel Project (NSABP) P1 trial randomly assigned 13,388 women at increased risk for breast cancer to either placebo or tamoxifen 20 mg/day for 5 years (35,36). Women were identified as having increased breast cancer risk if they were 60 years of age or older, or age 35 to 59 with a high predicted 5-year risk of breast cancer, or were any age with lobular carcinoma in situ (LCIS). A multivariable logistic regression algorithm (Gail model) (37) was used to quantify patients' risk and eligibility for participation. The investigators found that 5 years of tamoxifen significantly reduced the incidence of both invasive and noninvasive breast cancer, with more than 7 years of follow-up. Osteoporotic fractures were also significantly reduced, but the risk of thromboembolic disease, cataracts, and endometrial cancer was increased, with certain subsets of women, particularly BRCA2 mutation carriers, deriving a principal overall benefit from chemoprevention.

PROSTATE CANCER PREVENTION

The Selenium and Vitamin E Cancer Prevention Trial (SELECT) was a large trial that investigated whether selenium, vitamin E, or both could prevent prostate cancer (38). SELECT randomized more than 35,000 men from 427 participating sites in the United States, Canada, and Puerto Rico to four groups (selenium, vitamin E, selenium and vitamin E, or placebo) between August 2001 and June 2004. The planned follow-up was a minimum of 7 years. However, the trial was stopped in 2008 because selenium or vitamin E was shown to not prevent prostate cancer. Additional analysis on final data collected by the study sites through July 2011 revealed that vitamin E significantly increased the risk of prostate cancer by approximately 17%. A 2014 Cochrane review also found no convincing evidence that selenium supplements prevent cancer in humans.

Lycopene is a bright red carotene that contains protective properties that may play a role in preventing prostate cancer (39). This includes antioxidant properties, decreased lipid oxidation, and protection of lipoproteins and DNA. Lycopene is found in many red fruits and vegetables—tomatoes, red carrots, and watermelons. A few randomized controlled trials have examined the relationship between lycopene and prostate cancer progression and mortality. One study of 105 African American veterans found no significant decrease in prostate cancer risk for individuals who received 30 mg of tomato sauce every day over a course of 3 weeks (39). Another study reported identical declines in PSA levels for both lycopene and control groups after 1 month, but a return to baseline PSA levels 4 months after follow-up for both groups (40). A third study did not report a decrease in PSA levels among individuals administered lycopene (41). Overall, clinical trials have been generally limited by size and duration; current evidence does not provide strong support for or refutation of a link between lycopene and prostate cancer prevention.

CERVICAL CANCER PREVENTION

A trial (the results of which were published in 2015) investigated the efficacy and safety of the 9vHPV vaccine in 105 study sites across 18 countries—including Austria, Chile, Mexico, Germany, Thailand, and the United States (42). Between September 26, 2007 and December 18, 2009, a total of 14,215 women aged 16 to 26 years were randomly assigned to 9vHPV vaccine, Gardasil 9, or control vaccine. Eligible women had to be healthy, have no history of abnormal cervical cytology, no previous abnormal cervical biopsy results, and no more than four lifetime sexual partners. Women were followed for efficacy at preventing disease for up to 6 years after their first vaccine shots, and they were followed for production of infection-halting antibodies against the nine genotypes of HPV for more than 5 years. The HPV vaccine 9 showed 97.4% efficacy to prevent infections and disease caused by the nine HPV genotypes. This included the prevention of infection, cytological abnormalities, high-grade lesions, and cervical procedures. Furthermore, vaccine efficacy was sustained throughout the entire follow-up period of 6 years.

LUNG CANCER PREVENTION

Smoking Cessation Studies

Smoking rates among cancer patients are as high if not higher than in the general population (43). A systemic review on smoking cessation studies found that 14% to 58% of patients who smoked at diagnosis continue to smoke after cancer treatment (43). Continued tobacco use after cancer diagnosis results in lower survival, recurrent disease, decreased efficacy of cancer treatment, increased treatment-related complications, increased physical symptoms, and reductions in quality of life (43). Out of 19 primary intervention studies, 5 smoking cessation interventions had significant or marginally significant differences between the intervention and control group (44–48). Successful smoking cessations were characterized by high-intensity interventions, interventions that had at least six sessions, interventions that targeted multiple risk behaviors and/or used pharmacotherapy, behavioral counseling, and social support. In particular, advanced practice nurses have played a leading role in delivering smoking cessation interventions in the context of cancer care. More than half of the studies (10) tested the efficacy of nurse-delivered interventions. The study that showed the largest effect in promoting smoking cessation was a nurse-delivered intervention led by a nurse investigator (44). These findings highlight the impact nurses can have in promoting knowledge of smoking cessation interventions within cancer care.

Vitamins and Supplements

A 2012 systematic review sought to determine whether vitamins, minerals, and other potential agents, alone or in combination, reduce incidence of and mortality from lung cancer in healthy people (49). Eligible interventions included supplements of vitamins A, C, E, and selenium. The nine trials included in the systematic review compared these interventions to placebo. The studies were conducted from 1996 to 2010 and included healthy males and females of all ages. Five trials were in the United States, one in the United States, Canada, and Puerto Rico, one in China, and two in Europe. Four studies only included males and two only females. The type of supplements and doses varied across studies. Six included vitamin A, three vitamin C, one selenium supplements, and six studied combinations of two or more products. The primary outcomes were lung cancer incidence and lung cancer mortality. Overall, there was no evidence for recommending supplements of vitamins A, C, E, or selenium, either alone or in different combinations, for the prevention of lung cancer and lung cancer mortality.

DIETARY INTERVENTIONS TO PREVENT CANCER

A 2017 systematic review and meta-analysis of observational studies investigated adherence to a Mediterranean diet and its association with overall cancer mortality, incidence of different cancer types, and cancer mortality risk in cancer survivors (50). A Mediterranean diet is a diet that includes proportionally high consumption of olive oil, legumes, fruits, vegetables, fish, and wine. Study-specific estimates were pooled using a random effects model (see Chapters 11 and 28). A total of 56 observational studies in the United States and Europe were included for an overall patient population of 1,784,404. Adherence to a Mediterranean diet was significantly associated with a lower risk of all-cause cancer mortality, colorectal cancer, breast cancer, gastric cancer, prostate cancer, head and neck cancer, pancreatic cancer, and respiratory cancer. There was no significant association for esophageal, ovarian, endometrial, and bladder cancer. Finally, among cancer survivors, the association between adherence to a Mediterranean diet and the risk of cancer mortality and cancer recurrence was not statistically significant.

CONCLUSIONS

Screening and prevention trials play a critical role in establishing the impact of health interventions on the population. Many successful examples have led to lifestyle changes and primary care practice patterns that alter the natural history of cancer, and indeed prevent many people from suffering and dying from the disease. Carefully designed trials can have a significant public health impact, though many special considerations are needed, especially when introducing health interventions into large populations of asymptomatic and disease-free individuals.

GLOSSARY

primordial prevention: a type of activity that prevents future hazards to health.

primary prevention: activity that exerts its effects through cellular-level change.

secondary prevention: activity that reduces the impact of cellular-level change.

tertiary prevention: activity that aims to reduce the severity of disease after it has been diagnosed.

natural history: [of a disease] the course of a disease from its inception to its resolution.

reliability (precision): the ability of a screening test to give consistent results in repeated applications.

validity (accuracy): the ability of a test to measure what it purports to measure.

sensitivity: refers to the percentage of those with disease who will have a positive test result.

specificity: refers to the percentage of those without disease who will have a negative test result.

positive predictive value (PPV): the percentage of individuals with a positive screening test who truly have the disease.

negative predictive value (PPV): the percentage of individuals with a negative screening test who are truly disease free.

false positive rate (FPR): [of a test] refers to the probability of incorrectly identifying a tested individual as having the disease.

false negative rate (FNR): [of a test] refers to the probability of incorrectly identifying a tested individual as not having the disease.

likelihood ratio (LR): a critical property of a screening test that incorporates both its sensitivity and specificity; provides a direct estimate of how much a test result will change the odds of having disease.

positive LR (LR^+): indicates the extent to which the odds of having the disease increases when a test is positive.

negative LR (LR^-): indicates the extent to which the odds of having the disease decreases when a test is negative.

odds: the ratio of a probability to its complement.

probability: the cumulative relative frequency of an event for a given universe of possible outcomes.

pretest probability: probability of having a condition before a diagnostic test is performed.

Bayes theorem: mathematical formula used to determine conditional probability.

conditional probability: probability of an event in the presence of a given condition.

lead time: the amount of time gained by earlier detection of a cancer by screening compared to later detection after the appearance of symptoms.

lead time bias: occurs when screening detects disease, but does not ultimately change its course, leading to the false impression that screening increases life expectancy.

length time: the period of time a patient who has the disease will be asymptomatic.

length time bias: occurs when screening preferentially picks up disease that is progressing more slowly, leading to the false impression that screening increases life expectancy.

overdiagnosis bias: caused by improvements in imaging/disease detection; occurs when screening identifies an illness that would not have shown clinical symptoms.

Will Rogers effect: occurs when individuals are reclassified between categories and differences in outcomes are falsely attributed to improvements in therapy over time.

stage migration: tendency for new technologies to upstage patients over time.

volunteer bias: occurs in observational studies of screening efficacy when the decision to be screened is influenced by an individual's health awareness and related to his or her underlying morbidity.

enrichment: process that can help increase the specificity of the target population by identifying certain at-risk populations.

crossover contamination: a principal concern in evaluating results of randomized trials; occurs because patients in the control arm may feel uncomfortable forgoing or accepting reduced screening or prevention efforts, on the presupposition that such efforts are beneficial.

REFERENCES

1. Heidenreich A, Hofmann R, Engelmann UH. The use of bisphosphonate for the palliative treatment of painful bone metastasis due to hormone refractory prostate cancer. *J Urol*. 2001;165(1):136–140. doi:10.1097/00005392-200101000-00033
2. Feinstein AR, Sosin DM, Wells CK. The Will Rogers phenomenon. Stage migration and new diagnostic techniques as a source of misleading statistics for survival in cancer. *N Engl J Med*. 1985;312(25):1604–1608. doi:10.1056/NEJM198506203122504
3. Tabár L, Fagerberg CJ, Gad A, et al. Reduction in mortality from breast cancer after mass screening with mammography: randomised trial from the Breast Cancer Screening Working Group of the Swedish National Board of Health and Welfare. *Lancet*. 1985;325(8433):829–832. doi:10.1016/S0140-6736(85)92204-4
4. Andersson I, Sigfússon BF. Screening for breast cancer in Malmö: a randomized trial. In: Brünner S, Langfeldt B, eds. *Breast Cancer: Recent Results in Cancer Research*. Berlin, Heidelberg: Springer Publishing; 1987: vol 105.
5. Frisell J, Eklund G, Hellstrom L, et al. The Stockholm breast cancer screening trial: 5-year results and stage at discovery. *Breast Cancer Res Treat*. 1989;13(1):79–87. doi:10.1007/bf01806553
6. Bjurstam N, Bjorneld L, Duffy SW, et al. The Gothenburg Breast Cancer Trial: first results on the mortality, incidence, and mode of detection for women ages 39-49 years at randomization. *Cancer*. 1997;80:2091–2099. doi:10.1002/(SICI)1097-0142(19971201)80:11<2091::AID-CNCR8>3.0.CO;2-#
7. Roberts MM, Alexander FE, Anderson TJ, et al. The Edinburgh randomized trial of screening for breast cancer. *Br J Cancer*. 1984;47:1–6. doi:10.1038/bjc.1984.132
8. Miller AB, To T, Baines CJ, Wall C. Canadian National Breast Screening Study-2: 13-year results of a randomized trial in women aged 50-59 years. *J Natl Cancer Inst*. 2000;92(18):1940–1949. doi:10.1093/jnci/92.18.1490
9. Miller AB, To T, Baines CJ, Wall C. The Canadian National Breast Screening Study-1: breast cancer mortality after 11 to 16 years of follow-up: a randomized screening trial of mammography in women age 40 to 49 years. *Can Med Assoc J*. 1992;147(10):1459–1476. doi:10.7326/0003-4819-137-5_Part_1-200209030-00005

10. Shapiro S. *Periodic Screening for Breast Cancer: The Health Insurance Plan Project and Its Sequelae, 1963–1986*. Baltimore, MD: Johns Hopkins University Press; 1988.
11. U.S. Preventive Services Task Force. Final recommendation statement: Breast cancer. https://www.uspreventiveservicestaskforce.org/Page/Document/RecommendationStatementFinal/breast-cancer-screening1. 2016.
12. Thompson IM, Pauler DK, Goodman PJ, et al. Prevalence of prostate cancer among men with a prostate-specific antigen level < or = 4.0 ng per milliliter. *N Engl J Med*. 2004;350(22):2239–2246. doi:10.1056/NEJMoa031918
13. Martin RM, Donovan JL, Turner EL, et al. Effect of a low-intensity PSA-based screening intervention on prostate cancer mortality: the CAP randomized clinical trial. *JAMA*. 2018;319(9):883–895. doi:10.1001/jama.2018.0154
14. Schröder FH, Hugosson J, Roobol MJ, et al. Screening and prostate cancer mortality: results of the European randomized study of screening for prostate cancer— prostate cancer mortality at 13 years of follow-up. *Lancet*. 2014;384(9959):2027–2035. doi:10.1016/s0140-6736(14)60525-0
15. Andriole G, et al. Mortality results from a randomized prostate-cancer screening trial. *N Engl J Med*. 2009;360:1310–1319. doi:10.1016/s0140-6736(14)60525-0
16. U.S. Preventive Services Task Force. Recommendation statement: Prostate cancer screening. https://www.uspreventiveservicestaskforce.org/Page/Document/RecommendationStatementFinal/prostate-cancer-screening1. 2018.
17. Wright TC, Stoler MH, Behrens CM, et al. Primary cervical cancer screening with human papillomavirus: end of study results from the Athena study using HPV as the first-line screening test. *Gynecol Oncol*. 2015;136(2):189–197. doi:10.1016/j.ygyno.2014.11.076
18. U.S. Preventive Services Task Force. Draft recommendation statement: Prostate cancer screening. https://www.uspreventiveservicestaskforce.org/Page/Document/draft-recommendation-statement/cervical-cancer-screening2. 2017.
19. Aberle DR, Adams AM, Berg CD, et al. Reduced lung-cancer mortality with low-dose computed tomographic screening. *N Engl J Med*. 2011;365(5):395–409. doi:10.1056/nejmoa1102873
20. U.S. Preventive Services Task Force. Final update summary: Lung cancer screening. https://www.uspreventiveservicestaskforce.org/Page/Document/UpdateSummaryFinal/lung-cancer-screening. 2015
21. Mandel JS, Bond JH, Church TR, et al. Reducing mortality from colorectal cancer by screening for fecal occult blood. Minnesota Colon Cancer Control Study. *N Engl J Med*. 1993;328(19):1365–1371. doi:10.1056/NEJM199305133281901
22. Hardcastle JD, Chamberlain JO, Robinson MH, et al. Randomised controlled trial of faecal-occult-blood screening for colorectal cancer. *Lancet*. 1996;348(9040):1472–1477. doi:10.1016/s0140-6736(96)03386-7
23. Kronborg O, Fenger C, Olsen J, et al. Randomised study of screening for colorectal cancer with faecal-occult-blood test. *Lancet*. 1996;348(9040):1467–1471. doi:10.1016/s0140-6736(96)03430-7
24. Lindholm E, Brevinge H, Haglind E. Survival benefit in a randomized clinical trial of faecal occult blood screening for colorectal cancer. *Br J Surg*. 2008;95(8):1029–1036. doi:10.1002/bjs.6136
25. Thiis-Evensen E, Hoff GS, Sauar J, et al. Population-based surveillance by colonoscopy: effect on the incidence of colorectal cancer. Telemark Polyp Study I. *Scand J Gastroenterol*. 1999;34(4):414–420. doi:10.1080/003655299750026443
26. Hoff G, Grotmol T, Skovlund E, Bretthauer M. Risk of colorectal cancer seven years after flexible sigmoidoscopy screening: randomised controlled trial. *BMJ*. 2009;338:b1846. doi:10.1136/bmj.b1846
27. Atkin WS, Edwards R, Kralj-Hans I, et al. Once-only flexible sigmoidoscopy screening in prevention of colorectal cancer: a multicentre randomised controlled trial. *Lancet*. 2010;375(9726):1624–1633. doi:10.1016/S0140-6736(10)60551-X
28. Segnan N, Armaroli P, Bonelli L, et al. Once-only sigmoidoscopy in colorectal cancer screening: Follow-up findings of the Italian randomized controlled trial–SCORE. *J Natl Cancer Inst*. 2011;103(17):1310–1322. doi:10.1093/jnci/djr284
29. Schoen R, Pinsky P, Weissfield J, et al. Colorectal-cancer incidence and mortality with screening flexible sigmoidoscopy. *N Engl J Med*. 2012;366:2345–2357. doi:10.1056/NEJMoa1114635
30. U.S. Preventive Services Task Force. Final update summary: Colorectal cancer screening. https://www.uspreventiveservicestaskforce.org/Page/Document/UpdateSummaryFinal/colorectal-cancer-screening. 2015.
31. Pierce JP, Fearber S, Wright FA, et al. A randomized trial of the effect of a plant-based dietary pattern on additional breast cancer events and survival: the Women's Healthy Eating and Living (WHEL) Study. *Control Clin Trials*. 2002;23(6):728–56. doi:10.1016/S0197-2456(02)00241-6
32. Brown K. Breast cancer chemoprevention: risk-benefit effects of the anti-oestrogen tamoxifen. *Expert Opin Drug Saf*. 2002;1:253–267. doi:10.1517/14740338.1.3.253
33. Early Breast Cancer Trialists Collaborative Group. Tamoxifen for early breast cancer: an overview of the randomized trials. *Lancet*. 1998;351:1451–1467. doi:10.1016/S0140-6736(97)11423-4
34. Davies C, Pan H, Godwin J, et al. Long-term effects of continuing adjuvant tamoxifen to 10 years versus stopping at 5 years after diagnosis of estrogen receptor-positive breast cancer: ATLAS, a randomized trial. *Lancet*. 2013;381(9869):805–816. doi:10.1016/S0140-6736(12)61963-1
35. Fisher B, Costantino JP, Wickerham DL, et al. Tamoxifen for prevention of breast cancer: report of the National Surgical Adjuvant Breast and Bowel Project P-1 Study. *J Natl Cancer Inst*. 1998;90(18):1371–1388. doi:10.1093/jnci/90.18.1371
36. Fisher B, Costantino JP, Wickerham DL, et al. Tamoxifen for the prevention of breast cancer: current status of the National Surgical Adjuvant Breast and Bowel Project P-1 study. *J Natl Cancer Inst*. 2005;97(22):1652–1662. doi:10.1093/jnci/dji372
37. Gail MH, Brinton LA, Byar DP, et al. Projecting individualized probabilities of developing breast cancer for white females who are being examined annually. *J Natl Cancer Inst*. 1989;81:1879–1886. doi:10.1093/jnci/81.24.1879
38. Klein EA. Selenium and vitamin E cancer prevention trial. *Ann N Y Acad Sci*. 2006;1031(1):234–241. doi:10.1196/annals.1331.023
39. Van Breemen RB, Sharifi R, Viana M, et al. Antioxidant effects of lycopene in African-American men with prostate cancer or benign prostate hyperplasia: a randomized, controlled trial. *Cancer Prev Res*. 2011;4(5):711–718. doi:10.1158/1940-6207.CAPR-10-0288

40. Bunker CH, McDonald AC, Evans RW, et al. A randomized trial of lycopene supplementation in Tobago men with high prostate cancer risk. *Nutr Cancer*. 2007;57(2):130–137. doi:10.1080/01635580701274046
41. Schwarz S, Obermuller-Jevic UC, Hellmiss E, et al. Lycopene inhibits disease progression in patients with benign prostate hyperplasia. *J Nutr*. 2008;138(1):49–53. doi:10.1093/jn/138.1.49
42. Joura EA, Giuliano AR, Iversen OE, et al. A 9-valent HPV vaccine against infection and intraepithelial neoplasia in women. *N Engl J Med*. 2015;372:711–723. doi:10.1056/NEJMoa1405044
43. Cooley ME, Lundin R, Murray L. Smoking cessation interventions in cancer care: opportunities for oncology nurses and nurse scientists. *Annu Rev Nurs Res*. 2009;27:243–272. doi:10.1891/0739-6686.27.243
44. Duffy SA, Ronis DL, Valenstein M, et al. A tailored smoking, alcohol, and depression intervention for head and neck cancer patients. *Cancer Epidemiol Biomark Prev*. 2006;15(11):2203–2208. doi:10.1158/1055-9965.EPI-05-0880
45. Emmons KM, Puleo E, Park E, et al. Peer-delivered smoking counseling for childhood cancer survivors increases rate of cessation: the Partnership for Health study. *J Clin Oncol*. 2005;23(27):6516–6523. doi:10.1200/JCO.2005.07.048
46. Stanislaw AE, Wewers ME. A smoking cessation intervention with hospitalized surgical cancer patients: a pilot study. *Cancer Nurs*. 1994;17(2):81–86. doi:10.1097/00002820-199404000-00001
47. Hollen PJ, Hobbie WL, Finley SM. Testing the effects of a decision-making and risk-reduction program for cancer-surviving adolescents. *Oncol Nurs Forum*. 1999;26(9):1475–1486.
48. Cox CL, McLaughlin RA, Rai SN, et al. Adolescent survivors: a secondary analysis of a clinical trial targeting behavior change. *Pediatr Blood Cancer*. 2005;45(2):144–154. doi:10.1002/pbc.20389
49. Cortes-Jofre M, Rueda JR, Corsini-Munoz G, et al. Drugs for preventing lung cancer in healthy people. *Cochrane Database Syst Rev*. 2012;10:1–37. doi:10.1002/14651858.CD002141.pub2
50. Schwingshackl L, Schwedhelm C, Galbete C, Hoffmann G. Adherence to Mediterranean diet and risk of cancer: an updated systematic review and meta-analysis. *Nutrients*. 2017;9 (10);1–24. doi:10.3390/nu9101063

25

Imaging and Technology Trials

AARON B. SIMON ■ DANIEL R. SIMPSON ■ BRENT S. ROSE

Long before cancer was a disease defined by its genome, it was a disease defined by its anatomy, both where it began and where it spread. The early years of cancer treatment were marked by increasingly radical efforts to identify and eliminate all vestiges of cancer from the patient's body, a process that was limited by what a surgeon could see or feel, often with a scalpel as the only tool to permit him or her to peer beneath the skin's surface. The eradication of cancer remains the primary goal in oncology, albeit with a greater sensitivity to the morbidity that can accompany aggressive cancer therapy. It is not surprising, then, that advancements in imaging technology, which permit the physician to noninvasively identify and characterize tumors with increasing accuracy and to treat them with increasing precision, have generated enormous interest in the oncology community and rapidly transformed the standard of care in oncology practice.

Advancements in imaging technology can occur rapidly. In the field of MRI, for example, entirely novel image contrasts can be developed not just through costly and laborious hardware engineering but also through the clever manipulation of the pulse sequences available on a standard clinical scanner. Like their pharmaceutical counterparts, new imaging and treatment technologies must be carefully assessed in the laboratory and clinical settings to determine their safety and efficacy before they are incorporated into standard clinical practice. This chapter discusses the fundamental concepts of imaging and technology trials in oncology, with an emphasis on those that are unique to trials involving pharmaceuticals. Broadly, the chapter is subdivided into three sections, the first dealing with clinical trials designed specifically to test the utility of novel imaging technologies, the second dealing with clinical trials that use imaging metrics as endpoints to assess the utility of drugs or other therapeutic interventions, and the third dealing with clinical trials of image-guided interventions.

DIAGNOSTIC IMAGING

Like drugs or interventions, novel imaging technologies are born in the laboratory and gain acceptance in clinical practice through a series of trials or studies. What kind of trial is appropriate for a new imaging technology depends on where it is on the spectrum of bench to bedside. In the early 1990s, John Thornbury and Dennis Fryback described a hierarchical model of efficacy in diagnostic imaging that provides a conceptual framework for determining the necessary assessments to advance a particular technology given its level of maturity (1–3). This model consists of six sequential steps that take a new technology from prototype to standard of care. It is easy to think of these steps as occurring in a strictly linear order, though the reality of technological development is such that a particular technology may be undergoing both assessments of late-stage clinical efficacy as well as novel technical refinements at the same time. It may also be feasible to assess multiple steps within a single trial with multiple endpoints. In this section, we use this hierarchy to discuss common research questions that occur at every level of imaging technology development. Where it is helpful, we illustrate each level with representative examples from the literature.

LEVEL 1—TECHNICAL EFFICACY

The first level on this hierarchy is technical efficacy. This level is analogous to that of preclinical studies of drugs or molecular biomarkers. At this level the basic properties of an imaging system are assessed, typically by a physicist or engineer. Properties of interest could include signal-to-noise ratio, resolution, contrast, and artifacts of the imaging system (1,2). The interface of the system with the human technologist or physician who will interact with it may also be assessed.

With complex or functional imaging techniques, such as diffusion MRI, a significant body of work may be required simply to understand how the signal that is measured relates to the physiological or anatomical variable of interest (1,3–6). For techniques that are invasive, involve contrast agents or radiotracers, or otherwise have potential to cause harm, safety may also be assessed (7). Studies at this level could include animal models, phantom studies, and studies of normal humans. In addition, studies at this level may not be conducted with respect to a specific disease model if it is thought that the technology may be broadly applicable.

Note that there is no fixed achievement bar that a technology must surpass before it progresses to the next level of assessment. For example, when CT was first introduced into clinical practice in the 1970s, a typical slice was 8 to 13 mm thick and plotted on a grid of 80 × 80 to 160 × 160 voxels (8,9). Today this level of technical capability would be considered woefully inadequate, but at the time, it was sufficient to significantly impact the diagnosis of intracranial pathology (8).

LEVEL 2—DIAGNOSTIC ACCURACY

The second level on the hierarchy is *diagnostic accuracy*. By definition, studies conducted at this level must be disease oriented and conducted in a clinical population. The goal of level 2 studies is to determine how well a new imaging technology performs a diagnostic function in comparison to an accepted reference standard. Level 2 studies can be conducted either prospectively or retrospectively. Common metrics of interest in level 2 studies include the sensitivity and specificity of a technique for detection of a particular disease process, as well as the positive and negative predictive value of a diagnosis (Figure 25.1).

Recall that the **sensitivity** of a technique refers to the probability that it will yield a "positive" result in a disease-positive patient:

$$\text{Sensitivity} = \frac{\text{True positives}}{\text{True positives} + \text{False negatives}}$$

Specificity refers to the probability that a technique will yield a "negative" result in a disease-negative patient:

$$\text{Specificity} = \frac{\text{True negatives}}{\text{True negatives} + \text{False positives}}$$

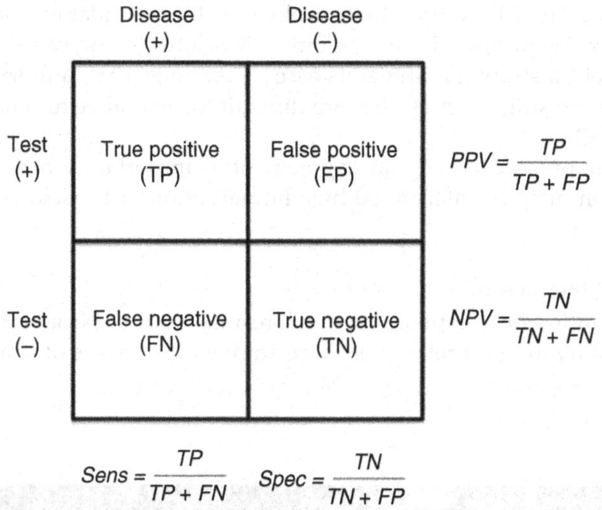
Disease (+)
Disease (−)
Test (+)
True positive (TP)
False positive (FP)
PPV = TP / TP + FP
Test (−)
False negative (FN)
True negative (TN)
NPV = TN / TN + FN
Sens = TP / TP + FN
Spec = TN / TN + FP

FIGURE 25.1 Fundamental metrics of diagnostic accuracy.
NPV, negative predictive value; PPV, positive predictive value; Sens, sensitivity; Spec, specificity.

If the prevalence of a particular disease within a population of interest is known, then the sensitivity and specificity of the technique can be used to estimate the **positive predictive value (PPV)** and **negative predictive value** (**NPV**) of a test, which the clinician ultimately uses to determine the probable accuracy of the test in ruling in or ruling out a disease:

$$\text{PPV} = \frac{\text{Sensitivity} \times \text{Prevalence}}{\text{Sensitivity} \times \text{Prevalence} + (1 - \text{Specificity}) \times (1 - \text{Prevalence})}$$

$$\text{NPV} = \frac{\text{Specificity} \times (1 - \text{Prevalence})}{(1 - \text{Sensitivity}) \times \text{Prevalence} + \text{Specificity} \times (1 - \text{Prevalence})}$$

For a given technology and a given disease, the sensitivity and specificity may depend on multiple variables related to the technical specifications of the system, the skill and interpretation of the human operators who perform and read the images (unless automated), the characteristics of the patient population studied, the reference standard to which the new technology will be compared, and (for quantitative techniques) the cut points at which a disease state will be defined. Understanding each of these factors is important in designing and analyzing a clinical trial at this level.

The first factor, technical specifications, is addressed to the extent possible by the level 1 studies that precede a clinical trial. A key question for the investigators proposing a level 2 study is whether the body of evidence from level 1 suggests that technical development is mature enough to warrant an investment in resources for a clinical study. Another key question is how strictly they will define the "technology" that they are assessing. A simple example is the question of how to assess the accuracy of diffusion MRI in detecting prostate cancer. Most diffusion MRI protocols have certain features in common (e.g., the employment of diffusion encoding gradients in multiple directions in order to produce Brownian motion–induced attenuation of the MR signal) (5). However, diffusion protocols can vary significantly across centers, in terms of magnetic field strength, scanner make and model, coil design, strength and number of diffusion gradients employed, slice thickness, echo time, repetition time, readout field of view and resolution, method of analysis, and so forth (10–13). A study that employs multiple similar technologies across centers will be more generalizable to clinical practice, but it risks introducing variability into the estimate of accuracy. Conversely, a study that limits its assessment to a strict, uniform protocol will likely produce a more precise result, but may be more difficult to generalize to centers without identical technology (Figure 25.2).

The second factor, operator ability and agreement, is important whenever the output of the technology in question must be interpreted by a human in order to yield a diagnosis. Important questions to consider are:

1. Who will interpret the images?
2. Does accurate operation or interpretation of the results require specialized training?
3. How much variability in interpretation is there among interpreters of similar skill and experience?

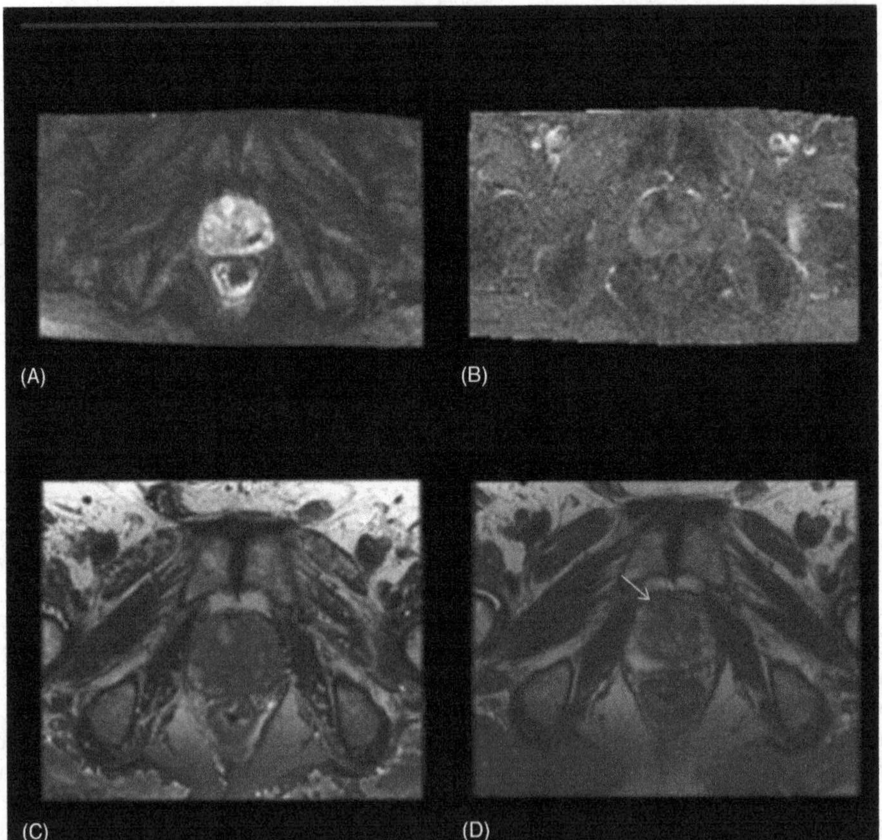

FIGURE 25.2 Methods of acquisition and analysis of diffusion MRI in prostate cancer. Diffusion MRI plays an increasingly important role in the diagnosis of prostate cancer; however, diffusion imaging can be performed and analyzed using several of methods that may differ in diagnostic accuracy. A to C show a lesion in the anteromedial prostate at the mid apex, at the border of the peripheral and transitional zones imaged using three different diffusion imaging techniques; (A) diffusion weighted imaging (DWI), (B) calculated apparent diffusion coefficient (ADC), and (C) restriction spectrum imaging (RSI), shown overlaid on a T2-weighted image. D Shows the T2-weighted image of the same lesion (arrow).

The first two questions can be addressed in both the design and analysis phases of a clinical study. It is important in the design phase of the study to have in mind who will be interpreting the results of the new technique. Will it be a subspecialized radiologist with significant previous experience in image interpretation and relevant anatomy and who will likely see numerous cases over the course of his or her career? Or will it be a more general practitioner who may be less experienced with diagnostic imaging and may use the technology less frequently? If the answer is the latter, then it may be important to include experts as well as more novice interpreters into the study in order to assess the importance of experience on the accuracy of the technique.

Multiple metrics can be used to quantify the agreement among multiple readers, whether of similar or disparate experience levels. A commonly used metric for assessing agreement amongst readers for categorical outcomes (e.g., presence vs. absence of disease) is the **kappa statistic**, whereas the **intraclass correlation coefficient** is often used for continuous outcomes (e.g., tumor diameter or volume) (3).

The third factor, study population, is an important concept when considering the external validity of a study. The accuracy of a diagnostic imaging technique may depend significantly on one or more characteristics of the patient population under study. For example, many imaging modalities will be more sensitive to detection of large, advanced tumors than small, early-stage lesions. Conversely, a novel imaging technique may be more specific for detection of recurrence after surgery than radiotherapy. Failure to recognize and account for differences between the study population and the population in which the technique will be employed can result in spectrum bias and artificially increase or decrease the estimated sensitivity and specificity of a technique. To avoid spectrum bias, care should be taken to recruit subjects broadly from the population of interest. When this is not possible, it is important to explicitly describe the subset of patients included in the study and how its characteristics may limit the generalizability of the results (3,14).

The fourth factor, reference standard, refers to the diagnostic modality to which a new imaging technique will be compared. Ideally, this standard would have as close to 100% sensitivity and specificity as possible. Examples of commonly utilized reference standards include surgical, autopsy, and pathology reports; other imaging modalities; and long-term clinical follow-up. In some cases it may be possible to construct a model or phantom system on which to test the accuracy of a new technique, thereby assuring that the "ground truth" is known with 100% certainty, at least within the limitations of the phantom. In other cases it may be difficult to find a "gold standard" against which to compare a new technique; under these conditions, a commonly used if imperfect reference standard may be employed, with the understanding that in cases of disagreement it may not be clear which modality is at fault and that in cases of agreement, it may be due to the limitations of both modalities. Kappa statistics may also be used to assess agreement between two imperfect systems as they are used to assess agreement among multiple observers (3,14).

For some imaging systems, especially those for which the output is quantitative rather than qualitative, a decision must be made about what level of the metric of interest to call "positive" and which to call "negative." Ideally, these two states separate cleanly along the metric's scale such that a cut point can be determined for which all of the positive subjects are one side and all of the negative subjects are on the other. Such a cut point would define a test with both 100% sensitivity and 100% specificity. Unfortunately, this case occurs only rarely, and in many instances there is not a unique, optimal cut point.

Under these conditions, it is useful to construct a **receiver operating characteristic (ROC) curve** (Figure 25.3). The ROC curve for a diagnostic test is a plot of the true-positive rate (sensitivity) against the false-positive rate (1-specificity) for a range of possible cut points. Typically the sensitivity is plotted on the y-axis and 1-specificity is plotted on the x-axis. The ROC curve for a diagnostic test is useful because it displays the trade-offs between sensitivity and specificity that must be made in determining what cut point will be used in clinical practice. The ROC curve also provides a metric of the performance of an imaging technique that can be compared against others.

For an ROC curve, the **area under the curve (AUC)** is a metric of the overall performance or accuracy of the test given all possible cut points and their relative effects on sensitivity and specificity. The AUC can be estimated in a number of ways, including simple approximation of the

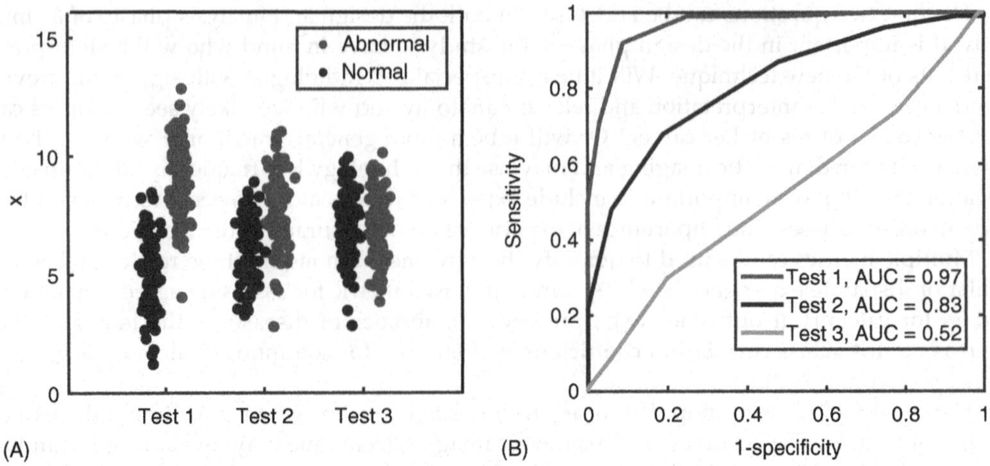

FIGURE 25.3 ROC curves. (A) Distribution of measurements from an abnormal and normal population for three hypothetical tests. In this example, there is relatively little overlap in x for Test 1, while for Test 3 the distributions are the same for the two groups. Test 2 is in between. (B) Corresponding ROC curves for the three tests. For Test 1, the AUC is nearly unity, meaning a cut point can be found that should provide both high sensitivity and specificity. For Test 3, AUC approaches 0.5, meaning use of this test is no better than random assignment.

AUC, area under the curve; ROC, receiver operating characteristic.

integral of the ROC curve using the trapezoidal rule. An alternative approach that is straightforward to calculate and has an intuitive interpretation is the calculation of the **Wilcoxon** or **Mann-Whitney statistic**. If the study population contains n_A abnormal subjects and n_N normal subjects and is to be classified based on the value x of the test in question (with higher values of x signifying abnormality), the Wilcoxon statistic can be expressed by the equation

$$W = \left(\frac{1}{n_A * n_N}\right) \Sigma_1^{n_A} \Sigma_1^{n_N} S(x_A, x_N), \text{where } S(x_A, x_N) = \begin{cases} 1 & x_A > x_N \\ \frac{1}{2} & x_A = x_N \\ 0 & x_A < x_N \end{cases}.$$

What this equation means intuitively is that the AUC for an ROC curve is equivalent to the probability that any randomly drawn sample x_A is greater than any randomly drawn sample x_N. The closer this probability is to unity, the easier it is to find a cut point for which no cases will be misclassified (perfect sensitivity and specificity). As this probability approaches 0.5, it becomes impossible to find a cut point that yields better performance than random guessing.

For a limited sample size, standard errors can also be calculated for the estimated AUC, and hypothesis tests can be constructed to determine whether the AUC of test A is greater than that of test B, given a common reference standard. These are described in detail in the referenced texts but are beyond the scope of this chapter (3,14,15).

LEVEL 3—DIAGNOSTIC THINKING EFFICACY

The third level on the hierarchy is *diagnostic thinking efficacy*. Diagnostic accuracy is an important feature of an imaging technology, but it is of little value if it does not affect the decision-making processes of the clinicians using it. The effect that a diagnostic test has on the decision-making process can be quantified and formalized in the likelihood ratio and the concepts of pretest and posttest probability.

The **likelihood ratio** is related to the sensitivity and specificity of a test. The **positive likelihood ratio** (LR^+) can be found by the equation LR^+ = sensitivity/(1-specificity). It indicates how much the likelihood of a subject having a disease increases with a positive test. Conversely, the **negative likelihood ratio** (LR^-) can be found by the equation LR^- = (1-sensitivity)/specificity. It indicates how much the likelihood of diseases decreases with a negative test.

The **pretest probability** (**P_{pre}**) refers to the probability that a subject has a disease prior to receiving a test. The pretest probability can be combined with the likelihood ratio to calculate the **posttest probability** (**P_{post}**), the likelihood that the disease is present after considering the new test (16). This calculation is carried out as follows:

First the pretest probability is converted to pretest odds by the equation $O_{pre} = P_{pre}/(1 - P_{pre})$. The pretest odds are then multiplied by the likelihood ratio to produce the posttest odds or $O_{post} = O_{pre}*LR(+/-)$. The posttest odds are then converted to posttest probability by the equation $P_{post} = O_{post}/(1 + O_{post})$.

For example, if a test has a sensitivity and specificity of 90%, then $LR^+ = 9$ and $LR^- = 0.11$. If a physician estimates a 50% chance of disease prior to ordering a test ($P_{pre} = 0.5$, $O_{pre} = 1$), then the posttest odds and probability after a positive test are $O_{post} = 9$ and $P_{post} = 90\%$ and the posttest odds and probability after a negative test are $O_{post} = 0.11$ and $P_{post} = 9\%$. In contrast, if the pretest probability is 80%, $O_{post} = 36$ and $P_{post} = 97\%$ for a positive test and $O_{post} = 0.44$ and $P_{post} = 30\%$ for a negative test.

The challenge of estimating the effect of a diagnostic test on decision making in this formal way lies in part in the estimation of the pretest probability. In the simplest case, this could be estimated as the prevalence of the disease in a population, and this may be a reasonable estimate for a screening test that will be administered very broadly and without much additional information gathering. However, in many cases, a diagnostic image is ordered after a physician has performed a history and physical exam, examined relevant laboratory data, and reviewed other imaging. Each of these pieces of information will change the pretest probability of a given condition in a physician's mind as he or she narrows the differential diagnosis. How much it changes may be difficult to quantify and may vary from physician to physician.

Similarly, the qualitative effect of a test on decision making may not be fully captured by the change in pretest and posttest probability. For example, a change in probability from 80% to 97% may be reassuring to a physician, but it might not change his or her top diagnosis on the differential. Conversely, a change in probability from 80% to 30% may cast significant doubt on a diagnosis, but if the condition is severe enough, a 30% probability may still not be low enough for a physician to comfortably consider it ruled out. Perhaps because of these ambiguities, there are relatively few clinical studies for which effect on decision making itself is the primary endpoint. Nevertheless, there are examples from the literature that illustrate how such a study can be conducted (14,17).

LEVEL 4—THERAPEUTIC EFFICACY

Perhaps a more intuitive and concrete measure of efficacy than how a diagnostic image affects physicians' thinking is how it affects their decisions. Level 4 on the hierarchy, *therapeutic efficacy*, is closely related to diagnostic thinking, with the addition of assessing how a technology changes the management of a patient. An interesting example of this comes from a study of how breast MRI affects surgical management of breast cancer patients.

The MONET trial was a randomized controlled trial in which 418 patients with nonpalpable Breast Imaging Reporting and Data System (BIRADS) three to five lesions on screening mammogram or ultrasound (i.e., possibly malignant or suspicious for malignancy, requiring further diagnostic workup) were randomly assigned to receive standard care, including mammography, ultrasound, and core needle biopsy versus standard care plus pre-biopsy MRI (18). Following biopsy, patients with invasive cancer or in situ disease were referred for surgery, with a choice of breast-conserving surgery (BCS) and adjuvant radiation versus mastectomy determined by the surgeon in conjunction with patient preference. The primary endpoint of the study was the rate of additional surgical procedures (re-excisions and mastectomies) after initial surgical management. Secondary endpoints included the primary BCS rate.

Interestingly, although the study found the rate of primary BCS to be similar in the MRI and control groups (68% vs. 66%, respectively), the number of re-excisions that were performed due to positive margins after BCS was significantly higher in the MRI group than in the control group (34% vs. 12%, $p = .008$). To understand this finding, they looked retrospectively at the size of the excision specimens from the BCSs and found that the median excision volume was 69.1 cm^3 in the MRI group versus 90.2 cm^3 in the control group. Among the patients who underwent MRI, they found that the excision volume in patients with negative MRIs was particularly low (median volume 40.3 cm^3) and the positive margin rate particularly high (64%). They concluded that preoperative MRI did not improve surgical management of breast cancer beyond usual care, given the equivalent rates of primary BCS, and that it could potentially lead to worse therapeutic outcomes, given that negative MRIs were associated with underestimation of the tumor volume at the time of surgery.

LEVEL 5—PATIENT OUTCOMES

At the fifth level of the hierarchy, *patient outcomes*, the outcomes of interest are the same as those in clinical trials of drugs and other interventions, including but not limited to progression-free and overall survival, quality of life, and complications and toxicity. As diagnostic images are not directly therapeutic, for them to affect these outcomes in meaningful ways, they must permit physicians to make superior therapeutic decisions.

As with clinical trials of pharmaceuticals and other interventions, the most reliable method of assessing the effect of an imaging technique on patient outcomes is through a prospective, randomized clinical trial. Depending on the outcome of interest, such a trial may require a small or large sample size and follow-up may be short term or long term. On the one hand, for trials like the MONET trial discussed earlier, a relatively small sample size and short-term follow-up may be adequate because the primary outcome—the need for repeat surgical procedures—can be quickly assessed and is closely related to imaging for surgical planning. On the other hand, a trial with an outcome of overall survival may require a very large sample size and many years of follow-up to assess, especially if the overall effect of the imaging technique is small. Such a study may be prohibitively expensive to conduct.

Nevertheless, there are a few notable examples of imaging trials that have demonstrated an overall survival benefit. One such example is the National Lung Screening Trial (19). In this trial, 53,454 people at high risk of lung cancer were enrolled from 33 U.S. medical centers between 2002 and 2004. Subjects were randomly assigned to undergo three annual screenings with either low-dose CT or chest radiography. All screening examinations were performed according to a standard protocol developed by the trial that specified acceptable characteristics of the machines and the acquisition parameters. Participating radiologists and technicians were certified by their respective agencies and were additionally trained in image acquisition, quality, and standardized interpretation. Images from the first round of screening were interpreted in isolation and images from subsequent rounds could be compared with these. Specific criteria for classifying an image as positive or "suspicious for lung cancer" were established for both CT and radiographs. Results and recommendations from the screening exams were communicated to the subjects and their healthcare providers; however, no standardized evaluation approach for positive findings was mandated.

Over the course of the study, 24.2% of low-dose CT scans were positive, as were 6.9% of radiographs. On follow-up evaluation, the false-positive rate was high in each arm (96.4% for CT and 94.5% for radiography). More lung cancers were diagnosed in the CT group than the radiograph group (1,060 vs. 941) and of these, a greater percentage was diagnosed after screening exam (61% vs. 30%). The percentage of stage IV cancer at time of diagnosis was lower in the CT group than the radiography group and the percentage of stage I cancers was higher. Ultimately, after follow-up of 144,103 person-years in the CT group and 143,368 person-years in the radiography group, low-dose CT screening demonstrated a significant reduction in lung cancer–specific mortality, with a relative risk reduction of 20.0% (p = .004) and number needed to treat (NNT) of 320. A relative risk reduction of 6.7% was also noted for death from any cause (p = .02). Overall complication rates from subsequent invasive diagnostic procedures were low in both arms; however, CT screening did lead to an increase in invasive procedures compared with radiography (19). This study highlights the significant resources required to conduct an imaging trial for which the outcome is overall survival. Many new imaging technologies enter clinical practice without demonstrating such results. Nevertheless, such randomized trials remain the gold standard in demonstrating efficacy in terms of meaningful, patient-centered outcomes. Observational and retrospective studies of the association between use of diagnostic techniques and patient-centered outcomes may also be conducted with considerably lower requirement for resources; however, these are subject to the same biases as other observational studies.

LEVEL 6—SOCIETAL EFFICACY

In levels 1 to 5, any improvement in outcome, whether at the level of technical implementation or up to the level of survival, is an unqualified success. In the final level of the hierarchy, *societal efficacy*, improvements in clinical outcomes are balanced against the costs—to patients, insurance providers, government entities, and so forth—required to achieve those improvements. The cost-effectiveness analysis is the tool most commonly used used to assess this balance and is discussed at length in Chapter 19 (1,3). Common metrics include quality-adjusted life years (QALYs), costs per person, and incremental cost-effectiveness ratios (ICERs). For the National Lung Screening Trial discussed earlier, screening with low-dose CT was estimated to cost an additional $1,631 per person and provided 0.0316 additional life years per person and 0.0201 QALYs per person. The estimated cost per QALY was $81,000 and the ICER was $52,000 per life year gained (20). There is no exact threshold above which an intervention becomes too costly for society to accept. For many years, $50,000 per QALY was taken as an acceptable cost, though recently some experts have suggested that a threshold of $100,000 to $150,000 per QALY is more appropriate (21).

IMAGING METRICS AS ENDPOINTS IN THERAPEUTIC CLINICAL TRIALS

In clinical trials of cancer therapy, determination of an appropriate endpoint is a challenging but critical task. Ideally, an endpoint is patient centered and highly clinically relevant, such as cancer-specific survival or quality of life. However, such endpoints may take years to become apparent, and the impact of a particular therapy may be obscured by the additional interventions and complications that occur in the course of a patient's life. For early-stage clinical trials designed to measure the antineoplastic activity of a novel therapy, endpoints that can be assessed serially and at relatively early time points are essential. Imaging, because of its minimally invasive nature and ability to assess changes in tumor anatomy and physiology throughout the body, has played an important role as a surrogate endpoint for therapeutic efficacy for many years (22). However, the implementation of imaging endpoints in clinical trials is not without challenges. In this section, we discuss some of the key questions that must be answered when one is using an imaging metric as a surrogate endpoint for a clinical trial in cancer and illustrate, wherever possible, with examples from the literature.

BIOLOGICAL UNDERSTANDING OF IMAGING ENDPOINTS

What criteria must be met before an imaging technique may be validated as a surrogate endpoint in a clinical trial? Perhaps the most fundamental criterion is that there is a firm understanding of the relationship between what an imaging technique measures and the physiological effect of the therapy in question. This idea is illustrated by the challenges encountered with utilization of contrast-enhanced MRI to assess treatment response in high-grade glioma and the subsequent development of the RANO criteria to address them (23).

In 1990, Macdonald et al. proposed a set of new criteria for assessment of high-grade gliomas for phase II trials (24). They noted that prior to this, clinical trials in neuro-oncology lacked the rigorous, standardized methods for radiographically assessing tumor response that were developing in other areas of medical oncology. At the time, contrast-enhanced CT and MRI were commonly used for monitoring gliomas and were incorporated into their imaging criteria for response assessment. The criteria that they developed were based on the World Health Organization (WHO) criteria for tumor response developed previously (25). Namely, they looked at changes in the size of the sum of the products of perpendicular diameters of all measureable enhancing lesions. A complete response required the disappearance of all disease for at least 4 weeks, partial response a ≥50% decrease in size, progressive disease a ≥25% increase in size, and stable disease not meeting criteria for any of the above. At that time, they understood that several factors, particularly steroid use, could affect the size of a contrast-enhancing lesion on CT or MRI and that case reports existed of transient changes after surgery or radiation that mimicked recurrent tumor (25,26).

However, with the exception of steroid use, they did not attempt to specifically account for these potential confounders in their imaging criteria. Despite these limitations, the "Macdonald Criteria" created a standardized set of imaging criteria for determining response or resistance to novel therapies that could be compared across trial centers or even clinical trials. In the years that followed, the Macdonald Criteria were utilized for numerous phase II clinical trials of efficacy in high-grade glioma (e.g., 27,28).

In the subsequent years, a number of limitations in the Macdonald Criteria were identified, including challenges with measuring irregular tumors, variability in measurements across readers, and issues with measuring nonenhancing, multifocal, and cystic tumors (29). In addition, especially after the incorporation of temozolomide and bevacizumab into the treatment of glioblastoma, it became apparent that the size of the enhancing tumor, even when accurately measured, was not always a good surrogate for tumor response or progression.

The term **pseudoprogression** refers to a phenomenon wherein the size of an enhancing glioblastoma transiently increases on MRI within the first 12 weeks of completion of radiation therapy. Pseudoprogression can only be distinguished from true disease progression through tissue biopsy or serial imaging, which will show spontaneous resolution in the case of pseudoprogression. Pseudoprogression was noted to be increasingly common after the introduction of temozolomide therapy and particularly common in patients with tumor MGMT promoter methylation; these are the patients who derive the most therapeutic benefit from temozolomide. It was hypothesized that rather than always representing tumor progression, increased enhancement could also represent transient blood–brain barrier breakdown in the setting of glioma cell killing (30).

In contrast, antiangiogenic agents such as bevacizumab were found to produce significant decreases in tumor enhancement, which did not subsequently lead to improvements in survival. In addition, a subset of patients with good initial responses in terms of tumor enhancement were subsequently found to have significant increases in nonenhancing tumor volume. The identification of these pseudoresponses led to the theory that antiangiogenic agents produced some of their radiographic effects not through tumor killing but through normalization of the leaky tumor vasculature. To address these issues and others, the Response Assessment in Neuro-Oncology Working Group introduced the RANO criteria, which made specific proscriptions against radiographically diagnosing "in-field" progression within the first 12 weeks of completion of chemoradiotherapy and also included specific criteria for diagnosing progression based on growth of nonenhancing disease in patients receiving antiangiogenic therapy (23).

STANDARDIZATION AND DISSEMINATION OF TECHNOLOGY

Assuming that the biological correlates of an imaging technique are well understood, the technology required to implement it must achieve a certain level of maturity such that it can be widely and uniformly implemented across potential clinical trial sites. As was discussed earlier in the chapter, at the early stages of development of a new technique, the optimal choice of certain technical parameters may be unclear; disparate centers may employ technologies from differing manufacturers that have not been rigorously compared; and protocols for acquiring, processing, and interpreting images may not be uniform. Each of these factors can have a significant effect on the performance of an imaging technique, even when the technique is quantitative. Because the performance of the technique will affect whether it leads the interpreting reader to call "response," "progression," or "stable disease," such variability in implementation will lead to increased variability in the endpoint across centers, reducing statistical power and potentially introducing systematic bias (4).

VALIDATION OF SURROGATE ENDPOINTS

Once a technique is well understood, standardized, and available for use in participating clinical trial sites, it should be validated against the more patient-centered, often phase III, outcome for which it is a proposed surrogate (e.g., survival). Prentice described a formal criterion for validating a **surrogate endpoint**. He suggested a surrogate endpoint should be "a response variable for which a test of the null hypothesis of no relationship to the treatment groups under comparison is also a valid test of the corresponding null hypothesis based on the true endpoint" (31). In other words, he required that the surrogate endpoint capture enough of the treatment effect that the true outcome of interest be statistically independent of the treatment, given knowledge of the surrogate endpoint (31).

This is a very strict criterion, one that requires the surrogate to capture essentially all of the treatment effect. Others have argued that a surrogate endpoint may still be valid if it explains only a large proportion of the treatment effect (e.g., Freedman et al. suggested a critical value of 0.5 or 0.75) (32,33). Nevertheless, the fundamental paradigm for validating surrogate endpoints as described by Prentice remains the cornerstone of endpoint validation for clinical trials today.

Ideally, validation studies for imaging endpoints are carried out in the context of prospective, randomized trials of treatment efficacy. Such trials allow for the assessment of the criteria necessary to validate an imaging endpoint, namely, (a) that the treatment improves the patient-centered outcome of interest (e.g., survival), (b) that the same treatment increases the "response" as measured by the surrogate, (c) that those who respond according to the surrogate also do better according to the patient-centered outcome, and (d) that the effect of the treatment on the patient-centered outcome is explained by the surrogate response (4,32,34). If a randomized trial is not feasible at the early stage of endpoint validation, then prospective, single-arm studies and even retrospective studies may still be useful to assess whether there is an association between the response to treatment in terms of the surrogate endpoint and the patient-centered outcome at the individual subject level, though without a control arm it may be difficult to determine definitively whether the association exists because the surrogate endpoint captures the treatment benefit or because both the surrogate and the patient-centered outcome are associated with an additional variable of prognostic significance (4).

Perhaps the best-validated imaging-based surrogate endpoint in oncology currently is RECIST 1.1. **RECIST (Response Evaluation Criteria in Solid Tumors)** is a set of criteria for measuring the response of solid tumors to therapy, typically with CT imaging, though in some instances MRI is permissible (22). RECIST is based on the simple biological assumption that the change in tumor burden in response to therapy is a marker of the efficacy of the treatment. However, determining the best way to assess a change in tumor burden radiographically is far from trivial.

Prior to RECIST, the most commonly used criteria for assessing changes in tumor burden were those developed by the WHO in 1981 (35). The WHO criteria classified treatment response into four categories: complete response—meaning disappearance of all lesions; partial response—meaning 50% decrease in total tumor burden; progressive disease—meaning a 25% increase in size in any lesion or development of new lesions; and stable disease—meaning all other responses. Individual tumor size was to be assessed by calculating the product of the longest diameter and the longest perpendicular diameter. Tumor burden was calculated as the sum of these products. Other, less detailed instructions were given for measurement of lesions that were more difficult to measure (e.g., bone lesions, pleural effusions).

However, in the years that followed the publication of the WHO criteria, differences in interpretation of these criteria led to fragmentation in their application, which was shown to potentially have a significant impact on the qualitative interpretation of clinical trials (36,37). Other work demonstrated that unidimensional measurement was equal to bidimensional measurement in terms of assessing tumor response and was less labor intensive to conduct (38). In response to this and other work, an international working group was established in the 1990s to develop a new set of criteria for assessing tumor response, which could be widely and uniformly applied to clinical trials. Their recommendations, the RECIST criteria, were published in 2000 and proposed a number of modifications to the WHO criteria, including unidimensional measurement, definitions of measurable and unmeasurable lesions, specific recommendations for evaluation of measurable and unmeasurable lesions, and specific recommendations and prescriptions for uses of various imaging modalities (e.g., x-ray, CT, MRI, ultrasound).

Following its publication, RECIST was widely adopted for use as a surrogate endpoint for efficacy in phase II clinical trials. Subsequently, numerous studies sought to validate the new criteria with varying disease sites and therapeutics. Overall, RECIST was found to perform well in numerous cancer subtypes, with the notable exceptions of mesothelioma and gastrointestinal stromal tumor (GIST) (39). Response to noncytotoxic, targeted therapies was also not well predicted by RECIST (22). Additional work led to better understanding of the response of pathological lymph nodes to cancer therapy (40) as well as the number of lesions needed to accurately sample the response to therapy (41). These findings and others were incorporated into RECIST 1.1, a revised set of criteria published in 2009. A full description is beyond the scope of this chapter; however, notable changes included a reduction of the number of target lesions, changes in the evaluation of lymph nodes, changes in the minimum size of target lesions, and specific guidance on the use of progression-free survival as an endpoint.

Notably, unidimensional measurement was not abandoned for volumetric measurement in the new criteria, due to lack of sufficient validation; nor were functional imaging techniques such as FDG-PET formally incorporated (4). In response to this, Wahl et al. developed a set of guidelines specifically designed to provide standardization both of implementation and assessment of FDG-PET response to cancer therapy, which they termed **PERCIST** 1.0 (42). The PERCIST criteria are currently being studied for correlation with clinical outcome in a number of disease sites, including small cell lung cancer, non-Hodgkin lymphoma, esophageal cancer, Ewing's sarcoma, and colorectal cancer (43).

A very recent adaptation of the RECIST 1.1 criteria is **iRECIST**, which was developed specifically to address the unique radiographic responses of some solid tumors to immunotherapies (44). As with chemoradiation for glioblastoma, some early immunotherapy investigators noted early changes in tumor burden that met criteria for progression that were followed by deep and durable responses at later time points. A number of guidelines were proposed to address the problem of immunotherapy-related pseudoprogression, and in response to the need for standardization and validation of these guidelines, the RECIST working group developed its own set of guidelines for handling clinical trials of immunotherapy.

The resulting guidelines, termed iRECIST and published in 2017, preserved many of the features of RECIST 1.1. One key change, however, was the division of the RECIST 1.1 category "progressive disease" into two categories, unconfirmed progressive disease (iUPD) and confirmed progressive disease (iCPD; the prefix *i* precedes all responses when iRECIST is utilized). Under RECIST 1.1, once a patient has met criteria for disease progression, a later response to therapy is precluded. Under iRECIST, if a patient meets criteria for disease progression (either by increase of tumor size or by development of new lesions), he or she is designated as iUPD. Confirmed progressive disease requires further growth or lesion development at the subsequent time point, typically 4 to 8 weeks later. If the burden of disease decreases at the subsequent time point, the patient can be designated as stable disease (iSD), partial response (iPD), or complete response (iCR), depending on the magnitude of response. Once a patient has been redesignated into one of these categories, the bar for progression is reset, and subsequent increases in tumor burden again have to be confirmed before the patient can be designated as having iCPD. This guideline has yet to be validated and the RECIST group is currently warehousing data from immunotherapy trials to serve this purpose. In the meantime, the authors of iRECIST urge caution in the application of those guidelines to clinical trials and recommend against using them in clinical practice (44).

CLINICAL TRIALS OF IMAGE-GUIDED INTERVENTIONS

As modern imaging modalities have been developed and become more widely accepted in recent years, there has been increasing interest in image-guided interventions (IGIs) such as surgery, percutaneous minimally invasive techniques, and radiation therapy, with the overarching goal of improving treatment accuracy. A wide array of imaging techniques has been employed for these purposes, including ultrasound, fluoroscopy, CT, MRI, and PET. Although IGIs have become pervasive throughout medicine, it is important to consider the process by which these technologies are introduced into clinical use. This section discusses some of the practical considerations for design, technical standards, and quality assurance for clinical trials of IGIs and provides examples of issues that may arise when conducting these studies. In order to be concise, this section focuses specifically on clinical trials involving image-guided radiation therapy (IGRT); however, the principles can be generalized to many types of IGIs. More comprehensive discussion of nonradiation therapy–related IGIs can be found elsewhere (3,45).

The traditional clinical trial paradigm largely evolved with the guidance of the Food and Drug Administration (FDA) in order to evaluate the safety and efficacy of pharmaceutical agents. In this paradigm, early (phase I) trials test the safety of a medication and often find the maximum tolerated dose (MTD) using a standard trial format. Intermediate-phase (phase II) trials demonstrate some measure of efficacy. The positive results of the prior phases lead to conducting a phase III randomized trial designed to test the superiority or noninferiority of the new agent compared to a current standard. If successful, this sequence of trials will lead to FDA approval of the agent and possibly inclusion of the agent in a new standard of care.

Clinical trials of IGIs are unique and differ from more traditional clinical trials in many ways. First, the safety of radiotherapy techniques is often not well assessed in a standard phase I trial, as the most concerning side effects tend to be relatively infrequent and develop at later time points. Second, radiotherapy innovation tends to require advanced technology, physics, and expertise that may not be widely available. Hence, the ability to disseminate the innovation to a broader community is a critical question that must be addressed. Additionally, the regulatory requirements for IGI and radiotherapy interventions are very different. Frequently, the IGI or radiotherapy technique is already approved or does not require approval. Thus, phase III trials may be difficult to conduct due to a lack of equipoise for investigators and patients and lack of funding—because phase III data are not routinely required to market the intervention or device. Finally, technology tends to advance faster than large trials can be performed. The techniques tested in large phase III trials may be obsolete by the time the results can be reported.

Due to clear limitations in applying the standard clinical trial paradigm, investigators need to approach clinical trials of IGI in an informed and thoughtful manner. It is important to note that although the framework may be somewhat different, it is still imperative that investigators proceed with high-quality clinical trials in order to develop these technologies, understand and demonstrate the safety and efficacy, and test the value of the intervention against the current standard of care.

EARLY PHASE CLINICAL TRIALS

The most common phase I clinical trial design is the 3 + 3 design (46). As discussed in Chapter 20, with this design, three patients are enrolled at a starting dose. If no patients experience a dose-limiting toxicity (DLT), the dose is escalated and three additional patients are treated at the higher dose level. If one patient experiences a DLT, three additional patients are accrued at that dose level. If no additional patients experience a DLT, the dose is increased again. If an additional patient experiences a DLT, the previous dose level is considered the MTD and will be recommended for the phase II trial. This trial design works relatively well for cytotoxic chemotherapy medications. However, there are multiple limitations for newer medications (46) and particularly for IGI trials (47).

Of particular concern for radiotherapy trials is the fact that severe toxicity is often relatively rare and can occur long after the conclusion of therapy. Stereotactic body radiotherapy (SBRT) for lung cancer is an important example of a breakthrough technology and the troubles that can delay its development (48,49). Early work in SBRT was done in a standard dose escalation fashion, using the canonical 3 + 3 paradigm. No acute DLTs were seen and the treatment was escalated to 6,000 cGy in three fractions (48).

However, in the subsequent phase II trial, 6 of 70 patients died from potential treatment-related side effects (49). Subsequent analysis found that the deaths occurred in patients with disease near the central airways. The median time to death for these patients was 12.4 months. Modifications were subsequently made to avoid high-dose SBRT to this area, which has greatly reduced the risk of fatal pulmonary hemorrhage from SBRT. The relative rarity and delay to onset of these toxicities demonstrates why the small numbers and short follow-up of a standard phase I trial are likely insufficient to assess severe late side effects of radiotherapy. An investigator who wishes to follow all patients through the late-effect time period before escalating the dose to the next dose level in a standard 3 + 3 model may find that the trial will take an impractically long time to complete and that the majority of patients will be treated at lower dose levels that may not be as effective (50).

As opposed to traditional "rule-based" phase I trial designs, toxicity "model-based" designs tend to be preferable for phase I IGI trials. Model-based designs include the continual reassessment method (CRM) and its derivatives (51–54), especially the **time to event CRM (TITE-CRM)** (50,55); these are discussed in detail in Chapter 16. The TITE-CRM requires the investigator to specify a predicted model of toxicity as a function of dose. Then patients are accrued and continually monitored for toxicity. After the expected number of patients per dose level is accrued, the trial advances to the next dose level without waiting until all patients have completed follow-up. As toxicities occur, the toxicity model is continually refined.

Advantages of the TITE-CRM model include faster accrual (50), more patients treated near the dose level the investigator expects to be effective (50), and a longer duration of follow-up for toxicity at the specified dose level (50). These models have been shown to provide accurate assessment of the MTD in a shorter period of time without increasing the risk to the patients (50). There is no one best methodology for phase I IGI trials, however. It is important to discuss the goals and statistical considerations with a trained biostatistician. In particular, the investigator should convey the level of concern for late toxicities and address methods to incorporate continued monitoring into the design of early and intermediate phase clinical trial designs.

INTERMEDIATE PHASE CLINICAL TRIALS

Intermediate (phase II) clinical trials for IGIs typically focus on demonstrating efficacy, with a component of continued safety and toxicity assessment. In this case, defining the endpoint of interest to assess efficacy is crucial. Because IGIs are often intended to improve the accuracy of a given locoregional therapy, it makes sense to analyze endpoints that evaluate the local treatment effects. These endpoints may focus on the target of the intervention—such as a tumor—or on adjacent organs that could potentially be damaged as a result of inaccurate treatment.

Endpoints may be technical in nature. For instance, investigators may seek to quantify the ability of an IGI to localize to a target by comparing the delivered treatment region to the intended region. This may be challenging, as it is sometimes difficult to define the treated tissues in vivo, due to uncertainty in real-time target and organ motion during treatment delivery. In such cases, clinical surrogate endpoints, such as local tumor control or adjacent organ injury, may be necessary to determine the accuracy of a given IGI. These clinical endpoints are often more clinically meaningful and also necessary when considering questions of comparative effectiveness.

However, the use of such clinical endpoints poses a timing issue. Many of these endpoints cannot be assessed immediately, instead often requiring years to decades to fully evaluate. This type of timeline is often problematic when assessing rapidly evolving IGIs. In such cases, it may be useful to employ early surrogate endpoints with imaging biomarkers such as tumor diameter on CT imaging or metabolic tissue response on posttreatment PET imaging. Trial endpoints will also vary depending on the intent of treatment. For instance, in a definitive therapy trial, early radiographic tumor response may serve as a convenient and quantifiable endpoint. However, in cases of adjuvant therapy in which there is no measurable target, other quantifiable parameters such as serologic markers may be more useful.

An important consideration for IGI trials is to assess the feasibility of the technique across institutions and providers with varying levels of technology and expertise. An important example of this is illustrated in the Radiation Therapy Oncology Group (RTOG) head and neck trial 0022. The purpose of this trial was to test the feasibility of **intensity-modulated radiation therapy (IMRT)** for the treatment of head and neck tumors. When this trial was designed, IMRT was a relatively novel technique that delivered radiation with much tighter dose gradients than more conventional radiation techniques. As such, IMRT allows more precise delivery of radiation therapy to head and neck tumors, with potential to spare surrounding sensitive normal tissues. However, this increased precision also increases the chance of missing the treatment target and thus requires greater care in ensuring treatment accuracy. This became evident to trial investigators when analyzing the locoregional failure outcomes. Although the overall rate of locoregional failure at 2 years was modest at 9%, the investigators found that two of the seven local failures were directly attributable to major deviations in treatment that led to inadequate tumor dose delivery (56). The investigators in this study were able to correctly recognize treatment inaccuracy as the source of poor clinical outcomes, but it is possible that one could draw an alternative conclusion that IMRT use leads to increased rates of local failure in head and neck cancer. Thus, this result raises the important consideration that experience and knowledge are critical to high-quality radiotherapy.

LATE PHASE CLINICAL TRIALS

Randomized phase III clinical trials are the cornerstone of evidence-based medicine. They provide the highest level of evidence of the effectiveness and safety of a treatment and establish its place within the standard of care. As such, testing an IGI in a phase III trial should ideally be performed prior to widespread adoption of the technique. That being said, there are several distinct difficulties in testing an IGI in a phase III trial.

As discussed earlier, most IGI or radiotherapy techniques will already have regulatory approval prior to completion of a phase III trial. Often, the technology appears clearly superior and therefore it may be unethical to enroll in a trial where one does not have equipoise. For example, proton therapy is a type of radiation therapy that frequently appears to have better radiation dose deposition (dosimetry) than photon radiotherapy, particularly in pediatric tumors. Many would argue that it is not ethical to randomize patients to what may be an inferior treatment that could lead to an increased rate of permanent, severe side effects and second cancers (57).

Another important consideration is cost. Randomized phase III trials can be incredibly expensive to conduct. In many pharmaceutical trials, a large company with significant financial backing would potentially earn the right to market the medication and hopefully earn a profit after a successful phase III trial. In contrast, IGI interventions are less likely to be supported by a large company, as many interventions are already marketable. Therefore, identifying funding sources can be a critical consideration for many late phase IGI trials. In some cases, the healthcare payor has a large financial incentive to test the value of a new intervention. For example, Canada and the United Kingdom have demonstrated exceptional leadership in clinical trials of shortened courses of radiotherapy (hypofractionated radiotherapy) for breast (58,59) and prostate cancer (60,61).

To successfully complete a randomized phase III trial of an IGI, an investigator needs to consider the most important principles. First, is a randomized phase III trial necessary to test the comparative effectiveness of the intervention and estimate its value to physicians, patients, regulatory agencies, and payors? Second, what endpoint should be used to assess the comparative effectiveness? Overall survival is often considered the gold standard for oncology trials, but it is worth considering whether a surrogate endpoint or cancer-specific endpoint would suffice to reduce the duration and cost of the clinical trial. Third, how common is the event of interest in the target population, and how large is the expected effect size of the intervention? Ideally, these questions will be informed by high-quality phase II trials. These factors will largely determine the required sample size for the trial. Fourth, will physicians and patients be willing to enroll on the trial (i.e., is there equipoise)? Fifth, are there sufficient patients at the investigator's institution, or will the trial have to be run through multiple institutions or a cooperative group setting? Finally, what funding source will support the trial?

To account for some of these potential issues in conducting IGI trials, numerous task groups have been formed to provide technical standards and guidelines for conducting clinical trials (62). The American Association of Physicists in Medicine (AAPM) recently published guidelines to define standards for various technical parameters involved in radiation therapy trials, including image acquisition, image registration, and motion assessment and management. Similarly, the Radiological Society for North America (RSNA) formed the Quantitative Imaging Biomarkers Alliance (QIBA) to develop standards for volumetric imaging including CT, PET, and MRI in clinical trials (63). The guidelines from these working groups provide important benchmarks that define acceptable amounts of variation in the technical parameters involved in IGIs used in clinical trials. These guidelines not only provide a useful template to follow for investigators looking to design new IGI trials, but also provide a helpful reference for scrutinizing previously published and emerging results of IGI clinical trials.

CONCLUSION

Imaging and IGIs are essential to the goal of eradicating cancer and maintaining quality of life for patients with the disease. The technologies that underlie these modalities continue to undergo exponential growth. However, the application of these technologies for human use requires a specialized set of skills. To succeed, investigators must understand both the fundamentals of their technologies and the science behind clinical trials. Fundamentally, the clinical trial is a critical mechanism that maintains the safety and well-being of patients throughout the process of developing new technologies with the capacity to help and to harm. Investigators need clinical trials to develop and refine their technologies, to establish the safety and efficacy of the modalities, and finally, to demonstrate their value and establish their place in the standard of care. No person can be an expert in all things, so successful investigations require close collaboration among engineers, physicists, physicians, statisticians, ethicists, regulatory agencies, and industry sponsors. There is no lack of technologic advancements in laboratories throughout the world. Hence, imaging and IGIs will remain at the forefront of cancer diagnosis and treatment as long as there are investigators with the skills and desire to continue to shape the future of the field.

GLOSSARY

sensitivity: refers to the probability that a technique will yield a positive result in a disease-positive patient.

specificity: refers to the probability that a technique will yield a negative result in a disease-negative patient.

positive predictive value (PPV):

$$PPV = \frac{\text{Sensitivity} \times \text{Prevalence}}{\text{Sensitivity} \times \text{Prevalence} + (1 - \text{Specificity}) \times (1 - \text{Prevalence})}$$

negative predictive value (NPV):

$$NPV = \frac{\text{Specificity} \times (1 - \text{Prevalence})}{(1 - \text{Sensitivity}) \times \text{Prevalence} + \text{Specificity} \times (1 - \text{Prevalence})}$$

kappa statistic: a commonly used metric for assessing agreement among readers for categorical outcomes.

intraclass correlation coefficient: a metric often used for assessing agreement among readers for continuous outcomes.

receiver operating characteristic (ROC) curve: for a diagnostic test, a plot of the true-positive rate (sensitivity) against the false-positive rate (1-specificity) for a range of possible cut points.

area under the curve (AUC): a metric of the overall performance or accuracy of ahe test given all possible cut points and their relative effects on sensitivity and specificity.

Wilcoxon statistic: an approach to estimating the area under the curve (AUC).

Mann-Whitney statistic: an approach to estimating the area under the curve (AUC).

likelihood ratio: ratio related to the sensitivity and specificity of a test.

positive likelihood ratio (LR+): indicates how much the likelihood of a subject having a disease increases with a positive test; can be found by the equation LR^+ = sensitivity/(1: specificity).

negative likelihood ratio (LR–): indicates how much the likelihood of a subject having a disease decreases with a negative test; can be found by the equation LR^- = (1: sensitivity)/specificity.

pretest probability (P_{pre}): refers to the probability that a subject has a disease prior to receiving a test.

posttest probability (P_{post}): the likelihood that the disease is present after considering the new test.

pseudoprogression refers to a phenomenon wherein the size of an enhancing glioblastoma transiently increases on MRI within the first 12 weeks of completion of radiation therapy.

surrogate endpoint: a response variable for which a test of the null hypothesis of no relationship to the treatment groups under comparison is also a valid test of the corresponding null hypothesis based on the true endpoint.

RECIST (Response Evaluation Criteria in Solid Tumors): a set of criteria for measuring the response of solid tumors to therapy.

PERCIST: a set of guidelines specifically designed to provide standardization of both implementation and assessment of FDG-PET response to cancer therapy.

iRECIST: an adaptation of the RECIST 1.1 criteria developed specifically to address the unique radiographic responses of some solid tumors to immunotherapies.

time to event CRM (TITE-CRM): method that requires the investigator to specify a predicted model of toxicity as a function of dose.

intensity-modulated radiation therapy (IMRT): a technique that delivers radiation with much tighter dose gradients than more conventional radiation techniques.

REFERENCES

1. Thornbury JR. Eugene W. Caldwell lecture. Clinical efficacy of diagnostic imaging: love it or leave it. *AJR Am J Roentgenol.* 1994;162(1):1–8. doi:10.2214/ajr.162.1.8273645
2. Fryback DG, Thornbury JR. The efficacy of diagnostic imaging. *Med Decis Making.* 1991;11(2):88–94. doi:10.1177/0272989X9101100203
3. Obuchowski NA, Gazelle GS. *Handbook for Clinical Trials of Imaging and Image-Guided Interventions.* Hoboken, NJ: John Wiley & Sons; 2016.
4. Sargent DJ, Rubinstein L, Schwartz L, et al. Validation of novel imaging methodologies for use as cancer clinical trial end-points. *Eur J Cancer.* 2009;45(2):290–299. doi:10.1016/j.ejca.2008.10.030
5. Basser PJ, Jones DK. Diffusion-tensor MRI: theory, experimental design and data analysis—a technical review. *NMR Biomed.* 2002;15(7–8):456–467. doi:10.1002/nbm.783
6. Assaf Y, Pasternak O. Diffusion tensor imaging (DTI)-based white matter mapping in brain research: a review. *J Mol Neurosci.* 2007;34(1):51–61. doi:10.1007/s12031-007-0029-0
7. Hao D, Ai T, Goerner F, et al. MRI contrast agents: basic chemistry and safety. *J Magn Reson Imaging.* 2012;36(5):1060–1071. doi:10.1002/jmri.23725
8. Baker HL, Houser OW, Campbell JK, et al. Computerized tomography of the head. *JAMA.* 1975;233(12):1304–1308. doi:10.1001/jama.1975.03260120066029
9. Hounsfield GN. Computerized transverse axial scanning (tomography): Part I. Description of system. *Br J Radiol.* 1973;46(552):1016–1022. doi:10.1259/0007-1285-46-552-1016
10. Kozlowski P, Chang SD, Jones EC, et al. Combined diffusion-weighted and dynamic contrast-enhanced MRI for prostate cancer diagnosis—correlation with biopsy and histopathology. *J Magn Reson Imaging.* 2006;24:108–113. doi:10.1002/jmri.20626
11. Haider MA, van der Kwast TH, Tanguay J, et al. Combined T2-weighted and diffusion-weighted MRI for localization of prostate cancer. *AJR Am J Roentgenol.* 2007;189(2):323–328. doi:10.2214/AJR.07.2211
12. Miao H, Fukatsu H, Ishigaki T. Prostate cancer detection with 3-T MRI: comparison of diffusion-weighted and T2-weighted imaging. *Eur J Radiol Open.* 2007;61(2):297–302. doi:10.1016/j.ejrad.2006.10.002
13. McCammack KC, Schenker-Ahmed NM, White NS, et al. Restriction spectrum imaging improves MRI-based prostate cancer detection. *Abdom Radiol.* 2016;41(5):946–953. doi:10.1007/s00261-016-0659-1
14. Zhou X-H, Obuchowski NA, McClish DK. *Statistical Methods in Diagnostic Medicine.* Hoboken, NJ: John Wiley & Sons; 2011.
15. Hanley JA, McNeil BJ. The meaning and use of the area under a receiver operating characteristic (ROC) curve. *Radiology.* 1982;143(1):29–36. doi:10.1002/9780470906514
16. Grimes DA, Schulz KF. Refining clinical diagnosis with likelihood ratios. *Lancet.* 2005;365(9469):1500–1505. doi:10.1016/S0140-6736(05)66422-7
17. Thornbury JR, Fryback DG, Edwards W. Likelihood ratios as a measure of the diagnostic usefulness of excretory urogram information. *Radiology.* 1975;114:561–565. doi:10.1148/114.3.561
18. Peters NHGM, van Esser S, van den Bosch MAAJ, et al. Preoperative MRI and surgical management in patients with nonpalpable breast cancer: the MONET–randomised controlled trial. *Eur J Cancer.* 2011;47:879–886. doi:10.1016/j.ejca.2010.11.035
19. The National Lung Screening Trial Research Team. Reduced lung-cancer mortality with low-dose computed tomographic screening. *N Engl J Med.* 2011;365:395–409. doi:10.1056/nejmoa1102873
20. Black WC, Gareen IF, Soneji SS, et al. Cost-effectiveness of CT screening in the National Lung Screening Trial. *N Engl J Med.* 2014;371(19):1793–1802. doi:10.1056/nejmoa1312547
21. Neumann PJ, Cohen JT, Weinstein MC. Updating cost-effectiveness—the curious resilience of the $50,000-per-QALY threshold. *N Engl J Med.* 2014;371(9):796–797. doi:10.1056/NEJMp1405158
22. Eisenhauer EA, Therasse P, Bogaerts J, et al. New response evaluation criteria in solid tumours: revised RECIST guideline (version 1.1). *N Engl J Med.* 2009;45(2):228–247. doi:10.1016/j.ejca.2008.10.026
23. Wen PY, Macdonald DR, Reardon DA, et al. Updated response assessment criteria for high-grade gliomas: response assessment in Neuro-Oncology Working Group. *J Clin Oncol.* 2010;28(11):1963–1972. doi:10.1200/JCO.2009.26.3541
24. Macdonald DR, Cascino TL, Schold SC, Cairncross JG. Response criteria for phase II studies of supratentorial malignant glioma. *J Clin Oncol.* 1990;8(7):1277–1280. doi:10.1200/JCO.1990.8.7.1277
25. Cascino TL, Kimmel DW, Dinapoli R. Report of four cases with a resolving syndrome which otherwise simulates recurrent brain tumor. In: Cascino TL, ed. *Neurology.* 1988;38:308.
26. Cairncross JG, Pexman JHW, Rathbone M. Post-surgical contrast enhancement mimicking residual tumor. *Can J Neurol Sci.* 1985;12(1):75. doi:10.1017/s031716710004664327.
27. Vredenburgh JJ, Desjardins A, Herndon JE II, et al. Bevacizumab plus irinotecan in recurrent glioblastoma multiforme. *J Clin Oncol.* 2007;25(30):4722–4729. doi:10.1200/JCO.2007.12.2440
28. Yung WK, Albright RE, Olson J, et al. A phase II study of temozolomide vs. procarbazine in patients with glioblastoma multiforme at first relapse. *Br J Cancer.* 2000;83(5):588–593. doi:10.1054/bjoc.2000.1316
29. Sorensen AG, Batchelor TT, Wen PY, et al. Response criteria for glioma. *Nat Clin Prac Oncol.* 2008;5(11):634–644. doi:10.1054/bjoc.2000.1316

30. Brandes AA, Franceschi E, Tosoni A, et al. MGMT promoter methylation status can predict the incidence and outcome of pseudoprogression after concomitant radiochemotherapy in newly diagnosed glioblastoma patients. *J Clin Oncol.* 2008;26(13):2192–2197. doi:10.1200/JCO.2007.14.8163
31. Prentice RL. Surrogate endpoints in clinical trials: definition and operational criteria. *Stat Med.* 1989;8(4):431–440. doi:10.1002/sim.4780080407
32. Freedman LS, Graubard BI, Schatzkin A. Statistical validation of intermediate endpoints for chronic diseases. *Stat Med.* 1992;11(2):167–178. doi:10.1002/sim.4780110204
33. Buyse M, Molenberghs G. Criteria for the validation of surrogate endpoints in randomized experiments. *Biometrics.* 1998;54(3):1014–1029. doi:10.2307/2533853
34. Bruzzi P, Del Mastro L, Sormani MP, et al. Objective response to chemotherapy as a potential surrogate end point of survival in metastatic breast cancer patients. *J Clin Oncol.* 2005;23(22):5117–5125. doi:10.1200/JCO.2005.02.106
35. Miller AB, Hoogstraten B, Staquet M, Winkler A. Reporting results of cancer treatment. *Cancer.* 1981;47(1):207–214. doi:10.1002/1097-0142(19810101)47:1<207::aid-cncr2820470134>3.0.co;2-6
36. Baar J, Tannock I. Analyzing the same data in two ways: a demonstration model to illustrate the reporting and misreporting of clinical trials. *J Clin Oncol.* 1989;7:969–978. doi:10.1200/JCO.1989.7.7.969
37. Tonkin K, Tritchler D, Tannock I. Criteria of tumor response used in clinical trials of chemotherapy. *J Clin Oncol.* 1985;3(6):870–875. doi:10.1200/JCO.1985.3.6.870
38. James K, Eisenhauer E, Christian M, et al. Measuring response in solid tumors: unidimensional versus bidimensional measurement. *J Natl Cancer Inst.* 1999;91:523–528. doi:10.1093/jnci/91.6.523
39. Therasse P, Eisenhauer EA, Verweij J. RECIST revisited: a review of validation studies on tumour assessment. *Eur J Cancer.* 2006;42(8):1031–1039. doi:10.1016/j.ejca.2006.01.026
40. Schwartz LH, Bogaerts J, Ford R, et al. Evaluation of lymph nodes with RECIST 1.1. *Eur J Cancer.* 2009;45(2):261–267. doi:10.1016/j.ejca.2008.10.028
41. Bogaerts J, Ford R, Sargent D, et al. Individual patient data analysis to assess modifications to the RECIST criteria. *Eur J Cancer.* 2009;45(2):248–260. doi:10.1016/j.ejca.2008.10.027
42. Wahl RL, Jacene H, Kasamon Y, Lodge MA. From RECIST to PERCIST: evolving considerations for PET response criteria in solid tumors. *J Nucl Med.* 2009;50(Suppl 1):122S–150S. doi:10.2967/jnumed.108.057307
43. Hyun J, Lodge MA, Wahl RL. Practical PERCIST: a simplified guide to PET response criteria in solid tumors 1.0. *Radiology.* 2016;280(2):576–584. doi:10.1148/radiol.2016142043
44. Seymour L, Bogaerts J, Perrone A, et al. iRECIST: guidelines for response criteria for use in trials testing immunotherapeutics. *Lancet Oncol.* 2017;18(3):e143–e152. doi:10.1016/S1470-2045(17)30074-8
45. Peters T, Cleary K, eds. *Image-Guided Interventions: Technology and Applications.* New York, NY; Springer; 2008.
46. Ivy SP, Siu LL, Garrett-Mayer E, Rubinstein L. Approaches to phase 1 clinical trial design focused on safety, efficiency and selected patient populations: a report from the Clinical Trial Design Task Force of the National Cancer Institute Investigational Drug Steering Committee. *Clin Cancer Res.* 2010;16:1726–1736. doi:10.1158/1078-0432.CCR-09-1961
47. Pijls-Johannesma M, van Mastrigt G, Hahn SM, et al. A systematic methodology review of phase I radiation dose escalation trials. *Radiother Oncol.* 2010;95:135–141. doi:10.1016/j.radonc.2010.02.009
48. Timmerman R, Papiez L, McGarry R, et al. Extracranial stereotactic radioablation: results of a phase I study in medically inoperable stage I non-small cell lung cancer. *Chest.* 2003;124:1946–1955. doi:10.1378/chest.124.5.1946.
49. Timmerman R, McGarry R, Yiannoutsos C, et al. Excessive toxicity when treating central tumors in a phase II study of stereotactic body radiation therapy for medically inoperable early-stage lung cancer. *J Clin Oncol.* 2006;24:4833–4839. doi:10.1200/JCO.2006.07.5937
50. Normolle D, Lawrence T. Designing dose-escalation trials with late-onset toxicities using the time-to-event continual reassessment method. *J Clin Oncol.* 2006;24:4426–4433. https://doi.org/10.1200/JCO.2005.04.3844
51. O'Quigley J, Pepe M, Fisher L. Continual reassessment method: a practical design for phase I clinical trials in cancer. *Biometrics.* 1990;46:33–48. doi:10.2307/2531628
52. O'Quigley J. Another look at two phase I clinical trial designs. *Stat Med.* 1999;18:2683–2690. doi:10.1002/(SICI)1097-0258(19991030)18:20<2683::AID-SIM193>3.0.CO;2-Z
53. Piantadosi S, Fisher J, Grossman S. Practical implementation of a modified continual reassessment method for dose-finding trials. *Cancer Chemother Pharmacol.* 1998;41:429–436. doi:10.1007/s002800050763
54. Goodman S, Zahurak M, Piantadosi S. Some practical improvements in the continual reassessment method for phase I studies. *Stat Med.* 1995;14:1149–1161. doi:10.1002/sim.4780141102
55. Cheung K, Chappell R. Sequential designs for phase I clinical trials with late-onset toxicities. *Biometrics.* 2000;56:1177–1182. doi:10.1111/j.0006-341X.2000.01177.x
56. Eisbruch A, Harris J, Garden AS, et al. Multi-institutional trial of accelerated hypofractionated intensity-modulated radiation therapy for early-stage oropharyngeal cancer (RTOG 00-22). *Int J Radiat Oncol Biol Phys.* 2010;76(5):1333–1338. doi:10.1016/j.ijrobp.2009.04.011
57. Sheehan M, Timlin C, Peach K, et al. Position statement on ethics, equipoise and research on charged particle radiation therapy. *J Med Ethics.* 2014;40:572–575. doi:10.1136/medethics-2012-101290
58. Whelan TJ, Pignol JP, Levine MN, et al. Long-term results of hypofractionated radiation therapy for breast cancer. *N Engl J Med.* 2010;362:513–520. doi:10.1056/NEJMoa0906260
59. Haviland JS, Owen JR, Dewar JA, et al. The UK Standardisation of Breast Radiotherapy (START) trials of radiotherapy hypofractionation for treatment of early breast cancer: 10-year follow-up results of two randomised controlled trials. *Lancet Oncol.* 2013;14:1086–1094. doi:10.1016/S1470-2045(13)70386-3
60. Dearnaley D, Syndikus I, Mossop H, et al. Conventional versus hypofractionated high-dose intensity-modulated radiotherapy for prostate cancer: 5-year outcomes of the randomised, non-inferiority, phase 3 CHHiP trial. *Lancet Oncol.* 2016;17:1047–1060. doi:10.1016/S1470-2045(16)30102-4

61. Catton CN, Lukka H, Gu CS, et al. Randomized trial of a hypofractionated radiation regimen for the treatment of localized prostate cancer. *J Clin Oncol.* 2017;35:1884–1890. doi:10.1200/JCO.2016.71.7397
62. Moran JM, Jeraj R, Molineu A, et al. *Guidance for the Physics Aspects of Clinical Trials: The Report of the AAPM Task Group 113.* https://www.aapm.org/pubs/reports/RPT_113.pdf. 2018.
63. Radiological Society of North America. Quantitative Imaging Biomarkers Alliance® (QIBA®). https://www.rsna.org/QIBA

26

Adaptive and Innovative Clinical Trial Designs

MARK CHANG ■ XUAN DENG ■ QIANG (ED) ZHANG

An **adaptive design** is a clinical trial design that allows adaptations or modifications to aspects of the trial after its initiation without undermining the validity and integrity of the trial (1,2). The PhRMA Working Group defines an adaptive design as a clinical study design that uses accumulating data to decide how to modify aspects of the study as it continues, without undermining the validity and integrity of the trial (3,4). Adaptive designs have been widely used in clinical trials, especially in oncology. During the course of adaptive design theory development, there have been many research advancements in design methodologies and numerous implementations of adaptive clinical trials. For reviews about adaptive designs, see Chow and Chang (5), Bauer et al. (6), Chang and Balser (7), Bhatt and Mehta, (8), Lin, Lin, and Sankoh (9), and Hatfield et al. (10).

TYPES OF ADAPTIVE DESIGNS

OVERVIEW

Types of adaptations may include, but are not limited to: (a) a group sequential design (GSD), (b) a sample-size adjustable design, (c) a drop-losers design, (d) an adaptive treatment allocation design, (e) an adaptive dose-escalation design, (f) a biomarker-adaptive design (BAD), (g) an adaptive treatment-switching design, (h) an adaptive dose-finding design, and (i) a combined adaptive design. An adaptive design usually consists of multiple stages. At each stage, data analyses are conducted, and adaptations are made based on updated information to maximize the probability of success. An adaptive design is also known as a *flexible design* (11).

An adaptive design has to preserve the trial's integrity and validity, both internal and external. **Integrity** involves creating a scientifically sound protocol design; minimizing operational bias; adhering firmly to the study protocol and standard operating procedures (SOPs); executing the trial consistently over time and across sites or countries; providing comprehensive analyses of trial data and unbiased interpretations of the results; and maintaining the confidentiality of the data. **Internal validity** is the degree to which we are successful in eliminating confounding variables and establishing a cause–effect relationship (treatment effect) within the study itself. **External validity** refers to the ability of a study's findings to be generalized to the population writ large.

From a regulatory perspective, the Food and Drug Administration (FDA) Center for Drug Evaluation and Research (CDER) and Center for Biologics Evaluation and Research (CBER) released a draft guidance on adaptive clinical trials for drugs and biologics in February 2010. In May 2016, the FDA Center for Devices and Radiological Heath (CDRH) and CBER issued the final guidance on adaptive medical device trials. The purpose of the final guidance is to provide clarity on how to plan and implement adaptive designs for clinical studies used in medical device development and to further encourage companies to use adaptive designs. Although both the device final guidance and drug and biologics draft guidance provided positive review of adaptive clinical trials, the final guidance position was stronger, stating that the FDA centers "further encourage companies to consider the use of ADs in their clinical trials." Both guidances emphasize the importance of preplanning to avoid type I error rate inflation, strict following of the plan to minimize operational bias, and frequent and early interactions with the FDA to ensure the success of planned adaptive clinical trials. Both guidances emphasize the utilities of clinical trial simulations (CTSs) in the design of adaptive clinical trials and in the analysis of adaptive trial data.

GROUP SEQUENTIAL DESIGN

A **group sequential design (GSD)** is an adaptive design that allows for premature termination of a trial due to efficacy or futility, based on the results of interim analyses. GSDs were originally developed to obtain clinical benefits under economic constraints. For a trial with a positive result, early stopping ensures that a new drug product can be exploited sooner. If a negative result is indicated, early stopping avoids waste of resources. Sequential methods typically lead to savings in sample size, time, and cost when compared with the classical design with a fixed sample size. Interim analyses also enable management to make appropriate decisions regarding the allocation of limited resources for continued development of a promising treatment. GSDs are one of the most commonly used adaptive designs in clinical trials.

Basically, there are three different types of GSDs: early efficacy stopping design, early futility stopping design, and early efficacy/futility stopping design. If we believe (based on prior knowledge) that the test treatment is very promising, then an early efficacy stopping design should be used. If we are very concerned that the test treatment may not work, an early futility stopping design should be employed. If we are not certain about the magnitude and direction of the effect size, a GSD permitting both early stopping for efficacy and futility should be considered. In practice, if we have a good knowledge regarding the effect size, then a classical design with a fixed sample size would be more efficient.

In general, the stopping rules in the interim of GSDs are given by:

- Stop for efficacy if $p_k \leq \alpha_k$
- Stop for futility if $p_k > \beta_k$
- Continue to the next stage if $\alpha_k < p_k \leq \beta_k$

where p_k is the p value at the kth interim analysis ($k = 1, \ldots, K$) in a GSD with K stages, α_k and β_k are the efficacy and futility **boundaries**, respectively, with $\alpha_k < \beta_k$ and $\alpha_k = \beta_k$, which satisfy the overall error rate control.

Commonly used boundaries include, but are not limited to: **Pocock boundary** (12), **O'Brien–Fleming boundary** (13), **Wang–Tsiatis boundary** (14), and **Lan–DeMets alpha spending function** (15). The Pocock boundary was designed for a test with the constant nominal alpha level at each interim analysis, and it only depends on the total number of planned interim analyses. The O'Brien–Fleming boundary is very conservative in the early analyses and the nominal test level increases as the study proceeds. Wang and Tsiatis proposed an approach with a shape parameter to allow several intermediate options between liberal (Pocock) and conservative (O'Brien–Fleming) boundaries. One of the shortcomings of those boundaries in GSDs is that they assume a fixed number of interim analyses with equally spaced information time, which could be violated in practice. Therefore, the alpha spending function was proposed to allow for more flexibilities, according to which the type I error is distributed as a function of information time, and the timing and number of analyses can be changed according to this prespecified spending function.

An example of the Pocock boundary was provided in a previous study (16). A trial was conducted in patients with non-Hodgkin lymphoma, in which two drugs, cytoxan–prednisone (CP) and cytoxan–vincristine–prednisone (CVP), were compared. The primary endpoint was binary response of presence/absence of tumor shrinkage. Patient accrual lasted over 2 years and 126 patients participated. Interim analyses were planned after approximately every 25 patients, resulting in five scheduled analyses. At each interim look, chi-square tests were performed; the corresponding p values are shown in Table 26.1. The trial was designed at 5% significance level, which produces the Pocock group sequential boundary of 0.0158 significance level at each analysis. Although the conventional significance value of 0.05 was exceeded in the fourth interim analysis, the efficacy boundary was not, so the trial continued. In the final stage, it did not lead to a statistically significant result with the Pocock boundary either.

A comprehensive review of these methods can be found in Jennison and Turnbull (17). Zhang, Freidlin, Korn, et al. (18) compared commonly used futility **stopping boundaries** using survival data from oncology trials.

SAMPLE SIZE REESTIMATION (SSR) DESIGN

SSR design refers to an adaptive design that allows for sample size adjustment or reestimation based on the review of interim analysis results (Figure 26.1). The sample size requirement for a trial is sensitive to the treatment effect and its variability. An inaccurate estimation of the effect size and its variability could lead to an underpowered or overpowered design, neither of which is desirable. If a trial is underpowered, it will not be able to detect a clinically meaningful difference, and consequently could prevent a potentially effective drug from being delivered to patients. In contrast, if a trial is overpowered, it could lead to unnecessary exposure of many patients to a potentially harmful compound when the drug, in fact, is not effective. In practice, it is often difficult to estimate the effect size and variability because of many uncertainties during protocol development. Thus, it is desirable to have the flexibility to reestimate the sample size in the middle of the trial.

TABLE 26.1 EXAMPLE OF POCOCK BOUNDARY

	Treatment Groups		
	CP	CVP	p value
Interim look 1	3/14	5/11	$p > .10$
Interim look 2	11/27	13/24	$p > .10$
Interim look 3	18/40	17/36	$p > .10$
Interim look 4	18/54	24/48	$.05 < p < .10$
Interim look 5	23/67	31/59	$.0158 < p < .10$

CP, cytoxan–prednisone; CVP, cytoxan–vincristine–prednisone.

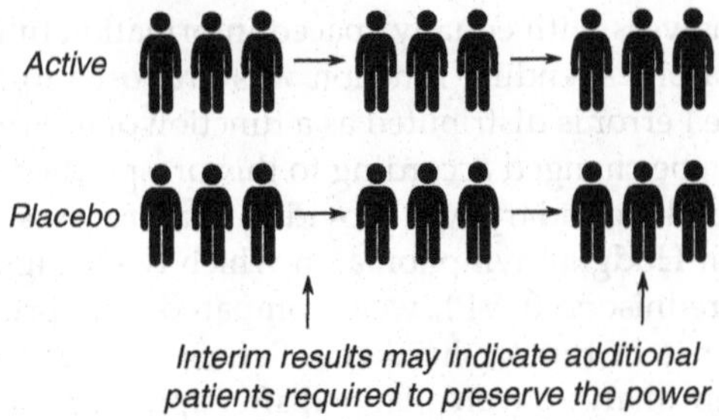

FIGURE 26.1 Sample size reestimation design.

There are two types of SSR procedures, namely, SSR based on **blinded data** and SSR based on **unblinded data**. In the first scenario, the sample size adjustment is based on the (observed) pooled variance at the interim analysis to recalculate the required sample size, which does not require unblinding the data. In this scenario, the type I error adjustment is practically negligible. In the second scenario, the effect size and its variability are reassessed, and sample size is adjusted based on the updated information. Note that the flexibility in SSR comes at the expense of a potential loss of power. Therefore, it is suggested that an SSR be used when there are no good estimates of the effect size and its variability. In the case where there is knowledge of the effect size and its variability, a classical design would be more efficient.

Here, we introduce two frequently used SSR methods: (a) SSR based on the observed effect size and (b) SSR based on the conditional power. The reestimated sample size based on the ratio of the initial estimate of effect size (E_0) to the observed effect size (E) is formulated as

$$N = \left|\frac{E_0}{E}\right|^2 N_0$$

where N_0 is the initial sample size based on E_0 to achieve the desired power in the classical clinical trial and N is the reestimated sample size based on the interim data E. In addition, the newly estimated sample size N should be smaller than the prespecified N_{max} according to the budget or the resources.

The **conditional power**, which is the probability of rejecting the null hypothesis at the end of the study given the observed interim data, is one crucial characteristic in an SSR design. The conditional power for a two-stage design is calculated by

$$cP = 1 - \Phi\left(B(\alpha_2, p_1) - \frac{\delta}{\sigma}\sqrt{\frac{n_2}{2}}\right), \alpha_1 < p_1 < \beta_1$$

where δ is the observed treatment difference and the B-function $B(\alpha_2, p_1)$ depends on the different methods used for the group sequential procedure (19). Then, the reestimated sample size for the following stage is given by

$$n_2^* = \begin{cases} \frac{2\sigma^2}{\delta^2}\left[B(\alpha_2, p_1) - \Phi^{-1}(1 - cP)\right]^2 & \text{if } \alpha_1 < p_1 < \beta_1 \\ 0, \text{otherwise} \end{cases}$$

When the sample size adjustment occurs in the interim, the traditional test statistic could lead to an inflation of the type I error rate. To prevent the error inflation, Cui et al. (20) proposed to use the Cui, Hung, and Wang (CHW) statistic instead of the conventional **Wald statistic**:

$$Z_{2,CHW}^{*} = \sqrt{\frac{n_1}{N_0}} Z_1 + \sqrt{\frac{n_2}{N_0}} Z_2$$

where n_1 and n_2 are the original sample sizes for the first and second stages, Z_1 and Z_2 are the Wald statistics based on the reestimated sample sizes n_1^* and n_2^* respectively. Other remedies to preserve the type I error in an SSR design are: (a) adjusting the stopping boundaries in the following stages through mathematical calculations (21) or simulations (22), and (b) adjusting the sample size only when the interim results are in the "promising zone" (23).

Consider the case study of the **V**osaroxin and **A**ra-C combination eva**L**uating **O**verall Survival in **R**elapsed/refractory acute myeloid leukemia (VALOR) trial using SSR in the promising zone presented by Cytel. The VALOR phase 3 trial was a double-blind, placebo-controlled, multinational trial with overall survival endpoint using a **two-stage promising zone design**. The study was designed to detect a hazard ratio of 0.71 requiring 375 events and 450 subjects with accrual of 19 per month. One interim analysis occurring at the information time of 0.5 takes place after 187 events with the adaption rule (also shown in Figure 26.2) as

- *Favorable*: stop early if there is overwhelming evidence of efficacy
- *Promising zone*: increase the number of events, sample size, and (if possible) rate of recruitment at the interim if results are promising
- *Unfavorable*: stop early for futility if the conditional power is low.

This way, the conventional CHW (20) weighted test statistic at the final stage can protect the type I error rate if the sample size adjustment only happens when the conditional power falls into the promising zone.

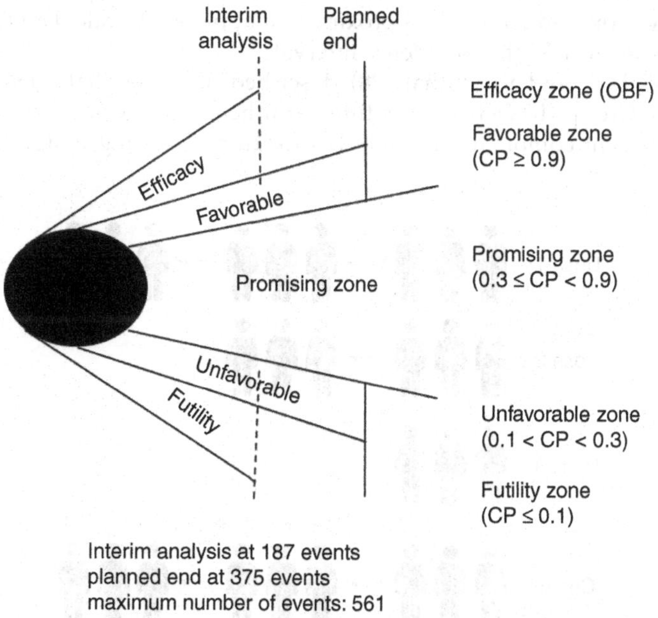

FIGURE 26.2 VALOR phase 3 trial: case study with promising zone design.

CP, cytoxan–prednisone; OBF, O'Brien–Fleming; VALOR, **V**osaroxin and **A**ra-C combination eva**L**uating **O**verall Survival in **R**elapsed/refractory acute myeloid leukemia.

DROP-THE-LOSER DESIGN

A **drop-the-loser design** (**DLD**) or **pick-the-winner design** is an adaptive design consisting of multiple stages. At each stage, interim analyses are performed and the losers (i.e., inferior treatment groups) are dropped based on prespecified criteria (Figure 26.3). Ultimately, the effective arm(s) are retained. If there is a control group, it is usually retained for comparison. This type of design can be used in phase II/III combined trials. Traditionally, a phase II trial is designed to test for treatment efficacy, and see if there is a significant treatment effect. Subsequently, the treatment will be tested in a phase III trial. This traditional approach is inefficient with respect to time and resources, however, because the phase II efficacy data are not pooled with data from phase III trials, which are useful for confirming efficacy. Therefore, it is desirable to combine phases II and III so that the data can be used efficiently, and the time required for drug development can be reduced.

Huang, Liu, and Hsiao proposed a seamless design to allow prespecifying probabilities of rejecting the drug at each stage to improve the efficiency of the trial (24,25). Posch, Maurer, and Bretz described two approaches to control the type I error rate in adaptive designs with sample size reassessment and/or treatment selection (26). The first method adjusts the critical value using a simulation-based approach that incorporates the number of patients at an interim analysis, the true response rates, the treatment selection rule, and so on. The second method is an adaptive **Bonferroni–Holm test** procedure (see also Chapter 11) based on conditional error rates of the individual treatment–control comparisons. They showed that this procedure controls the type I error rate, even if a deviation from a preplanned adaptation rule or the time point of such a decision is necessary.

Shun, Lan, and Soo considered a study starting with two treatment groups and a control group, with a planned interim analysis (27). In this design, the inferior treatment group is dropped after the interim analysis. Such an interim analysis can be based on the clinical endpoint or a biomarker. The unconditional distribution of the final test statistic from the "winner" treatment is skewed and requires numerical integration or simulations for the calculation. To avoid complex computations, they proposed a normal approximation approach to calculate the type I error, the power, the point estimate, and the confidence intervals.

Zhang, Wu, Harari, and Rosenthal (28) described a **phase II/III design** for Radiation Therapy Oncology Group (RTOG) 1216, a three-arm head and neck cancer trial in which the most effective treatment combination is selected for further testing if significant at the phase

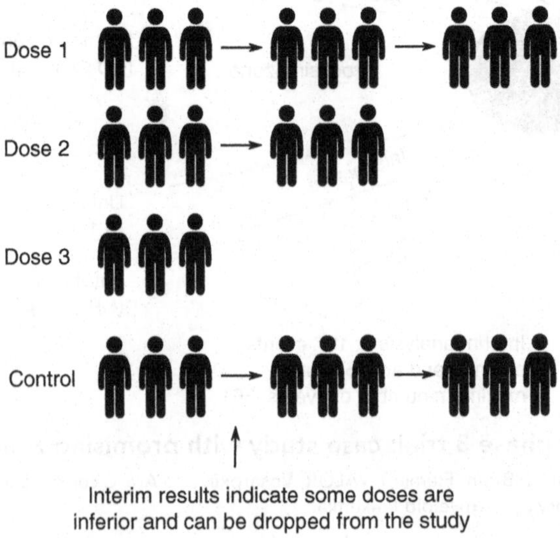
Dose 1
Dose 2
Dose 3
Control
Interim results indicate some doses are inferior and can be dropped from the study

FIGURE 26.3 Drop-the-loser design.

II final analysis. Progression-free survival and overall survival were the primary endpoints in phases II and III, respectively.

Heritier, Lo, and Morgan (29) studied the type I error control of **seamless unbalanced designs**, issues of noninferiority comparison, multiplicity of secondary endpoints, and covariance adjusted analyses. Further extensions of seamless designs that allow adaptive designs to continue seamlessly either in a subpopulation of patients or in the entire population based on data obtained from the first stage of a phase II/III design have also been developed. Jenkins, Stone, and Jennison (30) proposed a design that adds extra flexibility by allowing the trial to continue in all patients—but with both the subgroup and the full population as coprimary populations—when the phase II and III endpoints are different but correlated time-to-event endpoints (30). For a general *K*-group DLD, Chang and Wang (31) derived the distribution of the test statistic.

ADD-ARM DESIGN

In a pick-the-winner design, patients are randomized to all arms (doses) and at the interim analysis, inferior arms will be dropped. Compared to traditional dose-finding designs, this adaptive design can reduce the sample size by not carrying over all doses to the end of the trial or dropping the losers earlier. However, it does require that all the doses be explored. For unimodal response curves, Chang and Wang (31) proposed an effective adaptive dose-finding design that allows adding arms at the interim analysis. The trial design starts with two arms, and depending on the response of the two arms and the unimodality assumption, one can decide which are the new arms to be added. This design does not require exploration of all arms (doses) to find the best dose; therefore, it can further reduce the sample size compared to the DLD by as much as 20%.

Under a unimodal response, the Chang–Wang three-stage **add-arm design** is usually more powerful than the two-stage drop-arm design, primarily because the former takes advantage of the knowledge of unimodality of response. If the response is not unimodal, we can use that prior knowledge to rearrange the dose sequence so that it yields a unimodal response. In an add-arm design, all arms are usually selected with equal chance when all arms have the same expected response, but the probability of rejection is different even when all arms are equally effective. This feature allows us to effectively use the prior information to place more effective treatments in the middle, but at the same time the two arms in the first stage have a large enough separation in terms of response to increase the power. Moreover, dose levels do not have to be equally placed or based on the dose. The arms can be virtual dose levels or combinations of different drugs. Furthermore, the number of arms and the actual dose levels do not have to be prespecified; this can be decided after the interim analyses.

An add-arm design can further reduce the sample size from a pick-the-winner design, but it adds complexity to the trial: there are three stages in an add-arm design, but two stages in a pick-the-winner design. On the one hand, reducing the sample size will reduce the time for the trial. On the other hand, a staggered patient enrollment in three stages will take longer than enrolling patients for two stages.

An example of add-arm design for phase IV multiple-arm design in the multiple myeloma clinical trial was illustrated by Chang and Wang (31). Compared to the drop-arm design given the parameters they showed, the add-arm design requires 100 fewer subjects: a 17% savings in sample size. The authors also presented an application in a phase II dose-finding trial in iron deficiency anemia patients and an application of an add-arm design for a phase II/III seamless trial in asthma patients.

RESPONSE-ADAPTIVE RANDOMIZATION DESIGN

An **adaptive randomization/allocation design** (**ARD**) is a design that allows modification of randomization schedules during the conduct of the trial. In clinical trials, randomization is commonly used to ensure a balance with respect to patient characteristics among treatment groups. However, there is another type of ARD, called **response-adaptive randomization** (**RAR**), in which the allocation probability is based on the response of the previous patients.

RAR was initially proposed because of ethical considerations (i.e., to have a larger probability of allocating patients to a superior treatment group); however, response randomization can be considered a DLD with a seamless allocation probability of shifting from an inferior arm to a superior arm. The well-known response-adaptive models include the randomized **play-the-winner** (**RPW**) **model** (see Figure 26.4), an optimal model that minimizes the number of failures. Other RARs, such as utility-adaptive randomization, also have been proposed, which are combinations of response-adaptive and treatment-adaptive randomization (32). A more detailed review of this type of design can be found in Hu and Rosenberger (33). The two-arm RAR trial is not a popular design, however, due to power loss when the trial becomes imbalanced, and because of issues with unblinding (the randomization ratio indicates the effect size) and operation difficulties (too many analyses).

ADAPTIVE DOSE-FINDING DESIGN

Dose escalation is often considered in early phases of clinical development for identifying the **maximum tolerated dose (MTD)** for cancer patients. An *adaptive dose-finding* (or *dose-escalation*) *design* is a design in which the dose level used to treat the next-entered patient depends on the toxicity of previous patients, based on some traditional escalation rules. Many early dose-escalation rules are adaptive, but the adaptation algorithm is somewhat ad hoc. Recently, more advanced dose-escalation rules have been developed using modeling approaches (frequentist or Bayesian framework) such as the **continual reassessment method** (**CRM**) (32,34) and other accelerated escalation algorithms (see Chapter 20). These algorithms can reduce the sample size and overall toxicity in a trial and improve the accuracy and precision of the estimation of the MTD.

The CRM is a relatively monitor-intensive adaptive design, as it requires calculations to determine the next patient assignment based on the real-time data. When there is a delayed response, the efficiency of the design will be largely lost. The rule that no dose level can be skipped further reduces the efficiency of CRM designs. More sophisticated methods have been developed, including a model for dose finding for binary ordinal and continuous outcomes with monotone utility

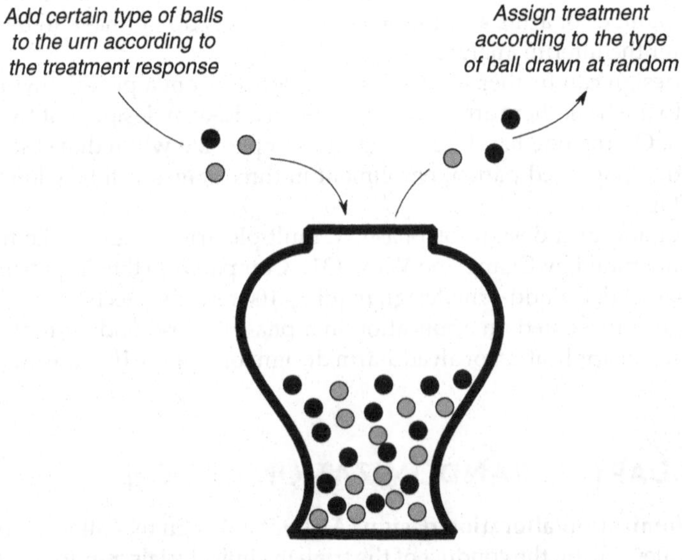

FIGURE 26.4 Response-adaptive randomization.

function (35), a method for cumulative cohort design for dose finding (36), a model calibration in the CRM (36,37), and CRM designs with efficacy–safety trade-offs (38–41). **Bayesian adaptive designs** with two agents in phase I oncology trials are studied by Thall et al. (42–44). Bayesian adaptive designs for different phases of clinical trials are also covered in the book by Berry, Carlin, Lee, and Muller (45).

BIOMARKER-ADAPTIVE DESIGN

A **biomarker-adaptive design (BAD)** refers to a design that allows for adaptations using information obtained from biomarkers. A **biomarker** is a characteristic that is objectively measured and evaluated as an indicator of normal biologic or pathogenic processes or pharmacologic response to a therapeutic intervention (46). A biomarker can be a **classifier** or **response** biomarker, and can be **prognostic** or **predictive** (see also Chapter 8).

A classifier biomarker is a test or assay that does not change over the course of the study. An example is 1p/19q codeletion, a prognostic molecular genetic signature in oligodendrogliomas. Classifier biomarkers can be used to select the most appropriate target population, or even for personalized treatment. It is often the case that a pharmaceutical company has to make a decision as to whether to target a highly selected population for whom the test drug likely works well, or to target a broader population for whom the test drug is less likely to work well. However, the size of the selected population may be too small to justify a benefit to the overall population. In this case, a BAD may be used, where the classifier can be used to determine which target populations to focus on.

A response biomarker may change over the course of the study. Often these may be blood tests; for example, Epstein–Barr virus (EBV) DNA in nasopharyngeal cancer. Elevated EBV DNA copy numbers both at baseline and posttreatment are associated with a poorer prognosis in this disease (47). The values of this biomarker may be used to assess response to therapy, and direct patients with persistently high levels after standard treatment to further risk-adapted therapy, such as in the NRG-HN001 trial design.

A prognostic biomarker informs the clinical outcomes, independent of treatment. One example is P16 positivity in oropharyngeal cancer, which tends to confer a better prognosis in this disease (48). Such biomarkers provide information about the natural course of the disease in individuals who have or have not received the treatment under study. Prognostic markers can be used to separate good- and poor-prognosis patients at the time of diagnosis. If expression of the marker clearly separates patients with an excellent prognosis from those with a poor prognosis, then the marker can be used to aid the decision about how aggressive the therapy should be.

A predictive biomarker informs the treatment effect on the clinical endpoint. A canonical example is the estrogen receptor (ER) in breast cancer, which is both prognostic (portends a more indolent natural history and superior prognosis) and predicts a benefit to the addition of ER blockade with tamoxifen and/or aromatase inhibitors.

Often response biomarkers are useful as surrogate endpoints. Compared to a gold-standard endpoint, such as overall survival, many biomarkers can be measured earlier, more easily, and more frequently. Imaging studies, such as positron emission tomography (PET), for example, can provide information about the metabolic activity of disease before and after treatment. Response on PET at 3 to 4 months post-therapy is a reliable marker of treatment failure in some diseases, such as cervical cancer (49). Surrogate response biomarkers can enable to decision making that is much faster than waiting for disease recurrence or mortality. In addition, surrogate biomarkers are less subject to noise from competing events and the cumulative impact of other treatment modalities. The consequence is a shorter time to accumulate events and larger effect sizes, which can substantially reduce trial sample size and cost. However, validating predictive biomarkers is often challenging.

The **biomarker-enrichment design** is discussed here as an example. The idea of such a design is to enroll all participants into the study regardless of their biomarker status, but an interim analysis will be conducted to identify whether the biomarker-positive patients react differentially to the treatment as compared to the biomarker-negative patients. If it appears that only the biomarker-positive patients are benefiting, then further enrollment would focus on the biomarker-positive subgroup. Otherwise, the overall patients would be recruited in the next stage. The final statistical analysis of the data would be based on information collected from the two stages with prespecified methods to prevent inflation of the type I error.

From the statistical perspective, let δ_+, δ_-, and δ denote the treatment difference between the test and control groups for biomarker-positive, biomarker-negative, and overall patients, respectively, and Z_+, Z_-, and Z denote the test statistics in these three groups. Then, we know that the test statistic in the overall population is

$$Z = Z_+\sqrt{\frac{n}{N}} + Z_-\sqrt{\frac{N-n}{N}}$$

where n and N are the sample sizes of the biomarker-positive patients and overall patients, and the correlation between Z and Z_+ is $\rho = \sqrt{\frac{n}{N}}$. For biomarker-enrichment design, the decision on whether the trial continues for the biomarker-positive patients or overall patients would depend on the information of Z_+, Z_-, and Z at the interim analysis. For more comprehensive information on biomarker-guided designs, see Wang, Chang, and Chow (50).

BASKET DESIGN

Cancer is a collection of diseases often defined by molecular subtypes with low prevalence. Thus, enrolling enough subjects for confirmatory trials with these indications is challenging. The current paradigm of "one indication at a time" in this instance is not sustainable. Patients may be better categorized by biomarker signatures than by tumor histology. However, such a shift to a molecular view of cancer requires a corresponding paradigm shift in drug development (51). For this reason, a new type of adaptive design, called a **basket design**, is being developed.

In a basket design, one drug is investigated for multiple disease indications—such as lung, breast, and colon cancers—in a single trial (52–56). A basket design trial consists of multiple stages and multiple tests for different disease indications; see, for example, a discussion of the DART trial (Chapter 9). Like the DLD, inactive indications (losers) are pruned at an interim analysis. Primary analysis is conducted in the pooled remaining population. A basket trial is ideal for testing if a drug is active in a subset of disease indications. Basket designs have been used in practice, but regulatory authorities deal with the design on a case-by-case basis. Type I error control is not necessarily strictly enforced by the regulatory agency in these cases. Rigorous statistical methodologies with type I control, however, are being developed (57).

CLINICAL TRIAL SIMULATION

CTS is a process that mimics clinical trials using computer programs. CTS is particularly important in adaptive designs for several reasons: (a) the statistical theory of adaptive design is complicated, with limited analytical solutions available under certain assumptions; (b) the concept of CTS is very intuitive and easy to implement; (c) CTS can be used to model very complicated situations with few assumptions and strongly controlled type I error; (d) using CTS, we can not only calculate the power of an adaptive design, but we can also generate many other important operating characteristics, such as expected sample size, conditional power, and repeated confidence interval (which ultimately leads to the selection of an optimal trial design or clinical development plan); (e) CTS can be used to study the validity and robustness of an adaptive design in different hypothetical clinical settings, or with protocol deviations; (f) CTS can be used to monitor trials, project outcomes, anticipate problems, and suggest remedies before it is too late; (g) CTS can be used to visualize the dynamic trial process from patient recruitment, drug distribution, treatment administration, and pharmacokinetic processes to biomarkers and clinical responses; and (h) CTS has minimal cost associated with it and can be done in a short time, compared with running a real clinical trial.

CONCLUSION

Adaptive trial designs represent a systematic approach to designing trials at different phases. The process streamlines and optimizes the development of novel therapeutics. In contrast, traditional methods typically comprise a weakly connected set of phase-wise processes. Adaptive trial design is a dynamic, decision-oriented process that permits real-time, sequential learning. It requires significant up-front planning and collaboration among the different parties involved in developing novel therapeutics. A major advantage is their flexibility, allowing for modifications that make them efficient, cost-effective, and robust against potential failures.

Adaptive designs are a revolution in pharmaceutical research and development that increases the probability of bringing successful treatments to market, with reduced cost. Bayesian designs and CTSs provide alternative, powerful tools for optimizing trial development. Together, this family of novel methodologies forms a powerful statistical instrument for the most successful development of new cancer therapies.

GLOSSARY

adaptive design (flexible design): a clinical trial design that allows adaptations or modifications to aspects of the trial after its initiation without undermining the validity and integrity of the trial.

integrity: in relation to a clinical trial, involves creating a scientifically sound protocol design; minimizing operational bias; adhering firmly to the study protocol and standard operating procedures (SOPs); executing the trial consistently over time and across sites or countries; providing comprehensive analyses of trial data and unbiased interpretations of the results; and maintaining the confidentiality of the data.

internal validity: the degree to which investigators are successful in eliminating confounding variables and establishing a cause–effect relationship (treatment effect) within the study itself.

external validity: the ability of a study's findings to be generalized to the population writ large.

group sequential design (GSD): an adaptive design that allows for premature termination of a trial due to efficacy or futility, based on the results of interim analyses.

boundaries: limits for decision making.

Pocock boundary: designed for a test with the constant nominal alpha level at each interim analysis; it only depends on the total number of planned interim analyses.

O'Brien–Fleming boundary: a boundary that is very conservative in the early analyses but increases the nominal test level as the study proceeds.

Wang-Tsiatis boundary: an approach with a shape parameter to allow several intermediate options between liberal and conservative boundaries.

Lan-DeMets alpha spending function: proposed to allow for more flexibilities in group sequential designs, according to which the type I error is distributed as a function of information time, and the timing and number of analyses can be changed according to this prespecified spending function.

stopping boundaries: points where clinical trials may be ended.

sample size reestimation (SSR) design: adaptive design that allows for sample size adjustment or reestimation based on a review of interim analysis results.

blinded data: data with information of subject treatment assignment.

unblinded data: data without information of subject treatment assignment.

conditional power: the probability of rejecting the null hypothesis at the end of the study given the observed interim data.

Wald statistic: a commonly used test statistic for a parametric test.

two-stage promising zone design: A sample size re-estimation design proposed by Mehta and Pocock in 2011, where sample-size is modified when the interim results are promising.

drop-the-loser design (DLD) (pick-the-winner design): an adaptive design consisting of multiple stages. At each stage, interim analyses are performed and the inferior treatment groups (losers) are dropped based on prespecified criteria.

Bonferroni–Holm test: A hypothesis test procedure that involves multiple hypothesis tests

phase II/III design: An adaptive design that combines a phase-II dose-find trial and a phase-III confirmatory trial.

seamless unbalanced design: An adaptive design that combines two different trials from two traditional phases.

add-arm design: adaptive trial design that takes advantage of the knowledge of unimodality of response.

adaptive randomization/allocation design (ARD): a trial design that allows modification of randomization schedules during conduct of the trial.

response-adaptive randomization (RAR): adaptive trial design in which the allocation probability is based on the response of the previous patients.

play-the-winner (RPW) model: an optimal adaptive design model that minimizes the number of failures.

maximum tolerated dose (MTD): The highest dose of a drug or treatment that does not cause unacceptable side effects. The maximum tolerated dose is determined in clinical trials by testing increasing doses on different groups of people until the highest dose with acceptable side effects is found.

continual reassessment method (CRM): an accelerated escalation algorithm that can reduce the sample size and overall toxicity in a trial and improve the accuracy and precision of the estimation of the maximum tolerated dose.

Bayesian adaptive designs: adaptive design that involve Bayesian statistical approach.

biomarker-adaptive design (BAD): a design that allows for adaptations using information obtained from biomarkers.

biomarker: a characteristic that is objectively measured and evaluated as an indicator of normal biologic or pathogenic processes or pharmacologic response to a therapeutic intervention.

classifier biomarker: a biomarker that does not change over the course of the study.

response biomarker: a biomarker that may change over the course of a study.

prognostic biomarker: biomarker that provides information about the natural course of the disease in individuals who have or have not received the treatment under study; informs the clinical outcomes, independent of treatment.

predictive biomarker: biomarker that informs the treatment effect on the clinical endpoint.

biomarker-enrichment design: a design in which all participants are enrolled into the study regardless of their biomarker status, but an interim analysis is conducted to identify whether the biomarker-positive patients react differentially to the treatment as compared to the biomarker-negative patients.

basket design: adaptive design that consists of multiple stages and multiple tests for different disease indications.

REFERENCES

1. Chang M. Adaptive clinical trial design. In: Janssen J, Lenca P. (eds.). *Proceedings of the XIth International Symposium on Applied Stochastic Models and Data Analysis.* Brest, France: École Nationale Supérieure des Télécommunications de Bretagne; 2005: 146.
2. Chow SC, Chang M, Pong A. Statistical consideration of adaptive methods in clinical development. *J Biopharm Stat.* 2005;15:575–591. doi:10.1081/BIP-200062277
3. Gallo P, Chuang-Stein C, Dragalin V, et al. Adaptive designs in clinical drug development. An executive summary of the PhRMA working group. *J Biopharm Stat.* 2006;16:275–283. doi:10.1080/10543400600614742
4. Dragalin V. Adaptive designs: terminology and classification. *Ther Innov Regul Sci.* 2006;40(4):425. doi:10.1177/216847900604000408
5. Chow CS, Chang M. Adaptive design methods in clinical trials—a review. *Orphanet J Rare Dis.* 2008;2(3):11. doi:10.1186/1750-1172-3-11
6. Bauer P, Bretz F, Dragalin V, et al. Twenty-five years of confirmatory adaptive designs: opportunities and pitfalls. *Stat Med.* 2016;35: 325–347. doi:10.1002/sim.6472
7. Chang M, Balser J. Adaptive design—recent advancement in clinical trials. *J Bioanal Biostat.* 2016;1–14.
8. Bhatt, DL, Mehta C. Adaptive designs for clinical trials. *N Engl J Med.* 2016;375:1. doi:10.1056/NEJMra1510061
9. Lin J, Lin LA, Sankoh S. A general overview of adaptive randomization design for clinical trials. *J Biom Biostat.* 2016;7:2. doi:10.4172/2155-6180.1000294
10. Hatfield I, Allison A, Flight L, et al. (2016). Adaptive designs undertaken in clinical research: a review of registered clinical trials. *Trials.* 2016;17:150. doi:10.1186/s13063-016-1273-9
11. EMEA European Medicines Agency. *Reflection Paper on Methodological Issues in Confirmatory Clinical Trials with Flexible Design and Analysis Plan. The European Agency for the Evaluation of Medicinal Products Evaluation of Medicines for Human Use.* London, UK; Author; 2006.
12. Pocock SJ. Group sequential methods in the design and analysis of clinical trials. *Biometrika.* 1977;64:191–199. doi:10.1093/biomet/64.2.191
13. O'Brien PC, Fleming TR. A multiple testing procedure for clinical trials. *Biometrika.* 1979;35:549–556. doi:10.2307/2530245
14. Wang SK, Tsiatis AA. Approximately optimal one-parameter boundaries for sequential trials. *Biometrics.* 1987;43:193–200. doi:10.2307/2531959
15. Lan KKG, DeMets DL. Discrete sequential boundaries for clinical trials. *Biometrika.* 1983;70:659. doi:10.2307/2336502
16. Pocock SJ. *Clinical Trials: A Practical Approach.* Chichester, UK; John Wiley & Sons; 1983.
17. Jennison C, Turnbull BW. (2000). *Group sequential tests with applications to clinical trials.* London/Boca Raton, FL: Chapman & Hall.
18. Zhang Q, Freidlin B, Korn EL, et al. Comparison of futility monitoring guidelines using completed phase III oncology trials. *Clin Trials.* 2017;14(1):48–58. doi:10.1177/1740774516666502
19. Chang, M. (2012). *Modern issues and methods in biostatistics.* New York, NY: Springer Publishing.
20. Cui L, Hung HM, Wang SJ. Modification of sample size in group sequential clinical trials. *Biometrics.* 1999; 55:853–857. doi:10.1111/j.0006-341X.1999.00853.x
21. Shun Z. Stopping boundaries adjusted for sample size reestimation and negative stop. *J Biopharm Stat.* 2002;12(4):485–502. doi:10.1081/BIP-120016232
22. Chang M. *Adaptive Design Theory and Implementation Using SAS and R.* 2nd ed. Boca Raton, FL: Chapman & Hall/CRC, Taylor & Francis; 2014.
23. Mehta CR, Pocock SJ. Adaptive increase in sample size when interim results are promising: a practical guide with examples. *Stat Med.* 2011;30(28):3267–3284. doi:10.1002/sim.4102
24. Bretz F, Schmidli H, Konig F, et al. Confirmatory seamless phase II/III clinical trials with hypotheses selection at interim: general concepts. *Biom J.* 2006;48:623–634. doi:10.1002/bimj.200510232
25. Huang WS, Liu JP, Hsiao CF. An alternative phase II/III design for continuous endpoints. *Pharm Stat.* 2011;10:105–114. doi:10.1002/pst.418
26. Posch M, Maurer W, Bretz F. Type I error rate control in adaptive designs for confirmatory clinical trials with treatment selection at interim. *Pharm Stat.* 2011;10:96–104. doi:10.1002/pst.413

27. Shun Z, Lan KK, Soo Y. Interim treatment selection using the normal approximation approach in clinical trials. *Stat Med.* 2008;27:597–618. doi:10.1002/sim.2990
28. Rosenthal DI, Zhang Q, Kies MS, et al. Seamless phase II/III trial design with survival and PRO endpoints for treatment selection: Case study of RTOG 1216 (abstr.). *J Clin Oncol.* 2013;31:15(suppl). doi:10.1200/jco.2013.31.15_suppl.tps6099
29. Heritier S, Lô SN, Morgan CC. An adaptive confirmatory trial with interim treatment selection: practical experiences and unbalanced randomisation. Stat Med. 2011;30:1541–1554. *doi:10.1002/sim.4179*
30. Jenkins M, Stone A, Jennison C. An adaptive seamless phase II/III design for oncology trials with subpopulation selection using correlated survival endpoints. *Pharm Stat.* 2011;10:347–356. doi:10.1002/pst.472
31. Chang M, Wang J. The add-arm design for unimodal response curve with unknown mode. *J Biopharm Stat.* 2015;25:1039–1064. doi:10.1080/10543406.2014.971164
32. Chang M, Chow SC. A hybrid Bayesian adaptive design for dose response trials. *J Biopharm Stat.* 2005;15:667–691. doi:10.1081/BIP-200062288
33. Hu F, Rosenberger WF. *The Theory of Response-Adaptive Randomization in Clinical Trials.* 1st ed. Hoboken, NJ: Wiley-Interscience; 2006.
34. O'Quigley J, Pepe M, Fisher L. Continual reassessment method: A practical design for phase I clinical trial in cancer. *Biometrics.* 1990;46:33–48. doi:10.2307/2531628
35. Ivanova A, Kim SH. Dose finding for continuous and ordinal outcomes with a monotone objective function: a unified approach. *Biometrics.* 2009;65:307–315. doi:10.1111/j.1541-0420.2008.01045.x
36. Ivanova A, Flournoy N, Chung Y. Cumulative cohort design for dosefinding. *J Stat Plan Inference.* 2007;137:2316–2317. doi:10.1016/j.jspi.2006.07.009
37. Lee SM, Cheung YK. Model calibration in the continual reassessment method. *Clin Trials.* 2009;6:227–238. doi:10.1177/1740774509105076
38. Thall PF, Cook JD. Dose-finding based on efficacy-toxicity trade-offs. *Biometrics.* 2004;60:684–693. doi:10.1111/j.0006-341X.2004.00218.x
39. Thall PF, Cook JD, Estey EH. Adaptive dose selection using efficacy/toxicity trade-offs: illustrations and practical considerations. *J Biopharm Stat.* 2006;16:623–638. doi:10.1080/10543400600860394
40. Yin G, Li Y, Ji Y. Bayesian dose-finding in phase I/II clinical trials using toxicity and efficacy odds ratios. *Biometrics.* 2006;62:777–784. doi:10.1111/j.1541-0420.2006.00534.x
41. Zhang W, Sargent DJ, Mandrekar S. An adaptive dose-finding design incorporating both toxicity and efficacy. *Stat Med.* 2006;25:2365–2383. doi:10.1002/sim.2325
42. Thall PF, Millikan RE, Muller P, Lee SJ. Dose-finding with two agents in phase I oncology trials. *Biometrics.* 2003;59:487–496. doi:10.1111/1541-0420.00058
43. Yin G, Yuan Y. A latent contingency table approach to dose finding for combinations of two agents. *Biometrics.* 2009;65:866–875. doi:10.1111/j.1541-0420.2008.01119.x
44. Yin G, Yuan Y. Bayesian dose finding in oncology for drug combinations by copula regression. *J R Stat Soc Ser C Appl Stat.* 2009;58:211–224. doi:10.1111/j.1467-9876.2009.00649.x
45. Berry SM, Carlin BP, Lee JJ, Muller P. *Bayesian Adaptive Methods for Clinical Trials.* Boca Raton, FL: Taylor and Francis Group/CRC Press; 2011.
46. Chakravarty A. Regulatory aspects in using surrogate markers in clinical trials. In: Burzykowski T, Molenberghs G, Buyse M, eds. *The Evaluation of Surrogate Endpoint.* New York, NY; Springer; 2005.
47. Lin JC, Wang WY, Chen KY, et al. Quantification of plasma Epstein-Barr virus DNA in patients with advanced nasopharyngeal carcinoma. *N Engl J Med.* 2004;350(24):2461–2470. doi:10.1056/NEJMoa032260
48. Ang KK, Harris J, Wheeler R, et al. Human papillomavirus and survival of patients with oropharyngeal cancer. *N Engl J Med.* 2010;363(1):24–35. doi:10.1056/nejmoa0912217
49. Schwarz JK, Siegel BA, Dehdashti F, Grigsby PW. Association of posttherapy positron emission tomography with tumor response and survival in cervical carcinoma. *JAMA.* 2007;298(19):2289–2295. doi:10.1001/jama.298.19.2289
50. Wang J, Chow SC, Chang M. Biomarker-driven adaptive design for precision medicine. *J Trans Biomarkers Diag.* 2016;2(1):15–24.
51. Chen C. *Two-Stage Adaptive Design of a Confirmatory Basket Trial.* Washington, DC: ENAR Spring Meetings; 2017.
52. Chen C, Li X, Yuan S, et al. Statistical design and considerations of a phase 3 basket trial for simultaneous investigation of multiple tumor types in one study. *Stat Biopharm Res.* 2016;8(3):248–257. doi:10.1080/19466315.2016.1193044
53. Beckman RA, Antonijevic Z, Kalamegham R, Chen C. Design for a basket trial in multiple tumor types based on a putative predictive biomarker. *Clin Pharmacol Ther.* 2016;100(6):617–625. doi:10.1002/cpt.446
54. Chen C. Two-stage Adaptive Design of a Confirmatory Basket Trial. ENAR Spring Meetings, 3/12-15, 2017, Washington, DC; 2017.
55. Simon R, Geyer S, Subramanian J. "The Bayesian Basket Design for Genomic Variant-Driven Phase II Trials." *Semin Oncol.* 2016;43:13–18.
56. Beckman RA, Antonijevic Z, Kalamegham R, Chen C. Adaptive design for a confirmatory basket trial in multiple tumor types based on a putative predictive biomarker. *Clin Pharmacol Ther.* 2016;100(6):617–625. doi:10.1002/cpt.446
57. Chen C, Li X, Yuan S, et al. Statistical design and considerations of a phase 3 basket trial for simultaneous investigation of multiple tumor types in one study. *Stat Biopharm Res.* 2016;8(3):248–257. doi:10.1080/19466315.2016.1193044

27

Noninferiority and Equivalence Trials

TIE-HUA NG

GOLD STANDARD FOR ASSESSING TREATMENT EFFICACY

A randomized double-blind placebo-controlled trial is usually considered the gold standard for assessing treatment efficacy. In such a trial, subjects are randomly assigned to either the test treatment or the placebo. "The purpose of randomization is to avoid selection bias and to generate groups which are comparable to each other" (1). Without randomization, the investigators could preferentially (either intentionally or unintentionally) enroll subjects into a particular group. With randomization, unobservable covariates that affect the outcome are also more likely to be distributed equally between the two groups; thus, randomization minimizes the allocation bias.

Double blinding means both the investigator/evaluator and the participant are unaware of the treatment assignment (i.e., experimental treatment or placebo). Without double blinding, the results may be subjected to potential bias, especially if the outcome variable is subjective. Whenever feasible, it is critical that randomization be properly executed and blinding be adequate, to ensure that any observed differences (beyond random chance) can be attributed to the experimental treatment. Lack of proper randomization and/or inadequate blinding may render the results uninterpretable due to various biases, which are very difficult, if not impossible, to assess and account for.

WHY ACTIVE-CONTROL TRIALS?

Equivalence trials as such emerged as early as 1973 (2,3). The term *noninferiority* began to emerge in the late 1990s, as indicated in Figure 27.1, which shows the number of publications appearing on PubMed referring to "noninferiority or non-inferiority," indicating the increasing research interest in this area over the past two decades.

When effective treatment is available in life-threatening disease such as cancer, **placebo-controlled trials** may be regarded as unethical (4). Therefore, an active control rather than placebo control is often used in such situations, with the objective to show that the experimental treatment produces the same benefit as the active control. The term **active control equivalence studies (ACESs)** is attributed to Makuch and Johnson (5). Note that equivalence trials might also be

The views expressed in Chapter 27 are those of the author and should not be construed to represent FDA's views or policies.

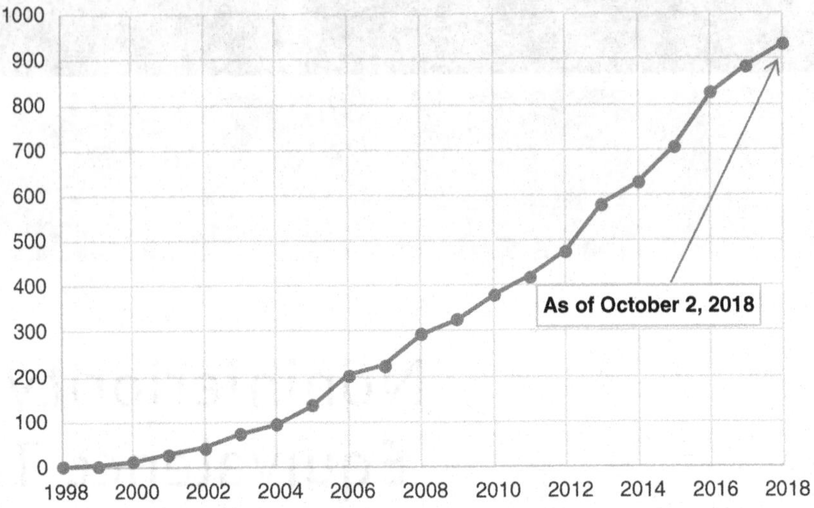

FIGURE 27.1 Numbers of publications by year.

conducted for other reasons (e.g., comparing two formulations). The objective of an ACES is to show there are no differences between the two treatments, that is, to rule out the possibility that the test treatment is worse or better than the control. It is, in some sense, two-sided. However, the intention of most ACESs is to rule out the possibility that the test treatment is worse than the control. It is, in some sense, one-sided.

PLACEBO CONTROL VERSUS ACTIVE CONTROL

For a placebo-controlled trial, the null hypothesis is that there is no difference between test treatment and placebo. This null hypothesis is usually tested at two-sided 0.05 or one-sided 0.025 significance level. Apart from randomization and blinding, there is an incentive to conduct high-quality studies, because poorly conducted studies (e.g., mixing up treatment assignment, poor compliance) are less likely to detect a true difference, due to increased variability and **bias toward the null**. Despite the many scientific merits of placebo-controlled trials, such trials have been controversial on ethical grounds, as more effective treatments are brought into the market. To wit, the Declaration of Helsinki (6) essentially called for an active-control trial rather than a placebo-controlled trial whenever effective treatments are available.

For an active-control trial, if the objective is to show the superiority of test treatment over the active control, the statistical principle in hypothesis testing is the same as that in the placebo-controlled trial. However, many issues arise if the objective is to show that the test treatment is similar to or not inferior to the active control, the so-called **equivalence/noninferiority trial**. These issues have been widely recognized in the literature since the early 1980s (7–12).

There is a consensus that the use of placebo should be prohibited when an intervention that has been shown to improve survival or decrease serious morbidity is available (13–15). Recognizing the inherent difficulties in an ACES, these authors elaborate on different scenarios in which the use of a placebo may be ethical, even when there is an effective treatment. Note that the current version of the declaration (16) allows the use of placebo (or no treatment) (a) when there is no effective treatment or (b) under certain scenarios even when there is an effective treatment (11).

These difficulties arise in an ACES but not in placebo-controlled trials (or superiority trials) as they relate to a property of studies called **assay sensitivity** (17). Assay sensitivity is defined as *the ability to distinguish an effective treatment from placebo*. A successful placebo-controlled trial has assay sensitivity, which is not the case for an ACES. Showing equivalence of the test treatment and the control may indicate that both treatments are equally ineffective. Therefore, an ACES requires external data to establish assay sensitivity, unless a placebo arm is also included in the study.

SAMPLE SIZE DETERMINATION

Sample size determination under conventional hypothesis testing in a *placebo-controlled* trial involves specifications of **type I** (α) and **type II** (β) **error** rates, and a **treatment effect** δ_0, where δ_0 is the assumed effect size at which the power (i.e., $1 - \beta$) is calculated. In practice, specification of α and β is based on convention. The value of δ_0 may be arbitrary; however, it is recommended that it be realistically chosen based on prior evidence of some potential difference.

Feinstein (18) noted, however, that

> *What often happens is that the statistician and investigator decide on the size of δ_0. The magnitude of the sample is then chosen to fit the two requirements (1) that the selected number of patients can actually be obtained for the trial and (2) that their recruitment and investigation can be funded.*

To specify δ_0, the paper continued: "In the absence of established standards, the clinical investigator picks what seems like reasonable value . . . . If the sample size that emerges is unfeasible, δ_0 gets adjusted accordingly, and so do α and β, until n comes out right." Spiegelhalter and Freedman (19) summarized this practice in the specification of δ_0 thus:

> *There is very little explicit guidance as to how to set δ_0, and in practice it seems likely that δ_0 is juggled until it is set at a value that is reasonably plausible, and yet detectable given the available patients.*

Others have referred to tinkering with statistical parameters to meet budgetary and time constraints as the "**sample size samba**" (20).

In the regulatory environment, α-level of one-sided 0.025 or two-sided 0.05 is the standard, and the study is typically powered at 80% or 90%. In reality, the estimate of the variability of the continuous endpoint or the background rate for the binary endpoint—or the number of events for the **time-to-event data** (see Chapter 16)—also plays a role in the sample size calculation. Once the sample size is determined and the study is completed, δ_0 does not play any role in the statistical analyses or inferences. The null hypothesis of equality is either rejected or not. No inference may be made about δ_0 when the null hypothesis is rejected, although point estimate and confidence interval provide information regarding the effect size.

It should be noted that a value of δ_0 that is too small would result in a very large sample size, which is a waste of valuable resources. Furthermore, this may lead to an undesirable outcome where the treatment difference is statistically significant but it is too small to be clinically meaningful. δ_0 is often set equal to a difference of undisputed clinical importance (i.e., **clinical significance**), which may be above the minimum difference of clinical interest by a factor of perhaps two or more. There may be scientific reasons to expect a treatment to have more than a minimal effect (21).

In contrast, the purpose of an ACES is to show that a given treatment is sufficiently similar to (or not too much worse than) the standard therapy, in order to be regarded as clinically indistinguishable (or noninferior). Therefore, the margin δ should be smaller than δ_0 (21–24). Jones et al. (21) suggest that δ be no larger than half of δ_0, leading to sample sizes roughly four times as large as those in similar placebo-controlled trials.

It should be noted that in the comparison of the test treatment against the standard therapy, showing **superiority** is harder than showing noninferiority, because the superiority is a stronger condition, in the sense that superiority implies noninferiority, but not vice versa. Therefore, under the same assumptions, the sample size for showing noninferiority is smaller than the sample size for showing superiority. This appears to be contrary to the preceding paragraph. However, the two scenarios are different. In the former scenario, noninferiority is in comparison with the standard therapy, whereas superiority is in comparison with placebo. In the latter scenario, both noninferiority and superiority are in comparison with the standard therapy.

NOTATIONS AND ASSUMPTIONS

In this chapter, T denotes the value of a primary event or metric of interest in the *test* or experimental group, S denotes the same value in the *standard* therapy (or the active control) group, and P denotes the value in the *placebo* group. Furthermore, assume that there is no concurrent placebo control, due to ethical reasons in life-threatening situations such as cancer trials. Note that T, S, and P could be the true mean responses for continuous outcomes, the true success rates (or proportions of successes) for binary outcomes, or the hazard function for time-to-event outcomes.

For an individual subject, the hazard function (or rate) at time t represents the instantaneous risk of an event at time t given that the subject has not had an event by time t (10); see Chapter 16 for further discussion. Assuming that the hazard functions for the two arms (T versus S; or S versus P) are proportional, the common ratio of the hazard functions is called the *hazard ratio*.

STATISTICAL HYPOTHESES

Although many, if not most, primary outcomes in cancer research are considered on the time-to-event scale, for ease and better understanding of the noninferiority concept, the majority of the discussion in this chapter considers mean differences, rather than hazard ratios. For example, tumor size may be a continuous endpoint of interest in cancer research, with the treatment effect expressed as the mean difference in tumor size. The mean ratio for the continuous outcomes and the hazard ratio for time-to-event outcomes are discussed later in this chapter. See Ng (11) for a discussion on binary outcomes.

STATISTICAL HYPOTHESES BASED ON THE MEAN DIFFERENCE

EQUIVALENCE HYPOTHESES (MEAN DIFFERENCE)

It is well recognized that it is not possible to show absolute equality of two means (9,24–27). Instead, hypotheses are formulated to show that the absolute mean difference is less than a prespecified $\delta > 0$. More specifically, the null hypothesis

$$H_0\colon\ |T - S| \geq \delta$$

is tested against the alternative hypothesis

$$H_A\colon\ |T - S| < \delta$$

Note the difference in the specification of the null hypothesis compared to a superiority trial (i.e., $H_0\colon |T - S| = 0$).

The **two one-sided tests procedure** (28–30) and the **confidence interval approach** are often used for testing this null hypothesis (11,25). Briefly, the aforementioned hypotheses may be decomposed into two one-sided hypotheses. If both of the decomposed null hypotheses are rejected at a significance level of a, then the original hypotheses will be rejected at the same significance level. This amounts to rejecting the original null hypothesis, if the $100(1 - 2a)\%$—*not* $100(1 - a)\%$—confidence interval for the difference $(T - S)$ completely falls inside the interval $(-\delta, \delta)$.

NONINFERIORITY HYPOTHESES (MEAN DIFFERENCE)

Assuming that a larger response corresponds to a better outcome, $T - S \geq 0$ means that the test treatment is at least as good as the standard therapy, or equivalently, the test treatment is not inferior to the standard therapy. However, it is not possible to show noninferiority literally in the sense

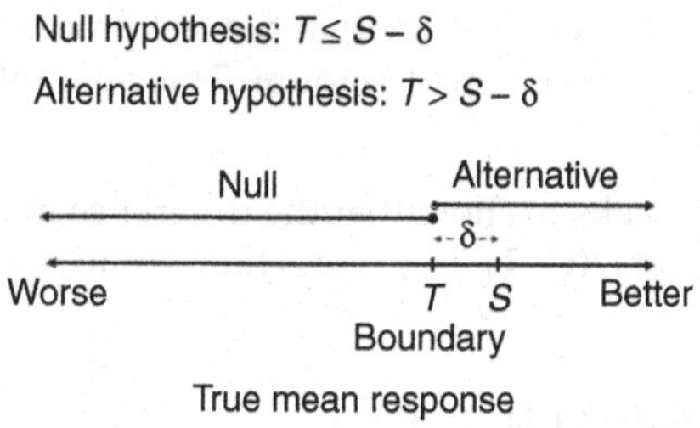

FIGURE 27.2 Hypotheses.

that $T - S \geq 0$, as the null hypothesis must include a boundary (11). Therefore, for noninferiority, we test the null hypothesis,

$$H_0: T - S \leq -\delta$$

against the alternative hypothesis,

$$H_A: T - S > -\delta$$

These hypotheses are shown graphically in Figure 27.2, where the axis is the true mean response, and the treatment gets better as we move to the right, and worse if we move to the left. At the boundary, we have $T = S - \delta$. The null hypothesis is to the left of this boundary inclusively, and the alternative hypothesis is to the right of the boundary. The noninferiority null hypothesis is rejected if the one-sided $100(1 - a)\%$ lower confidence limit for the difference $(T - S)$ exceeds $-\delta$.

NONINFERIORITY/EQUIVALENCE MARGIN δ

EQUIVALENCE MARGIN δ

A list of definitions of δ found in the literature is given by Ng (11). Many definitions relate δ to a clinical judgment or other benefits. The International Conference on Harmonization (ICH) E10 document (17) refers to δ as the *degree of inferiority* of the test treatment to the control, which the trial attempts to exclude statistically. It says exactly what the statistical inference does. The document then states that if the confidence interval for the difference between the test and control treatments excludes a degree of inferiority of the test treatment as large as, or larger than, the margin, the test treatment can be declared noninferior. There is no problem with this statement if δ is small, but it could be misleading if δ is too large (25).

The distinction between *equivalence* and *noninferiority* is a common point of confusion. In the 1990s, most ACESs were not recognized as a one-sided version of equivalence. For example, ICH E10 states the following (17):

> *Clinical trials designed to demonstrate efficacy of a new drug by showing that it is similar in efficacy to a standard agent have been called equivalence trials. Most of these are actually noninferiority trials, attempting to show that the new drug is not less effective than the control by more than a defined amount, generally called the margin.*

ICH E9 (23) distinguishes the **two-sided equivalence** as "equivalence" and **one-sided equivalence** as "noninferiority," with the categories distinguished by their differing objectives. Even so, the **noninferiority margin** is not used in ICH E9; the lower equivalence margin is used instead. This contrasts with two regulatory guidelines (12,31), where noninferiority is the primary focus. However, these documents do not define explicitly what δ is:

> "[A] noninferiority trial aims to demonstrate that the test product is not worse than the comparator by more than a pre-specified, small amount. This amount is known as the non-inferiority margin, or delta (Δ)" (31).
>
> "[T]he non-inferiority study seeks to show that the difference in response between the active control (C) and the test drug (T), (C–T), . . ., is less than some pre-specified, fixed non-inferiority margin (M) (12)."

However, neither do many authors (9,24–27,32).

CHOICE OF δ

How do you choose δ? Both ICH E10 (17) and the European Agency for the Evaluation of Medicinal Products (EMEA) (31) suggested that the determination of δ be based on both statistical reasoning and clinical judgment. This is supported by many authors (22,24). The "statistical reasoning" is due to dependence of δ on the effect size. For example, Suda et al. stated that "statistical reasoning takes into account previous placebo-controlled trials to identify an estimate of the active control effect" (24). A list of suggestions in the literature on the choice of δ is given by Ng (11). The majority of authors recommend that the margin depends on the effect size of the active control as compared to the placebo. Ng recommends that δ be a small fraction of the effect size (11,25,29,32).

There can be subtle differences in the wording and interpretation of *clinical judgment*. The following are two lists of such wordings, the key words in the first and second lists being "acceptable" and "important," respectively:

a. "**clinically acceptable difference**," "clinically irrelevant amount," "clinically irrelevant difference," "clinically meaningless difference," "irrelevantly different," "degree of acceptable inferiority"
b. "clinically important," "clinically meaningful difference," "clinically relevant difference," "**clinically significant**"

There are two approaches to set δ: (a) bottom up and (b) top down. The **bottom-up approach** starts with an extremely small difference that is "acceptable" and works up, whereas the **top-down approach** starts with a large difference that is "important" and works down. Ideally, these two approaches end in the same place, which becomes the δ. Treadwell et al. (33) refer to the top-down approach as identifying a threshold in terms of the *smallest value that would be clinically important*, and the bottom-up approach as identifying a threshold in terms of the *largest difference that is clinically acceptable.*

δ PROPOSED BY NG (29)

Choosing δ is a major question in testing for equivalence or noninferiority. To claim that the test treatment is equivalent—or noninferior—to the standard therapy, we want δ to be small relative to the effect size of the active control, that is, $S - P$. Mathematically, δ should be some small ε between 0 and 1, such as 0.2 times the true effect size; that is,

$$\delta = \varepsilon(S - P). \quad [1]$$

This proposal, although not stated explicitly as such, is in line with M_2 discussed in Food and Drug Administration (FDA) documents on noninferiority (12). At first blush, such a proposal appears to be useless, because the true effect size is unknown. However, the effect size can (and should) be estimated from historical data, either: (a) directly, where the active control was compared to the placebo, or (b) indirectly, where the active control was compared to another active control in a noninferiority/equivalence trial. If no such data exist, the active control should not be used as a control in the noninferiority trial, becauseince it is difficult to justify the noninferiority margin without such data.

For simplicity, we consider the situation where the effect size is estimated directly from historical data. The noninferiority margin given by equation [1] reduces to two smaller ones given in the following (divide-and-conquer strategy), which are more easily handled (32):

- How do you choose ε?
- How do you know the true effect size?

In answering the first question, we would have a better understanding of the rationale and interpretation of the noninferiority margin when the effect size is assumed to be known. Furthermore, this approach obviates worrying about different ways to estimate the effect size, and other issues (e.g., constancy assumption). Issues of estimating the effect size are discussed subsequently.

HOW DO YOU CHOOSE ε?

Recall we are testing the null hypothesis

$$H_0: T \leq S - \delta,$$

where $\delta = \varepsilon(S - P)$. At the boundary, we have $T = S - \delta = S - \varepsilon(S - P)$. Thus:

- If $\varepsilon = 0$, then $T = S$, so we would be testing for superiority against the standard therapy (i.e., $H_0: T = S$ vs. $H_A: T > S$).
- If $\varepsilon = 1$, then $T = P$, so we would be testing for efficacy as compared to putative placebo (i.e., $H_0: T = P$ vs. $H_A: T > P$).
- For $\varepsilon = 0.2$, it means that the test is 80% as effective as the standard therapy.

Figure 27.3 shows the hypotheses graphically with $\varepsilon = 0.2$ and 1.1, respectively. If we knew the true effect size, and the margin is less than or equal to the effect size (i.e., $\varepsilon \leq 1$), then we can conclude

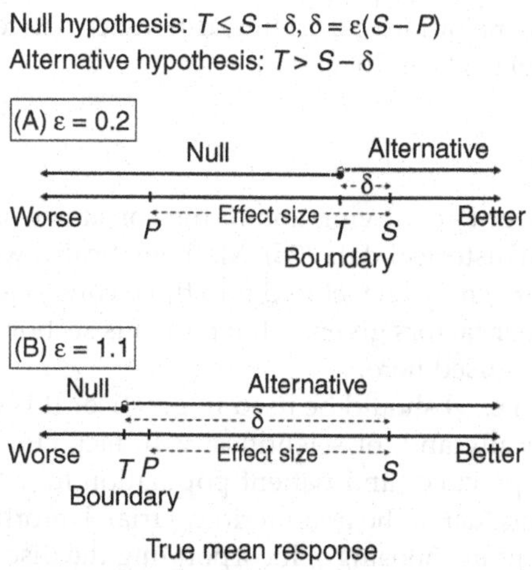

FIGURE 27.3 Choice of ε.

P, placebo; S, standard therapy; T, test.

that the test treatment is better than placebo when the null hypothesis is rejected because $T > S - \delta \geq S - (S - P) = P$ (Figure 27.3A). However, if the margin is greater than the effect size (i.e., $\varepsilon > 1$), then we cannot conclude that the test treatment is better than placebo, even when the null hypothesis is rejected, as shown in Figure 27.3B. Therefore, the margin must not be larger than the effect size.

It should be noted that when the null hypothesis is rejected with $\varepsilon = 0.2$, we would conclude that the test treatment preserves greater than 80% of the control effect, rather than at least 80% of the control effect. In many situations, a small ε would lead to a sample size that is impractical. In that case, we cannot show noninferiority. What we can do is use a larger δ and show the efficacy of the test treatment as compared to placebo.

The choice of ε depends on the study objective. If the objective is to establish the efficacy of the test treatment as compared to placebo through its comparison to the standard therapy, then ε can be as large as 1 (11,25,29,32). For example, in 1992, the FDA recommended using half of the effect size of the standard therapy as the noninferiority margin for trials with an objective to establish the efficacy of a test product (as compared to placebo), without claiming noninferiority (11). However, to claim equivalence or noninferiority, ε should be small. How small is small? This depends on other subjective determinations of benefits relative to the primary endpoint (e.g., better safety profiles).

HOW DO YOU KNOW THE TRUE EFFECT SIZE?

How do you know the effect size? This question is much more difficult than "How do you choose ε?", but easier than the original question "How do you choose δ?". The short answer is that we do not know the true effect size. It must be estimated from historical data—leading to a controversial issue called the **constancy assumption**.

CONSTANCY ASSUMPTION

For simplicity, assume that there is only one prior study of the active control compared to a placebo (see Ng (11) for discussion of the situations where there are multiple studies). The constancy assumption says that the effect size in the current noninferiority trial is equal to the effect size in the historical trial. This assumption allows one to estimate the effect size in the current trial using the historical data. Mathematically, the constancy assumption means

$$S - P = (S - P)_h$$

where $(S - P)_h \equiv S_h - P_h$ denotes the effect size in the historical trial, and S_h and P_h denote the mean responses for the standard therapy and placebo in the historical trial, respectively. The constancy assumption depends on three major factors: (a) time difference between the historical and current trials, (b) study design, and (c) trial conduct (11).

DISCOUNTING

One way to alleviate the concern about violation of the constancy assumption is to discount the effect size estimated from the historical data (25). Mathematically, we let $S - P = \gamma(S - P)_h$, where $0 < \gamma \leq 1$ is the **discount factor**. γ may be factored into three components, such as where γ_1, γ_2, and γ_3 correspond to the three major factors given in the previous section, respectively (11). Again, the divide-and-conquer strategy is used here.

How much discounting (i.e., γ) should be used in practice? It is difficult, if not impossible, to justify the choice of γ statistically and/or scientifically. In fact, choosing γ is more difficult than choosing ε, because medical practices and patient population may change over time, and γ also depends on the design and conduct of the noninferiority trial. Unfortunately, one may have to rely heavily on subjective judgment in choosing γ. Incorporating the discounting factor γ into noninferiority margin defined by equation [1] gives us

$$\delta = \varepsilon\gamma(S - P)_h \qquad [2]$$

As γ_3 depends on the conduct of the noninferiority trial, the constancy assumption cannot be fully assessed before the study is completed. At the design stage, a conservative approach is to build in a **safety margin** (e.g., $\gamma_3 = 0.95$) just in case, at the expense of a larger sample size.

NONINFERIORITY HYPOTHESES BASED ON THE MEAN RATIO

The hypotheses in terms of the mean ratio are more difficult conceptually. For the mean ratio, we test the null hypothesis,

$$H_0: T/S \leq 1/r$$

against the alternative hypothesis,

$$H_A: T/S > 1/r$$

where r (≥1) acts like the noninferiority margin. If $r = 1$, then it becomes testing for superiority against the standard therapy. In contrast, if $r = S/P > 1$ (assuming that $S > P$), it becomes testing for efficacy as compared to putative placebo and S/P acts like the effect size. If we knew this effect size, then a natural way to determine r would be to take this effect size and raise to a power of ε; that is, $r = (S/P)^{\varepsilon}$, for $0 \leq \varepsilon \leq 1$.

Although it is not intuitively clear if the proposed r makes sense, everything becomes clear after taking a log transformation. More specifically, we would test the null hypothesis,

$$H_0: \log(T) - \log(S) \leq -\log(r)$$

against the alternative hypothesis,

$$H_A: \log(T) - \log(S) > -\log(r)$$

where $\log(r) = \varepsilon\,[\log(S) - \log(P)]$. Note that the treatment difference and effect size are measured on the log scale. Again, the noninferiority margin is equal to ε times the effect size, on the log scale. Note that the null hypothesis can be rewritten as

$$H_0: T - S \leq -\delta$$

where $\delta = (1 - 1/r)S$. Hence, the noninferiority margin depends on S, as shown in Figure 27.4.

However, for testing the null hypothesis with a fixed constant r, it is not advisable to compare the lower confidence limit for $(T - S)$ with $-\delta$ computed using the point estimate of S, because

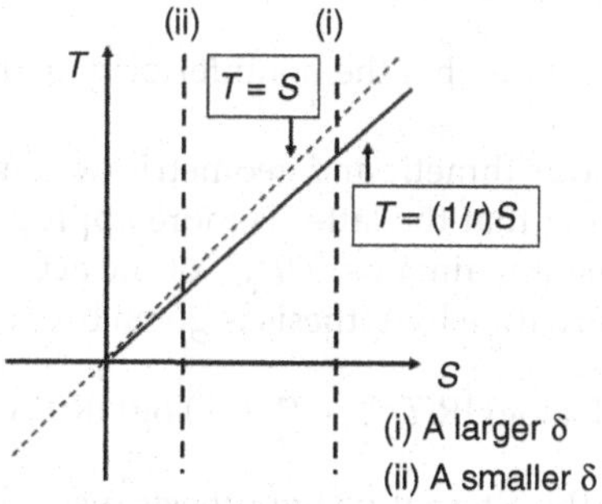

FIGURE 27.4 Mean ratio.

the variability of estimating S has not been taken into consideration in such a comparison. More importantly, S appears on both sides of the inequality, and the margin depends on S. Instead, the null hypothesis could be tested by comparing the lower confidence limit for T/S (with or without a log transformation) or $T - (1/r)S$ with the appropriate critical values. See Laster and Johnson (34) for further discussion on testing the null hypothesis for a fixed r.

NONINFERIORITY HYPOTHESES BASED ON HAZARD RATIO

As discussed in Chapter 16, time-to-event data are often collected in medical studies. Of particular interest in oncology and other medical disciplines is the effect of treatment on overall survival (OS). In randomized trials, OS is generally measured as the time from randomization to death due to any cause, or (if the data are censored) to the last time the subject was known to be alive. However, use of OS may require large samples with long-term follow-up, especially if the natural history of the disease course is lengthy (35). As a surrogate, progression-free survival (PFS) is typically defined in randomized trials as the time from randomization to disease progression or death from any cause. It should be noted, however, the success of using PFS depends heavily on the definition of *disease progression*.

Hazard ratios are frequently used in the analysis of time-to-event endpoints such as OS and PFS, with a lower hazard corresponding to a better outcome. This is different from the assumption for continuous data, where we assume that a larger value corresponds to a better outcome. Therefore, the noninferiority hypothesis based on the hazard ratio looks the opposite of a noninferiority hypothesis based on the mean ratio:

$$H_0: T/S \geq r$$

against the alternative hypothesis

$$H_A: T/S < r$$

where $r \geq 1$ acts like the noninferiority margin. Following the same ideas for the mean ratio discussed previously, we set

$$r = (P/S)^{\varepsilon}$$

for $0 \leq \varepsilon \leq 1$, if we know the effect size P/S (assuming that $S < P$). Taking a log transformation, we would test the null hypothesis,

$$H_0: \log(T) - \log(S) \geq \log(r)$$

against the alternative hypothesis,

$$H_A: \log(T) - \log(S) < \log(r)$$

where $\log(r) = \varepsilon\,[\log(P) - \log(S)]$. Note that the noninferiority margin is equal to ε times the effect size on the log scale.

Rothmann et al. (36) gave the arithmetic and geometric definitions of the proportion of active-control effect retained, recognizing that the latter is more appropriate than the former. They proposed to test whether the treatment maintains $100\delta_0\%$ of the active control, where $0 < \delta_0 < 1$. With the geometric definition, the alternative hypothesis is given by

$$H_A: \text{logHR}(T/C) < (1 - \delta_0)\text{logHR}(P/C)$$

which is essentially the same as the alternative hypothesis discussed previously with $\varepsilon = 1 - \delta_0$.

STATISTICAL APPROACHES FOR TESTING NONINFERIORITY

Although the discussion in this chapter is in the context of mean difference for a continuous endpoint, the concept can easily be adapted to the mean ratio for a continuous endpoint and the hazard ratio for a survival endpoint, as well as the odds ratio for a binary endpoint. Incorporating the noninferiority margin given by [2], we can test

$$H_0: T - S \leq -\varepsilon\gamma(S - P)_h$$

versus

$$H_A: T - S > -\varepsilon\gamma(S - P)_h$$

where $\varepsilon > 0$, $\gamma \leq 1$, and $(S - P)_h$ is the effect size in the historical trial. As noted previously, the choice of ε depends on the study objective and is related to **percent preservation** or **retention**. For example, for 60% preservation, $\varepsilon = 0.4$. Gamma (γ) is the discount factor discussed previously.

In general, there are two approaches in testing the noninferiority hypothesis given earlier. The first approach is known as the **fixed margin method (Appendix)**, because the noninferiority margin is considered a fixed constant, even though it is conditioned on the effect size estimated from the historical data (e.g., using the lower confidence limit for the effect size). The second approach is known as the **synthesis method (Appendix)** because it combines or synthesizes the data from the historical trials and the current noninferiority trial (12). In this approach, the effect size from the historical trial is considered as a parameter and the test statistic takes into account the variability of estimating this parameter from historical data. Therefore, it is *not* conditioned on the historical data. These two approaches have been discussed widely in the literature (25,37–39).

The conventional null hypothesis of equality is tested with a two-sided significance level a of 0.05. A statistically significant difference only in the "right" direction indicates the superiority of the test treatment against the control treatment, which could be a placebo or an active control. Therefore, the significant level of interest is effectively $a/2$ or 0.025. In contrast, the noninferiority hypothesis is one-sided in nature. To be consistent, however, the noninferiority hypothesis is also tested at $a/2$ significance level or 0.025.

ANALYSES OF RANDOMIZED CONTROLLED TRIALS

INTENTION-TO-TREAT PRINCIPLE

The phrase intention to treat (ITT) was coined by Sir Austin Bradford Hill and the term intent-to-treat is commonly used (10). Bradford-Hill (40) recommended that all participants should be "included in the comparison and thus measure the intention to treat in a given way rather than the actual treatment," as he noted that postrandomization exclusion of participants could affect the internal validity that randomization sought to achieve. As stated by Polit and Gillespie (41), "his advice was primarily aimed at researchers who deliberately removed subjects from the analysis."

The **intention-to-treat principle** (see also Chapter 10) asserts that the effect of a treatment can best be assessed by evaluating on the basis of the intention to treat a subject (i.e., the planned treatment regimen) rather than the actual treatment given. It has the consequence that subjects allocated to a treatment group should be followed up, assessed, and analyzed as members of that group irrespective of their compliance with the planned course of treatment (23).

INTENTION-TO-TREAT ANALYSIS

An ITT analysis includes all randomized subjects in the treatment groups to which they were originally randomized, regardless of whether they received or adhered to the assigned treatment. The fundamental idea behind ITT is that exclusion from the statistical analysis of some patients who were randomized to treatment may induce bias that favors one treatment group more than the other. Bias may also occur if patients are not analyzed as though they belonged to the treatment group originally intended by the randomization procedure, rather than the treatment actually received (42). Such an analysis preserves comparable treatment groups due to randomization and prevents bias resulting from postrandomization exclusions.

In theory, there is a consensus in the literature regarding the definition of an ITT analysis (33,43–49). In practice, however, a strict ITT analysis is often hard to achieve for two main reasons: **missing outcomes** for some participants, and **nonadherence** to the trial protocol (50). Different definitions of modified ITT analysis emerge due to nonadherence to the trial protocol by excluding some randomized patients. For example, randomized patients who never received treatment or who were never evaluated while receiving treatment are excluded in the modified ITT analysis (51).

To include all randomized patients in an ITT analysis, imputation methods are often used to deal with missing data. However, such methods require an untestable assumption of **missing at random**, to some degree. The best way to deal with the problem is to have as little missing data as possible (52,53). Strategies focused on preventing missing data during the conduct and management of clinical trials are preferable to relying on imperfect analytic methods. It is to be hoped that recent research efforts in the prevention and treatment of missing data in clinical trials can reduce the impact of missing data and improve the quality of future studies (53–55).

PER-PROTOCAL ANALYSIS

Although the ITT has been widely used as the primary analysis in superiority trials, it is often inadequately described and inadequately applied (56). For example, studies that claimed use of ITT did not indicate how missing outcomes or deviations from protocols were handled. In contrast to an ITT analysis, a **per-protocol analysis** includes only participants who adhere to or were treated according to the protocol (43,45,46,57,58). Some authors exclude only major protocol deviations from the analyses, but allow minor ones (44,59,60). However, this practice can open the door to subjective judgments as to (a) what constitutes minor or major protocol deviation, (b) what constitutes an acceptable amount of treatment, and (c) what constitutes minimal amount of follow-up.

ANALYSIS OF NONINFERIORITY AND EQUIVALENCE TRIALS

From a practical point of view, a strict ITT analysis including all randomized subjects may not be warranted. In fact, ICH E9 defines **full analysis set** as "the set of subjects that is as close as possible to the ideal implied by the ITT principle. It is derived from the set of all randomized subjects by minimal and justified elimination of subjects" (23).

The document presents three circumstances that might lead to excluding randomized subjects from the full analysis set:

1. The failure to satisfy major entry criteria (eligibility violations)
2. The failure to take at least one dose of trial medication
3. The lack of any data postrandomization

The document further states that such exclusions should always be justified. Peto and coworkers allow some inappropriately randomized patients to be excluded (61).

In the late 1980s, ITT analysis was endorsed by regulatory agencies as the primary, optimal way to analyze randomized controlled trial data (62,63). It is also recommended by the American Statistical Associations Group (64) and the Cochrane Collaboration (50). Note that such a recommendation is in the context of placebo-controlled trials as opposed to active-control trials (more specifically, noninferiority trials). However, ITT analysis plays a different role in noninferiority and equivalence trials, because the ITT analysis could be **anticonservative** in poorly conducted noninferiority trials. For example, mixing up treatment assignments would bias toward similarity of the two treatments when the test treatment is not effective or less effective than the active control (25). Extreme hypothetical examples are given by Schumi and Wittes (58), Lewis and Machin (43), and Brittain and Lin (65). Per-protocol analysis provides an alternative, which reflects the treatment difference that may exist by excluding noncompliant subjects. For this reason, use of the per-protocol population in the primary analysis in noninferiority trials became prominent in the early 2000s (66).

Many authors and regulatory agencies recommend performing both the ITT and per-protocol analyses in noninferiority trials (22,43,57,67–71). Others favor ITT analysis over the per-protocol analysis even in noninferiority trials (72). Nonadherence, withdrawals from therapy, missing data, violations in entry criteria, or other **protocol deviations** often reduce sensitivity to differences between regimens in an ITT analysis. Clearly, it is important to design and conduct trials in a manner to reduce the occurrence of protocol deviations (69–72).

CONCLUSION

There are three key aspects in the analysis of a noninferiority trial (or a randomized controlled trial, in general):

1. The participants are grouped according to the treatment to which they were randomized (as randomized) or the treatment that they actually received (as treated)
2. Whether or not to exclude protocol deviations
3. How to deal with missing data

Following the ITT principle, the analysis of a noninferiority trial should be as randomized rather than as treated.

Exclusion of subjects in the analysis should be minimal and justified (23). In principle, from regulatory and practical points of view, medical intervention should be shown to provide clinical benefits in a real-world setting; that is, showing **effectiveness** (i.e., net benefit) rather than **efficacy**. Therefore, noncompliant subjects should be included in the analysis and no adjustment for noncompliance is necessary. However, it should be noted that excessive noncompliance could render the results uninterpretable. Gillings and Koch (42) suggest that ideally, missing data due to errors and attrition should be kept below about 5%.

As missing data are unavoidable in clinical trials with human subjects, often one must resort to **imputation**. Methods for handling missing data are addressed in greater detail in Chapters 15 and 22, and in Rothmann, Wiens, and Chan (10). With improved quality of the trial conduct, hopefully protocol deviations and missing data can be minimized, to reduce the risk of falsely declaring noninferiority.

GLOSSARY

double blinding: study format in which both the investigator/evaluator and the participant are unaware of the treatment assignment.

placebo-controlled trials: studies in which the control is a placebo.

active control equivalence studies (ACESs): studies conducted to show there are no differences between the two treatments; that is, to rule out the possibility that the test treatment is worse or better than the control.

bias toward the null: bias that leads to a reduction of the treatment difference.

equivalence/noninferiority trial: study in which the objective is to show that the test treatment is similar to or not inferior to the active control.

assay sensitivity: the ability to distinguish an effective treatment from placebo.

type I (α) error: rejecting the null hypothesis when it is actually true.

type II (β) error: failing to reject the null hypothesis when it is actually false.

treatment effect: the assumed effect size at which the power (i.e., 1 – β) is calculated.

sample size samba: tinkering with statistical parameters to meet budgetary and time constraints.

time-to-event data: data that measures the length of time an event occurs.

clinical significance: a difference of undisputed clinical importance.

superiority: a stronger condition than noninferiority, in the sense that superiority implies noninferiority, but not vice versa.

two one-sided tests procedure: study method often used for testing for equivalence by testing two one-sided null hypotheses.

confidence interval approach: study method for testing the null hypothesis by using the confidence interval for an appropriate parameter.

two-sided equivalence: as equivalence.

one-sided equivalence: as noninferiority.

noninferiority margin: the degree of inferiority of the test treatments to the control that the trial will attempt to exclude statistically.

clinically acceptable difference: a treatment difference that is clinically acceptable.

bottom-up approach: starts with an extremely small difference that is "acceptable" and works up to identify a threshold in terms of the largest difference that is clinically acceptable.

top-down approach: starts with a large difference that is "important" and works down to identify a threshold in terms of the smallest value that would be clinically important.

constancy assumption: says that the effect size of the active control in the current noninferiority trial is equal to the effect size in the historical trial.

discount factor: factor to reduce to the effect size based on the historical trials.

safety margin: a built-in design element chosen in a conservative approach to dealing with the constancy assumption.

percent preservation: the effect of the test treatment in term of the percentage of the active control effect size. Thus a 100% preservation means the test treatment has the same effect as the active control.

percent retention: another terminology for percent preservation.

fixed margin method: an approach to testing the noninferiority hypothesis in which the margin is considered fix although it typically depends on the effect size from the historical data of the active control.

synthesis method: an approach to testing the noninferiority hypothesis in which the effect size from the historical trial is considered as a parameter and the test statistic takes into account the variability of estimating this parameter from historical data; thus, it is not conditioned on the historical data.

intention-to-treat principle: asserts that the effect of a treatment can best be assessed by evaluating on the basis of the intention to treat a subject (i.e., the planned treatment regimen) rather than the actual treatment given.

missing outcomes: unavailable study data.

nonadherence: not following a trial protocol.

missing at random: occurs if the missingness can be fully accounted for by variables where there is complete information.

per-protocol analysis: analysis that includes only participants who adhere to or were treated according to the protocol.

full analysis set: according to ICH E9, "the set of subjects that is as close as possible to the ideal implied by the intention-to-treat principle. It is derived from the set of all randomized subjects by minimal and justified elimination of subjects."

anticonservative: a statistical test is said to be anticonservative if the true null hypothesis is more likely to be rejected beyond the type I (α) error.

protocol deviations: sensitivity-reducing departures from a study protocol.

effectiveness: the benefit the treatment produces in routine clinical practice.

efficacy: the benefit a treatment produces under ideal conditions, often using carefully defined subjects in a research clinic.

imputation: method for handling missing data by imputing a value based on available data.

95%–95% method: fix-margin method where the margin is determined by the lower bound of the 95% confidence interval for the control effect size.

REFERENCES

1. Newell DJ. Intention-to-treat analysis: implications for quantitative and qualitative research. *Int J Epidemiol*. 1992:21:837–841. doi:10.1093/ije/21.5.837
2. Shaw TR, Raymond K, Howard MR, Hamer J. Therapeutic non-equivalence of digoxin tablets in the United Kingdom: correlation with tablet dissolution rate. *Br Med J*. 1973;4(5895):763–766. doi:10.1136/bmj.4.5895.763
3. Kline NS, Shah BK. Comparable therapeutic efficacy of tryptophan and imipramine: average therapeutic ratings versus "true" equivalence. An important difference. *Curr Ther Res Clin Exp*. 1973;15(7):484–487.
4. Lasagna L. Editorial: placebos and controlled trials under attack. *Eur J Clin Pharmacol*. 1979;15:373–374. doi:10.1007/BF00561733
5. Makuch R, Johnson M. Active control equivalence studies: Planning and interpretation. In: K. Peace, ed. *Statistical Issues in Drug Research and Development*. New York, NY: Marcel Dekker; 1990:238–246.
6. World Medical Association. *Declaration of Helsinki—Ethical Principles for Medical Research Involving Human Subjects*, 3rd revision. 1989. http://history.nih.gov/research/downloads/helsinki.pdf
7. Temple R. Government viewpoint of clinical trials. *Drug Inf J*. 1982;16:10–17. doi:10.1177/009286158201600102
8. Temple R. When are clinical trials of a given agent vs. placebo no longer appropriate or feasible? *Control Clin Trials*. 1997;18:613–620. doi:10.1016/S0197-2456(97)00058-5

9. Senn S. *Statistical Issues in Drug Development*. 2nd ed. Chichester, UK: John Wiley & Sons; 2007.
10. Rothmann MD, Wiens BL, Chan ISF. *Design and Analysis of Non-Inferiority Trials*. Boca Raton, FL: Chapman & Hall/CRC; 2011.
11. Ng, T-H. *Noninferiority Testing in Clinical Trials: Issues and Challenges*. Boca Raton, FL: Chapman & Hall/CRC; 2014. https://www.crcpress.com/Noninferiority-Testing-in-Clinical-Trials-Issues-and-Challenges/Ng/p/book/9781466561496
12. U.S. Food and Drug Administration. Guidance for industry: Non-inferiority clinical trials to establish effectiveness. 2016. http://www.fda.gov/downloads/Drugs/.../Guidances/UCM202140.pdf.
13. Temple R, Ellenberg SS. Placebo-controlled trials and active-control trials in the evaluation of new treatments. I. Ethical and scientific issues. *Ann Intern Med*. 2000;133:455–463. doi:10.7326/0003-4819-133-6-200009190-00014
14. Emanuel EJ, Miller FG. The ethics of placebo-controlled trials—A middle ground. *N Engl J Med*. 2001;345:915–919. doi:10.1056/NEJM200109203451211
15. Lyons DJ. Use and abuse of placebo in clinical trials. *Drug Inf J*. 1999;33:261–264. doi:10.1177/009286159903300129
16. World Medical Association. Declaration of Helsinki—ethical principles for medical research involving human subjects, 7th Revision. *JAMA*. 2013;310(20):2191–2194. doi:10.1001/jama.2013.281053. http://jama.jamanetwork.com/article.aspx?articleid=1760318
17. International Conference on Harmonization (ICH) E10 Guideline. Choice of Control Groups in Clinical Trials. 2001. http://www.fda.gov/downloads/Drugs/GuidanceComplianceRegulatoryInformation/Guidances/UCM073139.pdf
18. Feinstein AR. Clinical biostatistics XXXIV. The other side of 'statistical significance': alpha, beta, delta and the calculation of sample size. *Clin Pharmacol Ther*. 1975;18:491–505. doi:10.1002/cpt1975184491
19. Spiegelhalter DJ, Freedman LS. A predictive approach to selecting the size of a clinical trial, based on subjective clinical opinion. *Stat Med*. 1986;5:1–13. doi:10.1002/sim.4780050103
20. Schulz KF, Grimes DA. Sample size calculations in randomised trials: mandatory and mystical. *Lancet*. 2005;365:1348–1353. doi:10.1016/S0140-6736(05)61034-3
21. Jones B, Jarvis P, Lewis JA, Ebbutt AF. Trials to assess equivalence: the importance of rigorous methods. *BMJ*. 1996;313:36–39. doi:10.1136/bmj.313.7048.36
22. Kaul S, Diamond GA. Making sense of noninferiority: a clinical and statistical perspective on its application to cardiovascular clinical trials. *Prog Cardiovasc Dis*. 2007;49:284–299. doi:10.1016/j.pcad.2006.10.001
23. International Conference on Harmonization (ICH) E9 Guideline. Statistical Principles for Clinical Trials. 1998. http://www.fda.gov/downloads/Drugs/GuidanceComplianceRegulatoryInformation/Guidances/UCM073137.pdf
24. Suda KJ, Hurley AM, McKibbin T, Motl Moroney SE. Publication of noninferiority clinical trials: changes over a 20-year interval. *Pharmacotherapy*. 2011;31(9):833–839. doi:10.1592/phco.31.9.833
25. Ng T-H. Choice of delta in equivalence testing. *Ther Innov Regul Sci*. 2. 2001;35(4):1517–1527. doi:10.1177/009286150103500446
26. Piaggio G, Elbourne DR, Altman DG, et al. Reporting of noninferiority and equivalence randomized trials: an extension of the CONSORT statement. *JAMA*. 2006;295(10):1152–1160. doi:10.1001/jama.295.10.1152
27. Gülmezoglu AM, Widmer M, Merialdi1 M, et al. Active management of the third stage of labour without controlled cord traction: a randomized non-inferiority controlled trial. *Reproductive Health* (Open Access). 2009. http://www.reproductive-health-journal.com/content/6/1/2
28. Schuirmann DJ. A comparison of the two one-sided tests procedure and the power approach for assessing the equivalence of average bioavailability. *J Pharmacokinet Biopharm*. 1987;15:657–680. doi:10.1007/BF01068419
29. Ng T-H. A specification of treatment difference in the design of clinical trials with active controls. *Drug Inf J*. 1993;27:705–719. doi:10.1177/009286159302700313
30. Hauschke D. Choice of delta: a special case. *Drug Inf J*. 2001;35:875–879. doi:10.1177/009286150103500326
31. European Agency for the Evaluation of Medicinal Products, Committee for Proprietary Medicinal Products. Guideline on the Choice of the Non-Inferiority Margin EMEA/CPMP/EWP/2158/99. 2005. http://www.ema.europa.eu/docs/en_GB/document_library/Scientific_guideline/2009/09/WC500003636.pdf
32. Ng T-H. Noninferiority hypotheses and choice of noninferiority margin. *Stat Med*. 2008;27:5392–5406. doi:10.1002/sim.3367
33. Treadwell J, Uhl S, Tipton K, et al. Assessing equivalence and noninferiority. methods research report. (Prepared by the EPC Workgroup under Contract No. 290-2007-10063) AHRQ Publication No. 12-EHC045-EF. Rockville, MD: Agency for Healthcare Research and Quality; 2012. http://www.effectivehealthcare.ahrq.gov/ehc/products/365/1154/Assessing-Equivalence-and-Noninferiority_FinalReport_20120613.pdf
34. Laster LL, Johnson MF. Non-inferiority trials: the 'at least as good as' criterion. *Stat Med*. 2003;22:187–200. doi:10.1002/sim.1137
35. Gutman SI, Piper M, Grant MD, et al. *Progression-free survival: what does it mean for psychological well-being or quality of life? Methods Research Report (Prepared by the Blue Cross and Blue Shield Association Technology Evaluation Center Evidence-based Practice Center under Contract No. 290-2007-10058-I)* AHRQ Publication No.: 13-EHC074-EF. Rockville, MD: Agency for Healthcare Research and Quality; 2013.
36. Rothmann M, Li N, Chen G, et al. Design and analysis of non-inferiority mortality trials in oncology. *Stat Med*. 2003;22:239–264. doi:10.1002/sim.1400
37. Hauck WW, Anderson S. Some issues in the design and analysis of equivalence trials. *Drug Inf J*. 1999;33:109–118. doi:10.1177/009286159903300114
38. Tsong Y, Wang S-J, Hung H-MJ, Cui L. Statistical issues on objectives, designs and analysis of non-inferiority test active controlled clinical trials. *J Biopharm Stat*. 2003;13:29–41. doi:10.1081/BIP-120017724
39. Wang S-J, Hung H-MJ. Assessment of treatment efficacy in non-inferiority trials. *Control Clin Trials*. 2003;24:147–155. doi:10.1016/S0197-2456(02)00304-5
40. Bradford-Hill A. *Principles of Medical Statistics*. New York, NY: Oxford University Press; 1961.

41. Polit DF, Gillespie BM. Intention-to-treat in randomized controlled trials: recommendations for a total trial strategy. *Res Nurs Health*. 2010;33(4):355–368. doi:10.1002/nur.20386
42. Gillings D, Koch G. The application of the principle of intention-to-treat to the analysis of clinical trials. *Drug Inf J*. 1991;25:411–424. doi:10.1177/009286159102500311
43. Lewis JA, Machin D. Intention to treat—who should use ITT? *Br J Cancer*. 1993;68:647–650. doi:10.1038/bjc.1993.402
44. D'Agostino RB Sr, Massaro JM, Sullivan LM. Non-inferiority trials: design concepts and issues the encounters of academic consultants in statistics. *Stat Med*. 2003;22:169–186. doi:10.1002/sim.1425
45. Le Henanff A, Giraudeau B, Baron G, Ravaud P. Quality of reporting of noninferiority and equivalence randomized trials. *JAMA*. 2006;295:1147–1151. doi:10.1001/jama.295.10.1147
46. Sheng D, Kim MY. The effects of non-compliance on intent-to-treat analysis of equivalence trials. *Stat Med*. 2006;25:1183–1199. doi:10.1002/sim.2230
47. Gravel J, Opartny L, Shapiro S. The intention-to-treat approach in randomized trials: are authors saying what they do and doing what they say? *Clin Trials*. 2007;4:350–356. doi:10.1177/1740774507081223
48. Gonzalez CD, Bolaños R, de Sereday M. Editorial on hypothesis and objectives in clinical trials: superiority, equivalence and non-inferiority. *Thromb J*. 2009;7:3. doi:10.1186/1477-9560-7-3
49. Alshurafa M, Briel M, Akl EA, et al. Inconsistent definitions for intention-to-treat in relation to missing outcome data: systematic review of the methods literature. *PLoS One*. 2012;7(11):e49163. doi:10.1371/journal.pone.0049163
50. Moher D, Schulz KF, Altman DG. The CONSORT statement: revised recommendations for improving the quality of reports of parallel-group randomized trials. *Ann Intern Med*. 2001;134:657–662. doi:10.7326/0003-4819-134-8-200104170-00011
51. Hill CL, LaValley MP, Felson DT. Secular changes in the quality of published randomized clinical trials in rheumatology. *Arthritis Rheum*. 2002;46:779–784. doi:10.1371/journal.pone.0049163
52. Lachin JM. Statistical considerations in the intent-to-treat principle. *Control Clin Trials*. 2000;21(3):167–189. doi:10.1016/S0197-2456(00)00046-5
53. National Research Council, Panel on Handling Missing Data in Clinical Trials. Committee on National Statistics, Division of Behavioral and Social Sciences and Education.. *The Prevention and Treatment of Missing Data in Clinical Trials*. Washington, DC: National Academies Press; 2010. http://csph.ucdenver.edu/sites/kittelson/Bios6648-2013/Lctnotes/2013/NASmissingData.pdf
54. Dziura JD, Post LA, Zhao Q, et al. Strategies for dealing with missing data in clinical trials: from design to analysis. *Yale J Biol Med*. 2013;86:343–358.
55. Li T, Hutfless S, Scharfstein DO. Standards should be applied in the prevention and handling of missing data for patient-centered outcomes research: a systematic review and expert consensus. *J Clin Epidemiol*. 2014;67:15–32. doi:10.1016/j.jclinepi.2013.08.013
56. Hollis S, Campbell F. What is meant by intention to treat analysis? Survey of published randomised controlled trials. *BMJ*. 1999;319(7211):670–674. doi:10.1136/bmj.319.7211.670
57. Scott IA. Non-inferiority trials: determining whether alternative treatments are good enough. *Med J Aust*. 2009;190:326–330.
58. Schumi J, Wittes JT. Through the looking glass: understanding non-inferiority. *Trials*. 2011;12:106. doi:10.1186/1745-6215-12-106
59. Sanchez MM, Chen X. Choosing the analysis population in non-inferiority studies: per protocol or intent-to-treat. *Stat Med*. 2006;25:1169–1181. doi:10.1002/sim.2244
60. Wiens BL, Zhao W. The role of intention to treat in analysis of noninferiority studies. *Clin Trials*. 2007;4:286–291. doi:10.1177/1740774507079443
61. Peto R, Pike MC, Armitage P, et al. Design and analysis of randomized clinical trials requiring prolonged observation of each patient. I. Introduction and design. *Br J Cancer*. 1976;34:585–612. doi:10.1038/bjc.1976.220
62. U.S. Food and Drug Administration. *Guideline for the Format and Content of the Clinical and Statistical Sections of New Drug Applications*. Rockville, MD: U.S. Department of Health and Human Services; 1988.
63. Nordic Council on Medicine. *Good Clinical Practice: Nordic Guidelines*. Uppsala, Sweden: Author; 1989.
64. Fisher LD, Dixon DO, Herson J, et al. Intention to treat in clinical trials. In: Peace KE, ed. *Statistical Issues in Drug Research and Development*. New York, NY: Marcel Dekker; 1990:331–350.
65. Brittain E, Lin D. A comparison of intent-to-treat and per-protocol results in antibiotic noninferiority trials. *Stat Med*. 2005;24:1–10. doi:10.1002/sim.1934
66. Garrett AD. Therapeutic equivalence: fallacies and falsification. *Stat Med*. 2003;22:741–762. doi:10.1002/sim.1360
67. Ebbutt AF, Frith L. Practical issues in equivalence trials. *Stat Med*. 1998;17:1691–1701. doi:10.1002/(SICI)1097-0258(19980815/30)17:15/16<1691::AID-SIM971>3.0.CO;2-J
68. Gøtzsche PC. Lessons from and cautions about noninferiority and equivalence randomized trials. *JAMA*. 2006;295:1172–1174. doi:10.1001/jama.295.10.1172
69. Pocock SJ. Pros and cons of noninferiority trials. *Fundam Clin Pharmacol*. 2003;17:483–490. doi:10.1046/j.1472-8206.2003.00162.x
70. Pater C. Equivalence and noninferiority trials—are they viable alternatives for registration of new drugs? (III). *Curr Control Trials Cardiovasc Med*. 2004;5:8. doi:10.1186/1468-6708-5-8
71. Lesaffre E. Superiority, equivalence and non-inferiority trials. *Bull NYC Hosp Jt Dis*. 2008;66(2):150–154.
72. Fleming TR. Current issues in non-inferiority trials. *Stat Med*. 2008;27:317–332. doi:10.1002/sim.2855
73. Hung HMJ, Wang SJ, O'Neil RT. Issues with statistical risks for testing methods in noninferiority trial without a placebo arm. *J Biopharm Stat*. 2007;17:201–213. doi:10.1080/10543400601177343
74. Lawrence J. Some remarks about the analysis of active control studies. *Biom J*. 2005;47(5):616–622. doi:10.1002/bimj.200410145

APPENDIX

FIXED MARGIN METHOD

Using the fixed margin method, we replace $(S - P)_h$ by the lower limit of the two-sided $(1 - a^*)100\%$ (e.g., 95%) confidence interval—or the one-sided $(1 - a^*/2)100\%$ lower confidence limit—for $(S - P)_h$, that is

$$(\widehat{S-P})_h - z_{1-a^*/2}\,\mathrm{SD}(\widehat{S-P})_h,$$

where $z_{1-a^*/2}$ denotes the $(1 - a^*/2)100\%$ percentile of the standard normal distribution and $\mathrm{SD}(\widehat{S-P})_h$ denotes the standard deviation of the estimator $(\widehat{S-P})_h$. Therefore, the noninferiority margin is given by

$$\delta = \varepsilon\gamma\,[(\widehat{S-P})_h - Z_{1-a^*/2}\,\mathrm{SD}(\widehat{S-P})_h].$$

At a significance level of $a/2$, and if $a^* = a = 0.05$, then we reject H_0, if

$$\frac{(\widehat{T-S}) + \varepsilon\gamma(\widehat{S-P})_h}{\mathrm{SD}(\widehat{T-S}) + \varepsilon\gamma\mathrm{SD}(\widehat{S-P})_h} > z_{1-a/2} = 1.96.$$

See Ng (11; Section 5.3) for the detailed derivation. The fixed margin method is also referred to as the two-confidence-interval method, because two confidence intervals are used, one to estimate the effect size in the determination of the noninferiority margin, and the other one to test the null hypothesis, or more specifically, the **95%–95% method** (73). Because the lower bounds of the 95% confidence intervals are used, effective significance levels are 97.5%. For this reason, such a fixed margin method may be referred to as the 97.5%–97.5% method.

SYNTHESIS METHOD

Using the synthesis method, rewrite the hypotheses as

$$H_0: T - S + \varepsilon\gamma(S - P)_h \leq 0$$

and

$$H_A: T - S + \varepsilon\gamma(S - P)_h > 0,$$

respectively. At a significance level of $a/2$, we reject H_0, if the lower limit of the $(1 - a)100\%$ confidence interval—or the one-sided $(1 - a/2)100\%$ lower confidence limit—for $[(\underline{T} - S) + \varepsilon\gamma(S - P)_h]$ is greater than 0. That is

$$(\widehat{T-S}) + \varepsilon\gamma(\widehat{S-P})_h - Z_{1-a/2}\sqrt{\mathrm{Var}(\widehat{T-S}) + \varepsilon^2\gamma^2(\widehat{S-P})_h} > 0,$$

or equivalently,

$$\frac{(\widehat{T-S}) + \varepsilon\gamma(\widehat{S-P})_h}{\sqrt{\mathrm{Var}(\widehat{T-S}) + \varepsilon^2\gamma^2(\widehat{S-P})_h}} > Z_{1-a/2} = 1.96,$$

if $a = 0.05$, where "Var" stands for the variance.

FIXED MARGIN METHOD VERSUS SYNTHESIS METHOD

If the lower limit of the 95% confidence interval (or the one-sided 97.5% lower confidence limit) for the historical effect size is used in the determination of the noninferiority margin, then the denominator of the test statistic using the fixed margin approach, but viewing the historical data unconditionally is always larger than that of the test statistic using the synthesis method because:

$$\mathrm{SD}(\widehat{T-S}) + \varepsilon\gamma \mathrm{SD}(\widehat{S-P})_h \geq \sqrt{\mathrm{Var}(\widehat{T-S}) + \varepsilon^2\gamma^2(\widehat{S-P})_h}.$$

Therefore, it is easier to reject the null hypothesis using the synthesis method than using the fixed margin approach if the two-sided confidence level for estimating $(S - P)_h$ is at least 95%. However, that is not necessarily true if the confidence level for estimating $(S - P)_h$ is less than 95%. For example, at the extreme, if the point estimate of $(S - P)_h$ is used (corresponding to using 0% confidence interval, i.e., $a^* = 1$ and $z_{1-a^*/2} = 0$), then it is easier to reject the null hypothesis given using the fixed margin approach than using the synthesis method; see Ng (11).

The two approaches are intrinsically different although one can determine a^*, so that they are equivalent (11,37,73). The fixed margin method is conditioned on the historical data through the determination of the noninferiority margin and controls the conditional type I error rate in the sense of falsely rejecting the null hypothesis with the given noninferiority margin when the noninferiority trial is repeated (73). The synthesis method considers $(S - P)_h$ as the parameters and factors the variability into the test statistic; thus, it is unconditional and controls the unconditional type I error rate in the sense of falsely rejecting the null hypothesis when the historical trials and the noninferiority trial are repeated (74). Therefore, it is understood that the type I error rate is (a) conditional if the fixed margin method is used and (b) unconditional if the synthesis method is used. Ng concluded that, from a practical point of view, the fixed margin method rather than the synthesis method should be used (11).

ACKNOWLEDGMENTS

I thank Chunrong Cheng, Shiowjen Lee, and Qiang (Ed) Zhang for their review and helpful comments on the manuscript.

28

Systematic Reviews and Meta-Analyses

ENOCH CHANG ■ NICHOLAS G. ZAORSKY ■ HENRY S. PARK

As the number of scientific publications steadily increases, clinicians, patients, and policy makers benefit from succinct syntheses of the available evidence. Single studies could be underpowered (resulting in a failure to detect differences between interventions and the reporting of false-negative effects), or their findings might conflict with those of other similar studies. Systematic reviews can help address these issues by arbitrating differences between conflicting studies with a more objective and transparent approach compared to narrative reviews. They also serve to generalize findings across various studies that report on specific subgroups of patient populations. Moreover, when appropriate, they can aggregate findings through meta-analysis to report more precise treatment effects.

OVERVIEW OF TERMINOLOGY

A **systematic review** is a reproducible methodology that entails

1. Stating a clear objective to address a specific research question
2. Systematically identifying all relevant studies
3. Selecting eligible studies with predefined criteria
4. Assessing risk of bias
5. Extracting data
6. Presenting qualitative synthesis of included studies

Systematic reviews may contain an additional component if appropriate, called a **meta-analysis**, which summarizes and combines the results of independent studies that measure the effects of similar treatment approaches on similar patient populations through statistical methods (1). As discussed further in the following text, not all systematic reviews should include meta-analysis.

In this chapter, we describe the general steps required to perform a systematic review, which can be customized depending on the type of study design, data source, or statistical methodology.

We then discuss (a) narrative synthesis and the decision whether or not to combine data through meta-analysis; (b) the differences between systematic reviews of randomized controlled trials (RCTs) and of nonrandomized studies/observational studies; (c) the methodology of using aggregate data versus individual patient data (IPD); and (d) the differences between traditional meta-analysis and network meta-analysis.

STEPS TO PERFORM A SYSTEMATIC REVIEW

DEVELOPING A RESEARCH QUESTION

When planning a systematic review, the first step is to define the scope of the study in terms of **P**articipants, **I**nterventions, **C**omparisons, **O**utcomes, **S**tudy Design (PICOS). The scope can vary from broad (e.g., effects of chemotherapy and hormonal therapy on recurrence and survival for early-stage breast cancer patients) (2) to narrow (e.g., effect of adjuvant trastuzumab on recurrence, survival, brain metastases, and cardiotoxicity for HER-2-positive early-stage breast cancer patients) (3). A systematic review with a broad scope is advantageous because it comprehensively summarizes generalizable findings, but is also disadvantageous in that a synthesis of a wide variety of studies with different methodologies and patient populations may be difficult to interpret. Conversely, a systematic review with a narrow scope is more focused for both study authors and readers alike, but might not be generalizable if only a few studies are included (4).

FORMING A REVIEW TEAM

When planning a systematic review or meta-analysis, it is strongly recommended that one develop a detailed written protocol in collaboration with a research team. A team should include at least two individuals who have the appropriate skills, including clinical knowledge, statistics, and information retrieval.

REGISTERING A REVIEW PROTOCOL

A protocol outlining key details like background and context, inclusion and exclusion criteria with respect to PICOS, search strategy, data extraction, quality assessment, synthesis, subgroup and sensitivity analysis, and dissemination plans should be registered in an online database before carrying out a systematic review. A formal search strategy promotes a more transparent approach, helps prevent publication bias, and informs other researchers about work in progress. Protocols can be registered and published online for free at the PROSPERO database maintained by the Centre for Reviews and Dissemination (CRD) at the University of York: www.crd.york.ac.uk/prospero. Each protocol registered in PROSPERO is assigned a unique registration number that can be cited in publications, as recommended by reporting guidelines and publishers.

PERFORMING A LITERATURE SEARCH

The goal of the initial literature search is to identify relevant studies with high sensitivity and specificity.

Search Sources

At a minimum, the Cochrane Central Register of Controlled Trials (CENTRAL), MEDLINE, and EMBASE are three essential bibliographic databases to search for relevant studies. (Note: PubMed is the search engine that accesses primarily the MEDLINE database.) Subject-specific (biology, pharmacology, health promotion, international health, nursing, allied health, social science), national, and regional databases can also be included. Records of unpublished or ongoing studies can be found in national trial registries such as ClinicalTrials.gov or the World Health Organization International Trials Registry Platform Search Portal, pharmaceutical trial registries, or conference abstracts (e.g., ASCO: http://meetinglibrary.asco.org/browse-meetings). Reference lists of previously published systematic reviews or of identified subjects can serve as another source to look for additional studies. Researchers might also contact individual study authors regarding ongoing studies or missing data (5).

Formulating a Search Strategy

At this stage, it is highly recommended to seek the guidance of a healthcare librarian or information specialist. Generally, search strategies should only include the population and intervention of interest (and possibly study design if only including randomized clinical trials).

Indexers often assign standardized subject terms to studies that may use different terms to describe a particular concept. These sources are not necessarily all-inclusive, because they depend on indexers who may not necessarily be content experts. These terms—MeSH (Medical Subheading) in MEDLINE and EMTREE in EMBASE—can be expanded to include more specific terms automatically. For example, the MeSH term "radiotherapy" can be "exploded" to search for additional terms such as "brachytherapy," "chemoradiotherapy," "proton radiotherapy," and "radiosurgery." One way to identify these standardized MeSH or EMTREE terms is to examine a particular study in the database that meets the systematic review inclusion criteria and find the associated terms indexed with this study.

To maximize the sensitivity of the literature search, free text terms as well as standardized terms should be included (5). These words can be truncated: fractionat* (for fractionation or fractionated), or wildcards can be used: wom?n (for woman or women).

The Boolean operator "OR" can be used to combine all the relevant standardized subject terms and free text terms for both the population and intervention of interest. The operator "AND" can then be used to combine the combinations of population with the combination of interventions (5).

Example:
Here is a search strategy for Ovid MEDLINE, where the authors were interested in finding articles relevant to radiation therapy for craniopharyngiomas.

1 Craniopharyngioma/
2 rathke*.tw.
3 Craniopharyngioma*.tw.
4 1 or 2 or 3
5 exp Radiotherapy/
6 (fractionat* or Hypofractionat* or Gamma knife or gammaknife or cyber knife or cyberknife or linear accelerator* or linac or tomotherap*).tw.
7 proton*.tw.
8 heavy ion.tw.
9 intensity modulated.tw.
10 stereotactic.tw.
11 5 or 6 or 7 or 8 or 9 or 10
12 4 and 11
13 limit 12 to English language

Documenting the Search Strategy

The following information should be reported in the protocol: list of databases searched, dates searched, language or publication status restrictions, and additional sources searched. These details should be reported in the methods of the completed systematic review itself as well. In addition, the full electronic search strategy for at least one major database should be copied, pasted, and reported as an appendix or supplementary file of the completed systematic review to allow for transparency, replication of results, and future updates.

STUDY SELECTION

Study selection typically entails

1. Compiling all search results and removing duplicates using reference management software
2. Screening titles and abstracts according to predefined PICOS eligibility criteria. Screening should be performed by at least two independent reviewers, with the tendency to be overinclusive at this stage. Any discrepancies should be resolved through consensus by discussion, and if this is not possible, then by a third reviewer
3. Screening the full text of reports that pass title/abstract screening according to predefined PICOS eligibility criteria
   a. At this stage, multiple reports of the same study (identified by author or location in common) should be examined to identify the report from the most recent year, with the greatest number of participants, or with inclusion of the PICOS elements of interest. Only one report of each study should be included, to avoid counting duplicate studies.
   b. If necessary, contact study authors to determine inclusion eligibility.
   c. Document reasons for exclusion.
4. Note: It can be helpful to pilot the screening criteria for a small sample of reports to refine the criteria and ensure a consistent approach by all reviewers

Software resources like Covidence and EndNote help coordinate the process of reference management and study selection, making it easier for reviewers to collaborate electronically. The Preferred Reporting Items for Systematic Reviews and Meta-Analyses (**PRISMA**) guidelines were put together by a team of expert researchers, with a step-by-step guide along with explanations for writing of the manuscript of a systematic review and meta-analysis (6).

Figure 28.1 shows an example flow diagram reporting the study selection process according to the PRISMA guidelines (7).

DATA EXTRACTION

Data should be extracted from included studies using an electronic or paper data extraction form that is first piloted on a few studies. A "Characteristics of included studies" table and "Risk of bias" table should be drafted using the piloted data. The forms should be adjusted as necessary. At least two reviewers should extract data, resolving any disagreements through consensus, and possibly involving a third reviewer on any questions of interpretation. See Table 28.1 for a list of data items to include (8).

RISK OF BIAS ASSESSMENT

The risk of bias should be assessed for every included study to evaluate the likelihood that each study approximates some underlying true effect. Different biases can lead to variations in measured effects, leading to heterogeneity between studies.

Randomized controlled trials (RCTs) can be evaluated with Cochrane's "Risk of Bias" assessment tool along six domains (9):

1. *Selection bias:* due to lack of random sequence generation or inadequate allocation concealment
2. *Performance bias:* due to lack of blinding of participants and study personnel

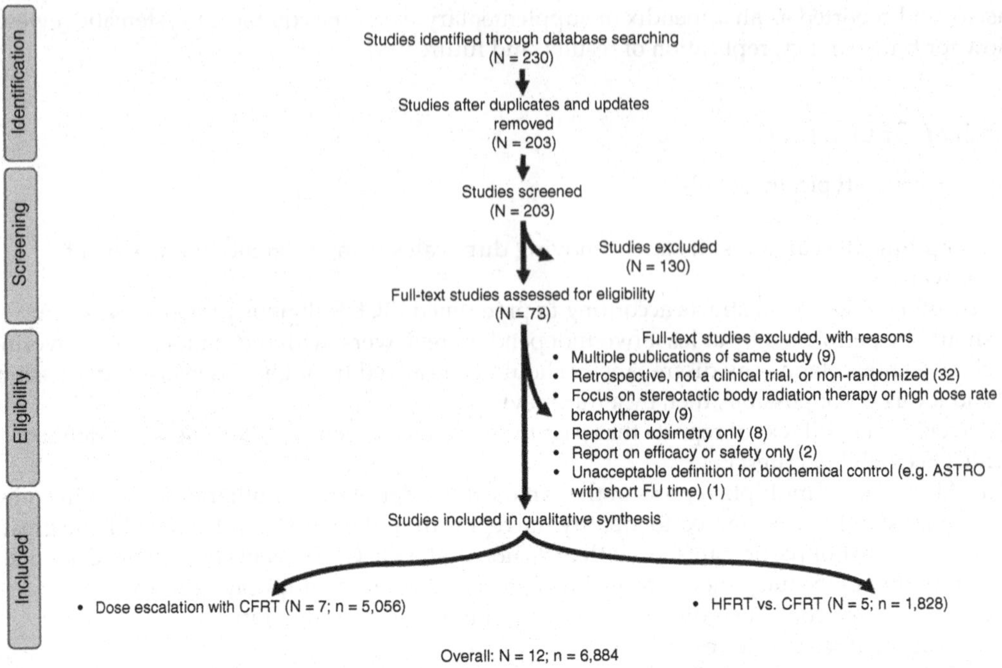

FIGURE 28.1 Example study selection flow diagram.

ASTRO, American Society for Radiation Oncology; CFRT, conventionally fractionated external beam radiation therapy; FU, follow-up; HFRT, hypofractionated external beam radiation therapy.

Source: Zaorsky NG, Keith SW, Shaikh T, et al. Impact of radiation therapy dose escalation on prostate cancer outcomes and toxicities. *Am J Clin Oncol.* 2016:1. doi:10.1097/coc.0000000000000285

3. *Detection bias*: due to knowledge of allocated interventions by outcome assessors
4. *Attrition bias*: due to incomplete outcome data collection
5. *Reporting bias*: due to selective outcome reporting
6. *Other bias*: due to any other additional sources

This tool guides reviewers to assess risk of bias in two steps:

1. Record relevant details for each study along the six domains listed.
2. Assign a judgment of "low," "high," or "unclear" risk of bias.

The criteria for judging low, high, or unclear risk of bias are summarized in Table 8.5.d "Criteria for Judging Risk of Bias in the 'Risk of Bias' Assessment Tool" of the Cochrane Handbook (found online at www.handbook.cochrane.org).

Theoretically, studies with higher risk of bias should be weighted less heavily in a meta-analysis. However, formal statistical methods have not yet been developed for this purpose, and so several strategies to incorporate risk of bias are proposed:

1. Only include studies with low or unclear risk of bias, performing a sensitivity analysis with high-risk studies included as well.
2. Present an estimated summary measure that includes all studies accompanied by a narrative discussion of risk of bias. This approach is recommended when all studies are assessed to have a certain level of risk, whether high, low, or unclear.

TABLE 28.1 LIST OF DATA ITEMS TO INCLUDE IN DATA EXTRACTION

Category	To Be Collected for All Reviews	Potentially Relevant to Some Reviews
Source	Study ID (created by review author) Report ID (created by review author) Review author ID (created by review author) Citation and contact details	
Eligibility	Confirm eligibility for each review Reason for exclusion	
Methods	Study design Total study duration Sequence generation Allocation sequence concealment Blinding Other concerns about bias	
Participants	Total number Setting Diagnostic criteria Age Sex Country	Comorbidity Sociodemographics Ethnicity Date of study
Interventions	Total number of intervention groups Specific intervention and details for each intervention or comparison	Integrity of intervention
Outcomes	Outcomes and time points collected and reported Outcome definition Unit of measurement Scales (upper and lower limits, whether high or low score is good)	
Results	Number of participants allocated to each intervention group Sample size Missing participants Summary data for each intervention group	Estimate of effect with confidence interval and *p* value Subgroup analyses
Miscellaneous	Funding source Study authors' key conclusion Study authors' miscellaneous comments References to other relevant studies Correspondence required Review authors' miscellaneous comments	

Source: Adapted from Higgins JPT, Deeks JJ (editors). Chapter 7: Selecting studies and collecting data. Table 7.3.a: Checklist of items to consider in data collection or data extraction. In: Higgins JPT, Green S, eds. *Cochrane Handbook for Systematic Reviews of Interventions*. Chichester, UK: John Wiley & Sons; 2008:157.

In the case of strategy 2, reviewers should discuss the summary assessments of risk of bias. (See the following text for discussion on nonrandomized studies.) Figure 28.2 shows an example risk of bias summary figure (10).

	Random sequence generation (selection bias)	Allocation concealment (selection bias)	Blinding (performance bias and detection bias): Survival	Blinding (performance bias and detection bias): Symptom control	Incomplete outcome data (attrition bias): Survival	Incomplete outcome data (attrition bias): Symptom control	Selective reporting (reporting bias)	Other bias
Abratt 1995	?	+	+	?	+	−	−	−
Bezjak 2002	?	?	+	?	+	−	+	+
Erridge 2005	?	+	+	−	+	+	+	−
Kramer 2005	?	?	+	+	+	?	+	+
MRC 1991	+	+	+	?	+	?	+	+
MRC 1992	+	+	+	?	+	−	+	+
MRC 1996	+	+	+	?	+	−	+	+
Nestle 2000	?	?	+	?	+	−	+	+
Rees 1997	?	?	+	?	+	+	+	−
Reinfuss 1999	?	?	+	?	+	?	−	?
Senkus-Konefka 2005	+	+	+	?	+	−	+	+
Simpson 1985	?	?	+	?	−	−	+	−
Sundstrom 2004	+	+	+	?	+	+	+	+
Teo 1988	+	?	+	?	?	?	−	?

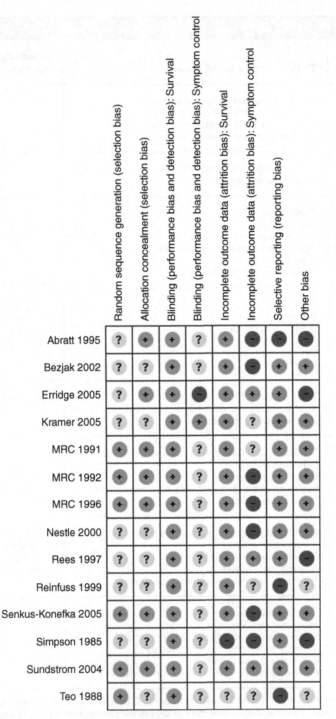

FIGURE 28.2 Example risk of bias summary figure.

Source: Stevens R, Macbeth F, Toy E, et al. Palliative radiotherapy regimens for patients with thoracic symptoms from non-small cell lung cancer. *Cochrane Database Syst Rev.* 2015;1:CD002143. doi:10.1002/14651858.cd002143.pub3

SYNTHESIS

Narrative synthesis entails a structured summary and discussion of the studies' characteristics and findings through words and text. Meta-analysis is the statistical combination of results from at least two separate studies.

The outcomes of two or more interventions on participants will usually be compared. The "effect," the "treatment effect," or the "intervention effect" measures difference in outcome between participants treated with different interventions. The Cochrane Handbook suggests this framework for both qualitative narrative synthesis and quantitative meta-analysis:

1. What is the direction of the effect?
2. What is the size of the effect?
3. Is the effect consistent across studies?
4. What is the strength of evidence for the effect?

If performing a subjective narrative synthesis when meta-analysis is not indicated (discussed in the following text), reviewers should systematically approach these questions with a prespecified approach. Such an approach avoids introducing bias resulting from overemphasizing the results of any particular study.

If performing quantitative meta-analysis, reviewers can approach questions 1 to 3 with statistical methods while assessing question 4 through exploration of study design, risk of bias, and statistical measures of uncertainty (11).

META-ANALYSIS: TO COMBINE OR NOT TO COMBINE DATA

Meta-analysis can be valuable due to its ability to (a) increase power, (b) improve precision, (c) evaluate consistency among a broader range of primary studies that are focused on more specific participant and intervention characteristics, and (d) facilitate formal statistical assessment of conflicting studies and exploration of reasons for divergent findings (11).

When deciding to combine data across studies, a common illustration is that researchers should avoid combining "apples with oranges," but rather seek to combine "just apples." The Cochrane Handbook lists three reasons not to perform meta-analysis (11):

1. Clinical differences between studies are too great. A mix of too many different comparators across individual studies can make it difficult to detect meaningful effects.
2. Meta-analysis will be skewed if combining studies with high risk of bias.
3. High publication and reporting bias can lead to inappropriate summary.

Study authors may choose not to calculate summary statistics because they believe statistical heterogeneity is too high. However, Ioannidis et al. found that in a comparison of systematic reviews with and without meta-analytic synthesis, the median heterogeneity of the synthesized studies was actually higher than that of the unsynthesized studies (12). Several methodological solutions to solve issues in quantitative synthesis were offered as shown in Table 28.2.

Knoll et al. published a helpful flowchart to decide whether to perform a narrative synthesis or a meta-analysis as shown in Figure 28.3 (13).

NARRATIVE SUMMARY

There are four stages of performing a narrative synthesis (14):

- Developing a theory of how the intervention works, why, and for whom
- Developing a preliminary synthesis of findings of included studies

TABLE 28.2 METHODOLOGICAL APPROACHES TO CONSIDER IN THE SYNTHESIS OF HETEROGENEOUS DATA

Problem	Possible Methodological Solution	Selected Key Caveats
High statistical heterogeneity*	Random effects Meta-regression	Does not explain heterogeneity, small study effects, limited data Choice of variables, ecological fallacy, limited data
	Bayesian meta-analysis	Prior specification
	Bayesian meta-regression	Similar to meta-regression and Bayesian meta-analysis
	Meta-analysis of individual level data	Unavailable individual level information
Different interventions compared	Merge intervention in same class	Unrecognized heterogeneity
	Network meta-analysis	Inconsistency in direct versus indirect comparisons
Different metrics of same outcome	Conversion formulas	Difficulties in clinical interpretation
Different outcomes, same construct	Standardised effects	Difficulties in clinical interpretation
Different outcomes	Meta-analysis of multiple outcomes	Specification of correlations
Observational data	Generalized evidence synthesis	Spurious precision, confounding, selective reporting
Cluster randomised trials	Account for clustering correlation	Unavailable sufficient information
Crossover trials	Account for period or carry-over effect	Unavailable sufficient information
Other study design issues	Same as for high statistical heterogeneity	As for high statistical heterogeneity above
Different participants or settings	Same as for high statistical heterogeneity	As for high statistical heterogeneity above
Many counts per participant	Meta-analysis of multiple period or follow-up	Unavailable sufficient information
Limited data	Standard meta-analysis methods	Caution needed as for any meta-analysis

Note: Popular software such as RevMan can accommodate only random-effects calculations, while Comprehensive Meta-Analysis also accommodates simple meta-regressions. Bayesian models and models of multiple treatments or outcomes can be run in WinBugs. Most models can also be run in STATA or R.

*The approach used for high statistical heterogeneity may also be applicable to situations where clinical heterogeneity is considered high because of differences in interventions, metrics, outcomes, designs, participants, or settings.

Source: Ioannidis JP, Patsopoulos NA, Rothstein HR. Reasons or excuses for avoiding meta-analysis in forest plots. *BMJ.* 2008;336(7658):1413–1415. doi:10.1136/bmj.a117

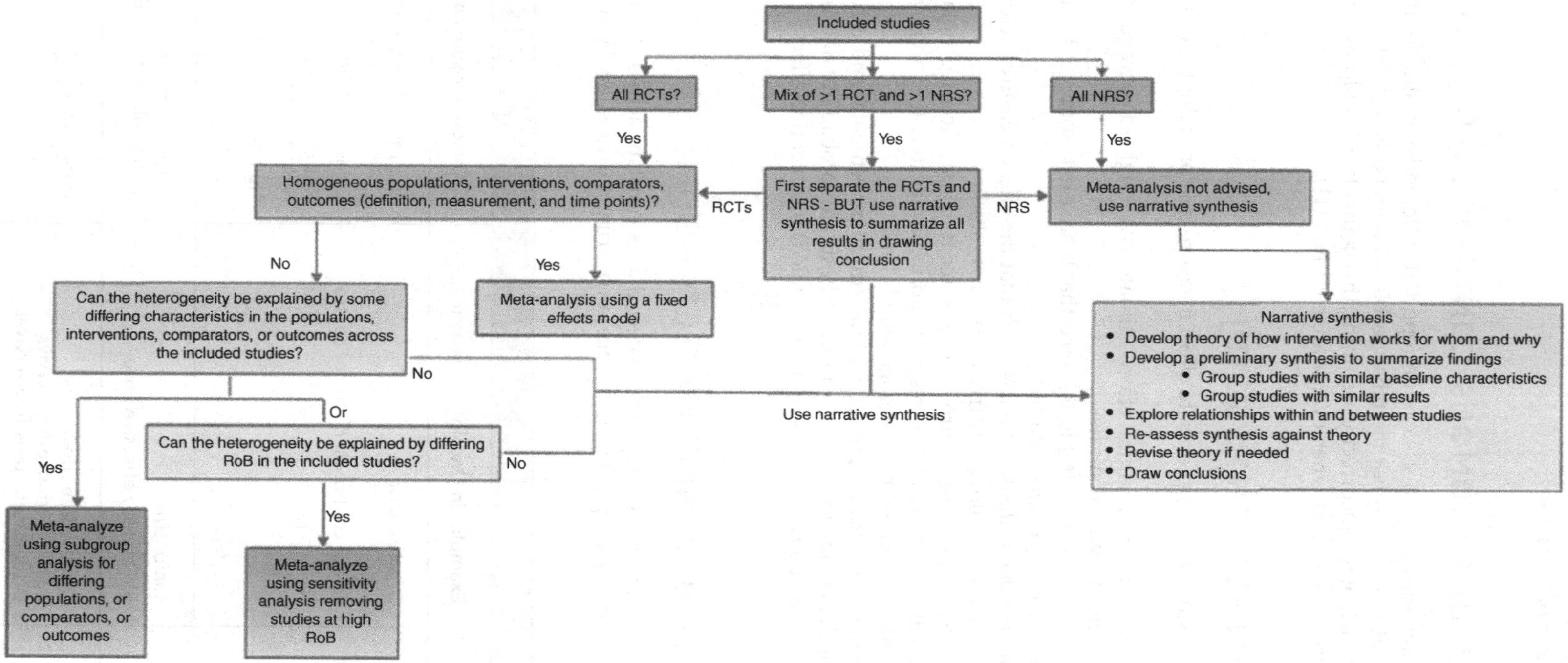

FIGURE 28.3 Flowchart to decide whether to perform a narrative synthesis or a meta-analyze.

NRS, nonrandomized studies; RCT, randomized controlled trials; RoB, risk of bias.

Source: Knoll T, Omar MI, Maclennan S, et al. Key steps in conducting systematic reviews for underpinning clinical practice guidelines: methodology of the European Association of Urology. *Eur Urol*. 2018;73:290–300. doi:10.1016/j.eururo.2017.08.016

- Exploring relationships in the data
- Assessing the robustness of the data

EFFECT MEASURES: DICHOTOMOUS, CONTINUOUS, TIME TO EVENT

Depending on the outcome measure, effects can be reported differently, as shown in Table 28.3. It is important to note that risk ratio is not interchangeable with an odds ratio, though these are often misinterpreted for each other. Incorrectly assuming this equivalence could overestimate the observed intervention effect, especially when events are common (11).

STEPS TO PERFORM META-ANALYSIS (11)

1. Calculate summary statistic of the appropriate effect measure (see preceding text) for each individual study.
2. Calculate a summary (pooled) intervention effect estimate as a weighted average of the effects measures estimated in the individual studies.
   a. Perform a *fixed-effects meta-analysis* if it is assumed that there exists some underlying "true" effect measure that is constant across studies.
   b. Perform *random-effects meta-analysis* if it is assumed that the effect measures across studies are not the same but actually follow a distribution across studies.
   c. Perform a *mixed-effects meta-analysis* to provide more accurate variances for meta-estimates when the heterogeneity among studies is high, or more conservative (i.e., somewhat inflated) variance estimates when the heterogeneity is low.
3. Derive a confidence interval (indicates precision of the summary estimate) and calculate a p value (indicates strength of evidence against null hypothesis and probability of false-positive results) based on the standard error of the summary (pooled) intervention effect.
4. Assess *heterogeneity*.

FIXED-EFFECTS VERSUS RANDOM-EFFECTS MODEL

A *fixed-effects model* assumes an underlying "true" effect that is constant across studies and that any differences between studies are a product of chance, answering the question: "What is the best

TABLE 28.3 COMMON EFFECTS MEASURES

Type of Effect Measure	Examples in Oncology Research	Common Measures of Effect
Dichotomous	Dead vs. alive Tumor control vs. no tumor control	Risk ratio / Relative risk (RR) Odds ratio (OR) Risk difference / Absolute risk reduction (RD) Number needed to treat (NNT)
Continuous	Tumor size Biologically effective dose	Mean difference Standardized mean difference
Time to Event	Disease-free survival Local recurrence-free survival Distant metastasis-free survival	Hazard ratio

estimate of the intervention effect?" (11). Meta-analysis of dichotomous outcomes can be carried out using three fixed-effects methods: Mantel-Haenszel, Peto, and inverse variance. The Mantel-Haenszel method is used most commonly because its versatility allows it to be applied to different effect measure types (risk ratio, odds ratio, risk difference) (11). For continuous and time-to-event outcomes, the inverse-variance method can be used for both fixed- and random-effects models (see the Cochrane Handbook 9.4.3, "A generic inverse-variance approach to meta-analysis" for more information).

A *random-effects model*, such as the DerSimonian and Laird method, assumes that effect measures vary across different populations in some unknown underlying distribution, answering the question: "What is the average intervention effect?" (11). The random-effects model will mirror the fixed-effects model when there is no heterogeneity. However, if heterogeneity is present, a random-effects model will estimate a wider confidence interval around an estimated effect measure than a fixed-effects model will, leading to more conservative claims of statistical significance. A disadvantage, however, is that a random-effects model will place greater weight on a smaller study compared to a fixed-effects model, allowing a smaller study to affect the overall effect estimate. Smaller studies can be susceptible to publication bias and overestimate treatment effects, skewing the results of meta-analysis when using a random-effects model. Thus, one option is to compare using a random-effects model initially, then construct a fixed-effects model as a sensitivity analysis (15).

Finally, meta-analysis with a *mixed-effects model* is sometimes preferable to one with fixed effects in the context of patient care decision making (16,17). In general, if the estimates are consistent between trials, then a fixed-effects model might be appropriate. The mixed-effects model includes random and fixed effects, and it tends to provide more accurate variances for meta-estimates when the heterogeneity among studies is high and somewhat inflated variance estimates when the heterogeneity is low. For example, there may be clear evidence of heterogeneity for certain results and less so for others. When analyzing outcomes from a considerable number of studies, assuming heterogeneity and applying one consistent robust approach may be somewhat conservative for highly consistent data. In general, the use of the mixed-effects regression model does not have strong or adverse impacts on the conclusions drawn. If researchers use a mixed-effects model and analyze a dependent versus independent variable (e.g., outcome versus dose) (7,18), the width of the confidence intervals generated by the mixed modeling approach accounts for the degree of heterogeneity seen in the data and appropriately represents the level of uncertainty in parameter estimates.

HETEROGENEITY

Statistical heterogeneity is the variability in effects measures across different studies due to clinical diversity (differences in participants, intervention, and outcomes) and methodological diversity (differences in study design and risk of bias).

One way to evaluate heterogeneity is to visually inspect a **forest plot** as shown in Figure 28.4. Forest plots display the effects measures and confidence intervals for a particular outcome of interest from both individual studies and the combined overall estimate from meta-analysis (19). Generally, studies are listed on the left side chronologically by author and date. On the right, a graph and a table with specific data values for effects measures are presented. In the graph, a solid vertical line indicates the line of no effect. For each individual study, the value of the effect measure is plotted as a square whose area represents the weight assigned to that study. Through this square, a horizontal line is plotted, usually representing the 95% confidence interval. A diamond is plotted at the bottom to represent the pooled estimate, with horizontal lines extending to its 95% confidence interval. A dotted vertical line runs through the center of the diamond at the value of the pooled estimate. If the diamond does not intersect with the line of no effect, the pooled estimate is considered statistically significant (20).

Reviewers can also include the results of the **Cochran's Q test** for heterogeneity with the associated p value in a forest plot. The Cochran's Q test whether the differences between individual

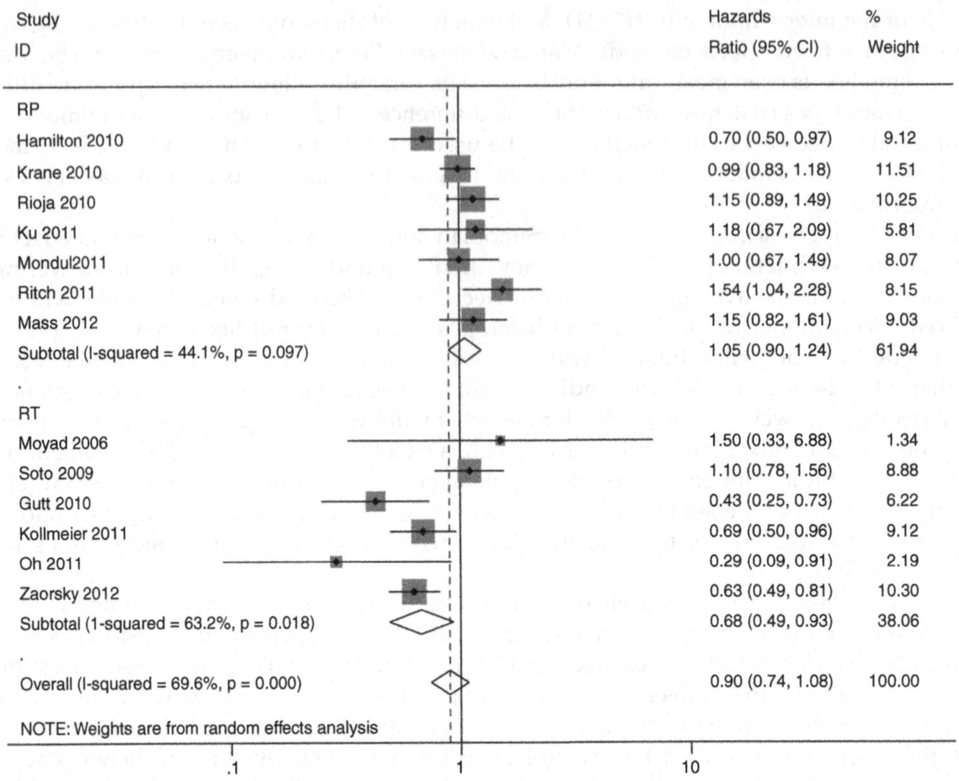

FIGURE 28.4 Example forest plot. Meta-analysis of studies investigating association of statins with RFS, stratified by primary treatment modality. Hazard ratios (HRs) and 95% confidence intervals (CIs) are reported on a logarithmic scale. Pooled estimates are from a random-effects model.

RFS, recurrence-free survival; RP, radical prostatectomy; RT, radiotherapy.

Source: Park HS, Schoenfeld JD, Mailhot RB, et al. Statins and prostate cancer recurrence following radical prostatectomy or radiotherapy: a systematic review and meta-analysis. *Ann Oncol.* 2013;24(6):1427–1434. doi:10.1093/annonc/mdt077

studies' effect measures and the common effect are attributable to more than a product of chance. A significant Cochran's Q test indicates the presence of statistical heterogeneity. Because a low number of studies might be underpowered to detect statistically significant heterogeneity and a high number of studies might be too sensitive, researchers often use an alpha of 0.10 to detect heterogeneity when only a few studies are included (21).

Instead of merely detecting the presence of heterogeneity (which is likely to exist), reviewers can also quantify inconsistency based on the impact of heterogeneity on meta-analysis. One such measure is I^2, which is based on the Cochran's Q test statistic and the degrees of freedom. Generally, I^2 values of 25%, 50%, and 75% are considered to represent low, moderate, and high amounts of heterogeneity, respectively (22). These cutoffs can be arbitrary, so reviewers might judge heterogeneity at their own discretion.

If statistical heterogeneity is detected, options include the following:

1. Verify data (e.g., standard errors might be entered mistakenly as standard deviation).
2. Avoid performing meta-analysis.
3. Explore heterogeneity to determine potential causes by conducting subgroup analyses or meta-regression.
4. Ignore heterogeneity, as in fixed-effects meta-analysis.

5. Perform random-effects or mixed-effects meta-analysis to account for heterogeneity that cannot be explained.
6. Change the effect measure; for example, standardized mean difference instead of mean difference if continuous data use different scales or units.
7. Exclude studies that have an apparent reason for causing an outlying result. There is a risk of bias here because an outlying characteristic can be isolated in almost any individual study, but it is reasonable to consider this strategy in sensitivity analyses (11).

SUBGROUP ANALYSIS

Interaction is the variation on intervention effect observed with different populations or intervention characteristics such as dose or timing.

Reviewers can investigate interaction through **subgroup analysis**—separating the overall study population by characteristics such as age, sex, tumor stage, treatment modality, and geography. Unless reviewers have access to individual patient data (to be discussed in the following text), it is less likely that they will be able to perform subgroup analysis on subsets of participants within studies. Quantitative interaction occurs when an intervention benefits various subgroups to different degrees. Though this occurs uncommonly, qualitative interaction can occur if an intervention is beneficial for one subgroup but is harmful for another subgroup.

Subgroup analysis should be treated carefully because it is typically performed retrospectively, and there is a risk of false-negative or false-positive findings (23). Thus, reviewers should document any planned subgroup analysis in the protocol beforehand to minimize selective reporting and identify any post hoc subgroup analyses in the final report.

If comparing only two subgroups, reviewers can infer that there is a statistically significant difference between the subgroups if the confidence intervals do not overlap, in general. Reviewers can perform subgroup analysis using Cochrane's RevMan software by testing for heterogeneity across subgroups as opposed to individual studies.

META-REGRESSION

Meta-regression allows the exploration of continuous characteristics in addition to categorical characteristics across studies and should only be considered if including at least 10 studies for each characteristic modelled. In meta-regression, reviewers examine the influence of an explanatory variable—a *covariate* (a characteristic of the included study)—on an outcome variable (an effect estimate such as mean difference, risk difference, log odds ratio, log risk ratio). A meta-regression differs from simple regression in that larger studies are weighted more heavily than smaller studies. A regression coefficient describing the linear relationship between the outcome and explanatory variables can be obtained (11).

Example: Zaorsky et al. examined the effect of increasing biologically equivalent dose of external radiation therapy on various patient outcomes (such as overall survival, distant metastasis, cancer-specific mortality, and genitourinary and gastrointestinal toxicities) through the use of mixed-effects meta-regression models (7).

SENSITIVITY ANALYSIS

To show that the summary findings are not a product of unclear or arbitrary inclusion of studies, **sensitivity analyses** can be performed by repeating the meta-analysis with different subsets of the included studies. Examples include

- Comparing only studies with similar dosing schedules (24)
- Including only studies with sufficient follow-up (25)
- Using a fixed-effects model if a random-effects model was used initially (11)

These analyses can be planned a priori in the protocol, but can also be designed during the review process. Furthermore, it is recommended that the results of sensitivity analyses be reported in a summary table or figure, rather than presenting individual forest plots. Reviewers can be more certain of their findings if the combined effect measure does not vary much on various sensitivity analyses.

It should be noted that sensitivity analyses differ from subgroup analyses in that only the effect measure is estimated for the included studies. The effect of the newly excluded studies is not estimated. In subgroup analysis, studies in each subgroup would be evaluated. Moreover, sensitivity analyses do not require the same formal statistical comparisons as are required by prespecified subgroup analyses.

REPORTING BIAS

Reporting bias occurs because studies reporting positive findings are more likely to be published, published more quickly, published in higher impact journals, cited more often, and published in English, compared to those reporting negative findings (15). One way to address this bias is to include "gray literature," or studies not published by commercial publishers. However, this can introduce more bias, because gray literature is not peer-reviewed and might have lower methodological quality (26).

A **funnel plot**, as shown in Figure 28.5, helps detect potential bias through a scatter plot of intervention effect estimates on the horizontal scale and some measure of precision or study size on the vertical scale. The funnel shape is observed as effect estimates converge with increased precision as the study size increases. Effect estimates will be more widely spread out at the base of the plot where study size is smaller (15). Asymmetrical funnel plots may indicate the presence of publication bias, differences in study quality, true heterogeneity, or chance. When at least 10 studies are included, a statistical test like **Egger's regression asymmetry test** (27) can be performed to evaluate funnel plot asymmetry. Other tests of asymmetry have been developed, so it may be helpful to consult a statistician regarding the appropriate test (15).

SYSTEMATIC REVIEWS OF NONRANDOMIZED STUDIES

Traditionally, many have subscribed to a hierarchy of study designs based on methodological quality, with RCTs considered the highest quality, followed by cohort studies, then case–control

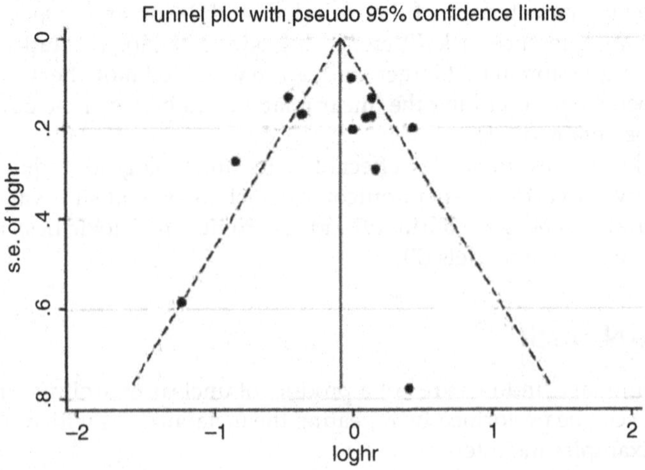

FIGURE 28.5 Example funnel plot.

Source: Park HS, Schoenfeld JD, Mailhot RB, et al. Statins and prostate cancer recurrence following radical prostatectomy or radiotherapy: a systematic review and meta-analysis. *Ann Oncol.* 2013;24(6):1427–1434. doi:10.1093/annonc/mdt077

studies, then case series/reports. In Figure 28.6, the wavy lines indicate that each type of study design has its own methodological limitations or strengths on an individual study basis. For example, an RCT might be inadequately concealed and blinded, whereas a nonrandomized observational study might be of high methodological quality (28).

REASONS TO PERFORM A SYSTEMATIC REVIEW OF NONRANDOMIZED STUDIES

Although systematic reviews of RCTs usually provide less biased information compared with reviews that include other study designs, there are certain circumstances in which reviewers should consider including nonrandomized studies that might be moderately susceptible to bias. Some reasons include

1. Evaluating the limitations of currently available nonrandomized studies and consequently highlighting the need for higher quality RCTs while identifying potential subgroups for RCT design
2. Synthesizing the available body of knowledge on interventions that cannot be randomized (e.g., risk of lung cancer from those exposed to secondhand smoke)
3. Reporting on the effects that cannot be studied in RCTs, such as long-term outcomes, rare outcomes, or previously unknown outcomes (29)
4. Summarizing existing evidence on rare conditions (e.g., craniopharyngiomas) that are unlikely to be studied in RCTs
5. Understanding effects of therapy on populations like children, pregnant women, or the elderly, who are often excluded from RCTs (30). Nonrandomized studies of a wider population might help to generalize study findings. However, the Cochrane Handbook cautions that increased bias associated with nonrandomized studies could lead to misleading conclusions in RCTs and might not necessarily serve the aim of generalization (29)

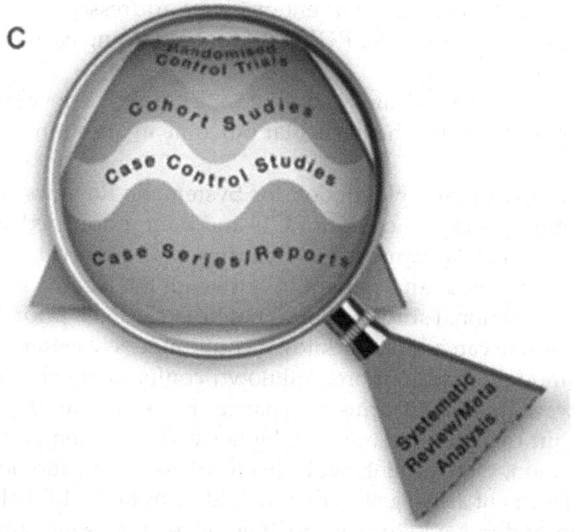

FIGURE 28.6 "The revised pyramid: systematic reviews are a lens through which evidence is viewed (applied)."

Source: Murad MH, Asi N, Alsawas M, Alahdab F. New evidence pyramid. *Evid Based Med.* 2016;21(4):125–127. doi:10.1136/ebmed-2016-110401

However, issues with performing systematic reviews of nonrandomized studies include selection bias and confounding (31), which can affect summary measures when combining data across studies, and can lead to greater heterogeneity (29).

CONSIDERATIONS FOR PERFORMING SYSTEMATIC REVIEWS OF NONRANDOMIZED STUDIES

Though much of the basic structure for performing systematic reviews of nonrandomized studies is shared with that for reviewing RCTs, some key points are important to consider:

Protocol: In the protocol, the reasoning for including nonrandomized studies should be documented (29).

Eligibility criteria: When prespecifying study designs in the eligibility criteria, reviewers may plan to include nonrandomized studies if too few RCTs are found. If this occurs, the Cochrane group recommends that nonrandomized studies and RCTs be presented separately (29). Another possibility is to include RCTs to evaluate benefits of an intervention, while including nonrandomized studies to report on harms of an intervention. For example, rare instances of an adverse effect might not be detected during the follow-up period of RCTs, but could be presented in case series or case–control studies (29).

Risk of bias assessment: The Cochrane Bias Methods Group and Cochrane Non-Randomized Studies Methods Group developed the **ROBINS-I** tool for evaluating the risk of bias in nonrandomized studies of interventions (32). The ROBINS-I tool similarly evaluates across several domains, but also incorporates the evaluation of confounding. Additional background information and templates can be found online at www.riskofbias.info.

During systematic review protocol development, reviewers should list potential confounders and co-interventions that might affect outcomes. Then, for each included study and every outcome assessed, reviewers should

1. Document how confounders and cointerventions were addressed
2. Answer guided questions listed in the ROBINS-I tool regarding each bias domain, recording textual support from each study
3. Judge the risk of bias for each domain according to the answers developed in steps 1 and 2
4. Assess the overall risk of bias for the particular outcome in question

Synthesis: Although the Cochrane Handbook for Systematic Reviews of Interventions advises against combining evidence from RCTs and nonrandomized studies (29), others have made the case that "advantages of including both observational studies and randomized studies in a meta-analysis could outweigh the disadvantages in many situations and that observational studies should not be excluded a priori" (33). Shrier et al. make the case that one can adjust for known confounders in observational studies by using statistical models. Furthermore, unknown confounders should theoretically be allocated between treatment arms by chance. For example, if researchers are unaware that a certain treatment results in a higher toxicity when patients have a preexisting heart condition, then patients with this heart condition should be randomly assigned between treatment arms, just as they would be in RCTs. RCTs have been found to contradict nonrandomized studies, but they have also been contradicted by other RCTs (34). Studies comparing RCTs with high-quality nonrandomized studies examining the same question have found similar results (35–38). Shrier et al. conclude that study design can be explored as an explanatory variable, requiring an assessment of whether or not study design is the reason for discrepancies between studies.

INDIVIDUAL PATIENT DATA

Individual patient data (IPD) (as opposed to literature-based) meta-analysis is considered the "gold standard" approach, because it entails collecting original research data from individual study authors instead of merely extracting published summary data. The steps for performing an IPD review are similar to those for other systematic reviews through the study selection stages and only differ at the data collection, verification, and analysis stages. Usually, a team performing an IPD review includes the researchers contributing study data, individuals managing the project, and, potentially, an advisory group.

Some advantages of IPD reviews, especially in cancer research, are that they incorporate unpublished data, allow for better time-to-event analyses when evaluation time periods vary across studies, offer an opportunity for researchers to provide more updated data, enable more detailed subgroup analysis than can be carried out within studies themselves, and allow for further exploration of specific patient characteristics as prognostic factors. However, IPD reviews generally require more effort to contact individual trial authors to persuade them to collaborate and share data.

Example: In a large systematic review and meta-analysis of IPD from 194 randomized trials, the Early Breast Cancer Trialists' Collaborative Group (EBCTCG) studied the effects of various adjuvant chemotherapy or hormone therapy treatments on breast cancer survival and recurrence (2). The study authors compared outcomes for several subgroups according to age, type of chemotherapy regimen, presence or absence of hormone therapy, hormone receptor status, nodal status, and period of follow-up, identifying favorable treatment plans for a range of patient characteristics.

NETWORK META-ANALYSIS

A network meta-analysis compares multiple interventions for the same disease and outcomes (39). Whereas standard meta-analyses usually only study two interventions that have been compared directly, network meta-analyses evaluate two separate interventions that have never been compared head-to-head in a study through a common comparator that has been studied directly (e.g., combining studies of A vs. B with studies of B vs. C to compare the effects of A vs. C).

Example: An IPD network meta-analysis studying the best treatment for nasopharyngeal carcinoma combined data from 20 trials of 5,144 patients who were treated with seven different permutations of adjuvant chemotherapy, induction chemotherapy, and radiotherapy (40). Through network meta-analysis, the authors were able to evaluate the effect of different timings of concomitant chemotherapy that had not been directly compared before.

CONCLUSION

Systematic reviews and meta-analyses are useful in synthesizing the results of individual studies, and thus can lead to greater power and precision in summary estimates, leading in turn to potentially practice-changing findings. However, it is critical to perform these analyses in a methodical fashion to ensure the validity and generalizability of the results, acknowledging that the limitations of the conclusions depend on the quality of the extracted data. We hope that this chapter serves as a helpful starting point for researchers working to perform these analyses.

HELPFUL RESOURCES

1. CRD. Systematic Reviews: CRD's Guidance for Undertaking Reviews in Healthcare. CRD, University of York; 2009.

2. Higgins J, Green S, (editors). Cochrane Handbook for Systematic Reviews of Interventions Version 5.1.0 [updated March 2011]. The Cochrane Collaboration, 2011: Available from www.handbook.cochrane.org
3. Liberati A, Altman DG, Tetzlaff J, et al. The PRISMA statement for reporting systematic reviews and meta-analyses of studies that evaluate health care interventions: explanation and elaboration. *PLoS Med*. 2009;6(7):e1000100.

GLOSSARY

Cochran's Q test: tests whether the differences between individual studies' effect measures and the common effect are attributed to more than a product of chance. A significant Cochran Q test indicates the presence of statistical heterogeneity.

Egger's regression asymmetry test: a statistical test to evaluate funnel plot asymmetry.

forest plot: graphic display of the effect measures and confidence intervals for a particular outcome of interest from both individual studies and the combined overall estimate from meta-analysis.

funnel plot: helps detect potential bias through a scatter plot of intervention effect estimates on the horizontal scale and some measure of precision or study size on the vertical scale. The funnel shape is observed as effect estimates converge with increased precision as the study size increases.

sensitivity analysis: repeating a meta-analysis with different subsets of included studies and estimating effect measures only for these included studies.

statistical heterogeneity: the variability in effect measures across different studies due to clinical diversity (differences in participants, intervention, and outcomes) and methodological diversity (differences in study design and risk of bias).

subgroup analysis: separating the overall study population by characteristics such as age, sex, tumor stage, treatment modality, or geography, and estimating effect measures for each group.

systematic review: a reproducible methodology that entails

1. Stating a clear objective to address a specific research question
2. Systematically identifying all relevant studies
3. Selecting eligible studies with predefined criteria
4. Assessing risk of bias
5. Extracting data
6. Presenting qualitative synthesis of included studies

meta-analysis: a review that summarizes and combines the results of independent studies that measure the effects of similar treatment approaches on similar patient populations through statistical methods.

PRISMA: the **P**referred **R**eporting **I**tems for **S**ystematic **R**eviews and **M**eta-**A**nalyses guidelines, which were put together by a team of expert researchers, along with a step-by-step guide to and explanations for writing the manuscript of a systematic review and meta-analysis.

ROBINS-I tool: developed by the Cochrane Bias Methods Group and Cochrane Non-Randomized Studies Methods Group for evaluating the risk of bias in nonrandomized studies of interventions.

REFERENCES

1. Green S, Higgins J. Preparing a Cochrane review. In: Higgins J, Green S, eds. *Cochrane Handbook for Systematic Reviews of Interventions*. Version 5.1.0. London, UK: The Cochrane Collaboration; 2011:11–30. http://handbook-5-1.cochrane.org/
2. Early Breast Cancer Trialists' Collaborative Group. Effects of chemotherapy and hormonal therapy for early breast cancer on recurrence and 15-year survival: an overview of the randomised trials. *Lancet*. 2005;365(9472):1687–1717. doi:10.1016/s0140-6736(05)66544-0
3. Viani GA, Afonso SL, Stefano EJ, et al. Adjuvant trastuzumab in the treatment of her-2-positive early breast cancer: a meta-analysis of published randomized trials. *BMC Cancer*. 2007;7:153. doi:10.1186/1471-2407-7-153
4. O'Connor D, Green S, Higgins J. Defining the review question and developing criteria for including studies. In: Higgins J, Green S, eds. *Cochrane Handbook for Systematic Reviews of Interventions*. Version 5.1.0. London, UK: The Cochrane Collaboration; 2011:83–94. http://handbook-5-1.cochrane.org
5. Lefebvre C, Manheimer EJG. Chapter 6: Searching for studies. In: Higgins J, Green S, eds. *Cochrane Handbook for Systematic Reviews of Interventions*. Version 5.1.0. London, UK: The Cochrane Collaboration; 2011:95–150. http://handbook-5-1.cochrane.org
6. Liberati A, Altman DG, Tetzlaff J, et al. The PRISMA statement for reporting systematic reviews and meta-analyses of studies that evaluate health care interventions: explanation and elaboration. *PLoS Med*. 2009;6(7):e1000100. doi:10.1371/journal.pmed.1000100
7. Zaorsky NG, Keith SW, Shaikh T, et al. Impact of radiation therapy dose escalation on prostate cancer outcomes and toxicities. *Am J Clin Oncol*. 2018;41(4):409–415.
8. Higgins JPT, Deeks JJ, (editors). Chapter 7: Selecting studies and collecting data. Table 7.3.a: Checklist of items to consider in data collection or data extraction. In: Higgins JPT, Green S, eds. *Cochrane Handbook for Systematic Reviews of Interventions*. Chichester, UK: John Wiley & Sons; 2008:157.
9. Higgins JP, Altman DG, Gotzsche PC, et al. The Cochrane Collaboration's tool for assessing risk of bias in randomised trials. *BMJ*. 2011;343:d5928. doi:10.1136/bmj.d5928
10. Stevens R, Macbeth F, Toy E, et al. Palliative radiotherapy regimens for patients with thoracic symptoms from non-small cell lung cancer. *Cochrane Database Syst Rev*. 2015;1:CD002143. doi:10.1002/14651858.cd002143.pub3
11. Deeks J, Higgins J, Altman DG. Analysing data and undertaking meta-analyses. In: Higgins J, Green S, eds. *Cochrane Handbook for Systematic Reviews of Interventions*. Version 5.1.0. London, UK: The Cochrane Collaboration; 2011:243–296. http://handbook-5-1.cochrane.org
12. Ioannidis JP, Patsopoulos NA, Rothstein HR. Reasons or excuses for avoiding meta-analysis in forest plots. *BMJ*. 2008;336(7658):1413–1415. doi:10.1136/bmj.a117
13. Knoll T, Omar MI, Maclennan S, et al. Key steps in conducting systematic reviews for underpinning clinical practice guidelines: methodology of the European Association of Urology. *Eur Urol*. 2018;73:290–300. doi:10.1016/j.eururo.2017.08.016
14. Popay J, Roberts H, Sowden A, et al. Guidance on the conduct of narrative synthesis in systematic reviews. *ESRC Methods Programme*. 2006.
15. Sterne JA, Egger M, Moher D. Addressing reporting biases. In: Higgins J, Green S, eds. *Cochrane Handbook for Systematic Reviews of Interventions*. Version 5.1.0. London, UK: The Cochrane Collaboration; 2011:335–358. http://handbook-5-1.cochrane.org
16. Ades AE, Lu G, Higgins JP. The interpretation of random-effects meta-analysis in decision models. *Med Decis Making*. 2005;25(6):646–654. doi:10.1177/0272989x05282643
17. Fleiss JL, Gross AJ. Meta-analysis in epidemiology, with special reference to studies of the association between exposure to environmental tobacco smoke and lung cancer: a critique. *J Clin Epidemiol*. 1991;44(2):127–139. doi:10.1016/0895-4356(91)90261-7
18. Zaorsky NG, Lee CT, Zhang E, et al. Hypofractionated radiation therapy for basal and squamous cell skin cancer: A meta-analysis. *Radiother Oncol*. 2017;125(1):13–20. doi:10.1016/j.radonc.2017.08.011
19. Lewis S, Clarke M. Forest plots: trying to see the wood and the trees. *Brit Med J*. 2001;322(7300):1479–1480. doi:10.1136/bmj.322.7300.1479
20. Park HS, Schoenfeld JD, Mailhot RB, et al. Statins and prostate cancer recurrence following radical prostatectomy or radiotherapy: a systematic review and meta-analysis. *Ann Oncol*. 2013;24(6):1427–1434. doi:10.1093/annonc/mdt077
21. Deeks JJ, Altman DG, Bradburn MJ. Statistical methods for examining heterogeneity and combining results from several studies in meta-analysis. In: Egger M, Smith GD, Altman D, eds. *Systematic Reviews in Health Care: Meta-Analysis in Context*. London, UK: BMJ Books; 2001:285–312.
22. Higgins JP, Thompson SG, Deeks JJ, Altman DG. Measuring inconsistency in meta-analyses. *BMJ*. 2003;327(7414):557–560. doi:10.1136/bmj.327.7414.557
23. Davey Smith G, Egger M, Phillips AN. Meta-analysis. Beyond the grand mean? *BMJ*. 1997;315(7122):1610–1614. doi:10.1136/bmj.315.7122.1610
24. Fairchild A, Harris K, Barnes E, et al. Palliative thoracic radiotherapy for lung cancer: a systematic review. *J Clin Oncol*. 2008;26(24):4001–4011. doi:10.1200/jco.2007.15.3312
25. Mauguen A, Le Pechoux C, Saunders MI, et al. Hyperfractionated or accelerated radiotherapy in lung cancer: an individual patient data meta-analysis. *J Clin Oncol*. 2012;30(22):2788–2797. doi:10.1200/jco.2012.41.6677
26. Egger M, Juni P, Bartlett C, et al. How important are comprehensive literature searches and the assessment of trial quality in systematic reviews? Empirical study. *Health Technol Assess*. 2003;7(1):1–76.
27. Egger M, Davey Smith G, Schneider M, Minder C. Bias in meta-analysis detected by a simple, graphical test. *BMJ*. 1997;315(7109):629–634. doi:10.1136/bmj.315.7109.629

28. Murad MH, Asi N, Alsawas M, Alahdab F. New evidence pyramid. *Evid Based Med.* 2016;21(4):125–127. doi:10.1136/ebmed-2016-110401
29. Reeves B, Deeks J, Higgins J, Wells GA. Including non-randomized studies. In: Higgins J, Green S, eds. *Cochrane Handbook for Systematic Reviews of Interventions.* Version 5.1.0. London, UK: The Cochrane Collaboration; 2011:391–432. http://handbook-5-1.cochrane.org
30. Hutchins LF, Unger JM, Crowley JJ, et al. Underrepresentation of patients 65 years of age or older in cancer-treatment trials. *N Engl J Med.* 1999;341(27):2061–2067. doi:10.1056/nejm199912303412706
31. Giordano SH, Kuo YF, Duan Z, et al. Limits of observational data in determining outcomes from cancer therapy. *Cancer.* 2008;112(11):2456–2466. doi:10.1002/cncr.23452
32. Sterne JA, Hernan MA, Reeves BC, et al. ROBINS-I: a tool for assessing risk of bias in non-randomised studies of interventions. *BMJ.* 2016;355:i4919. doi:10.1136/bmj.i4919
33. Shrier I, Boivin JF, Steele RJ, et al. Should meta-analyses of interventions include observational studies in addition to randomized controlled trials? A critical examination of underlying principles. *Am J Epidemiol.* 2007;166(10):1203–1209. doi:10.1093/aje/kwm189
34. Ioannidis JP. Contradicted and initially stronger effects in highly cited clinical research. *JAMA.* 2005;294(2):218–228. doi:10.1001/jama.294.2.218
35. Concato J, Shah N, Horwitz RI. Randomized, controlled trials, observational studies, and the hierarchy of research designs. *N Engl J Med.* 2000;342(25):1887–1892. doi:10.1056/NEJM200006223422507
36. MacLehose RR, Reeves BC, Harvey IM, et al. A systematic review of comparisons of effect sizes derived from randomised and non-randomised studies. *Health Technol Assess.* 2000;4(34):1–154. doi:10.3310/hta4340
37. Benson K, Hartz AJ. A comparison of observational studies and randomized, controlled trials. *N Engl J Med.* 2000;342(25):1878–1886. doi:10.1056/NEJM200006223422506
38. Ioannidis JP, Haidich AB, Pappa M, et al. Comparison of evidence of treatment effects in randomized and nonrandomized studies. *JAMA.* 2001;286(7):821–830. doi:10.1001/jama.286.7.821
39. Mills EJ, Thorlund K, Ioannidis JP. Demystifying trial networks and network meta-analysis. *BMJ.* 2013;346:f2914. doi:10.1136/bmj.f2914
40. Ribassin-Majed L, Marguet S, Lee AWM, et al. What is the best treatment of locally advanced nasopharyngeal carcinoma? an individual patient data network meta-analysis. *J Clin Oncol.* 2017;35(5):498–505. doi:10.1200/JCO.2016.67.4119

29 Future Directions in Clinical Cancer Research

BRANDON E. TURNER ■ AADEL A. CHAUDHURI

The future of cancer research is a rapidly changing space that is increasingly defined by multiple, converging technological trends. Advances in engineering are facilitating the development of experimental techniques that sensitively probe molecular information that was previously inaccessible or prohibitively expensive to develop. These methods often generate enormous amounts of data, requiring new strategies and infrastructure for rapidly storing, querying, and retrieving information for researchers to study. New analytical techniques have risen in parallel to enable researchers to combine and extract biological and clinical insights from this exploding collection of information.

This chapter explores many of the emerging tools and concepts that are essential to future cancer research. These analyses are referred to as "**omics**" because they capture information about the genome, transcriptome, metabolome, or other "-omes." Omics analyses require unique toolsets, and each is frequently the sole focus of entire textbooks. The goal for this chapter is to introduce the critical background for understanding each of these topics, provide a conceptual overview of the typical tools and analytic techniques required to perform the analyses, and highlight some of the example applications and emerging trends in cancer research and clinical practice.

GENOMICS

The **central dogma** of molecular biology states that the flow of information in biological systems starts at the level of nucleic acids and flows toward proteins (1). The classic, more granular simplification of this dogma asserts DNA → RNA → proteins → phenotype. The **genome** comprises all the coding and noncoding DNA within a biological system. Genomic instability is one of the hallmarks of cancer and an important part of the mechanism by which cancer cells accumulate mutations that permit proliferative capabilities such as sustained angiogenesis, evasion of the immune system, and resistance to cell death (2). Whereas early studies of cancer genetics examined individual or panels of genes, genomic studies assess the entire genome to analyze all genes concurrently. At their core, genomic studies seek to understand how genome sequence variants give rise to specific phenotypes and endpoints (e.g., cancer, survival, response to therapy).

The first effort to sequence the entire 3 billion base-pair human genome was an unprecedented challenge, the immense scale of which was matched only by the $3 billion effort required to complete it in 2003 (3). The first two full genomes were sequenced using Sanger sequencing and shotgun sequencing, both accurate but difficult to scale for large cohorts (4,5). Modern high-throughput sequencing methods have dramatically increased the speed of sequencing while simultaneously decreasing the cost. **Next-generation sequencing** (**NGS**) is currently the most popular high-throughput genomics technique, though there are others such as **DNA microarrays** and **optical mapping** (6). NGS can refer to several distinct sequencing approaches (e.g., pyrosequencing, sequencing by synthesis, sequencing by ligation, ion semiconductor sequencing), with sequencing by synthesis being by far the most popular. However, almost all NGS methods share a similar core framework: (a) Extracted nucleic acids are processed to add **adapter** sequences for template or "library" preparation; (b) the adapter-ligated material then undergoes clonal amplification; (c) finally, the resulting product undergoes repeated rounds of massively parallel sequencing by addition and detection of synthetically altered nucleotides (6,7).

Alignment of detected sequences to the reference genome is crucial for biological interpretation and is accomplished using several established algorithms (8,9). By comparing these new sequences to the corresponding reference sequence, one can identify biologic variants including **single nucleotide variants** (**SNVs**), **insertions and deletions** (**indels**), **inversions**, **copy number variants** (**CNVs**), and **translocations**. There are also several less accurate algorithms that permit de novo genome assembly when a reference genome is unavailable or undesired (10,11).

Per sequencing read, NGS platforms are less accurate than traditional Sanger sequencing platforms, with the error rate for any given base pair (bp) being ~0.1% (6). Massively parallel sequencing ameliorates this issue by providing significant "coverage" (or "depth") at each nucleotide position resulting from multiple overlapping reads. Thus, the final consensus sequence is less susceptible to the effects of sporadic errors. Particular attention is also growing for NGS platforms that produce long reads, which are often >3,000 bp long and therefore able to span uninterrupted across repetitive or complex genomic regions (12). Such regions are normally challenging for short-read methods, which produce shorter continuous reads (~50–700 bp) that are difficult to localize accurately within repetitive or complex genomic regions (13). Compared to **whole genome sequencing** (**WGS**), **whole exome sequencing** (**WES**) methods further simplify this problem by using targeted probes to isolate only DNA fragments from the ~20,300 protein-coding genes. This "capture" method results in selectively sequencing only ~1% of the genome, which dramatically reduces cost, sequencing time, and mapping complexity. Although WES is less comprehensive than WGS, an estimated 85% of disease-causing mutations occur within exons, thus giving WES great utility and efficiency in clinical applications (14).

In the typical genomics workflow (Figure 29.1), DNA is first extracted from a sample (e.g., tumor biopsy; healthy tissue; peripheral blood mononuclear cells [PBMCs]). The DNA is fragmented and library preparation is performed before subsequently conducting NGS. The consensus sequence output is used to detect genome variants in the sample (e.g., SNVs, indels, CNVs). These variants are analyzed to identify significant genomic features that elucidate important biology. Some statistical analyses, such as **genome-wide association studies** (**GWAS**), are unique to genomic investigations. However, many other genomic analyses rely on **machine learning** and **bioinformatics** pipelines to extract valuable insights (15,16). Because genome sequencing can be time-consuming and expensive, studies often initially use NGS with small patient cohorts to identify promising gene candidates and subsequently track these genes across large cohorts using cheaper, targeted gene panels.

Genomics is the oldest "omic" and has already been used in a large number of applications to help refine our understanding of cancer. Cancers have originally been understood in terms of their tissues of origin—breast cancer, lung cancer, colon cancer, and so forth. Later work resulted in additional classification based on histology (e.g., adenocarcinoma vs. small-cell carcinoma), anatomical spread (i.e., TNM staging), and later molecular status (e.g., $EGFR^{+/-}$, $ER^{+/-}$, $PR^{+/-}$, $HER^{+/-}$). Genomic studies have taken this strategy further by analyzing and clustering cancers based on

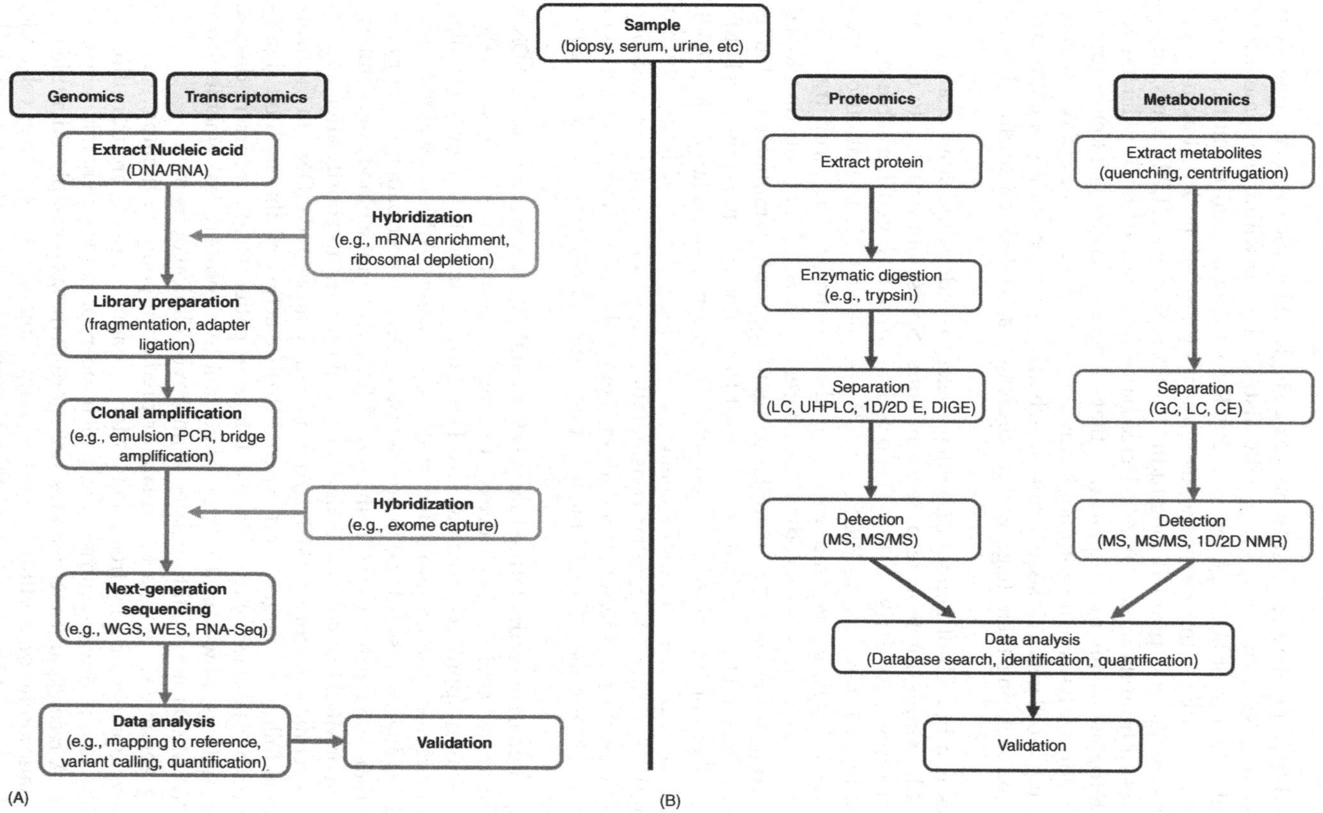

FIGURE 29.1 Sample workflows for omics techniques. (A) Simplified schematic for next-generation sequencing of nucleic acids. Hybridization step is optional, but selective probes may be used during WES to isolate and selectively sequence protein-coding DNA. For RNA-Seq, probes can bind rRNA for ribosomal depletion or can bind polyadenylated tail of mRNA for mRNA enrichment. (B) Simplified workflow schematic for both bottom-up "shotgun" proteomics and untargeted metabolomics. During metabolomics, a quenching reaction is performed to freeze metabolism and prevent further consumption of metabolites.

CE, capillary electrophoresis; DIGE, differential image gel electrophoresis; GC, gas chromatography; LC, liquid chromatography; MS, mass spectrometry; MS/MS, tandem mass spectrometry; NMR, nuclear magnetic resonance; RNA-Seq, RNA sequencing; UHPLC, ultrahigh-performance liquid chromatography; WES, whole exome sequencing; WGS, whole genome sequencing; 1D/2D E, one-/two-dimensional electrophoresis.

their entire genomes. A recent study of 10,000 samples from 33 different cancer types identified 28 distinct molecular subtypes (17). Though the cell of origin remained the most dominant determinant of which subtype a tumor was clustered into, many clusters included tumors from different cancers and many tumors from the same cancer type were dispersed across clusters. The molecular heterogeneity between tumors is now understood to be a major source of tumor resistance to therapy.

It is now understood that the view of most tumors as a single, if unique, molecular entity is also inaccurate. Studies using NGS on multiple, spatially distinct regions within the same tumor have revealed significant intra-tumor heterogeneity (18–20). Rather than a uniform entity, tumors can instead be compared to a tree with heterogeneous branches (or subclones) that accumulate diverse driver mutations when also profiled longitudinally through time (21,22). Thus, many treatment failures may result from therapies, often selected based on a single biopsy, which inadequately address the heterogeneous mixture of pathways that are perturbed across different tumor subclones. Higher resolution analyses of intra-tumor heterogeneity will likely depend on the continued development of single-cell genomic sequencing, which involves mechanically or enzymatically dissociating cells and isolating them (e.g., with fluorescence-activated cell sorting [FACS]) before sequencing (23).

Pharmacogenomics is a branch of genomics, which seeks to understand how analysis of genome-wide variants like **single nucleotide polymorphisms (SNPs)** can be used to explain patients' response to treatment. As early as 1956, reports had already noted heritable differences in drug response (24,25). Leveraging WGS or WES has enabled identification of complex relationships between drugs, genes, and various pathways that govern drug transport and metabolism (26–28). For example, observed racial differences in which patients developed toxicities to mercaptopurine, an essential antineoplastic agent for acute lymphoblastic leukemia (ALL), were revealed through GWAS analyses to result from inherited mutations in TPMT and NUDT15—both members of the pathway responsible for thiopurine metabolism (29,30). Pharmacogenomics for cancer presents a unique challenge because of the need to account for both somatic and germline variants (31). Similar considerations are also relevant for radiation genomics, which seeks to explain response to radiation therapy based on the patient/tumor genome (32,33). Identifying biomarkers for treatment response represents one of the major goals for genomic applications.

One such promising biomarker is **circulating tumor DNA (ctDNA)**, which is the result of DNA shed into the blood by tumors where it can be detected using highly sensitive NGS approaches (34). Targeted hybrid capture-based approaches such as CAPP-Seq can be used to achieve very high depth within the genomic region of interest to detect mutations (35,36); CAPP-Seq was shown to reliably detect minimal residual disease (MRD) in nonmetastatic lung cancer patients after radiotherapy months earlier than standard-of-care CT imaging (37). ctDNA in the blood was similarly shown to enable detection of MRD in colon cancer and breast cancer patients shortly after surgery, and correlated with worse clinical outcomes (38,39). Another study measured ctDNA in the urine of bladder cancer patients following surgery and showed that detection by this method significantly preceded detection by standard-of-care urine cytology in patients with recurrent disease (40). These are exciting findings; however, it will be important to rigorously test whether early intervention at the ctDNA MRD time point translates to improved clinical outcomes.

In addition to using genome-wide data to explain or predict response to therapy, genomic data can help guide development of new treatments. Many genomic studies are transitioning from a gene-specific view to a pathway-centric view, which incorporates the dynamic networks between multiple genes. A recent pan-cancer analysis of more than 9,000 samples identified 64 common patterns of somatic alterations within 10 canonical signaling pathways such as cell cycle, Myc, and RTK-RAS pathways (41). Their analysis further determined that 57% of tumors carried a potentially actionable alteration that could be targeted even using current drugs. Amid the recent proliferation and success of immunotherapies, analyses of tumor samples have also demonstrated how somatic aberrations influence the tumor microenvironment, including infiltrating leukocyte levels and the specific immune subtypes activated (16).

TRANSCRIPTOMICS

Although the accumulation of mutations and genomic instability are hallmark features of cancer, DNA variants ultimately must alter gene expression to influence phenotype. DNA variants (including noncoding regions) may influence both the types of RNA that are expressed and the level at which they are expressed. Unlike DNA, mRNA transcripts are transient and the half-life for mRNA degradation is on the order of minutes to hours (42). Thus, sequencing RNA transcripts provides a better real-time depiction of intracellular activity and thus phenotype within a biological system.

Strictly speaking, the genome refers to the collection of DNA, while the transcriptome comprises the total collection of RNA transcripts in a cell at a point in time. However, *genomics* is sometimes imprecisely used to refer to any large-scale study of nucleic acids. Early **transcriptomics** studies relied on tools like microarrays to quantify the transcriptome. Here mRNA transcripts are reverse-transcribed into cDNA before fragmentation and hybridization to oligonucleotide probes on an ordered microarray. Though high throughput and inexpensive, microarrays suffer from poor resolution and require large amounts of RNA to function effectively (43,44). Newer developments have improved microarray resolution (~5–20 bp); however, they still suffer from high background noise levels and a limited dynamic range when comparing expression levels between different genes (up to a few-hundredfold) (45). RNA sequencing (RNA-Seq) is an NGS method that has largely supplanted microarrays in transcriptomic analyses. As with other NGS techniques, RNA-Seq resolves sequences at a single-base level while requiring small amounts of RNA. RNA-Seq's dynamic range is also >8,000-fold. The experimental considerations for RNA-Seq are similar to those reviewed for NGS in the previous section.

A unique challenge to transcriptomic analysis is the inherent instability and fragility of RNA compared to DNA. This restricts the types of samples suitable for transcriptomic analyses and necessitates strict sample preparation protocols to preserve the reliability of quantitative analyses. For RNA-Seq analyses, RNA is first extracted from the biological sample. However, because most transcriptomic analyses are focused on mRNA, other types of RNA must be excluded during library preparation. This can be achieved by using oligonucleotide probes that bind rRNA sequences for rRNA depletion or that bind the polyadenylated (poly-A) tails of mRNA for mRNA enrichment (45). NGS also provides the capacity to sequence **noncoding RNA (ncRNA)** such as miRNA and siRNA. This process, though less precise, can be accomplished through a modified library preparation, which performs both 3′ and 5′ adapter ligation, polymerase chain reaction (PCR) amplification, and purification for short RNA fragments (~20–30 nt) using gel electrophoresis (46–48). Whichever method is chosen, after the RNA depletion, enrichment, or purification steps, the resulting library can be sequenced consistent with other NGS practices.

The transcriptomic workflow (Figure 29.1) often resembles the genomic procedures reviewed earlier. However, the biology of gene expression and the abundance of available transcriptomic data have permitted the development of many unique toolsets at the data analysis stage. Transcriptomics likely has the most robust applications out of all the omics. For example, RNA-Seq may be used to detect DNA-level mutations such as SNVs, gene fusions, and other structural variants—though genomic data remain more reliable and may also detect mutations in promoters, enhancers, and introns (46,47).

One of the first applications of transcriptomic data was to look for **differentially expressed genes (DEGs)** between two groups of clinical interest (e.g., normal vs. cancer tissue; responders vs. nonresponders). A classic early example of this approach identified >400 DEGs after estradiol binding in ER-positive breast cancer cells (49). Another investigation identified 30 genes that become abnormally expressed in pancreatic cancer cells (50). Most early studies analyzed genes independently, but in reality, gene expression is often highly correlated within shared pathways and regulatory networks. This paradigm can be exploited by analyses that look for differential activation of entire gene sets, coexpression networks, or modules, rather than individual genes (51–53). Construction of these modules can vary and is usually based on domain knowledge or experimental data. Whether individual genes or pathways, clinically relevant patterns can guide development of drugs to modulate the relevant target.

Expression signatures (Figure 29.2) have also been used to classify tumors molecularly. Several cancer subtypes were originally discovered through the application of unsupervised clustering (a machine learning technique) to gene expression data (54,55). For example, the original classification of GBM subtypes (proneural, neural, classical, and mesenchymal) was discovered through clustering of gene expression profiles (56). RNA-Seq has also been used (often in combination with exome sequencing) to classify tumors based on their expression of patient-specific mutant epitopes, also called *neoantigens* (57). These neoantigens are being explored as possible biomarkers for immunotherapy response and as potential targets for cancer vaccines or other novel therapeutic approaches (57,58).

Discovery of expression-based biomarkers remains one of the dominant pursuits of transcriptomic analyses. Such biomarkers have multiple potential clinical applications, such as cancer screening and diagnosis, assessment of patient risk and prediction of treatment response for therapy selection, and post-therapy monitoring for disease relapse. Many gene expression signatures have already been identified for a variety of these purposes in practically every cancer (59–68). For radiation therapy, a radiation sensitivity index (RSI) was developed, which established a gene expression signature that distinguished cells that were intrinsically sensitive to radiation from others (69–70). This was subsequently clinically extended to create a genomic-adjusted radiation dose (GARD) tool, which could predict clinical outcome by calculating a patient-specific radiation dose (71).

Single-cell RNA-Seq (scRNA-Seq) has arisen as a powerful new tool for dissecting the intratumoral heterogeneity that often undercuts single-sample transcriptomic studies. There are multiple approaches for performing scRNA-Seq on a specimen. In the most common protocol, rather than extracting RNA directly from a bulk sample, cells are first dissociated (chemically or mechanically) and subsequently sorted (e.g., with FACS) before NGS. Several studies have demonstrated the utility of scRNA-Seq for characterizing the **tumor microenvironment** based on the diverse cell phenotypes harbored in tumor samples (72,73). The enumeration (and characterization) of immune cells is of particular interest, given recent findings that infiltration of immune cells plays a significant role in determining response to immunotherapy (74,75). Other studies have demonstrated the capacity for scRNA-Seq to assist in the identification of cancer stem cells or clonal hierarchy (76,77). Similar approaches can also be helpful in identifying resistant subclonal populations within tumors (78). The sensitivity of single-cell methods is also uniquely suited for the detection and profiling of **circulating tumor cells (CTCs)** whose signals are often too small to be detected through bulk approaches (79).

Continued development of single-cell sequencing methods is positioned to revolutionize the field over the next decade. However, several steps in the pipeline will have to be improved for clinically viable insights to thrive. For example, cell-cycle effects have been identified as a source of systematic bias in the expression patterns captured by single-cell methods (80,81). Additionally, dissociation of bulk samples likely perturbs the distribution (and expression patterns) of the phenotypes that are sequenced (81,82). The emergence of deconvolution algorithms, such as CIBERSORT, has enabled the enumeration of cell phenotypic populations, such as tumor-infiltrating leukocytes, within bulk samples (using RNA-Seq) without the need to physically dissociate the sample (83).

PROTEOMICS

The proteome consists of all the proteins within a cell at a point in time. Because proteins collectively control nearly all the processes within a cell, the proteome captures a dynamic snapshot of the cell's functional state. The information embedded in the proteome is only weakly correlative with the transcriptome and thus hints at the unique functional insights provided by the proteome (84). Conventional methods of protein detection rely on targeted antibodies (e.g., Western blotting, protein microarrays, immunohistochemistry) and consequently are able to assess only

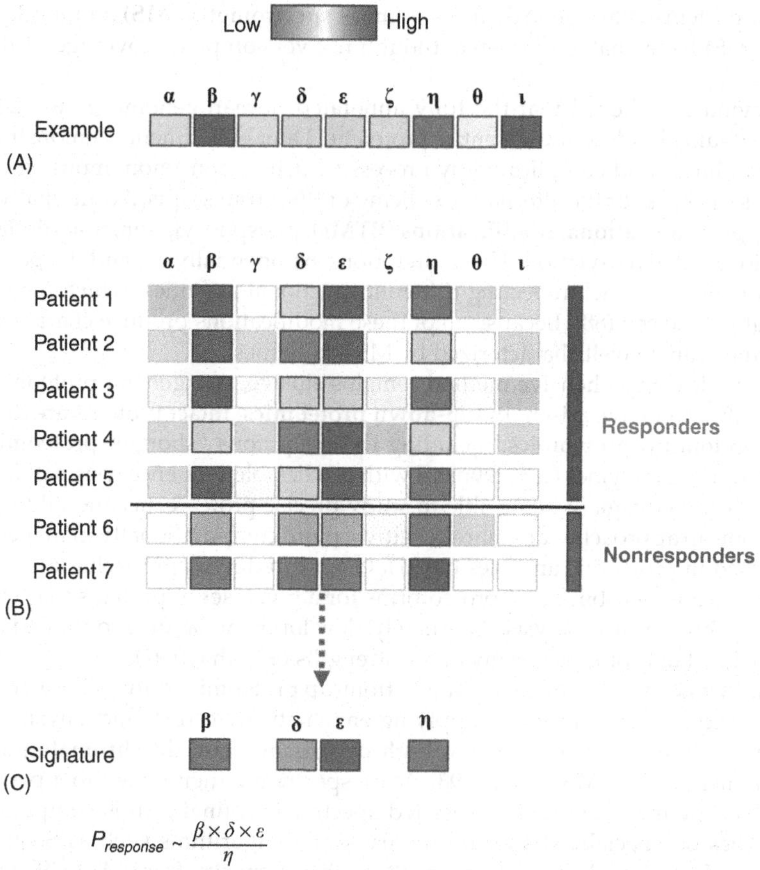

FIGURE 29.2 Conceptual construction of an omics signature for treatment response. (A) Example row of data for a single patient. The labeled columns α, β, ..., ι can represent any type of data. For example, in a transcriptomic study, each column might represent a gene (e.g., CTLA4, PDCD1) and the shading indicates how many mRNA transcripts were detected for that gene by RNA-Seq. In a proteomic study, each column might represent a different protein (NTM, NCAN, HAPLN1) and the shading indicates how many of each protein was detected by MS/MS spectra. (B) Example data matrix where each row represents a distinct patient sample and each column again represents a particular omic data element (e.g., change in gene expression after exposure to a given drug). (C) A signature can be calculated when there are certain data elements that demonstrate a consistent, quantifiable pattern across the cohort of patients. In this toy example, the columns corresponding to β, δ, and ε are consistently high across all responders and low in nonresponders, while the column η is consistently low in responders and high in nonresponders. The remaining columns do not demonstrate a consistent pattern, so they are dropped. The resulting four-element signature can then be used to make predictions of response. For example, if our columns represented gene expression data, our four-gene signature might be helpful for investigating the probability of responding to immunotherapy based on the measured expression level of genes β, δ, ε, and η. Most real signatures are more complex and require data from multiple types of patients and statistical testing for significance. However, the general principle is the same.

MS/MS, tandem mass spectrometry; RNA-Seq, RNA sequencing.

a limited set of proteins at a time. Advances in **mass spectrometry (MS)** and tandem mass spectrometry (MS/MS) have enabled massive, though not yet complete, coverage of the entire proteome (85–87).

It was previously believed that the fully annotated human genome (now ~20,300 protein-coding genes) should also describe the entire proteome. Later experiments demonstrated that gene expression is nonlinear and complicated by processes such as nonsynonymous single nucleotide polymorphisms (nsSNPs) or the alternative splicing of RNA transcripts. Additionally, proteins can undergo many **posttranslational modifications (PTMs)**: phosphorylation, ubiquitylation, acetylation, methylation, and glycosylation. These alterations exponentially expand the potential number of unique "proteoforms," each reflecting different functional activities, which may influence the phenotypic state of the cell (88). Because all of these modifications produce characteristic shifts in protein mass, they can be well characterized by MS techniques.

Though a single comprehensive method remains elusive, two general proteomic approaches to protein identification have arisen. In **top-down proteomics**, intact proteins are directly studied using MS. In **bottom-up proteomics**, including the ubiquitous "shotgun proteomics," peptides are first digested using enzymes (e.g., trypsin) with predictable sequence lysis patterns. Top-down methods have the advantage of being able to study precise proteoforms and all their PTMs (89). However, bottom-up approaches are more sensitive, more computationally manageable, and thus more widely used in proteomic analyses (90,91). Often top-down approaches are utilized to precisely characterize the distribution of proteoforms for a given set of proteins that were originally identified using a bottom-up analysis. Alternately, development has also continued on a "middle-down" approach, which combines many of the strengths of both (90,92).

The general workflow (Figure 29.1) for a bottom-up proteomic analysis involves taking a biological sample, extracting the proteins, applying enzymatic digestion, and physically separating the complex peptide mixtures (e.g., using **high-performance liquid chromatography [HPLC]**) before measurement of MS/MS spectra (93). Mass spectra are then linked to a peptide sequence within a database by matching their associated spectra. This final step is computationally challenging and relies on specialized spectral library search algorithms such as Sequest or Mascot (94–96). In spite of continued progress, more than 70% of spectra from MS/MS experiments are never matched to a peptide; peptide spectral matching remains an unresolved and active area of research (97,98). The identity and quantity of various proteins can be studied using statistical models to determine if any proteins are associated with clinical response.

Analyzing protein networks is one major application of proteomics. The dynamic activity of proteins is facilitated by a host of interactions with both other proteins and separate macromolecules. Many of the newest proteomic techniques attempt to capture this modular biology. Interaction proteomics uses a pull-down assay featuring **bait proteins** followed by affinity-purification mass spectrometry (AP-MS) to characterize protein–protein interactions (PPIs) as part of an **interactome** (99,100). Chemical cross-linking of residues combined with MS (XL-MS) is another technique that enables the characterization of protein interactions and protein assemblies by exploiting the distance constraints imposed by the size and shape of the cross-linking reagent (101,102). These types of tools can potentially be leveraged to uncover the binding partners (both intended and unintended) of chemotherapeutic drugs or reveal conformational changes induced by ligand binding on a proteomic scale. More broadly, they also provide a mechanism for studying how interaction networks are perturbed in pathologic states (103,104).

The proteins identified through proteomic studies can also be investigated as potential **biomarkers**. Because proteomic workflows can be time-consuming and challenging to analyze, clinically viable studies often are split into a "discovery" phase and a "validation" phase. The discovery phase is exploratory and employs high-performance MS/MS and bioinformatics techniques to identify potential protein candidates. These efforts are then scaled to larger patient cohorts using more targeted panels (e.g., immunohistochemistry or enzyme-linked immunosorbent assay [ELISA]) for validation. However, selected reaction monitoring (SRM) is an alternative but highly sensitive and specific method that utilizes tandem MS to selectively quantify a set of protein compounds within a complex mixture (105). In addition to protein expression, modification events (most commonly phosphorylation, glycosylation, or acetylation) are crucial to cancer signaling and can be monitored across the proteome as potential signs of carcinogenesis or drug response (106,107).

Multiple proteomic studies, including phase II/III trials, have identified **signatures** and Food and Drug Administration (FDA)-approved biomarkers that help predict prognosis or guide treatment selection (108–112). Several isolated protein marker candidates were originally identified in proteomic studies (113). However, large successes overall have been limited. Current proteomic efforts have had greater success in explaining tumor biology than in actual biomarker or drug discovery (114–117). MS/MS methods have been held back by limited reproducibility and large fluctuations based on sample preparation and technique (118,119). Because proteomic studies can be laborious and analytically challenging, many research groups also report only discovery phase results and do not perform validation analyses. Recent global efforts to increase transparency, codify data protocols, and create accessible public repositories for proteomics data have laid the groundwork for more rigorous and systematic analysis (and reanalysis) of highly complex proteomic data (120,121).

METABOLOMICS

Metabolomics is one of the newest omics and concerns the study of all the metabolites within a biological system. Metabolites are traditionally defined as any small molecule in a cell, organ, or organism with a molecular weight <1,500 daltons (122). For reference, the average weight of a single DNA base pair is 650 daltons, and insulin, one of the smallest peptides in the human body, is >5,800 daltons. The analysis of the metabolome has several attractive properties. Though genes and proteins carry the potential for various actions, much of the actual downstream activity is at the metabolite level (e.g., cell communication, signaling, energy conversion). Thus, the metabolome represents the closest real-time manifestation of the cancer "cellular phenotype." Additionally, because metabolites can capture both the intermediate and final downstream products of both gene expression and protein catalytic activity, metabolomic changes are often magnified compared to concomitant changes in the transcriptome or proteome (123).

Unfortunately, whereas the transcriptome and proteome encapsulate fundamentally homogeneous forms of biological information (nucleic acids and peptides, respectively), the exceptional diversity of metabolites has made it challenging to develop biochemical techniques that perform accurately and consistently across the entire metabolome. Unlike the genome and transcriptome, which can be entirely sequenced, the number of potentially measurable metabolites is not yet known (though it continues to grow) (124).

Metabolomic data are commonly taken from various **biofluids** (serum, plasma, urine, cerebrospinal fluid, seminal fluid, synovial fluid, amniotic fluid, etc.). Cells or tissue extracts can also be used. The available techniques for extracting metabolomic data from biological samples are still in early development. The first step is typically a separation technique: **liquid chromatography (LC)**, **gas chromatography (GC)**, or the less common **capillary electrophoresis (CE)**. Coupled to these is a compound detection method: either MS or **nuclear magnetic resonance** (NMR) **spectroscopy**. As with proteomics, MS is the dominant technique for analyzing sample compounds. However, while MS is extremely sensitive, able to detect metabolites at the femtomolar to attomolar range, a major weakness of MS is its inability to quantify the levels of metabolites using MS signal intensities. NMR has the opposite weaknesses: NMR is able to precisely quantify the abundance of various compounds; however, its sensitivity is orders of magnitude weaker than MS (125). NMR is often preferred in spite of its shortcomings because it has great reproducibility and can be performed using intact tissue samples (126).

Several improvements are being developed to improve the sensitivity of NMR, for example, using higher field strength superconducting magnets, miniaturized radiofrequency coils, and cryogenically cooled probe technology (125,127,128). Despite advances in NMR sensitivity, its utility as a general untargeted method for detecting metabolites remains more potential than certain. There currently exists no method or assay that can measure even the known metabolome, and in practice, most metabolomic studies have quantified fewer than 100 metabolites per sample (129). The most promising results in the near future will likely come from the methods that combine both MS and NMR (130,131).

Metabolomic studies may be targeted or untargeted, but the analysis of metabolomic data always requires parsing spectra from MS/NMR. Targeted studies must filter down to a set of known metabolites. Untargeted studies are ideal because they are unconstrained by prior knowledge of which metabolites, and thus which spectral regions, are important (analogous to a selected gene panel vs. a whole genome analysis). Identifying metabolites within MS/NMR spectra is, at present, a severe bottleneck for the field. Only 1.8% of recognized peaks in untargeted metabolomic experiments can be identified, with the vast majority comprising unknown molecules (132). This metabolic "dark matter" suggests that a significant proportion of information from these experiments is currently unexploited. The 2018 release of the Human Metabolome Database (HMDB) has begun to create libraries that collect the associated MS/NMR spectra for each metabolite (124). Experimentally deriving each of these spectra is costly and parallel efforts are underway to create in silico simulated MS/NMR spectra for a given chemical structure using a combination of informatics techniques (124,133–135).

In the typical metabolomic workflow (Figure 29.1), biological samples are acquired, separated (using LC, GC, or CE), and then analyzed (using MS or NMR). Spectra between two cohorts of interest (e.g., case vs. control; tumor vs. normal; treated vs. untreated) are compared using multivariable statistical techniques such as **principal components analysis (PCA), orthogonal projections to latent structures (OPLS)**, or **partial least squares-discriminant analysis (PLS-DA)** (130,136). These are used to identify the regions of the spectra that differ and subsequently identify which metabolites match the divergent spectral patterns. Metabolites can be analyzed independently, but the analyses are more powerful when combined with knowledge of metabolic pathways. For example, modest, scattered increases across a few metabolites may appear insignificant until one projects them onto a metabolic map to reveal multiple intermediates along a single pathway, which is being upregulated.

Though metabolomics has not yet produced huge breakthroughs in cancer-related biomarkers, several studies have shown its early promise. A few examples follow, though there are many more. In breast cancer, metabolomic studies of patient tissue samples have identified metabolites such as glycerophosphocholine and lactate, which are associated with treatment response and survival (137–139). Other studies were able to identify prognostic metabolites from patients' blood and urine samples (140–142). Gastric patients' urine levels of 2-hydroxyisobutyrate, 3-indoxylsulfate, and alanine have been used to build a highly sensitive and specific (AUC = 0.95) discriminatory model for distinguishing gastric cancer from benign gastric disease (143). A hallmark analysis of data from four pancreatic cancer prospective cohort studies also revealed that elevated plasma levels of branched-chain amino acids more than doubled the risk of future pancreatic cancer, even when the samples were obtained 2 to 5 years prior to cancer diagnosis (85).

These findings showcase the potential for metabolomic techniques to capture subclinical diseases years before they become detectable. Additionally, though many studies understandably focus on early detection and diagnosis of cancers, it should not be forgotten that the metabolome also provides mechanistic insights, for example, from metabolic pathways that can become drug targets (85).

RADIOMICS

Since the first clinical x-ray was performed in 1896, interpretation of medical images has been limited to human observation of recognizable visual patterns. Imaging (e.g., CT, MRI, PET) is particularly crucial to many aspects of clinical oncology: (a) visualizing malignancies for diagnosis and staging; (b) defining target volumes and adjacent normal structures for treatment planning; and (c) monitoring response to therapy and potential recurrence. **Radiomics** is a field of study that seeks to use algorithms and mathematical models to quantify and extract critical features from images. These features are often difficult or impossible to detect from human visualization alone.

Radiomics is a unique "omic" in that it does not directly measure the molecular components that manifest biological phenotype. In fact, radiomic studies often begin by measuring visual phenotype and working backward to infer molecular correlates. There are several subfields and applications of radiomics. In general, most radiomic analyses follow a typical workflow that has been commonly summarized into the following four steps (144):

1. Acquiring images (e.g., CT, MRI, PET)
2. Identifying volumes of interest (e.g., tumor, critical organs) and delineating borders of the volumes (e.g., tumor vs. normal tissue)
3. Extracting, qualifying, and tabulating descriptive features from the volume
4. Combining other information (e.g., clinical, genomic, demographic) as needed and applying various models to begin predicting outcomes of interest (e.g., gene expression, disease status, treatment response)

Each of these steps has the potential to advance both cancer research and clinical practice and is explored further in the following text.

INTEGRATING MULTIMODALITY IMAGING

In addition to improving the resolution of well-established tomographic images, advances in radiomics also seek to maximize the diverse information captured by separate modalities. Full-body PET/CT has become the standard of care for screening oncology patients for FDG-avid tumors (145). In contrast, the optimal clinical use and acquisition of PET/MRI remains a challenge (146). Simultaneously integrating the metabolic information from PET with the structural and physiologic information from MRI is difficult for the human eye but represents a promising application of preclinical and clinical radiomics.

Early approaches have shown that diffusion weighted MRI (DW-MRI), which can capture differences in cellular density, may be combined with dynamic contrast-enhanced MRI (DCE-MRI), which can capture blood flow dynamics, to derive valuable prognostic and pathophysiological signatures (147). In a separate context, combining multimodal multiparametric imaging (e.g., PET/MRI) with machine learning feature extraction has been used in animal models to demonstrate the potential for imaging-based noninvasive molecular profiling of heterogeneous tumors (148,149). More generally, these imaging techniques can be used to identify distinct intra-tumor "habitats," which are discussed further in the following text.

VOLUME DELINEATION

Volume segmentation is crucial to radiomic analyses because it bounds the region from which features will be extracted. Delineating volumes is also an important step of radiation therapy to ensure that radiation dose is precisely delivered to the tumor, while minimizing dose to normal tissues. Manual volume delineation can be challenging, subjective, and a time-consuming component of radiotherapy planning (150). Contouring tumors is particularly challenging because their intra-tumor and inter-tumor physiological heterogeneities result in a similarly heterogeneous visual morphology, whereas normal healthy structures tend to be fairly consistent. Previous work has also shown that there is significant inter-rater variability in manually delineated volumes and that this can affect the clinical accuracy of the downstream features

(151,152). Thus, reproducible, automatic volume delineation represents both a valuable goal and a crucial step of future radiomic analysis.

There are currently three main approaches to automatic volume delineation—**atlas methods**, machine learning methods, and statistical **shape model** (SSM) or statistical appearance model (SAM) methods. Atlas methods utilize a reference image (called an *atlas*) with manually delineated structures and attempt to find the optimal transformation between the atlas image and test images using image processing algorithms (153,154). A deficiency of this approach is the frequent occurrence of new patient images that are not sufficiently similar to atlas images. Machine learning methods commonly employ tools like **random forests** or **convolutional neural networks** (**CNNs**) to automatically learn how to classify voxels into various types of tissue (155,156). These methods require enormous amounts of training data, are computationally intensive—frequently requiring special **graphical processing units** (**GPUs**)—and are markedly affected by differences between training and test images (e.g., image quality, anatomic variation, or deformations resulting from prior therapies). SSM/SAM methods combine patient-derived training images with theory-driven geometric constraints that force generated volumes to assume anatomically plausible shapes (e.g., the colon must appear tubular) (157,158). SSM/SAM methods are challenging to truly automate because they often require proper prealignment of the model to the target image and also restrict the final volume to a limited range of shapes.

These tools work best when combined into a multilayered process (e.g., using SSM/SAM to constrain output from a neural network). In practice, truly automated volume generation is not yet accurate and a "semiautomatic" approach is used such that automated volumes are generated and subsequently adjusted by an experienced observer (150,156). There are several commercial software packages, already in clinical use, which offer automatic and semiautomatic volume delineation (153,159,160).

RADIOMIC FEATURE EXTRACTION

After volumes have been identified, features are extracted for use in downstream modeling. Sometimes subvolumes, or **habitats,** are identified within a volume based on spatially distinct regions (e.g., heterogeneous tumors with areas of necrosis vs. edema vs. angiogenesis). Unique features can thus be extracted from each of these habitats for greater precision. There are two main types of volume features. **Semantic features** are defined by practitioners and often have clear interpretability: shape, size, spiculation, and so forth. Nonsemantic or **agnostic features** are mathematically derived abstractions that quantify voxel attributes that often have no lexical interpretation: the **kurtosis** of voxel intensity distributions, texture relationships between voxels, wavelet transformations of the image, and so forth (161,162). Semantic and nonsemantic features capture both related and distinct phenotypic attributes and can be combined to produce thousands of features for the final analysis (161,163). Selecting the optimal subset of these features for the final model building is a critical step that is performed using machine learning techniques, prior analyses, or domain expertise.

RADIOMIC APPLICATIONS

Once features have been extracted, they can be correlated with molecular and clinical data derived from the patient. Radiogenomic analyses can, for example, be used to molecularly profile tumors, using enhancement texture (entropy) to predict ER/PR/HER2 mutation status in breast cancer (164). One of the earliest radiogenomic applications demonstrated the ability to reconstruct 78% of global gene expression profiles in liver cancer using radiographic features in CT scans (165). Example applications in cancer diagnostics include automatically computing prostate Gleason scores with up to 93% accuracy and classifying benign versus malignant pulmonary nodules with over 80% accuracy (166,167).

Another exciting application is the creation of **radiomic signatures** with potential to predict prognosis or treatment response (168–171). The recent emergence of **deep learning** techniques such as CNNs are allowing researchers to skip volume segmentation and feature extraction entirely, for example, classifying benign versus malignant lung nodules using raw CT data (172). Such approaches represent a major evolution of the field and may eliminate much of the time and effort currently spent extracting volumes and features for modeling.

CONCLUSION

Many of the omics studies in the literature rely on the identification of signatures that associate with clinical outcomes of interest. Despite the plethora of signatures with promising results published in large, well-cited studies, validation attempts in independent patient cohorts have shown that most tested signatures consistently fall short. In one lung cancer outcomes study, every single published prognostic gene signature the investigators examined failed to reproduce a significant effect when tested in a different dataset from the original publication (173). In fact, the authors demonstrated that by creating 5,000 completely random mock genes, they were able to discover "significant" signatures that appeared to predict lung cancer outcomes but that subsequently failed when tested on a held-out population. Similar analyses have demonstrated that the majority of published breast cancer outcome signatures were outperformed by randomly generated signatures (173).

Lack of reproducibility often results from weaknesses in study design, such as failure to use held-out test data, failure to compare signatures to previously known risk factors, and failure to demonstrate utility of signatures in clinically realistic scenarios. Many signatures are published with statistical significance but with unknown or contradictory biological interpretability (173). Analytic tools such as **meta-analysis** or batch correction can offset these weaknesses by helping to eliminate noise and extract the most reliable signal present in multiple independent studies. However, poor study methodologies will always confer some bias to the data. Inadequate experimental design and validation are not unique to gene expression studies (174–176). Concerns regarding reproducibility are indeed common to all omics studies and remain pernicious challenges for omics analyses, which depend on datasets that commonly contain 10 to 100 times more variables than observations (144,177–179).

Each omics method has unique strengths and weaknesses (Table 29.1). There are other emerging omics areas we did not profile in this chapter, including **epigenomics** (the study of all epigenetic modifications to the genetic material) and **microbiomics** (the study of the genomes of microorganisms that make up the gut flora). The study of unstructured data within **electronic health records** (**EHRs**; see Chapter 18) is another important area of future cancer research. These areas of study are less established, but represent exciting additions to a rapidly expanding constellation of precision medicine frameworks.

Perhaps the largest frontier is the integration of these many omics frameworks into single analyses. A lack of data is probably one of the biggest obstacles; there are few datasets in which patient samples are profiled using multiple omics. **The Cancer Genome Atlas** (**TCGA**) is by far the largest repository that includes data from multiple sources, including DNA NGS, RNA-Seq, and clinical data (200). Several studies can also serve as examples of possible approaches to robust omics integration (201,202). However, overall the field of multi-omics remains relatively untapped. The considerable cost of acquiring multi-omics datasets, the analytical complexity of interpreting such diverse and massive data, and the nontrivial challenge of deploying experimental protocols to process limited biological samples for multi-omic analyses will likely make multi-omics integration one of the most formidable but exciting challenges in all of cancer research.

TABLE 29.1 COMPARISON OF THE MAJOR OMICS METHODS

	Genome	Transcriptome	Proteome	Metabolome	Radiome
Known Size in *Homo sapiens*	• 3 billion base pairs • ~20,300 protein-coding genes	• ~20,900 mRNA (180) • ~40,700 long ncRNA • ~11,200 short ncRNA • ~2,000 miRNA (181)	• ~20,300 protein-coding genes • ~70,000 proteins, given splice variants (182) • Potentially millions of unique isoforms	• ~114,000 metabolites (124) • 1,500–2,500 compounds with experimental NMR/MS spectra	NA
Advantages	• Performs well with small amounts of DNA • Captures fundamental mutations and driver mutations for cancer biology • DNA is highly stable and well suited for molecular diagnostics • NGS able to comprehensively sequence near entirety of the genome • Mature analytic tools with large amounts of publicly available data	• Performs well with small amounts of RNA • Can capture both coding and noncoding RNA • Captures dynamic cellular phenotype • Can resolve much of the tumor microenvironment • NGS able to comprehensively sequence near entirety of the transcriptome	• Captures dynamic cellular phenotype • Newer methods have high sensitivity • Can be performed easily on varied biofluids • Direct capture of protein–protein interactions (PPIs) • Helps identify potential drug targets (including off-site reactions that could lead to side effects)	• Extremely sensitive • Closest representation of cellular phenotype • Can be performed easily on varied biofluids • Able to provide metabolic pathway information	• Completely noninvasive • Ubiquitous clinical infrastructure already available (CT, MRI, etc.) • Tracking changes with longitudinal measurements is easy • Captures entire tumor (less impacted by intra-tumoral heterogeneity) • Imaging data not subject to physical degradation over time

(continued)

TABLE 29.1 COMPARISON OF THE MAJOR OMICS METHODS (*continued*)

	Genome	Transcriptome	Proteome	Metabolome	Radiome
Weaknesses	• Genomic variants are not always expressed and thus do not fully correlate with phenotype • Often more effective at explaining biology of tumor than providing actionable targets • Insufficient data to resolve multiple phenotypes • Unable to assess most dynamic phenotypic changes	• RNA degrades easily, sensitive to preparation and storage, making it a challenge for molecular diagnostics • Extraction methods (especially scRNA-Seq) likely perturb expression	• Difficult to capture the full proteome • Not able to match full MS spectra to peptide sequences • Post-translational modifications (PTMs) only variably accounted for • Reproducibility is inconsistent • Experiments and analyses can be laborious and time-consuming	• No laboratory method able to capture full metabolome • Large diversity of measurable structures makes biological interpretation challenging • Not able to match full MS/NMR spectra to chemical structures	• Limited to correlative interpretation, cannot capture fundamental molecular biology • Not all relevant tumor features are expressed in visually distinct patterns • Sophisticated computational tools required to process and analyze images
Public Data Repositories	• GDC/TCGA (183) • 1000 Genomes Project (184) • International Cancer Consortium (185)	• GEO (186) • miRBase (181)	• PRIDE Database (184) • ProteomeXchange (187) • PeptideAtlas (188)	• HMDB (124) • KEGG (189) • METLIN (190) • MassBank (191)	• TCIA (192) • XNAT Central (193) • IDA (194) • QIDW (195)
Example Commercial Clinical Uses	CANCERPLEX Assay (DNA capture NGS method to sequence extract from FFPE) (196)	FoundationOne Heme test (integrated DNA/RNA capture NGS method to sequence extract from FFPE, fresh blood, or bone marrow) (182)	OVA1 Test (multi-protein assay originally identified with MS proteomic study) (197)	Citrate (reimbursable test in diagnosis of prostate cancer, but not discovered in a metabolomic study) (198)	MIM Maestro 6+ (radiotherapy imaging software providing automated image segmentation, uses Atlas-based method) (199)

Note: Advantages and weaknesses are relative to other omics methods.

FFPE, formalin fixed paraffin embedded; GDC, Genomic Data Commons; GEO, Gene Expression Omnibus; HMDB, Human Metabolome Database; IDA, the Image & Data Archive; KEGG, Kyoto Encyclopedia of Genes and Genomes; METLIN, METabolite LINk; MS, mass spectrometry; NGS, next-generation sequencing; NMR, nuclear magnetic resonance; PRIDE, PRoteomics IDEntifications Database; QIDW, Quantitative Imaging Data Warehouse; TCGA, The Cancer Genome Atlas; TCIA, The Cancer Imaging Archive; XNAT, Extensible Neuroimaging Archive Toolkit.

GLOSSARY

omics: analyses that capture information about the genome, transcriptome, proteome, metabolome, or other "-omes."

central dogma (of molecular biology): states that the flow of information in biological systems starts at the level of nucleic acids and flows toward proteins.

genome: comprises all the coding and noncoding DNA within a biological system.

next-generation sequencing (NGS): currently the most popular high-throughput genomics technique.

DNA microarrays: a high-throughput genomics technique.

optical mapping: a high-throughput genomics technique.

adapter: short synthetic oligonucleotide that is ligated to the end of a DNA or RNA molecule that enables next-generation sequencing.

single nucleotide variants (SNVs): a single nucleotide that is altered in the DNA sequence.

insertions and deletions (indels): the addition or deletion of one or more nucleotides in a DNA sequence; the second most common type of genetic variation in human genomes.

inversions: the reversal of the DNA sequence within a section of the chromosome (often results when two breaks occur in one section of the chromosome).

copy number variants (CNVs): variation between individuals in the number of copies of a specific region of DNA.

translocations: a major genomic variant whereby one section of chromosome is displaced onto another section of the same or nearby chromosome.

whole genome sequencing (WGS): sequencing the entire DNA sequence of nucleotides, including both coding and noncoding regions, such as introns.

whole exome sequencing (WES): a method for sequencing all of the protein-coding genes in a genome.

genome-wide association studies (GWASs): statistical analyses of genetic variants across the entire genome of different individuals to determine if any are associated with a disease or trait of interest.

machine learning: a branch of artificial intelligence that explores the construction of algorithms that are able to automatically learn from and make predictive models of data.

bioinformatics: scientific discipline of analyzing large amounts of biological data, such as omics data, using computational approaches.

pharmacogenomics: a branch of genomics which seeks to understand how analysis of genomewide variants like single nucleotide polymorphisms (SNPs) can be used to explain patients' response to treatment.

single nucleotide polymorphisms (SNPs): variation in a single nucleotide that occurs in at least 1% of the population; the most common type of genetic variation in human genomes.

circulating tumor DNA (ctDNA): A promising biomarker which is the result of DNA shed into the blood by tumors where it can be detected using highly sensitive NGS approaches.

transcriptomics: field of study and quantification of the transcriptome, which comprises the total collection of RNA transcripts in a cell at a point in time.

noncoding RNA (ncRNA): RNA type that includes miRNA and siRNA.

differentially expressed genes (DEGs): groups of genes of clinical interest, the search for which was one of the first applications of transcriptomic data.

single-cell RNA-Seq (scRNA-Seq): a powerful tool for dissecting the intra-tumoral heterogeneity that often undercuts single-sample transcriptomic studies.

tumor microenvironment: the network of surrounding of cellular (e.g. immune cells, fibroblasts, endothelial cells) and noncellular (e.g. extracellular matrix) material both within and immediately adjacent to the tumor.

circulating tumor cells (CTCs): cells whose signals are often too small to be detected through bulk approaches.

mass spectrometry (MS): tool that has enabled massive, though not yet complete, coverage of the entire proteome.

posttranslational modifications (PTMs): changes in proteins such as phosphorylation, ubiquitylation, acetylation, methylation, and glycosylation.

top-down proteomics: one of two general proteomic approaches to protein identification, in which intact proteins are directly studied using MS.

bottom-up proteomics: one of two general proteomic approaches to protein identification, in which peptides are first digested using enzymes (e.g., trypsin) with predictable sequence lysis patterns.

high-performance liquid chromatography (HPLC): a form of column chromatography that optimizes detection of components in a mixture, most often by using a pressurized solvent, smaller column particle sizes, and highly sensitive detection methods.

bait proteins: used in interaction proteomics pull-down assays to characterize protein–protein interactions.

interactome: the entire set of molecular interactions in a particular cell (most often between proteins).

biomarker: a substance that acts as a signal or "flag" of a condition or status.

signature: a characteristic pattern of biologic data (e.g. a particular set of DNA nucleotides or mRNA transcripts) that is strongly associated with a feature of interest, often to predict prognosis or guide treatment selection.

biofluids: serum, plasma, urine, cerebrospinal fluid, seminal fluid, synovial fluid, amniotic fluid, and other substances from which metabolomic data are commonly taken.

Liquid chromatography (LC): see definition for high performance liquid chromatography (HPLC).

gas chromatography (GC): an analytical chemistry technique for separating and quantifying a mixture by vaporizing it and injecting it into a carrier gas stream moving through a liquid or solid stationary phase.

capillary electrophoresis (CE): an analytical technique that applies a voltage and separates ions based on their electrophoretic mobility within submillimeter diameter capillaries.

nuclear magnetic resonance (NMR) spectroscopy: a technique that gives details on molecular structure by using radio waves to induce nuclear excitation which is then detected and quantified.

principle components analysis (PCA): a statistical technique that reduces the complexity of high-dimensional data by extracting a smaller subset of new variables that are linearly independent from each other.

orthogonal projections to latent structures (OPLS): a modified version of partial least squares regression that reduces the complexity of high-dimensional data by separating true sample variance (that is correlated with a factor of interest) from variance due to systematic bias that is not correlated with a factor of interest.

partial least squares-discriminant analysis (PLS-DA): a statistical technique that is often used for analyzing high-dimensional data to perform classification into discrete groups, or identifying important variables associated with different groups, by optimizing the orthogonal separation between data from samples in each group.

radiomics: a field of study that seeks to use algorithms and mathematical models to quantify and extract critical features from images.

atlas method: utilize a reference image (an atlas) with manually delineated structures to attempt to find the optimal transformation between the atlas image and test images using image processing algorithms.

statistical shape model (SSM): a method for representing and detecting biological shapes within images by combining example shape data from multiple patients to create a more representative model.

random forests: a machine learning algorithm that creates classifications or predictions by aggregating multiple decision trees that capture important relationships between variables in a set of data.

convolutional neural networks (CNNs): a deep-learning technique that utilizes multiple layers of artificial neural networks to process an initial piece of data, often image data, and make a decision or prediction.

graphical processing units (GPUs): a piece of computer hardware, often used for processing visual data, that can perform thousands of simple calculations in parallel.

habitats: subvolumes identified within a volume based on spatially distinct regions.

semantic features: radiomic features defined by practitioners that often have clear interpretability: shape, size, spiculation, and so forth.

agnostic (nonsemantic) features: mathematically derived abstractions that quantify voxel attributes that are associated with no lexical interpretation of semantic features.

kurtosis: a method for quantifying asymmetry in a set of data.

radiomic signatures: signatures derived from imaging that predict prognosis or treatment response.

deep learning: a subset of machine learning that involves use of many layers of artificial neural networks to mimic biological neuronal system architecture and automatically learn important classification, prediction, and decision tasks.

meta-analysis: a statistical approach for combining results of multiple independent studies to identify strongly conserved signals and effects.

epigenomics: the study of all epigenetic modifications to the genetic material.

microbiomics: the study of the genomes of microorganisms that make up the gut flora.

The Cancer Genome Atlas (TCGA): the largest repository that includes data from multiple sources, including DNA NGS, RNA-Seq, and clinical data.

REFERENCES

1. Crick F. Central dogma of molecular biology. *Nature.* 1970;227(5258):561–563. doi:10.1038/227561a0
2. Hanahan D, Weinberg RA. Hallmarks of cancer: the next generation. *Cell.* 2011;144(5):646–674. doi:10.1016/j.cell.2011.02.013
3. Collins FS, Morgan M, Patrinos A. The human genome project: lessons from large-scale biology. *Science.* 2003;300(5617):286–290. doi:10.1126/science.1084564
4. Lander ES, Linton LM, Birren B, et al. Initial sequencing and analysis of the human genome. *Nature.* 2001;409(6822):860–921. doi:10.1038/35057062
5. Venter JC, Adams MD, Myers EW, et al. The sequence of the human genome. *Science.* 2001;291(5507):1304–1351. doi:10.1126/science.291.5507.1155d
6. Goodwin S, McPherson JD, McCombie WR. Coming of age: ten years of next-generation sequencing technologies. *Nat Rev Genet.* 2016;17(6):333–351. doi:10.1038/nrg.2016.49
7. Reuter JA, Spacek DV, Snyder MP. High-throughput sequencing technologies. *Mol Cell.* 2015;58(4):586–597. doi:10.1016/j.molcel.2015.05.004
8. Li H, Durbin R. Fast and accurate short read alignment with Burrows-Wheeler transform. *Bioinformatics.* 2009;25(14):1754–1760. doi:10.1093/bioinformatics/btp324
9. Langmead B, Trapnell C, Pop C, Salzberg SL. Ultrafast and memory-efficient alignment of short DNA sequences to the human genome. *Genome Biol.* 2009;10(3):R25. doi:10.1186/gb-2009-10-3-r25
10. Li R, Zhu H, Ruan J, et al. De novo assembly of human genomes with massively parallel short read sequencing. *Genome Res.* 2010;20(2):265–272. doi:10.1101/gr.097261.109
11. Zerbino DR, Birney E. Velvet: algorithms for de novo short read assembly using de Bruijn graphs. *Genome Res.* 2008;18(5):821–829. doi:10.1101/gr.074492.107
12. Chaisson MJP, Huddleston J, Dennis MY, et al. Resolving the complexity of the human genome using single-molecule sequencing. *Nature.* 2014;517(7536):608–611. doi:10.1038/nature13907
13. Lam ET, Hastie A, Lin C, et al. Genome mapping on nanochannel arrays for structural variation analysis and sequence assembly. *Nat Biotechnol.* 2012;30(8):771–776. doi:10.1038/nbt.2303
14. Choi M, Scholl UI, Ji W, et al. Genetic diagnosis by whole exome capture and massively parallel DNA sequencing. *Proc Natl Acad Sci.* 2009;106(45):19096–19101. doi:10.1073/pnas.0910672106
15. Way GP, Sanchez-Vega F, La K, et al. Machine learning detects pan-cancer ras pathway activation in the cancer genome atlas. *Cell Rep.* 2018;23(1):172–180.e3. doi:10.1016/j.celrep.2018.03.046
16. Ellrott K, Bailey MH, Saksena G, et al. Scalable open science approach for mutation calling of tumor exomes using multiple genomic pipelines. *Cell Syst.* 2018;6(3):271–281.e7. doi:10.1016/j.cels.2018.03.002
17. Hoadley KA, Yau C, Hinoue T, et al. Cell-of-origin patterns dominate the molecular classification of 10,000 tumors from 33 types of cancer. *Cell.* 2018;173(2):291–304.e6. doi:10.1016/j.cell.2018.03.022
18. Hiley C, de Bruin EC, McGranahan N, Swanton C. Deciphering intratumor heterogeneity and temporal acquisition of driver events to refine precision medicine. *Genome Biol.* 2014;15(8):453. doi:10.1186/s13059-014-0453-8
19. Gerlinger M, Rowan AJ, Horswell S, et al. Intratumor heterogeneity and branched evolution revealed by multiregion sequencing. *N Engl J Med.* 2012;366(10):883–892. doi:10.1056/NEJMoa1113205
20. Yap TA, Gerlinger M, Futreal PA. Intratumor heterogeneity: seeing the wood for the trees. *Sci Transl Med.* 4(127):127ps10. doi:10.1126/scitranslmed.3003854
21. Jiang Y, Qiu Y, Minn AJ, Zhang NR. Assessing intratumor heterogeneity and tracking longitudinal and spatial clonal evolutionary history by next-generation sequencing. *Proc Natl Acad Sci U S A.* 2016;113(37):E5528–E5537. doi:10.1073/pnas.1522203113
22. de Bruin EC, McGranahan N, Mitter R, et al. Spatial and temporal diversity in genomic instability processes defines lung cancer evolution. *Science.* 2014;346(6206):251–256. doi:10.1126/science.1253462
23. Gawad C, Koh W, Quake SR. Single-cell genome sequencing: current state of the science. *Nat Rev Genet.* 2016;17(3):175–188. doi:10.1038/nrg.2015.16
24. Kalow W. Familial incidence of low pseudocholinesterase level. *Lancet.* 1956;268(6942):576–577. doi:10.1016/S0140-6736(56)92065-7
25. Evans DA, Manley KA, McKusick VA. Genetic control of isoniazid metabolism in man. *Br Med J.* 1960;2(5197):485–491. doi:10.1136/bmj.2.5197.485
26. Evans WE, McLeod HL. Pharmacogenomics—drug disposition, drug targets, and side effects. *N Engl J Med.* 2003;348(6):538–549. doi:10.1056/NEJMra020526
27. Thorn CF, Klein TE, Altman RB. Pharmacogenomics and bioinformatics: PharmGKB. *Pharmacogenomics.* 2010;11(4):501–505. doi:10.2217/pgs.10.15
28. Thorn CF, Klein TE, Altman RB. PharmGKB: the Pharmacogenomics Knowledge Base. *Methods Mol Biol.* 2013;1015:311–320. doi:10.1007/978-1-62703-435-7_20

29. Yang JJ, Landier W, Yang W, et al. Inherited NUDT15 variant is a genetic determinant of mercaptopurine intolerance in children with acute lymphoblastic leukemia. *J Clin Oncol.* 2015;33(11):1235–1242. doi:10.1200/JCO.2014.59.4671
30. Dean L. Mercaptopurine therapy and TPMT genotype. In: Pratt V, McLeod H, Rubinstein W, et al., eds. *SourceMedical Genetics Summaries*. Bethesda, MD: National Center for Biotechnology Information; 2012:5–7.
31. McLeod HL. Cancer pharmacogenomics: early promise, but concerted effort needed. *Science.* 2013;339(6127):1563–1566. doi:10.1126/science.1234139
32. BratmanSV, Milosevic MF, Liu F-F, Haibe-Kains B. Genomic biomarkers for precision radiation medicine. *Lancet Oncol.* 2017;18(5):e238. doi:10.1016/S1470-2045(17)30263-2
33. West CM, Barnett GC. Genetics and genomics of radiotherapy toxicity: towards prediction. *Genome Med.* 2011;3(8):52. doi:10.1186/gm268
34. Chaudhuri AA, Binkley MS, Osmundson EC. Predicting radiotherapy responses and treatment outcomes through analysis of circulating tumor DNA. *Semin Radiat Oncol.* 2015;25(4):305–312. doi:10.1016/j.semradonc.2015.05.001
35. Newman AM, Bratman SV, To J, et al. An ultrasensitive method for quantitating circulating tumor DNA with broad patient coverage. *Nat Med.* 2014;20(5);548–554. doi:10.1038/nm.3519
36. Newman AM, Lovejoy AF, Klass DM, et al. Integrated digital error suppression for improved detection of circulating tumor DNA. *Nat Biotechnol.* 2016;34(5):547–555. doi:10.1038/nbt.3520
37. Chaudhuri AA, Chabon JJ, Lovejoy AF, et al. Early detection of molecular residual disease in localized lung cancer by circulating tumor DNA profiling. *Cancer Discov.* 2017;7(12):1394–1403. doi:10.1158/2159-8290.CD-17-0716
38. Tie J, Wang Y, Tomasetti C, et al. Circulating tumor DNA analysis detects minimal residual disease and predicts recurrence in patients with stage II colon cancer. *Sci Transl Med.* 2016;8(346):346ra92. doi:10.1126/scitranslmed.aaf6219
39. Garcia-Murillas I, Schiavon G, Weigelt B, et al. Mutation tracking in circulating tumor DNA predicts relapse in early breast cancer. *Sci Transl Med.* 2015;7(302):302ra133. doi:10.1126/scitranslmed.aab0021
40. Springer SU, Chen CH, Pena MDCR, et al. Non-invasive detection of urothelial cancer through the analysis of driver gene mutations and aneuploidy. *Elife.* 2018;7:e32143. doi:10.7554/eLife.32143
41. Sanchez-Vega F, Mina M, Armenia J, et al. Oncogenic signaling pathways in The Cancer Genome Atlas. *Cell.* 2018;173(2):321–337.e10. doi:10.1016/j.cell.2018.03.035
42. Shamir M, Bar-On Y, Phillips R, Milo R. SnapShot: timescales in cell biology. *Cell.* 2016;164(6):1302–1302.e1. doi:10.1016/j.cell.2016.02.058
43. David L, Huber W, Granovskaia M, et al. A high-resolution map of transcription in the yeast genome. *Proc Natl Acad Sci U S A.* 2006;103(14):5320–5325. doi:10.1073/pnas.0601091103
44. Cheng J, Kapranov P, Drenkow J, et al. Transcriptional maps of 10 human chromosomes at 5-nucleotide resolution. *Science.* 2005;308(5725):1149–1154. doi:10.1126/science.1108625
45. Wang Z, Gerstein M, Snyder M. RNA-Seq: a revolutionary tool for transcriptomics. *Nat Rev Genet.* 2009;10(1):57–63. doi:10.1038/nrg2484
46. Illumina. Customize a short end-to-end workflow guide with the Custom Protocol Selector TruSeq® Small RNA Library Prep Reference Guide. 2016. https://support.illumina.com/content/dam/illumina-support/documents/documentation/chemistry_documentation/samplepreps_truseq/truseqsmallrna/truseq-small-rna-library-prep-kit-reference-guide-15004197-02.pdf
47. Dard-Dascot C, Naquin D, Aubenton-Carafa Y–D, et al. Systematic comparison of small RNA library preparation protocols for next-generation sequencing. *BMC Genomics.* 2018;19(1):118. doi:10.1038/nrg2484
48. Raabe CA, Tang T–H, Brosius J, Rozhdestvensky TS. Biases in small RNA deep sequencing data. *Nucleic Acids Res.* 2014;42(3):1414–1426. doi:10.1093/nar/gkt1021
49. Frasor J, Danes JM, Komm B, et al. Profiling of estrogen up- and down-regulated gene expression in human breast cancer cells: insights into gene networks and pathways underlying estrogenic control of proliferation and cell phenotype. *Endocrinology.* 2003;144(10):4562–4574. doi:10.1210/en.2003-0567
50. Yamamoto H, Itoh F, Nakamura H, et al. Genetic and clinical features of human pancreatic ductal adenocarcinomas with widespread microsatellite instability. *Cancer Res.* 2001;61(7):3139–3144. http://cancerres.aacrjournals.org/content/61/7/3139.long
51. Subramanian A, Tamayo P, Mootha VK, et al. Gene set enrichment analysis: a knowledge-based approach for interpreting genome-wide expression profiles. *Proc Natl Acad Sci U S A.* 2005;102(43):15545–15550. doi:10.1073/pnas.0506580102
52. Mitrea C, Taghavi Z, Bokanizad B, et al. Methods and approaches in the topology-based analysis of biological pathways. *Front Physiol.* 2013;4:278. doi:10.3389/fphys.2013.00278
53. Ackermann M, Strimmer K. A general modular framework for gene set enrichment analysis. *BMC Bioinformatics.* 2009;10(1):47. doi:10.1186/1471-2105-10-47
54. Alizadeh AA, Eisen MB, Eric Davis R, et al. Distinct types of diffuse large B-cell lymphoma identified by gene expression profiling. *Nature.* 2000;403(6769):503–511. doi:10.1038/35000501
55. Yeoh E-J, Ross ME, Shurtleff SA, et al. Classification, subtype discovery, and prediction of outcome in pediatric acute lymphoblastic leukemia by gene expression profiling. *Cancer Cell.* 2002;1(2):133–143. doi:10.1016/S1535-6108(02)00032-6
56. Verhaak RGW, Hoadley KA, Purdom E, et al. Integrated genomic analysis identifies clinically relevant subtypes of glioblastoma characterized by abnormalities in PDGFRA, IDH1, EGFR, and NF1. *Cancer Cell.* 2010;17(1):98–110. doi:10.1016/j.ccr.2009.12.020
57. van Rooij N, van Buuren MM, Philips D, et al. Tumor exome analysis reveals neoantigen-specific T-cell reactivity in an ipilimumab-responsive melanoma. *J Clin Oncol.* 2013;31(32):e439–e442. doi:10.1200/JCO.2012.47.7521
58. Schumacher TN, Schreiber RD. Neoantigens in cancer immunotherapy. *Science.* 2015;348(6230): 69–74. doi:10.1126/science.aaa4971
59. Schwartz DR, Kardia SLR, Shedden KA, et al. Gene expression in ovarian cancer reflects both morphology and biological behavior, distinguishing clear cell from other poor-prognosis ovarian carcinomas. *Cancer Res.* 2002;62(16):4722–4729. http://cancerres.aacrjournals.org/content/62/16/4722

60. Bloomston M, Frankel WL, Petrocca F, et al. MicroRNA expression patterns to differentiate pancreatic adenocarcinoma from normal pancreas and chronic pancreatitis. *JAMA*. 2007;297(17):1901. doi:10.1001/jama.297.17.1901
61. Budhu A, Forgues M, Ye Q-H, et al. Prediction of venous metastases, recurrence, and prognosis in hepatocellular carcinoma based on a unique immune response signature of the liver microenvironment. *Cancer Cell*. 2006;10(2):99–111. doi:10.1016/j.ccr.2006.06.016
62. Lu Y, Lemon W, Liu P-Y, et al. A gene expression signature predicts survival of patients with stage I non-small cell lung cancer. *PLoS Med*. 2006;3(12):e467. doi:10.1371/journal.pmed.0030467
63. Chang HY, Sneddon JB, Alizadeh AA, et al. Gene expression signature of fibroblast serum response predicts human cancer progression: similarities between tumors and wounds. *PLoS Biol*. 2004;2(2):e7. doi:10.1371/journal.pbio.0020007
64. Cuzick J, Swanson GP, Fisher G, et al. Prognostic value of an RNA expression signature derived from cell cycle proliferation genes in patients with prostate cancer: a retrospective study. *Lancet Oncol*. 2011;12(3):245–255. doi:10.1016/S1470-2045(10)70295-3
65. Lamb J, Crawford ED, Pecket D, et al. The Connectivity Map: using gene-expression signatures to connect small molecules, genes, and disease. *Science*. 2006;313(5795):1929–1935. doi:10.1126/science.1132939
66. Salazar R, Roepman P, Capella G, et al. Gene expression signature to improve prognosis prediction of stage II and III colorectal cancer. *J Clin Oncol*. 2010;29:17–24. doi:10.1200/JCO.2010.30.1077
67. Del Rio M, Molina F, Bascoul-Mollevi C, et al. Gene expression signature in advanced colorectal cancer patients select drugs and response for the use of leucovorin, fluorouracil, and irinotecan. *J Clin Oncol*. 2007;25(7):773–780. doi:10.1200/JCO.2006.07.4187
68. van de Vijver MJ, He YD, van't Veer LJ, et al. A gene-expression signature as a predictor of survival in breast cancer. *N Engl J Med*. 2002;347(25):1999–2009. doi:10.1056/NEJMoa021967
69. Torres-Roca JF, Eschrich S, Zhao H, et al. Prediction of radiation sensitivity using a gene expression classifier. *Cancer Res*. 2005;65(16):7169–7176. doi:10.1158/0008-5472.CAN-05-0656
70. Eschrich S, Zhang H, Zhao H, et al. Systems biology modeling of the radiation sensitivity network: a biomarker discovery platform. *Int J Radiat Oncol*. 2009;75(2):497–505. doi:10.1016/j.ijrobp.2009.05.056
71. Scott JG, Berglund A, Schellet MJ, et al. A genome-based model for adjusting radiotherapy dose (GARD): a retrospective, cohort-based study. *Lancet Oncol*. 2017;18(2):202–211. doi:10.1016/S1470-2045(16)30648-9
72. Venteicher AS, Tirosh I, Hebert C, et al. Decoupling genetics, lineages, and microenvironment in IDH-mutant gliomas by single-cell RNA-seq. *Science*. 2017;355(6332):eaai8478. doi:10.1126/science.aai8478
73. Tirosh I, Izar B, Prakadan SM, et al. Dissecting the multicellular ecosystem of metastatic melanoma by single-cell RNA-seq. *Science*. 2016;352(6282):189–196. doi:10.1126/science.aad0501
74. Dave SS, Wright G, Tan B, et al. Prediction of survival in follicular lymphoma based on molecular features of tumor-infiltrating immune cells. *N Engl J Med*. 2004;351(21):2159–2169. doi:10.1056/NEJMoa041869
75. Taube JM, Klein A, Brahmer JR, et al. Association of PD-1, PD-1 ligands, and other features of the tumor immune microenvironment with response to anti-PD-1 therapy. *Clin Cancer Res*. 2014;20(19):5064–5074. doi:10.1158/1078-0432.CCR-13-3271
76. Tirosh I, Venteicher AS, Hebert C, et al. Single-cell RNA-seq supports a developmental hierarchy in human oligodendroglioma. *Nature*. 2016;539(7628):309–313. doi:10.1038/nature20123
77. Patel AP, Tirosh I, Trombetta JJ, et al. Single-cell RNA-seq highlights intratumoral heterogeneity in primary glioblastoma. *Science*. 2014;344(6190):1396–1401. doi:10.1126/science.1254257
78. Haque A, Engel J, Teichmann SA, Lönnberg T. A practical guide to single-cell RNA-sequencing for biomedical research and clinical applications. *Genome Med*. 2017;9(1):75. doi:10.1186/s13073-017-0467-4
79. Zhu S, Qing T, Zheng Y, et al. Advances in single-cell RNA sequencing and its applications in cancer research. *Oncotarget*. 2017;8(32):53763–53779. doi:10.18632/oncotarget.17893
80. White AK, VanInsberghe M, Petrivet OI, et al. High-throughput microfluidic single-cell RT-qPCR. *Proc Natl Acad Sci U S A*. 2011;108(34):13999–14004. doi:10.1073/pnas.1019446108
81. Stegle O, Teichmann SA, Marioni JC. Computational and analytical challenges in single-cell transcriptomics. *Nat Rev Genet*. 2015;16(3):133–145. doi:10.1038/nrg3833
82. Yuan GC, Cai L, Elowitz M, et al. Challenges and emerging directions in single-cell analysis. *Genome Biol*. 2017;18(1):84. doi:10.1186/s13059-017-1218-y
83. Newman AM, Liu CL, Green MR, et al. Robust enumeration of cell subsets from tissue expression profiles. *Nat Methods*. 2015;12(5):453–457. doi:10.1038/nmeth.3337
84. Vogel C, Marcotte EM. Insights into the regulation of protein abundance from proteomic and transcriptomic analyses. *Nat Rev Genet*. 2012;13(4):227–232. doi:10.1038/nrg3185
85. Mayers JR, Wu C, Clish CB, et al. Elevation of circulating branched-chain amino acids is an early event in human pancreatic adenocarcinoma development. *Nat Med*. 2014;20(10):1193–1198. doi:10.1038/nm.3686
86. Wilhelm M, Schlegl J, Hahne H, et al. Mass-spectrometry-based draft of the human proteome. *Nature*. 2014;509(7502):582–587. doi:10.1038/nature13319
87. Kim M-S, Pinto SM, Getnet D, et al. A draft map of the human proteome. *Nature*. 2014;509(7502):575–581. doi:10.1038/nature13302
88. Smith LM, Kelleher NL, The Consortium for Top Down Proteomics. Proteoform: a single term describing protein complexity. *Nat Methods*. 2013;10(3):186–187. doi:10.1038/nmeth.2369
89. Tran JC, Zamdborg L, Ahlf DR, et al. Mapping intact protein isoforms in discovery mode using top-down proteomics. *Nature*. 2011;480(7376):254–258. doi:10.1038/nature10575
90. Zhang Y, Fonslow BR, Shan B, et al. Protein analysis by shotgun/bottom-up proteomics. *Chem Rev*. 2013;113(4):2343–2394. doi:10.1021/cr3003533
91. Yates JR, Ruse CI, Nakorchevsky A. Proteomics by mass spectrometry: approaches, advances, and applications. *Annu Rev Biomed Eng*. 2009;11(1):49–79. doi:10.1146/annurev-bioeng-061008-124934

92. Cristobal A, Marino F, Post H, et al. Toward an optimized workflow for middle-down proteomics. *Anal Chem.* 2017;89(6):3318–3325. doi:10.1021/acs.analchem.6b03756
93. Richards AL, Merrill AE, Coon JJ. Proteome sequencing goes deep. *Curr Opin Chem Biol.* 2015;24:11–17. doi:10.1016/j.cbpa.2014.10.017
94. Eng JK, McCormack AL, Yates JR. An approach to correlate tandem mass spectral data of peptides with amino acid sequences in a protein database. *J Am Soc Mass Spectrom.* 1994;5(11):976–989. doi:10.1016/1044-0305(94)80016-2
95. Perkins DN, Pappin DJC, Creasy DM, Cottrell JS. Probability-based protein identification by searching sequence databases using mass spectrometry data. *Electrophoresis.* 1999;20(18):3551–3567. doi:10.1002/(SICI)1522-2683(19991201)20:18<3551::AID-ELPS3551>3.0.CO;2-2
96. Colinge J, Bennett KL. Introduction to computational proteomics. *PLoS Comput Biol.* 2007;3(7):e114. doi:10.1371/journal.pcbi.0030114
97. Chick JM, Kolippakkam D, Nusinow DP, et al. A mass-tolerant database search identifies a large proportion of unassigned spectra in shotgun proteomics as modified peptides. *Nat Biotechnol.* 2015;33(7):743–749. doi:10.1038/nbt.3267
98. Griss J, Perez-Riverol Y, Lewis S, et al. Recognizing millions of consistently unidentified spectra across hundreds of shotgun proteomics datasets. *Nat Methods.* 2016;13(8):651–656. doi:10.1038/nmeth.3902
99. Dunham WH, Mullin M, Gingras A-C. Affinity-purification coupled to mass spectrometry: basic principles and strategies. *Proteomics.* 2012;12(10):1576–1590. doi:10.1002/pmic.201100523
100. Hein M, Hubner NC, Poser I, et al. A human interactome in three quantitative dimensions organized by stoichiometries and abundances. *Cell.* 2015;163(3):712–723. doi:10.1016/j.cell.2015.09.053
101. Liu F, Rijkers DTS, Post H, Heck AJR. Proteome-wide profiling of protein assemblies by cross-linking mass spectrometry. *Nat Methods.* 2015;12(12):1179–1184. doi:10.1038/nmeth.3603
102. Leitner A, Faini M, Stengel F, Aebersold R. Crosslinking and mass spectrometry: an integrated technology to understand the structure and function of molecular machines. *Trends Biochem Sci.* 2016;41(1):20–32. doi:10.1016/j.tibs.2015.10.008
103. Huttlin EL, Bruckner RJ, Paulo JA, et al. Architecture of the human interactome defines protein communities and disease networks. *Nature.* 2017;545(7655):505–509. doi:10.1038/nature22366
104. Kolch W, Pitt A. Functional proteomics to dissect tyrosine kinase signalling pathways in cancer. *Nat Rev Cancer.* 2010;10(9):618–629. doi:10.1038/nrc2900
105. Addona TA, Abbatiello SE, Schilling B, et al. Multi-site assessment of the precision and reproducibility of multiple reaction monitoring–based measurements of proteins in plasma. *Nat Biotechnol.* 2009;27(7):633–641. doi:10.1038/nbt.1546
106. Mann M, Jensen ON. Proteomic analysis of post-translational modifications. *Nat Biotechnol.* 2003;21(3):255–261. doi:10.1038/nbt0303-255
107. Pierobon M, Wulfkuhle J, Liotta L, Petricoin E. Application of molecular technologies for phosphoproteomic analysis of clinical samples. *Oncogene.* 2015;34(7):805–814. doi:10.1038/onc.2014.16
108. Tsai T-H, Song E, Zhu R, et al. LC-MS/MS-based serum proteomics for identification of candidate biomarkers for hepatocellular carcinoma. *Proteomics.* 2015;15(13):2369–2381. doi:10.1002/pmic.201400364
109. Jones RP, Sutton P, Greensmith RMD, et al. Hepatic activation of irinotecan predicts tumour response in patients with colorectal liver metastases treated with DEBIRI: exploratory findings from a phase II study. *Cancer Chemother Pharmacol.* 2013;72(2):359–368. doi:10.1007/s00280-013-2199-5
110. Gregorc V, Novello S, Lazzari C, et al. Predictive value of a proteomic signature in patients with non-small-cell lung cancer treated with second-line erlotinib or chemotherapy (PROSE): a biomarker-stratified, randomised phase 3 trial. *Lancet Oncol.* 2014;15(7):713–721. doi:10.1016/S1470-2045(14)70162-7
111. Yanagisawa K, Tomida S, Shimada Y, et al. A 25-signal proteomic signature and outcome for patients with resected non–small-cell lung cancer. *JNCI J Natl Cancer Inst.* 2007;99(11):858–867. doi:10.1093/jnci/djk197
112. Høgdall C, Fung ET, Christensen Ib J, et al. A novel proteomic biomarker panel as a diagnostic tool for patients with ovarian cancer. *Gynecol Oncol.* 2011;123(2):308–313. doi:10.1016/j.ygyno.2011.07.018
113. Panis C, Pizzatti L, Souza GF, Abdelhay E. Clinical proteomics in cancer: where we are. *Cancer Lett.* 2016;382(2):231–239. doi:10.1016/j.canlet.2016.08.014
114. Zhang Z, Chan DW. Cancer proteomics: in pursuit of "true" biomarker discovery. *Cancer Epidemiol Biomarkers Prev.* 2005;14(10):2283–2286. doi:10.1158/1055-9965.EPI-05-0774
115. Hanash SM. Why have protein biomarkers not reached the clinic? *Genome Med.* 2011;3(10):66. doi:10.1186/gm282
116. Dias MH, Kitano ES, Zelanis A, Iwai LK. Proteomics and drug discovery in cancer. *Drug Discov Today.* 2016;21(2):264–277. doi:10.1016/j.drudis.2015.10.004
117. Diamandis EP. The failure of protein cancer biomarkers to reach the clinic: why, and what can be done to address the problem? *BMC Med.* 2012;10(1):87. doi:10.1186/1741-7015-10-87
118. Mischak H, Apweiler R, Banks RE, et al. Clinical proteomics: a need to define the field and to begin to set adequate standards. *Proteom Clin Appl.* 2007;1(2):148–156. doi:10.1002/prca.200600771
119. Tabb DL, Vega-Montoto L, Rudnick PA, et al. Repeatability and reproducibility in proteomic identifications by liquid chromatography-tandem mass spectrometry. *J Proteome Res.* 2010;9(2):761–776. doi:10.1021/pr9006365
120. Vaudel M, Verheggen K, Csordas A, et al. Exploring the potential of public proteomics data, *Proteomics.* 2016;16(2):214–225. doi:10.1002/pmic.201500295
121. Martens L, Vizcaíno JA. A golden age for working with public proteomics data. *Trends Biochem Sci.* 42(5):333–341. doi:10.1016/j.tibs.2017.01.001
122. Wishart DS. Current progress in computational metabolomics. *Brief Bioinform.* 2007;8(5):279–293. doi:10.1093/bib/bbm030
123. Urbanczyk-Wochniak E, Luedemann A, Kopka J, et al. Parallel analysis of transcript and metabolic profiles: a new approach in systems biology. *EMBO Rep* 2003;4(10):989–993. doi:10.1038/sj.embor.embor944
124. Wishart DS, Feunang YD, Marcu A, et al. HMDB 4.0: the human metabolome database for 2018. *Nucleic Acids Res.* 2018;46(D1):D608–D617. doi:10.1093/nar/gkx1089

125. Veenstra TD. Metabolomics: the final frontier? *Genome Med*. 2012;4(4):40. doi:10.1186/gm339
126. Günther UL. Metabolomics biomarkers for breast cancer. *Pathobiology*. 2015;82(3–4):153–165. doi:10.1159/000430844
127. Felli IC, Brutscher B. Recent advances in solution NMR: fast methods and heteronuclear direct detection. *ChemPhysChem*. 2009;10(9–10):1356–1368. doi:10.1002/cphc.200900133
128. Kentgens APM, Bart J, van Bentum PJM, et al. High-resolution liquid- and solid-state nuclear magnetic resonance of nanoliter sample volumes using microcoil detectors. *J Chem Phys*. 2008;128(5):52202. doi:10.1063/1.2833560
129. Wolahan SM, Hirt D, Glenn TC. *Translational Metabolomics of Head Injury: Exploring Dysfunctional Cerebral Metabolism with Ex Vivo NMR Spectroscopy-Based Metabolite Quantification*. Boca Raton, FL: CRC Press/Taylor & Francis; 2015.
130. Marshall DD, Powers R. Beyond the paradigm: combining mass spectrometry and nuclear magnetic resonance for metabolomics. *Prog Nucl Magn Reson Spectrosc*. 2017;100:1–16. doi:10.1016/j.pnmrs.2017.01.001
131. Bingol K, Bruschweiler-Li L, Yu C, et al. Metabolomics beyond spectroscopic databases: a combined MS/NMR strategy for the rapid identification of new metabolites in complex mixtures. *Anal Chem*. 2015;87(7):3864–3870. doi:10.1021/ac504633z
132. da Silva RR, Dorrestein PC, Quinn RA. Illuminating the dark matter in metabolomics. *Proc Natl Acad Sci U S A*. 2015;112(41):12549–12550. doi:10.1021/ac504633z
133. Gao J, Ellis LBM, Wackett LP. The University of Minnesota Biocatalysis/Biodegradation Database: improving public access. *Nucleic Acids Res*. 2010;38(suppl 1):D488–D491. doi:10.1093/nar/gkp771
134. Jeffryes JG, Colastani RL, Elbadawi-Sidhu M, et al. MINEs: open access databases of computationally predicted enzyme promiscuity products for untargeted metabolomics. *J Cheminform*. 2015;7(1):44. doi:10.1186/s13321-015-0087-1
135. Rathahao-Paris E, Alves S, Junot C, Tabet J-C. High resolution mass spectrometry for structural identification of metabolites in metabolomics. *Metabolomics*. 2016;12(1):10. doi:10.1007/s11306-015-0882-8
136. Gromski PS, Muhamadali H, Elliset DI, et al. A tutorial review: Metabolomics and partial least squares-discriminant analysis – —a marriage of convenience or a shotgun wedding. *Anal Chim Acta*. 2015;879:10–23. doi:10.1016/j.aca.2015.02.012
137. Sitter B, Bathen TF, Singstad TE, et al. Quantification of metabolites in breast cancer patients with different clinical prognosis using HR MAS MR spectroscopy. *NMR Biomed*. 2010;23(4):424–431. doi:10.1002/nbm.1478
138. Cao MD, Sitter B, Bathenet Tone F, et al. Predicting long-term survival and treatment response in breast cancer patients receiving neoadjuvant chemotherapy by MR metabolic profiling. *NMR Biomed*. 2012;25(2):369–378. doi:10.1002/nbm.1762
139. Choi JS, Baek H-M, Kim S, et al. Magnetic resonance metabolic profiling of breast cancer tissue obtained with core needle biopsy for predicting pathologic response to neoadjuvant chemotherapy. *PLoS One*. 2013;8(12):e83866. doi:10.1371/journal.pone.0083866
140. Tenori L, Oakman C, Claudino WM., et al. Exploration of serum metabolomic profiles and outcomes in women with metastatic breast cancer: a pilot study. *Mol Oncol*. 2012;6(4):437–444. doi:10.1016/j.molonc.2012.05.003
141. Wei S, Liu L, Zhanget J, et al. Metabolomics approach for predicting response to neoadjuvant chemotherapy for breast cancer. *Mol Oncol*. 2013;7(3):297–307. doi:10.1016/j.molonc.2012.10.003
142. Yu L, Jiang C, Huang S, et al. Analysis of urinary metabolites for breast cancer patients receiving chemotherapy by CE-MS coupled with on-line concentration. *Clin Biochem*. 2013;46(12):1065–1073. doi:10.1016/j.clinbiochem.2013.05.049
143. Chan AW, Mercier P, Schiller D, et al. 1H-NMR urinary metabolomic profiling for diagnosis of gastric cancer. *Br J Cancer*. 2016;114(1):59–62. doi:10.1038/bjc.2015.414
144. Gillies RJ, Kinahan PE, Hricak H. Radiomics: images are more than pictures, they are data. *Radiology*. 2016;278(2):563–577. doi:10.1148/radiol.2015151169
145. Heusch P, Nensa F, Schaarschmidt B, et al. Diagnostic accuracy of whole-body PET/MRI and whole-body PET/CT for TNM staging in oncology. *Eur J Nucl Med Mol Imaging*. 2015;42(1):42–48. doi:10.1007/s00259-014-2885-5
146. Bailey DL, Pichler BJ, Gückel B, et al. Combined PET/MRI: multi-modality multi-parametric imaging is here: summary report of the 4th International Workshop on PET/MR imaging. *Mol Imaging Biol*. 2015;17(5):595–608. doi:10.1007/s11307-015-0886-9
147. Vandenberghe S, Marsden PK. PET-MRI: a review of challenges and solutions in the development of integrated multimodality imaging. *Phys Med Biol*. 2015;60(4):R115–R154. doi:10.1088/0031-9155/60/4/r115
148. Schmitz J, Schwab J, Schwenck J, et al. Decoding intratumoral heterogeneity of breast cancer by multiparametric in vivo imaging: a translational study. *Cancer Res*. 2016;76(18):5512–5522. doi:10.1158/0008-5472.CAN-15-0642
149. Gillies RJ, Raghunand N, Karczmar GS, Bhujwalla ZM. MRI of the tumor microenvironment. *J Magn Reson Imaging*. 2002;16(4):430–450. doi:10.1002/jmri.10181
150. Rios Velazquez E, Aerts HJWL, Gu Y, et al. A semiautomatic CT-based ensemble segmentation of lung tumors: comparison with oncologists' delineations and with the surgical specimen. *Radiother Oncol*. 2012;105(2):167–173. doi:10.1016/j.radonc.2012.09.023
151. Weiss E, Hess CF. The impact of gross tumor volume (GTV) and clinical target volume (CTV) definition on the total accuracy in radiotherapy. *Strahlentherapie und Onkol*. 2003;179(1):21–30. doi:10.1007/s00066-003-0976-5
152. Huang Q, Lu L, Dercle L, et al. Interobserver variability in tumor contouring affects the use of radiomics to predict mutational status. *J Med Imaging*. 2017;5(1):1. doi:10.1117/1.jmi.5.1.011005
153. Sharp G, Fritscher KD, Pekar V, et al. Vision 20/20: perspectives on automated image segmentation for radiotherapy. *Med Phys*. 2014;41(5):50902. doi:10.1118/1.4871620
154. Sabuncu MR, Yeo BTT, Van Leemput K et al. A generative model for image segmentation based on label fusion. *IEEE Trans Med Imaging*. 2010;29(10):1714–1729. doi:10.1109/TMI.2010.2050897
155. Geremia E, Clatz O, Menze BH, et al. Spatial decision forests for MS lesion segmentation in multi-channel magnetic resonance images. *Neuroimage*. 2011;57(2):378–390. doi:10.1016/j.neuroimage.2011.03.080
156. Lustberg T, van Soest J, Gooding M, et al. Clinical evaluation of ATLAS and deep learning based automatic contouring for lung cancer. *Radiother Oncol*. 2018;126(2):312–317. doi:10.1016/j.radonc.2017.11.012

157. Heimann T, Meinzer H-P. Statistical shape models for 3D medical image segmentation: a review. *Med Image Anal.* 2009;13(4):543–563. doi:10.1016/j.radonc.2017.11.012
158. Fritscher KD, Grünerbl A, Schubert R. 3D image segmentation using combined shape-intensity prior models. *Int J Comput Assist Radiol Surg.* 2007;1(6):341–350. doi:10.1007/s11548-007-0070-z
159. Chaney EL, Pizer S, Joshi S, et al. Automatic male pelvis segmentation from CT images via statistically trained multi-object deformable m-rep models. *Int J Radiat Oncol.* 2004;60(1):S153–S154. doi:10.1016/j.ijrobp.2004.06.067
160. Haas B, Coradi T, Scholz M, et al. Automatic segmentation of thoracic and pelvic CT images for radiotherapy planning using implicit anatomic knowledge and organ-specific segmentation strategies. *Phys Med Biol.* 2008;53(6):1751–1771. doi:10.1088/0031-9155/53/6/017
161. Parekh V, Jacobs MA. Radiomics: a new application from established techniques. *Expert Rev Precis Med Drug Dev.* 2016;1(2):207–226. doi:10.1080/23808993.2016.1164013
162. O'Connor JPB, Rose CJ, Waterton JC, et al. Imaging intratumor heterogeneity: role in therapy response, resistance, and clinical outcome. *Clin Cancer Res.* 2015;21(2):249–257. doi:10.1158/1078-0432.CCR-14-0990
163. Yip SSF, Liu Y, Parmar C, et al. Associations between radiologist-defined semantic and automatically computed radiomic features in non-small cell lung cancer. *Sci Rep.* 2017;p7(1):3519. doi:10.1038/s41598-017-02425-5
164. Li H, Zhu Y, Burnside ES, et al. Quantitative MRI radiomics in the prediction of molecular classifications of breast cancer subtypes in the TCGA/TCIA data set. NPJ *Breast Cancer.* 2016;2(1):16012. doi:10.1038/npjbcancer.2016.12
165. Segal E, Sirlin CB, Ooi C, et al. Decoding global gene expression programs in liver cancer by noninvasive imaging. *Nat Biotechnol.* 2007;25(6):675–680. doi:10.1038/nbt1306
166. Ma J, Wang Q, Ren Y, et al. Automatic lung nodule classification with radiomics approach. Paper presented at: Medical Imaging 2016: PACS and Imaging Informatics: Next Generation and Innovations; Apr 5, 2016; San Diego, CA; 9789:978906.
167. Fehr D, Veeraraghavan H, Wibmer A, et al. Automatic classification of prostate cancer Gleason scores from multiparametric magnetic resonance images. *Proc Natl Acad Sci U S A.* 2015;112(46):E6265–E6273. doi:10.1073/pnas.1505935112
168. Gevaert O, Mitchell LA, Achrol AS, et al. Glioblastoma multiforme: exploratory radiogenomic analysis by using quantitative image features. *Radiology.* 2014;273(1):168–174. doi:10.1148/radiol.14131731
169. Teruel JR, Heldahl MG, Goa PE, et al. Dynamic contrast-enhanced MRI texture analysis for pretreatment prediction of clinical and pathological response to neoadjuvant chemotherapy in patients with locally advanced breast cancer. *NMR Biomed.* 2014;27(8):887–896. doi:10.1002/nbm.3132
170. Kuo MD, Gollub J, Sirlin CB, et al. Radiogenomic analysis to identify imaging phenotypes associated with drug response gene expression programs in hepatocellular carcinoma. *J Vasc Interv Radiol.* 2007;18(7):821–830. doi:10.1016/j.jvir.2007.04.031
171. Aerts HJWL, Velazquez ER, Leijenaar RTH, et al. Decoding tumour phenotype by noninvasive imaging using a quantitative radiomics approach. *Nat Commun.* 2014;5:4006. doi:10.1038/ncomms5006
172. Ciompi F, Chung K, van Riel SJ, et al. Towards automatic pulmonary nodule management in lung cancer screening with deep learning. *Sci Rep.* 2017;7:46479. doi:10.1038/srep46479
173. Subramanian J, Simon R. Gene expression-based prognostic signatures in lung cancer: ready for clinical use? *JNCI J Natl Cancer Inst.* 2010;102(7):464–474. doi:10.1093/jnci/djq025
174. Rhodes DR, Yu J, Shanker K, et al. Large-scale meta-analysis of cancer microarray data identifies common transcriptional profiles of neoplastic transformation and progression. *Proc Natl Acad Sci.* 2004;101(25):9309–9314. doi:10.1073/pnas.0401994101
175. Wirapati P, Sotiriou C, Kunkel S, et al. Meta-analysis of gene expression profiles in breast cancer: toward a unified understanding of breast cancer subtyping and prognosis signatures. *Breast Cancer Res.* 2008;10(4):R65. doi:10.1186/bcr2124
176. Bin Goh WW, Wang W, Wong L. Why batch effects matter in omics data, and how to avoid them. *Trends Biotechnol.* 2017;35(6):498–507. doi:10.1016/j.tibtech.2017.02.012
177. Bernau C, Riester M, Boulesteix A-L, et al. Cross-study validation for the assessment of prediction algorithms. *Bioinformatics.* 2014;30(12):i105–i112. doi:10.1093/bioinformatics/btu279
178. Ransohoff DF. Lessons from controversy: ovarian cancer screening and serum proteomics. *JNCI J Natl Cancer Inst.* 2005;97(4):315–319. doi:10.1093/jnci/dji054
179. Townsend MK, Clish CB, Kraft P, et al. Reproducibility of metabolomic profiles among men and women in 2 large cohort studies. *Clin Chem.* 2013;59(11):1657–1667. doi:10.1373/clinchem.2012.199133
180. Pertea M. The human transcriptome: an unfinished story. *Genes.* 2012;3(3):344–360. doi:10.3390/genes3030344
181. Griffiths-Jones S, Grocock RJ, van Dongen S, et al. miRBase: microRNA sequences, targets and gene nomenclature. *Nucleic Acids Res.* 2006;34(90001):D140–D144. doi:10.1093/nar/gkj112
182. He J, Abdel-Wahab O, Nahas MK, et al. Integrated genomic DNA/RNA profiling of hematologic malignancies in the clinical setting. *Blood.* 2016;127(24):3004–3014. doi:10.1182/blood-2015-08-664649
183. Grossman RL, Heath AP, Ferretti V, et al. Toward a shared vision for cancer genomic data. *N Engl J Med.* 2016;375(12):1109–1112. doi:10.1056/NEJMp1607591
184. Auton A, The 1000 Genomes Project Consortium, Boerwinkle E, et al. A global reference for human genetic variation. *Nature.* 2015;526(7571):68–74. doi:10.1038/nature15393
185. Zhang J, Baran J, Cros A, et al. International Cancer Genome Consortium Data Portal--a one-stop shop for cancer genomics data. *Database.* 2011;2011:bar026. doi:10.1093/database/bar026
186. Edgar R, Domrachev M, Lash AE. Gene expression omnibus: NCBI gene expression and hybridization array data repository. *Nucleic Acids Res.* 2002;30(1):207–210. doi:10.1093/nar/30.1.207
187. Vizcaíno JA, Deutsch EW, Wang R, et al. ProteomeXchange provides globally coordinated proteomics data submission and dissemination. *Nat Biotechnol.* 2014;32(3):223–226. doi:10.1038/nbt.2839

188. Farrah T, Deutsch EW, Hoopmann MR, et al. The state of the human proteome in 2012 as viewed through PeptideAtlas. *J Proteome Res*. 2013;12(1):162–171. doi:10.1021/pr301012j
189. Kanehisa M, Goto S. KEGG: Kyoto Encyclopedia of Genes and Genomes. *Nucleic Acids Res*. 2000;28(1):27–30. doi:10.1093/nar/28.1.27
190. Smith CA, O' Maille G, Want EJ, et al. METLIN: a metabolite mass spectral database. *Ther Drug Monit*. 2005;27(6):747–751. doi:10.1097/01.ftd.0000179845.53213.39
191. Horai H, Arita M, Kanaya S, et al. MassBank: a public repository for sharing mass spectral data for life sciences. *J Mass Spectrom*. 2010;45(7):703–714. doi:10.1002/jms.1777
192. Clark K, Vendt B, Smith K, et al. The Cancer Imaging Archive (TCIA): maintaining and operating a public information repository. *J Digit Imaging*. 2013;26(6):1045–1057. doi:10.1007/s10278-013-9622-7
193. Herrick R, Horton W, Olsen T, et al. XNAT Central: open sourcing imaging research data. *Neuroimage*. 2016;124:1093–1096. doi:10.1016/j.neuroimage.2015.06.076
194. Crawford KL, Neu SC, Toga AW. The image and data archive at the laboratory of neuro imaging. *Neuroimage*. 2016;124:1080–1083. doi:10.1016/j.neuroimage.2015.04.067
195. Radiological Society of North America. Quantitative Imaging Data Warehouse (QIDW). 2018. https://www.rsna.org/QIDW
196. Eifert C, Pantazi A, Sun R, et al. Clinical application of a cancer genomic profiling assay to guide precision medicine decisions. *Per Med*. 2017;14(4):309–325. doi:10.2217/pme-2017-0011
197. Fung ET. A recipe for proteomics diagnostic test development: the OVA1 test, from biomarker discovery to FDA clearance. *Clin Chem*. 2010;56(2):327–329. doi:10.1373/clinchem.2009.140855
198. Costello LC, Franklin RB, Narayan P. Citrate in the diagnosis of prostate cancer. *Prostate*. 1999;38(3):237–245. doi:10.1002/(SICI)1097-0045(19990215)38:3<237::AID-PROS8>3.0.CO;2-O
199. Hu K, Lin A, Young A, et al. Timesavings for contour generation in head and neck IMRT: multi-institutional experience with an ATLAS-based segmentation method. *Int J Radiat Oncol*. 2008;72(1):S391. doi:10.1016/j.ijrobp.2008.06.1261
200. Tomczak K, Czerwińska P, Wiznerowicz M. The Cancer Genome Atlas (TCGA): an immeasurable source of knowledge. *Contemp Oncol*. 2015;19(1A):A68–A77. doi:10.5114/wo.2014.47136
201. Chaudhary K, Poirion OB, Lu L, Garmire LX. Deep learning-based multi-omics integration robustly predicts survival in liver cancer. *Clin Cancer Res*. 2018;24(6):1248–1259. doi:10.1158/1078-0432.CCR-17-0853
202. Rohart F, Gautier B, Singh A, Lê Cao K-A. Mixomics: an R package for 'omics feature selection and multiple data integration. *PLOS Comput Biol*. 2017;13(11):e1005752. doi:10.1371/journal.pcbi.1005752

Index

Printed in the United States
By Bookmasters